ORTHODONTICS AND DENTOFACIAL ORTHOPEDICS

James A McNamara Jr DDS PhD

*Thomas M and Doris Graber Endowed Professor of Dentistry,
   Department of Orthodontics and Pediatric Dentistry, School of Dentistry;
Professor of Cell and Developmental Biology, School of Medicine; and,
Research Scientist, Center for Human Growth and Development
The University of Michigan
Ann Arbor, Michigan*

William L Brudon

*Associate Professor Emeritus, Department of Art; and,
Associate Professor Emeritus, Department of Medical and Biological Illustration
The University of Michigan
Ann Arbor, Michigan*

With: **Vincent G Kokich DDS MS**

*Professor, Department of Orthodontics
School of Dentistry
The University of Washington*

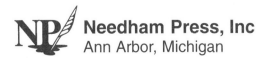 **Needham Press, Inc**
Ann Arbor, Michigan

Published by
Needham Press, Inc.
P.O. Box 130530
Ann Arbor, MI 48113-0530
Phone: 734-668-6666
Fax: 734-668-8339
E-mail: needhamp@izzy.net
www.needhampress.com

First printing, April 2001

Copyright © 2001 by Needham Press, Inc.

All rights reserved. No part of this publication may be reproduced, stored in a retrieval system, or transmitted, in any form or by any means, electronic, mechanical, photocopying, recording, or otherwise, without prior written permission from the publisher.

Printed in the United States of America

Library of Congress Cataloguing in Publication Data
Orthodontics and dentofacial orthopedics/ by James A. McNamara, Jr, William L. Brudon
    Includes bibliographical references and index
        ISBN 0-9635022-3-9 (hardcover)

DEDICATION

To Charlene, Laurie and David

To Margaret

COLLABORATORS

Tiziano Baccetti DDS PhD
    Research Associate
    Department of Orthodontics
    University of Florence, Italy; and,
    Thomas M Graber Visiting Scholar
    The University of Michigan

Donald R Burkhardt DDS MS
    Private practice of orthodontics
    Okemos and Ann Arbor, Michigan

Lorenzo Franchi DDS PhD
    Research Associate
    Department of Orthodontics
    University of Florence, Italy; and,
    Thomas M Graber Visiting Scholar
    The University of Michigan

Paul A Gange, President
    Reliance Orthodontic Products
    Itasca, Illinois

James J Hilgers DDS MS
    Private practice of Orthodontics
    Mission Viejo, California; and,
    Visiting Clinical Professor,
    Department of Growth and
      Development,
    University of California, San Francisco

Scott A Huge, President
    Specialty Appliances
    Norcross, Georgia

Cherie R Lovett RDA
    Treatment Coordinator
    Drs McNamara, Nolan, West, and
      Burkhardt
    Ann Arbor, Michigan

David P Mathews DDS
    Specialist in Periodontics
    Tacoma, Washington

Patrick J Nolan DDS MS
    Private practice of Orthodontics
    Canton and Ann Arbor, Michigan; and,
    Department of Orthodontics and
      Pediatric Dentistry
    The University of Michigan

Jeffrey P Okeson DMD
    Professor
    Department of Oral Health Practice, and
    Director, Orofacial Pain Center
    College of Dentistry
    University of Kentucky
    Lexington, Kentucky

Valmy Pangrazio-Kulbersh DDS MS
    Professor, Department of Orthodontics
    University of Detroit Mercy
    Detroit, Michigan

Donald A Seligman DDS
    Adjunct Assistant Professor
    Section of Orofacial Pain and Occlusion
    School of Dentistry
    University of California Los Angeles

Michael L Swartz DDS MS
    Director, Orthodontic Continuing Education
    Ormco Corporation
    Orange, California

Frans PGM van der Linden DDS PhD
    Professor and Chairman, Emeritus
    Department of Orthodontics
    University of Nijmegen
    The Netherlands

Kristine S West DDS MS
    Private practice of Orthodontics
    Okemos and Ann Arbor, Michigan; and,
    Department of Orthodontics and
      Pediatric Dentistry
    The University of Michigan

TABLE OF CONTENTS

Preface		ix
Acknowledgments		xi
Chapter 1.	Introduction: and Overview	1
Chapter 2.	The Clinical Examination With *Patrick J Nolan, Kristine S West* and *Cherie L Lovett*	13

GENERAL TREATMENT STRATEGIES

Chapter 3.	Dentitional Development	31
Chapter 4.	Tooth-Size/Arch-Size Discrepancies	39
Chapter 5.	Class II Malocclusion With *Lorenzo Franchi* and *Tiziano Baccetti*	63
Chapter 6.	Class III Malocclusion With *Tiziano Baccetti* and *Lorenzo Franchi*	85
Chapter 7.	Transverse Dimension	97
Chapter 8.	Vertical Dimension With *Frans PGM van der Linden*	111

CLINICAL MANAGEMENT

Chapter 9.	Comprehensive Fixed Appliance Therapy With *Michael L Swartz*	149
Chapter 10.	Orthodontic Bonding With *Paul A Gange*	169
Chapter 11.	Utility Arches	187
Chapter 12.	Transpalatal Arch	199
Chapter 13.	Rapid Maxillary Expansion	211
Chapter 14.	The Schwarz Appliance	233
Chapter 15.	The Twin Block Appliance	243
Chapter 16.	The Function Regulator (FR-2) of Fränkel	265
Chapter 17.	The Herbst Appliance With *Donald R Burkhardt* and *Scott A Huge*	285
Chapter 18.	The Bionator With *Valmy Pangrazio-Kulbersh* and *Scott A Huge*	319
Chapter 19.	The Jasper Jumper	333

Chapter 20.	The Pendulum and Other Molar Distalizing Appliances With *James J Hilgers*	343
Chapter 21.	Extraoral Traction	361
Chapter 22.	The Facial Mask With *Lorenzo Franchi* and *Tiziano Baccetti*	375
Chapter 23.	The Function Regulator (FR-3) of Fränkel	387
Chapter 24.	Impacted Teeth: Orthodontic and Surgical Considerations By *Vincent G Kokich* and *David P Mathews*	395
Chapter 25.	Managing Orthodontic-Restorative Treatment of the Adolescent Patient By *Vincent G Kokich*	423
Chapter 26.	Finishing and Retention With *Patrick J Nolan* and *Kristine S West*	453
Chapter 27.	Invisible Retainers and Aligners	475
Chapter 28.	Cephalometric Evaluation	487
Chapter 29.	Orthodontics, Occlusion and Temporomandibular Disorders With *Donald A Seligman* and *Jeffrey P Okeson*	519
Chapter 30.	Study Models	545

PREFACE

I have known and worked with my good friend and colleague Bill Brudon for over thirty years. This book is the natural outgrowth of our collaboration that began in the Department of Anatomy* in 1968. Bill retired from the faculty of The University of Michigan Medical School in 1985, but if anything, our collaboration has increased since then. We have spent literally hundreds and hundreds of hours together developing the illustrations for this book.

Our first formal joint effort was the publication of *Orthodontic and Orthopedic Treatment in the Mixed Dentition* in 1993. Bill had provided illustrations for most of my publications on topics in orthodontics and craniofacial biology before that time. In fact, some of the illustrations originally were created during the 1970s, when I was involved in basic and applied research in non-human primates. Concurrently, I was learning the nuances of orthodontic and orthopedic treatment within a private practice setting.

We have had many discussions concerning whether the current book should be considered a second edition of our earlier text. We have decided against it, because the current volume is much broader in focus and includes the contributions of Vince Kokich, as well as the collaborative efforts of 15 other colleagues, none of whom (at least formally) contributed to the earlier volume. The book considering mixed dentition treatment is out of print, but we have incorporated slenderized and updated versions of the essential material from that text.

Throughout the text, the editorial "we" often is used. The meaning of "we" varies according to the chapter. Since I wrote or rewrote virtually all of the text, with the exception of the two Kokich chapters, the "we" always includes me. In the chapters that address specific protocols from the practice of Drs. McNamara, Nolan, West, and Burkhardt, the "we" refers to the four partners. If a chapter had contributions from one or more collaborators, generally the "we" refers to them as well. I know this may seem confusing at first, but I chose to insert some personal opinion (and, of course, bias) into most of the chapters. The opinions expressed are based, in part, on clinical and/or basic biological data, as well as over thirty-five years of clinical experience.

You will note that at the end of nearly every chapter, a section appears entitled "Concluding Remarks." In these paragraphs, I have attempted to summarize the chapter briefly and to give a few pertinent comments regarding how the material covered in the chapter relates to the rest of the book and to orthodontic practice.

The material covered in this volume must be considered a "work in progress." Although most of the appliances and protocols have been incorporated into our private practice for many years, we still attempt to "kaizen" our orthodontic and orthopedic treatment on an ongoing basis. "Kaizen" is a Chinese word that means "small but continuing improvements in a process or system." Thus, we continually attempt to improve every aspect of our practice (*e.g.*, treatment protocols, practice management procedures, staff interactions, external and internal marketing) every day. The careful reader of our earlier book and now this one will notice many subtle changes in the recommendations that we make regarding specific treatment protocols.

We also have taken the liberty of introducing several "new technologies" within the text. Technological advancements, such as self-ligating brackets, the Invisalign® System, and the Distal Jet appliance are examples of methodologies with which we have had some positive experience, but on which only limited data exists as to their effectiveness and efficiency. Similarly, we also are presenting for the first time a method of determining the maturational status of the patient, based on stages of development of the cervical vertebrae visible in the lateral headfilm. These advancements are presented as just that, new technology and methodology that are to be evaluated on their own merits.

In this text, an attempt has been made to present an

---

*The Department of Anatomy has been renamed the Department of Cell and Developmental Biology, a sign of changing times.

approach to routine orthodontic and orthopedic treatment, primarily in the growing patient. Specific recommendations are made regarding fixed appliances, as well as various orthopedic therapies. If the reader searches for a topic and finds it missing, this probably means that we do not use that treatment approach in our practice.

There are several limitations to this book, most of which are intentional. First, and perhaps most important, very few case studies are presented. This book is long enough in its present form. It would have been relatively easy to double the size of the book by presenting patient after patient with excellent treatment outcomes, but the Brudon illustrations are worth "a thousand case reports." In this instance, conciseness is considered a virtue.

In addition, no chapter exists on the specific treatment of surgical orthodontic patients or of patients with craniofacial anomalies. While we participate in the care of these types of patients on a routine basis, the diagnosis and treatment planning of orthognathic surgical patients can be found in Chapter 28 (cephalometric analysis), and virtually all of the mechanics used in these patients are part of the routine orthodontic and orthopedic treatments described throughout the volume.

Distracting reflections have been removed from most of the intraoral photographs by way of Photoshop™ to improve the quality of the illustration. In no instance, however, was the anatomy altered or the basic content of the photograph enhanced in any way.

In closing, I take full responsibility for any errors or omissions. It is my hope that this work will provide the orthodontist with a reasonable approach to routine orthodontic and orthopedic treatment applicable in the 21st century. Just as our approach to clinical treatment has changed greatly during the last decade, it is assumed that many of the protocols outlined in this volume will be modified and refined in the years to come.

James A McNamara
January, 2001
Ann Arbor

ACKNOWLEDGMENTS

No book of this nature could be written without the unselfish help of many individuals. We thank them for their efforts and recognize them here.

First, this book became more of a family effort than anyone could have anticipated. We thank Charlene McNamara for her efforts in all aspects of the publication process, including reading every chapter many times and making appropriate critical suggestions. We also thank dental student Laurie McNamara for her review of most of the chapters in this book. Laurie also is recognized for her help in converting the references to Endnote™ format. We also thank David McNamara, scanner extraordinaire, for his energy in scanning and rescanning much of the original artwork and slides used to produce the illustrations.

We thank Margaret Croup Brudon, an award-winning medical illustrator in her own right, for her help in the preparation of many of the illustrations used in this text.

We also thank graphic artist Chris Jung for designing the cover of the book as well as for the preparation of many of the graphs and cephalometric tracings. His advice on the intricacies of Photoshop™ was very helpful in the preparation of many of the halftones and line drawings.

Many thanks to computer guru John Ellis, who kept the computers, scanners, printers, and network alive and well throughout this process. John saved us at many inopportune moments. We also thank Susan Rigterink from *Needham Press* and K.C. Steiner and Yvonne Robinson from *Huron Valley Graphics* for all their efforts in preparing this manuscript for publication.

We recognize the photographic expertise of Per Kjeldsen and Keary Campbell for helping prepare many of the photographs found within this book. We thank Ruth Dames for transcribing the initial versions and for proofreading many of the chapters. Lorenzo Franchi, Tiziano Baccetti, Libby Kutcipal, and Brenda Brightman also reviewed many chapters. We also thank Frans van der Linden for his formatting suggestions.

Many of the chapters also were proofread by many of our orthodontic residents and postdocs, including Rebecca Rubin, Mark Berkman, Brian Reyes, Scott Schultz, Mo Gupta, Derek Straffon, Sylvie Sarment, Pat Chiu, T. J. Robinson, Lainie Shapiro, Laura Edwards, Abbie Schaefer, Paul O'Grady, Thais Carvalho, Renata Johnson, Manuel Vasquez, and Yu-kyung Kim.

Most of the chapters were written with the input and critical review of fellow orthodontic colleagues from around the world, as well as from friends from within the orthodontic industry who provided technical expertise. In addition, we received valuable, practical input from members of our own orthodontic staff, who made sure that what was said in the chapters was a reflection of what actually occurred in our practice on a day-to-day basis. We are grateful for all their contributions. They are recognized below:

Chapter 2 (Initial Examination): We acknowledge the role of Charlene White, practice management consultant, for assisting us in streamlining our practice protocols and for helping us define the role of the treatment coordinator. We also thank our office manager, Liz Maxbauer, for establishing many of the protocols associated with the function of the front office staff and for her thorough review of this chapter.

Chapter 6 (Class III): The authors recognize the assistance of Rolf Fränkel, Kuniaki Miyajima, and Eli Berger.

Chapter 8 (Vertical Dimension): We thank Lysle Johnston, Rolf Fränkel, Bill Proffit, Lloyd Pearson, Tom Graber, and Fred Preis for reviewing this chapter and for making helpful suggestions.

Chapter 9 (Fixed Appliances): We acknowledge the contributions of Dwight Damon and of Michael Larrain from *Ormco Corporation*. We also thank Barry Mollenhauer for providing the anonymous quote at the beginning of the chapter.

Chapter 10 (Orthodontic Bonding): We thank Robert Gange for providing some of the photographs used in this chapter. We also recognize orthodontic staff members Pam Dennison, Cherie Lovett, and Sandy Potoczak for their critical review of the protocols outlined in this and other chapters.

Chapter 11 (Utility Arches): We thank Robert Ricketts and Ruel Bench for introducing us to the multiple uses of utility arches.

Chapter 12 (Transpalatal Arches): Much of our early experience using the transpalatal arch was based on interactions with the late Bob Goshgarian and Norman Cetlin. Their help in this regard is greatly appreciated. In addition, we thank dental hygienist Nancy Cleland for suggesting the use of indicator wires.

Chapter 13 (Rapid Maxillary Expansion): We recognize the technical expertise of Paul Gange of *Reliance Orthodontics* and Brian Willison of *Great Lakes Orthodontic Laboratory*.

Chapter 15 (Twin Block): We acknowledge Bill Clark for helping us gain an understanding of the nuances of clinical management of this appliance. His many trips to Ann Arbor are appreciated greatly. We also thank Doug Willison of *Great Lakes Orthodontic Laboratory* and Forbes Leishman for their technical assistance. In addition, we recognize David Sarver for suggesting the development of the Triad™ reactivation technique for the Twin Block.

Chapter 16 (FR-2): We thank Rolf Fränkel for the many hours of discussion of his technique during the last 25 years. We also acknowledge the contributions of his daughter Christine Fränkel, Scott Huge, Raymond Howe, Mike Dierkes, Tom Laboe, Nelson Diers, Bob Scholz, Hans Eirew, Hans-Jürgens Kaufmann, and the late Billy West in helping with many of the technical aspects of FR appliance management.

Chapter 17 (Herbst): We recognize Hans Pancherz for introducing us to the Herbst appliance and Jim Hilgers for reviewing this chapter in detail. Many of his suggestions are incorporated within the text. We also thank Terry Dischinger, Joe Mayes, Bob Smith, and Bob Chastant for their help in the clinical management of the stainless steel crown Herbst appliance. We also recognize Ray Howe and Mike Dierkes for co-developing with us the acrylic splint Herbst design.

Chapter 18 (Bionator): The authors value the contributions of Bob Scholz and F. G. Sander.

Chapter 19 (Jasper Jumper): An earlier version of this chapter was written in collaboration with my classmate at UCSF, J. J. Jasper.

Chapter 20 (Distalizing Appliances): We acknowledge the contributions of Aldo Carano, Jay Bowman, and Tony Gianelly for the clinical management suggestions presented. We also thank Scott Huge, Tim Bussick, Don Burkhardt, and Max Hall of *AOA/Pro Laboratory* for their assistance in preparing this chapter.

Chapter 21 (Extraoral Traction): We acknowledge John Kloehn for his in depth discussion of the facebow as developed by his father, Silas. We also recognize Jim Vaden, Wick Alexander, Jack Hickham, and Eli Berger for their help.

Chapter 22 (Facial Mask): We thank Henri Petit for introducing us to the concept of heavy force orthopedic facial mask therapy.

Chapter 23 (FR-3): Rolf Fränkel, Christine Fränkel, and Scott Huge from *Specialty Appliance* contributed to this chapter.

Chapter 26 (Finishing and Retention): We thank Scott Huge again.

Chapter 27 (Invisible Retainers and Aligners): Ross Miller, Ben Kuo, and Amir Abolfathi from *Align Technology* were very helpful in providing the details of the Invisalign™ process.

Chapter 29 (Temporomandibular Disorders): Christian Stohler must be recognized for his encouragement and help in putting together a global review of this most controversial topic.

Chapter 30 (Study Models): We thank John Jankowiak and the staff of *Great Lakes Orthodontics Laboratory* for providing the basic protocols described in this chapter and Rich Johnson for his helpful suggestions.

Chapter 1
INTRODUCTION AND OVERVIEW

It is our intent to synthesize a rational approach to orthodontics and dentofacial orthopedics, incorporating the wide variety of new treatments and protocols that have evolved during the last decade.

In this volume, we discuss how orthodontic patient care is delivered, the rationale behind it, and the clinical and experimental evidence supporting this overall approach. This is not a theoretical discussion, however. This book reflects the practical experience gained during 30 years of providing patient care in both solo and group private practice, combined with teaching and conducting clinical and experimental studies within a university setting. The expertise of collaborators, each drawing from a varied background, is incorporated into the text as well.

One of the challenges in writing a book such as this, which presents in detail an array of diagnostic and treatment protocols, is to make the material covered relevant to the reader. We realize that each reader brings a level of didactic expertise and orthodontic clinical experience that varies widely, from the seasoned clinician to the first year orthodontic resident, from the non-orthodontic specialist to the family practitioner, from the orthodontic staff member to the interested lay person. It is hoped that this text will provide something of value for each reader, regardless of background.

Some will choose to read the first few chapters and then glance through the rest of the book to see what is new in orthodontics and what is emphasized, simply to gain an overview of major concepts. Others will want to understand the detailed nuances of many of the specific techniques discussed later in the volume in an attempt to improve or expand options of orthodontic patient care. Still others will be interested in the numerous references presented throughout the text that provide documentation for the techniques and protocols described.

TREATMENT OPTIONS

This book starts at the beginning, that is with the initial examination. Although each orthodontic practitioner develops his or her style of interacting with a new patient family, there are specific ingredients that should be part of any initial examination, regardless of the age or chief concern of the patient. Our examination protocol, including the role of the treatment coordinator, is described in the next chapter. We have found that establishing the position of treatment coordinator within our practice has enabled us to shorten our workday, while providing more "quality time" for the first contact with the patient and family. This style of examination eliminates the need for a follow-up consultation appointment in most instances. The specifics of the medical and dental history as well as a protocol for the routine evaluation of the temporomandibular joint region are described.

A general discussion of the development of the dentition is presented next, basic material that is helpful in understanding the management of tooth-size/ arch-size discrepancies. The subsequent chapters present overviews of the treatment options available for specific challenges that occur in routine orthodontic and orthopedic treatment, including the management of sagittal

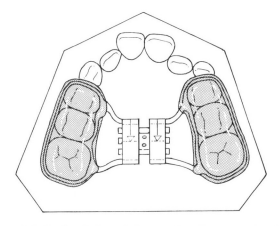

Figure 1-1. Occlusal view of the acrylic splint expander. This appliance is used frequently in the mixed dentition to widen the two parts of the maxilla. Other treatment effects are produced as well.

malocclusion (Class I, Class II, Class III) as well as problems in the transverse and vertical dimensions. Much has been written about the diagnosis and treatment of the classifications of anteroposterior malocclusion, less so about problems in the other dimensions. Summaries of the various treatment methods available for each category of malocclusion comprise these chapters.

Of special interest is the chapter concerning the vertical dimension, in which this complex subject is considered from several perspectives, including the relationship of upper airway obstruction to normal and abnormal craniofacial growth.

The next four chapters describe routine fixed appliance therapy, the "bread and butter" of any orthodontic practice. This discussion of *ordinary orthodontics*[1] may be one of the most important aspects of this book, in that it describes what we do routinely for virtually every patient at some point in their treatment. The orthodontic practitioner is advised to read these chapters closely, in that much of the success of fixed appliance treatment is in the details of clinical management. Topics covered include bracket and band placement, archwire selection and sequencing, as well as self-ligating brackets, a new technology increasing in popularity during the last few years. In addition, an in-depth discussion of orthodontic bonding in a variety of situations is presented.

The manipulation of utility arches and transpalatal arches (TPA), both integral parts of our routine fixed appliance protocol, are described in detail. We use utility arches in many ways, including as a primary method of incisor intrusion and retraction, and less frequently for incisor protraction. Utility arches minimize the need for patient compliance, as is required when J-hook headgears are used for incisor retraction and intrusion.

Soldered transpalatal arches are incorporated into the treatment of well over 90% of our patients, a much higher percentage than found in most other practices. It is very important for the reader to understand exactly how these relatively simple auxiliary archwires are adjusted in a sequential manner, so that prescribed movements of the maxillary first molars are achieved within the first few months of treatment. The incorporation of the transpalatal arch as a routine part of fixed appliance therapy has reduced our reliance on extraoral traction significantly.

Chapter 13 describes the details of three types of rapid maxillary expansion (RME) appliances (Hyrax, Haas, and acrylic splint types; Fig 1-1). RME has become the orthopedic cornerstone of our treatment of growing patients, and this procedure is indicated in some adults if accompanied by a surgical assist. The following chapter considers the removable lower Schwarz appliance, an appliance that is most effective when used in the mixed dentition. Both of these types of appliances produce treatment effects primarily in the transverse dimension, with the forces generated primarily orthodontic* in the mandible and orthopedic** in the maxilla in growing patients.

RME can be used in a variety of situations other than for the correction of crossbite,[3] including gaining additional arch perimeter, especially in the maxillary dental arch (our rate of extraction of permanent teeth other than third molars during orthodontic treatment now is about 10–15%). This orthopedic technique also can be used in instances of maxillary canine impaction, before functional jaw orthopedics in Class II patients, and during facial mask therapy to mobilize the maxillary sutural system in Class III individuals. RME also is indicated in patients with pronounced buccal corridors (*i.e.*, black spaces at the corners of the mouth) to broaden the smile.

Aside from dental crowding and/or protrusion, the most commonly occurring clinical problem in orthodontics in the United States today is Class II malocclusion,[4,5] a situation in which, simply stated, the mandibular dentition is located posterior to its normal orientation relative to the maxillary dentition. This type of malocclusion can have many etiologies (*e.g.*, maxillary and/or mandibular; skeletal and/or dentoalveolar). The variety of appliances used in the correction of Class II malocclusion can be divided arbitrarily into

---

* Force applied to the teeth for the purpose of effecting tooth movement, generally having a magnitude lower than an orthopedic force.[2]
** Higher magnitude of force delivered via the teeth for 12-16 hours or more per day that produces skeletal effect on the maxillofacial complex.[2] In the instance of RME, the two halves of the maxilla are separated.

INTRODUCTION AND OVERVIEW

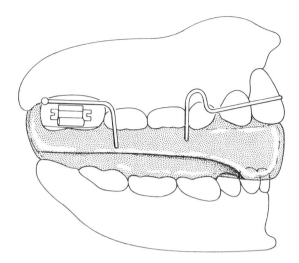

Figure 1-2. Lateral view of a Shaye-LSU activator. This appliance is representative of the activator-type of appliance that has been used in the treatment of Class II malocclusion for nearly a century. When the appliance is worn, the mandible is carried in a downward and forward position. In this type of activator, the appliance is retained by way of clasps that contact bands placed on the maxillary first molars.

two general categories, enhancing appliances and distalizing appliances.

The primary intent of so-called *enhancing* appliances is to promote increased growth of the lower jaw, at least over the short-term. Some forward movement of the lower dentition, which may be an unfavorable outcome in many patients, can occur as well. This general category encompasses functional jaw orthopedic (FJO) treatment, removable or fixed appliances that create a forward posturing of the mandible during function in a growing patient.* Such appliances include activator (Fig. 1-2), the twin block, the function regulator (FR-2) of Fränkel, several varieties of the Herbst appliance, and the bionator. Most clinical studies of FJO treatment indicate that the length of the mandible can be increased modestly over the short-term in comparison to untreated Class II controls; the long-term outcome of such treatment, however, remains controversial.

Distalizing appliances have their main effect on maxillary dentoalveolar and skeletal structures. The primary treatment effect of a number of appliances, many of which have been developed during the last decade, simply is to move the maxillary teeth posteriorly. Treatment approaches that minimize the need for patient compliance include the Pendulum and Pendex (Fig. 1-3), the Distal Jet, Niti coils combined with a Nance holding arch, as well as the Jasper Jumper™. The Wilson distalizing arch, the use of which also leads to Class II molar correction but relies on significant patient cooperation concerning elastic wear, can be used occasionally as a primary treatment appliance. In our experience, however, the Wilson arch is most useful as an auxiliary appliance for residual Class II correction near the end of active fixed appliance treatment.

Perhaps the most widely used method of Class II correction worldwide is extraoral traction (*i.e.*, facebows, headgears; Fig. 1-4). Such appliances not only are effec-

---

*There are virtually no data to support the concept that FJO appliances are effective in producing clinically relevant skeletal changes in adults.

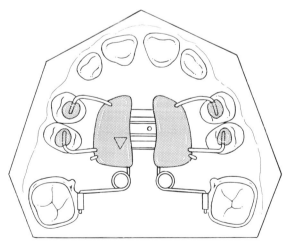

Figure 1-3. The Pendex appliance is representative of a new family of appliances that produce distalization of the maxillary molars without requiring significant patient coopration. In this example, the midline screw has been expanded and both maxillary molars have moved posteriorly.

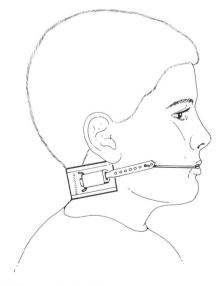

Figure 1-4. The cervical-pull facebow perhaps is the most frequently used method of Class II correction wordwide.

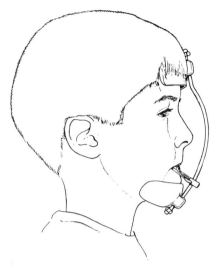

Figure 1-5. The orthopedic facial mask of Petit can be combined with bonded acrylic splint expander to mobilize the maxillary sutural system in young patients with Class III malocclusion. Forward movement of the maxilla and the maxillary dentition is observed as is a downward rotation of the mandible. This protocol is effective in managing young patients with anterior crossbite.

tive in distalizing maxillary molars, but they also afford the clinician the opportunity of restricting the downward and forward development of the maxillary complex, depending on the direction of force application. Extraoral traction is used in a number of ways in both extraction and non-extraction therapy, according to the particular philosophy of the practitioner (*e.g.*, Tweed-Merrifield, Bioprogressive, Cetlin, Alexander).

The next two chapters describe the treatment of Class III malocclusion with two of the most commonly used orthopedic/orthodontic treatment approaches: the facial mask (Fig. 1-5) combined with the acrylic splint expander, and the FR-3 appliance of Fränkel. Both of these approaches produce treatment effects that are spread throughout the skeletal and dentoalveolar structures of the craniofacial region. Early treatment of developing Class III malocclusion is stressed.

Chapters 24 and 25 address topics of major interdisciplinary interest. A unique chapter on the management of impactions has been written by orthodontist Vincent Kokich and periodontist David Matthews. These two clinicians provide a detailed discussion of a wide variety of impactions that are encountered in orthodontic patients, some common, some not. Many case examples are presented to illustrate specific clinical situations. The subsequent chapter by Kokich describes the orthodontic-restorative interface for the adolescent patient. Topics include the management of congenitally missing and malformed incisors, missing premolars, and retained deciduous molars, all perplexing clinical situations for the interdisciplinary team. Dental implants, conventional and resin bonded bridges, and porcelain fused to metal crowns are examples of the types of treatment options discussed.

Two types of retention protocols are considered in Chapter 26: simple and complex. Simple protocols often involve the removal of the fixed appliances and the delivery of a removable wire and acrylic retainer, such as a Hawley retainer. Active orthodontic treatment, however, does not always terminate with the removal of fixed appliances. In fact, we consider the end of fixed appliance therapy and the initial stages of active retention as a continuous process. Protocols that are more complex may involve a number of finishing and stabilizing procedures, including circumferential supracrestal fiberotomy, esthetic gingivectomy, enamoplasty and interproximal reduction, bonded lingual retainers, vertical finishing elastics, tooth positioners, and invisible retainers.

A new technology on which only limited scientific information is available in the literature, but which has had significant exposure in the lay media, is the Invisalign® System, developed by Align Technology. This approach generally is consistent with our use of invisible retainers, a type of clear retainer that we have used in a much more limited fashion for the past 30 years. The Invisalign® process, which has brought the invisible retainer into the 21st century by means of CAD/CAM technology, is discussed in the chapter on invisible retainers and aligners.

Chapter 28 presents a method of cephalometric appraisal developed by the senior author nearly 25 years ago. This analysis can be used effectively in the evaluation of a single pretreatment lateral headfilm. This evaluative approach also can be used to determine the serial cephalometric changes in the growth of an individual, with or without treatment. The chapter updates and expands on the original article that appeared in the *American Journal of Orthodontics*.[6]

Finally, one of the most controversial topics in dentistry in general and orthodontics in particular during the last 15 years is the relationship between orthodontics, occlusal factors, and temporomandibular disorders. The current literature on this subject is reviewed thoroughly in a attempt to distinguish between fact and fiction concerning this often hotly debated subject.

TREATMENT POSSIBILITIES

Historically, orthodontic treatment was provided mainly for adolescents. Fixed appliance therapy in the United States, for example, usually was deferred until after the second molars had erupted, so that a single phase of comprehensive treatment was rendered in an efficient manner. Adult treatment was limited, and therapy initiated in the mixed dentition often consisted of guidance of eruption and serial extraction protocols, as well as extraoral traction in instances of Class II malocclusion.

Adult Treatment

Interest in both adult and juvenile treatment has blossomed during the last two or three decades. The number of adults seeking orthodontic treatment, in general, has increased substantially during the past twenty years. These patients often present with complex dental and orthodontic problems for which treatment options are limited, due in part to a lack of substantive future craniofacial growth and/or concurrent periodontal, surgical and restorative needs.[7] For example, the use of dental implants has increased dramatically during the last decade, so that implants often are the treatment of choice for single or multiple tooth replacement. In addition, the use of implants and onplants for orthodontic anchorage has broadened the treatment options for adults.

Similarly, the development of more sophisticated periodontal surgical techniques (*e.g.*, guided tissue regeneration, guided bone regeneration, esthetic gingivectomy) makes satisfying the functional and esthetic needs of the adult patient easier to attain. Further, the refinement of orthognathic surgical procedures makes possible the manipulation of the skeletal elements of late adolescent and adult patients in all three planes of space.

Mixed Dentition Treatment

During the last two decades, increased interest has been expressed in early treatment by a ponderable segment of the orthodontic community. This interest has been stimulated by a number of seemingly diverse but interrelated factors. For example, the lay population seeks treatment for their children at an earlier age, in part due to a general rise in the level of consciousness concerning preventive dentistry and medicine. In addition, a significant segment of the dental community, including both generalists and specialists, has shown interest not only in correcting existing problems but also in intercepting or modifying abnormal orofacial conditions as they are recognized.

Just as the interest in early treatment has increased, so have the treatment options for the growing patient, especially in the mixed dentition and early permanent dentition.[8-11] Certainly not all orthodontic therapy delivered under the guise of "early treatment," however, is good treatment. We have seen many instances of young patients being treated for extended periods, with regimens that have ill-defined goals and unpredictable outcomes. There have been problems not only with patient compliance, but also with parent dissatisfaction and clinician and patient/parent fatigue.

Thus, the concept of early treatment must be defined further within the context of overall orthodontic intervention to derive principles to guide the clinician in providing effective early treatment. The provider must have a thorough understanding of craniofacial growth and of the development of the dental arches in order to deliver to the patient the most effective and efficient regimen of treatment. Most of these protocols have been in existence for a decade or longer, however, so now we can judge the effectiveness of these protocols in patients treated in the mixed dentition who now are young adults.

Traditionally, mixed dentition treatment has not been taught effectively in most graduate programs in orthodontics. Part of the reason for this is that a two or three year graduate orthodontic curriculum does not lend itself easily to the management of early treatment patients. The therapy for young patients often encompasses five or more years from the beginning of intervention to the final removal of the fixed appliances, after the second molars have erupted and the permanent dentition has been aligned. Thus, such protocols generally have not evolved within a university environment, but rather have tended to arise out of the needs of the individual practitioner.

PHASES OF TREATMENT

The orthodontic treatment protocols applied to growing patients generally can be divided into two categories: one-phase treatment and two-phase treatment. Both approaches have strong and vocal advocates. Nevertheless, this is not an "either/or" discussion. In our opinion, some patients benefit from a single phase of comprehensive treatment, whereas the orthodontic problems of others are managed better if treatment is initiated in the early mixed dentition. The challenge is to select the proper treatment and the appropriate time of intervention for each patient.

One-Phase Treatment

Those individuals who advocate one phase of treatment do so because of several sound arguments. First, one-phase treatment is more efficient, in that it usually allows for a circumscribed treatment period, typically 18-30 months in duration. Often comprehensive fixed appliance therapy is not begun until all the deciduous teeth have been lost and the second premolars and second molars have erupted. A number of orthopedic options remain for these patients, including rapid maxillary expansion, extraoral traction, and functional jaw orthopedics. Patients are treated with or without the extraction of permanent teeth.

Employing a one-phase treatment approach also allows for the growth potential of the patient to be known before orthodontic intervention is initiated. One of the best examples of this approach to treatment concerns the patient who obviously is a candidate for orthognathic surgery. The argument can be made that the patient's skeletal abnormality should be allowed to progress until the rate of growth is minimal, so that the full magnitude of the problem is known before surgical intervention in undertaken. Regardless of the severity of the problem, usually a patient can be managed by orthodontics alone or by a combination of orthodontics and surgery within a two- or three-year period.

One of the problems associated with single-phase treatment, however, is cooperation, especially in patients of high school age.[12] Adolescent patients often exhibit difficulties with compliance, not only with instructions concerning treatment (*e.g.,* elastic and headgear wear), but also with basic oral hygiene procedures (*e.g.,* proper brushing and flossing). Deficiencies in these areas may prolong the treatment and/or compromise the outcome. Scheduling appointments for high school patients also has proved to be more difficult than for children in elementary or middle school.

Further, if treatment is not begun until the eruption of the permanent teeth is completed, the clinician cannot take advantage of the leeway space that usually is gained during the transition from the second deciduous molars to the second premolars in both arches. The maintenance of this increase in arch perimeter (by means of a transpalatal arch and lower lingual arch) may dictate if the patient can be treated with or without the extraction of permanent teeth. The maintenance of the leeway space is an important goal in our overall approach to treatment.

Two-Phase Treatment

Two-phase treatment involves an initial intervention in the early or middle mixed dentition followed by an interim (*i.e.,* resting, transitional) period, during which the patient is wearing some type of simple retainer full- or part-time, or later not at all. After the transition to the permanent dentition occurs, a second phase of comprehensive fixed appliance therapy is completed.

Two-phase treatment is advocated in an attempt to minimize or eliminate skeletal, dental, and/or neuromuscular problems identified in the mixed dentition (*e.g.,* dental crowding, crossbite, hyperactive mentalis muscle with lips-apart posture). Typically, an initial phase of treatment, defined in scope and limited in duration, is undertaken, the goal of which is to provide an environment that promotes an unimpeded optimal eruption of the permanent dentition, as well as the elimination of skeletal and neuromuscular imbalances. A second phase of comprehensive fixed appliance therapy usually is required to align and detail the permanent dentition. Occasionally ($< 5\%$), Phase II treatment is deemed unnecessary because a reasonable alignment of the dentition occurs without further intervention.

Early treatment advocates state that a treatment is needed for a number of reasons including the following (with our comments in italics):

- Reduces the need for the extraction of permanent teeth *(probably so)*
- Reduces treatment time in the adolescent years *(probably so)*
- Reduces the need for patient cooperation (*e.g.,* headgear) *(probably so)*
- Makes scheduling easier *(definitely yes)*
- Improves long-term stability *(the jury still is out on this one)*

One of the major goals of our approach to early treatment is to have the majority of patients complete the final fixed appliance phase before the first day of high school. In our community, there is a major difference between scheduling a patient during elementary and middle school hours as opposed to scheduling a patient in high school. In fact, we have found that by initiating treatment, the speed of the eruption of teeth in some early mixed dentition patients appears to be accelerated.

Our experience has shown that it is very important, when initiating various early treatment protocols, to avoid prolonged Phase I treatments with ill-defined goals and of unknown duration. Each protocol should be established so that the length of treatment is predictable and should be known to the patient and the parent before treatment begins. Our initial treatment protocols generally average about one year in duration, with the intent of providing both efficient and effective treatment. Perhaps Dr. Alvin W. Nolan, a New Orleans orthodontist who practiced for nearly 50 years, said it best regarding early treatment, with the admonition, "Do not treat from the womb to the tomb."

TREATMENT TIMING

So, when is the optimal time to begin orthodontic treatment? Which is better, one-phase treatment or two-phase treatment? Articles concerning these questions have appeared in major lay publications such as *Newsweek*, *Time*, *The Wall Street Journal*, and *The New York Times* within the last two years. The topic of the 2001 Moyers Symposium, "Treatment Timing: Orthodontics in Four Dimensions," also points to the relevance of these issues today. Yet, there is no simple answer to either of the aforementioned questions.

It is our contention that there is no one "best time" to treat all orthodontic patients. Rather, the decision concerning when to treat depends on the nature of the patient's problems and concerns; the needs of each patient must be evaluated individually. Therefore, only general comments can be made regarding the efficacy of a specific treatment protocol administered at a specific stage of maturational development. That said, we still will venture our opinion concerning a general scheme of treatment timing that is based not only our clinical experience, but also on the outcomes of the many clinical studies described in detail later in this volume. Intervention at various stages of development is discussed below.

Deciduous Dentition

We often are referred very young patients for evaluation who have significant skeletal and/or dental abnormalities. It is very unusual for us to see patients before the age of three years. By this time, the complete deciduous dentition has erupted. The problems that appear most often in very young patients are Class III malocclusion (often characterized by mandibular prognathism) as well as patients with increased vertical development and often an accompanying anterior open bite. Other open bites may be associated with a persistent digital (*i.e.*, thumb, finger) sucking habit. We sometimes are referred patients with unilateral posterior crossbite who have a significant lateral shift of the mandible to one side during closure. Less frequently, patients with craniofacial anomalies (*e.g.*, cleft lip and palate, hemifacial microsomia, Crouzon's syndrome) are seen by us as part of an interdisciplinary work-up.

Unless there is a significant skeletal abnormality or asymmetry that obviously will cause further harm to the patient, generally we do not intervene until the patient is in the early mixed dentition. We do not begin treatment until this time for several reasons, the first of which is patient cooperation. Often a three or four year old patient simply is not capable of understanding what is required and thus, in spite of the wishes and encouragement of well-meaning parents, is not compliant. We do not want to run the risk of harming the orthodontist-patient relationship by insisting that the patient do something that could be handled easily later.

An example of such a situation is the elimination of a digital sucking habit. Our usual approach to this problem is to tell the parent that not much irreversible harm will occur in the skeletal regions of the face until the time of eruption of the upper and lower permanent central incisors. At this point, especially for a child with a reasonable level of psychological maturation, an aggressive approach to the management of the digital habit (including the implementation of a "thumb contract;" see Chapter 8) is undertaken.

A similar timing of the management of Class III malocclusion is recommended. Treatment is initiated at about the time of the eruption of the upper central incisors. Even though the parents or family dentist may notice the appearance of an anterior crossbite at a very young age, we prefer to coordinate treatment in most instances so that all permanent first molars are erupted and the maxillary central incisors are near eruption or just beginning to erupt.

We have found that perhaps the most important factor in the maintenance of the correction of a Class III malocclusion is establishing adequate vertical overlap (*i.e.*, overbite) of the permanent incisors. Usually, when treatment of underbite is initiated in the deciduous dentition, a satisfactory resolution of the problem can be attained, especially if the patient wears an orthopedic facial mask as directed. Much difficulty is encountered, however, in maintaining the correction if the patient is in the deciduous dentition, because of the lack of interdigitation of the flat primary teeth.

The prognosis for the success of treatment of Class III malocclusion depends on a number of factors, including the severity of the problem, the age of the patient at the orthodontic examination, a family history of Class III skeletal problems, and the presence of etiological factors that may promulgate the Class III relationship (*e.g.*, upper airway obstruction). Upper airway obstruction may also be a concern in patients with problems in the vertical dimension (*e.g.*, skeletal open bite). In instances of apparent airway obstruction, observed either clinically or radiographically, referral to a medical specialist may be indicated.

Early Mixed Dentition

Tooth-size/arch-size discrepancy problems often are handled efficiently and effectively in the early mixed dentition. Perhaps the most common aged patient referred to our practice for examination and possible treatment is the eight or nine year old child who is in the second or third grade. These patients usually present with crowding and rotation of the maxillary and/or mandibular incisors and often a lack of space for the eruption of the maxillary lateral incisors. Less frequently, the patients may have a unilateral or bilateral posterior crossbite.

In instances of a severe arch length discrepancy (*i.e.*, >6 mm of crowding in the mandibular arch), a serial extraction protocol is recommended, by which deciduous teeth are removed sequentially to allow space for the eruption of the permanent dentition. The implementation of this protocol usually results in the removal of four first premolars combined with a single phase of fixed appliance therapy after the rest of the permanent teeth have erupted (excluding third molars). This approach to treatment is undertaken infrequently, because patients in the early mixed dentition with severe tooth-size/arch-size problems are not seen too often; however, serial extraction is appropriate in such patients.

We have had much success over the last twenty years in managing patients with mild to moderate arch length problems by way of an orthopedic expansion protocol, with or without prior orthodontic "decompensation" of the mandibular arch. The bonded acrylic splint expander (Fig. 1-1) has been our appliance of choice in patients with transverse constriction of the maxilla (*e.g.*, intermolar width of <31 mm). Whereas the extraction of permanent teeth still is necessary in about 10% of patients in whom this protocol is undertaken (often the extraction of two maxillary first premolars in Class II patients with reasonably well-balanced facial profiles), long-term stability of the treated result has been observed.[13]

Treatment with a bonded acrylic splint expander has many other positive treatment effects in addition to increasing maxillary arch length, such as the correction of unilateral and bilateral posterior crossbites. Further, we have observed the spontaneous correction of many borderline Class III malocclusions characterized by anterior crossbite. Typically, the acrylic splint expander has a bite opening effect because of the posterior occlusal coverage that opens the vertical dimension slightly, facilitating anterior crossbite correction.

Paradoxically, rapid maxillary expansion also may lead to a spontaneous correction of borderline Class II malocclusion. The maxilla is widened so that when active treatment is finished, the maxillary dentition is wider than the mandibular dentition. The patient often postures the mandible slightly forward after the expander has been removed and a simple removable palatal plate has been delivered. In contrast to the spontaneous correction of Class III malocclusion that may occur within the first few weeks or months of expander treatment, spontaneous Class II correction, if it occurs, appears during the retention period.

Late Mixed Dentition

The opportunity to treat Class II malocclusion successfully exists at many stages of dentitional development. A search of the literature reveals that various orthodontic and orthopedic treatments are undertaken by orthodontists worldwide from the late deciduous dentition to adulthood. Therefore, when is the optimal time to treat Class II problems, especially those characterized by mandibular skeletal retrusion?

In the selection of treatment modalities, particularly in the treatment of Class II malocclusion, the admonition of Hippocrates (roughly translated, "Above all, do no harm") should be kept in mind. It may have been that many of the more recently developed techniques and protocols were devised in response to unfavorable treatment outcomes that were seen in the past, such as the treatment response of the patient shown in Figure 1-6. This patient was treated in the 1970s with extraoral traction and the removal of four first premolars. An unfavorable change in his soft tissue profile resulted, even though he had a satisfactory occlusion at the end of treatment. This patient probably would have been managed far differently today, given our better understanding of diagnostic criteria and the increased number of treatment methods available, including functional jaw orthopedics and orthognathic surgery.

In contrast, the selection of an appropriate treatment protocol, such as that used in the treatment of an eight-year-old patient with significant mandibular skeletal retrusion camouflaged in part by a decreased lower anterior facial height (Fig. 1-7), can result in a satisfactory functional and esthetic outcome.

We have found that an efficient time to initiate treatment of Class II malocclusion is during the late mixed or early permanent dentition. Both clinical and experimental evidence demonstrates that Class II treatment is more effective in the circumpubertal growth period than at an earlier time.[14-17] Thus, in patients with reasonably well-balanced faces and mild-to-moderate overjet, deferring a definitive correction of Class II until the end of the mixed dentition period may be prefer-

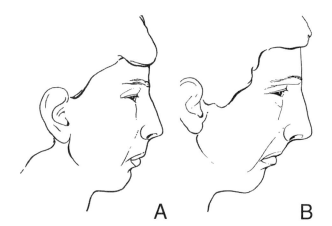

Figure 1-6. Facial outline of a patient treated by way of extraoral traction and the removal of four first premolars. Note the negative facial changes that occurred, including the backward slant of the upper lip and the opening of the nasolabial angle. *A.* Before treatment. *B.* After treatment.

able. For example, a twin block or FR-2 appliance of Fränkel can be used effectively during this period of development to treat patients whose major anteroposterior problem is mandibular skeletal retrusion. On the other hand, patients with maxillary prognathism can be treated effectively with extraoral traction.

It should be noted, however, that the majority of Class II patients present with a transverse discrepancy of the maxilla relative to the mandible.[18] In addition, many Class II patients present with interarch discrepancies between tooth size and available arch perimeter. Frequently, crowding in one or both arches is superimposed on the sagittal problem. If this is the situation, early orthodontic and orthopedic intervention is recommended in the early mixed dentition to facilitate the correction of intraarch problems; definitive correction of the Class II relationship is deferred until later.

Permanent Dentition

The management of some orthodontic problems is best left to the early permanent dentition, for example, interdental spacing. Many maxillary midline diastemas improve after the permanent canines erupt, especially if excess soft tissue is not present in the region of the diastema. Spacing problems in general are treated effectively after the permanent teeth have erupted, and earlier intervention may necessitate prolonged retention of the achieved result. For these patients, a circumferential supracrestal fiberotomy[19] or frenectomy[20] may be indicated after space closure is completed.

Most mild-to-moderate crowding problems also are handled satisfactorily in the early permanent dentition. Treatment can involve an initial phase of rapid maxillary expansion to widen the maxilla, creating additional space for the eruption and alignment of the maxillary dentition. A modest amount of additional arch space can be gained in the mandibular dental arch as well. The mandibular teeth of patients with a constricted maxilla often are tipped lingually. After RME, the teeth in the lower arch can be uprighted with fixed appliances into a stable position.

An alternative method of managing mild-to-moderate arch length problems is to perform judicious interproximal reduction, particularly in the canine and premolar regions. If larger tooth-size/arch-size problems are present, the extraction of permanent teeth (usually first or second premolars) is indicated. Fixed appliances are used to fine detail the occlusion.

Most types of surgical impactions are handled in the permanent dentition. First, it is important to monitor retained deciduous teeth carefully. As a rule, as soon as the same tooth on the opposite side is lost, the retained or ankylosed tooth (assuming a permanent successor is present) should be removed. If the impaction of a maxillary canine is noted, rapid maxillary expansion at the beginning of the comprehensive phase of treatment has been shown to be helpful in facilitating canine eruption.

Finally, the management of patients with missing, misshapen or malposed teeth pose particular problems for the orthodontist. In these instances, an interdisciplinary team should be formed to manage such problems prospectively. It is far better for everyone concerned to establish a written set of objectives on which everyone involved agrees, rather than simply "see what happens" when the orthodontist tries to solve the problem alone

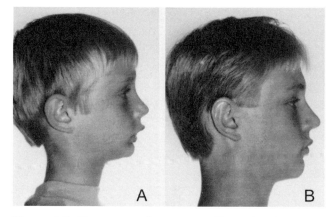

Figure 1-7. Treatment of a young Class II patient with mandibular skeletal retrusion and a short lower anterior facial height. *A.* Initial lateral photograph. *B.* After treatment with the FR-2 appliance of Fränkel followed by comprehensive fixed appliance therapy. Note the improvement in the soft tissue profile.

and then consults the family dentist or specialist after orthodontic treatment has been completed.

CONCLUDING REMARKS

In a lecture given to junior dental students at the University of Michigan, Lee W. Graber discussed the method of Class III correction with the orthopedic facial mask. He described the treatment effects in simple and straightforward terms, *i.e.*, "A little bit here, a little bit there." In many respects, his comment may summarize the orthopedic treatment of both Class III and Class II malocclusion.

In fact, the same conclusions were reached in our studies of functional protrusion in non-human primates some 25 years ago.[21-23] The treatment results were not due to a change in a specific craniofacial structure or region. Rather, the change in molar relationship was due to both pronounced and subtle adaptations throughout the craniofacial complex.

We have been involved in clinical and experimental studies of growth modification now for nearly 35 years. Our expectations regarding clinically relevant orthodontic and orthopedic intervention have changed over the years, as both short-term and long-term experimental and clinical data become available. With regard to sagittal malocclusion, in general our expectations are more limited than they were some years ago. There is no question that functional jaw orthopedics and facial mask therapy can have a positive effect compared to what would have occurred without intervention. Over the long-term, however, the responses are more muted, with part of the achieved skeletal effect incorporated into the further anteroposterior and vertical craniofacial growth of the patient.

One of the critical factors in correcting anteroposterior malocclusions is to achieve an optimal interdigitation of the permanent teeth. Even though some or most of the orthopedic treatment effect may not be detectable at the end of adolescence (depending on the specific appliance used), the establishment of an interlocking occlusion leads to a stable treatment result over the long-term.

From our perspective, the single most useful orthopedic appliance that has broad application is the rapid maxillary expander, an appliance that is used to treat deficiencies in maxillary development. Signs of maxillary deficiency include far more than just anterior and posterior crossbite as well as crowding of the maxillary dentition. In fact, the signs of maxillary deficiency are such that they often appear together, as in what might be termed "maxillary deficiency syndrome."[3] This topic will be discussed in more detail in subsequent chapters.

REFERENCES CITED

1. McNamara JA, Jr. Ordinary orthodontics: Starting with the end in mind. World J Orthod 2000;1:45-54.
2. Daskalogiannakis J. Glossary of orthodontic terms. Chicago: Quintessence, 2000.
3. McNamara JA, Jr. Maxillary transverse deficiency. Amer J Orthod Dentofac Orthop 2000;117:567-570.
4. Brunelle JA, Bhat M, Lipton JA. Prevalence and distribution of selected occlusal characteristics in the US population, 1988-91. J Dent Res 1996;75:706-713.
5. Proffit WR, Fields HW, Moray LJ. Prevalence of malocclusion and orthodontic treatment need in the United States: Estimates from the N-HANES III survey. Int J Adult Orthod Orthogn Surg 1998;13:97-106.
6. McNamara JA, Jr. A method of cephalometric evaluation. Am J Orthod 1984;86:449-69.
7. McNamara JA, Jr, Kelly KA. Frontiers in dental and facial esthetics. Ann Arbor: Monograph 38, Craniofacial Growth Series, Center for Human Growth and Development and Department of Orthodontics and Pediatric Dentistry, The University of Michigan, 2001.
8. Graber TM, Swain BF. Orthodontics: current principles and techniques. St. Louis: CV Mosby, 1985.
9. Graber TM, Rakosi T, Petrovic AG. Dentofacial orthopedics with functional appliances. St. Louis: C.V. Mosby Co., 1985.
10. Proffit WR, Fields HW, Jr. Contemporary orthodontics, 2nd edition. St Louis: Mosby Year Book, 1993.
11. McNamara JA, Jr, Brudon WL. Orthodontic and orthopedic treatment in the mixed dentition. Ann Arbor: Needham Press, 1993.
12. Trotman CA, McNamara JA, Jr, eds. Creating the compliant patient. Ann Arbor: Monograph 33, Craniofacial Growth Series, Center for Human Growth and Development, The University of Michigan, 1997.
13. Geran RG. The long-term effects of rapid maxillary expansion in the early mixed dentition. Ann Arbor: Department of Orthodontics and Pediatric Dentistry, The University of Michigan, 1998.
14. Petrovic A, Stutzmann JJ, Oudet C. Control process in the postnatal growth of the condylar cartilage. In: McNamara JA, Jr, ed. Determinants of mandibular form and growth. Ann Arbor: Monograph 4, Craniofacial Growth Series, Center for Human Growth and Development, The University of Michigan, 1975:
15. McNamara JA, Jr, Bookstein FL, Shaughnessy TG. Skeletal and dental changes following functional regulator therapy on Class II patients. Am J Orthod 1985;88:91-110.
16. Baccetti T, Franchi L, Toth LR, McNamara JA, Jr. Treatment timing for twin block therapy. Am J Orthod Dentofac Orthop 2000
17. Baccetti T, Franchi L. Maximizing esthetic and functional changes in Class II treatment by appropriate treatment timing. In: McNamara JA, Jr, Kelly KA, eds. Frontiers of

dental and facial esthetics. Ann Arbor: Monograph 38, Craniofacial Growth Series, Center for Human Growth and Development and Department of Orthodontics and Pediatric Dentistry, The University of Michigan, 2001.
18. Tollaro I, Baccetti T, Franchi L, Tanasescu CD. Role of posterior transverse interarch discrepancy in Class II, Division 1 malocclusion during the mixed dentition phase. Am J Orthod Dentofacial Orthop 1996;110:417-22.
19. Edwards JG. A long-term prospective evaluation of the circumferential supracrestal fiberotomy in alleviating orthodontic relapse. Am J Orthod Dentofac Orthop 1988;93:380-7.
20. Edwards JG. The diastema, the frenum, the frenectomy: a clinical study. Am J Orthod 1977;71:489-508.
21. McNamara JA, Jr. Neuromuscular and skeletal adaptations to altered function in the orofacial region. Am J Orthod 1973;64:578-606.
22. McNamara JA, Jr, Carlson DS. Quantitative analysis of temporomandibular joint adaptations to protrusive function. Am J Orthod 1979;76:593-611.
23. McNamara JA, Jr, Bryan FA. Long-term mandibular adaptations to protrusive function: an experimental study in *Macaca mulatta*. Am J Orthod Dentofac Orthop 1987;92:98-108.

Chapter 2
THE CLINICAL EXAMINATION

With Patrick J. Nolan, Kristine S. West and Cherie R. Lovett

One of the most elementary yet critical procedures in every orthodontic practice is the initial clinical examination, the style of which varies widely among clinicians. The purpose of this chapter is to describe in detail the step-by-step protocol that is used in our private practice. This sequence of events has evolved since one of us (JAMc) entered the private practice of orthodontics in Ann Arbor in 1971. We remained a solo practice until 1989, at which time a partnership was formed. At present, four orthodontists share the care of virtually all patients.

PRACTICE DEMOGRAPHICS

We are very fortunate to practice in a fully restored and modernized 1889 Victorian residence of the Queen Anne style (Fig. 2-1), a historic landmark (the Reuben Kempf house) in Ann Arbor. We feel that the physical appearance of a practitioner's office building makes a statement to the community about the quality of orthodontics provided, and we have made every effort to make our building warm and friendly to our patient families, providing 21st century orthodontics in a 19th century structure.

Considering the three above ground floors, as well as the lower level, the building occupies about 6,000 square feet, 3,800 square feet of which is devoted to our orthodontic practice. The foyer, reception area (Fig. 2-2), business office, and main operatory are located on the first floor. There are five chairs in the main operatory, four in an open bay arrangement (Fig. 2-3) and one in a smaller private treatment room that is used for mini-consultations as well as for routine treatment. In addition, we have a large initial examination room and a records room on the second floor. In the lower level are the laboratory, staff lounge and kitchen area, staff meeting room, and space for model storage.

Our practice has evolved over the years to include a substantial number of young children (Table 2-1). The percentage of adults has dropped somewhat during the last two decades from nearly 30% to 17% currently, not necessarily because the number of adult patients is less, but rather that referrals of patients in the mixed dentition have risen sharply. Patients who might be considered traditional orthodontic age (11–16 years) now comprise only slightly more than a quarter of our patients beginning active treatment.

Patients with tooth-size arch-size discrepancies are seen most commonly, with their malocclusions due primarily to crowding or protrusion problems, although a third present with Class II malocclusion (Table 2-2). Six percent of patients are treated for various types of Class III malocclusion.

Most of the treatment protocols used routinely in our practice are described in detail throughout this text. For mixed dentition patients, arch development protocols are most common, but we also undertake protocols involving guidance of eruption and serial extraction. Most functional jaw orthopedics is performed during the late mixed and early permanent dentition stages, although earlier orthopedic intervention sometimes is indicated in patients with severe skeletally based malocclusions.

Surgical orthodontic protocols are prescribed for late

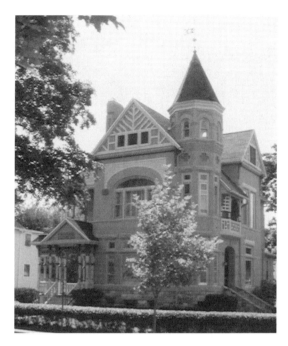

Figure 2-1. Our orthodontic practice is located in an 1889 Victorian building in the Queen Anne style, a historic landmark in Ann Arbor.

Table 2-1. Percentage of patients according to chronological age at the start of treatment.

Group	Age Range	Percentage
Adult	> 16 years	17%
Adolescent	11–16 years	28%
Juvenile	< 11 years	55%

Table 2-2. Distribution of patients currently in active treatment according to the Angle classification of malocclusion.

Classification	Percentage
Class I	59%
Class II, Division 1	28%
Class II, Division 2	7%
Class III	6%

adolescent and adult patients with significant skeletal discrepancies, and we work closely with colleagues from other disciplines in the treatment of dentally compromised patients. Typically, we refer patients with temporomandibular joint problems to their family dentist or another dental specialist for primary treatment, and intervene orthodontically only after their symptoms have subsided. Virtually all patients treated by us undergo at least one phase of comprehensive fixed appliance treatment.

INITIAL CONTACT WITH OFFICE

It is our aim to conduct the initial examination as part of a routine practice day, rather than at the beginning or end of the day or on specific days set aside for "practice growth." Thus, we have designated one of our senior staff members as the "treatment coordinator," whose responsibility it is to coordinate all aspects of the initial patient examination. During the examination, the treatment coordinator functions in a manner somewhat similar to a "physician's assistant" in a medical practice.

One of the most obvious attributes of a successful treatment coordinator is the ability to communicate effectively and efficiently with patients, parents, and referring dentists regarding all aspects of orthodontic, orthopedic, and surgical treatments. The treatment coordinator assumes primary responsibility for conducting the initial examination, after having been

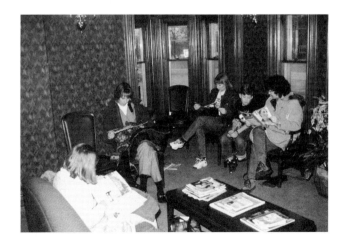

Figure 2-2. Reception room.

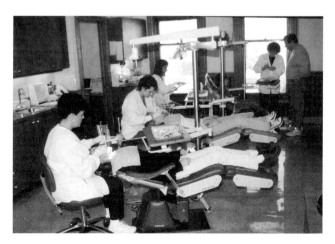

Figure 2-3. Main operatory.

trained appropriately by the orthodontist. In addition, the orthodontists must calibrate the treatment coordinator to make sure that the specific orofacial measurements and evaluations to be described below are obtained correctly and in a reproducible manner.

It is our objective to provide our patient families and their referring practitioners with as much information as possible during the initial examination. We have found that in well over 90% of our initial meetings, the patient and their families are provided with sufficient information (*e.g.*, differential diagnosis, treatment options, treatment recommendations, length and cost of treatment) to allow them to determine whether they wish to pursue treatment in our office. We choose to make the initial examination a "one-step exam," in most instances, avoiding the necessity of a formal consultation later.

Telephone Interaction

As with most orthodontic practices, the vast majority of initial contacts with our business office are made by telephone (Fig. 2-4). Our office staff consists of the office manager, the appointment coordinator, and an office assistant. Each of these individuals is capable of registering a patient for an initial examination visit.

We try to leave nothing to chance regarding the initial office interaction, and we have a script that is followed by our office personnel. A log is kept regarding each phone call. If there is anything unusual about the patient, including preexisting conditions, this information is noted in the log and later is made available to the treatment coordinator before she sees the patient.

The person calling is questioned regarding whether the patient has been seen in our office previously and whether the patient has been seen before by another orthodontist. If the answer to the second question is in the affirmative, the staff member discusses with the caller the nature of the interaction and whether orthodontic treatment has been rendered previously.

A modest fee is charged for a routine orthodontic examination; we do not provide our services without fee. If the patient is seeking a second opinion or has a problem involving temporomandibular disorders (TMD), the examination usually is more complicated, and a slightly higher fee for the examination is charged.

If a patient has a complicated history of temporomandibular joint problems, the patient is asked to bring a written chronology of his or her condition to the initial examination, including a description of the symptoms, the onset and duration of the symptoms, and a list of the names, addresses, and telephone numbers of any of the dental and medical practitioners seen in the past for the condition.

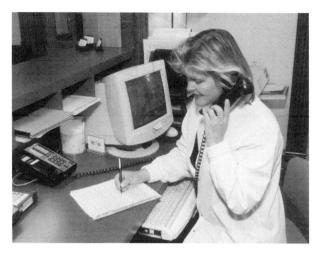

Figure 2-4. The initial contact with the office is via telephone.

The caller will be offered several appointment times and then will be asked which day and time is most convenient (we do not offer weekend or evening appointments). The staff member schedules the appointment and then obtains the appropriate demographic information concerning the patient. She then describes the sequence of events that will occur during the initial examination, including the role of the treatment coordinator.

The caller is told that we routinely obtain a panoramic radiograph at the beginning of the appointment. If the family dentist has taken a panoramic radiograph recently, the family is asked to bring a copy of the radiograph with them to the initial examination. It usually is not necessary for us to retake the panoramic radiograph, unless the radiograph from the family dentist is more than one year old or is not of diagnostic quality.

The caller is informed that, although the new patient will be examined by one of the orthodontic partners at the initial examination, patient care is shared by all orthodontists. It has been our experience that if a family is informed of this style of practice from the beginning, little difficulty is encountered with this arrangement. In fact, most patients and their families appreciate having an orthodontist on-call whom they know and have interacted with previously in case of emergency.

The office staff member will thank the caller for contacting the practice, ask if there are any further questions (including a need for directions to the office), and then tells the caller that she looks forward to meeting their family in the near future.

New Patient Letter

Following the gathering of demographic information from the patient or parent if the patient is a minor, a personalized letter is sent to the family, welcoming them to our office. In the letter, the date and time of the examination is listed. In addition, we provide written information about our practice, including office hours and practice policies (*e.g.,* no long appointment after 3:30 p.m., patients seen by multiple orthodontists).

Health History

In addition to the new patient letter, each patient is sent a health history (Fig. 2-5) that has been customized either for a child or an adult patient. Each health history requests demographic information, as well as a listing of the family dentist, family physician, and the source of referral. We also inquire about family history, medical history, respiratory history, and dental and temporomandibular joint history. Finally, we ask the patient about their primary concerns and their expectations regarding orthodontic treatment.

The introductory letter and health history are mailed the day the appointment is made. We ask that the health history be filled out and sent back to us two weeks prior to the initial examination appointment.[1] This time interval allows the office staff to make the chart in advance and check insurance benefits prior to the patient's appointment. The office staff also have sufficient time to call the family dentist to see if they have a recent panoramic radiographic or to determine whether records are available if the examination is a second opinion. If a dental condition exists, specific information can be obtained from the family practitioner or specialist (*e.g.,* vitality of evulsed tooth, specific concerns about implant placement, information about treatment for temporomandibular disorders.) If there is a medical condition, it also is possible to contact the patient's physician for any required information (*e.g.,* premedication).

One of the front office staff will contact the patient or patient's parent if the health history has not been returned to our office within the specified period. If the health history still has not been returned by the appropriate date, the patient will be asked to arrive at the office early. This request is made when one of the office staff calls to confirm the initial examination appointment.

INITIAL EXAMINATION

At the start of each practice day, we conduct what is called the "huddle,"[2] a brief staff meeting held at the beginning of each practice day. The staff and orthodontist gather in the main operatory five minutes prior to the first scheduled appointment time. The staff has checked

Table 2-3. Items considered at the "huddle," the brief staff meeting held at the beginning of each practice day.

- Number and type of initial examinations and consultations
- Record reviews and treatment evaluations
- Patients with extended treatment times
- Problem patients
- Patients scheduled for immediate appliances
- Routine appointment rotations (number of weeks between appointments)
- Staff person "on deck" for the day
- Last person to leave the office at the end of the day (responsible for closing the office)
- Upcoming schedule alerts

in and is ready to deliver patient care. This brief meeting is organized and conducted by the office manager.

Although the meeting time is short, a variety of items are considered, including the topics listed in Table 2-3. The office manager will tell the orthodontist about the patients scheduled for an initial examination, mentioning if they are relatives of current patients and if they have any unusual problems or concerns (*e.g.,* craniofacial malformation, TMD problem, restorative issue).

We feel that the huddle is very important for sustaining office morale and for setting the tone for the day. It allows us not only to deal with patient issues, but with staff concerns as well. In effect, the huddle serves as a mini staff meeting.

Arrival of Patient at Office

For the purpose of this example, we will be describing the initial examination of a 10-year old male patient accompanied by his mother. After the patient family enters the office (Fig. 2-6), immediate eye contact is made by one or more of the staff members, and the patient and parent are greeted as soon as possible (Fig. 2-7). Usually the new arrivals are carrying the new patient packet, so identifying them is not difficult. At the corner of the reception desk is a framed list of the names of new patients that will be seen on that day (Fig. 2-8). We find that the use of this type of notification is another form of welcoming that is appreciated, especially by younger patients.

The patient is instructed on the method of using the "On-Deck™" feature of the Ortho II computer system (Ortho II™ Computer Systems, Ames IA). A terminal and keyboard are located on a table in the foyer of the office. The patient simply types his or her last name on the keyboard and, if the patient has an appointment on that day, their complete name will appear with the question, "Is this you?" The patient then responds by indicating "yes" or by typing his or her name if it is not.

CLINICAL EXAMINATION

ORTHODONTIC PATIENT INFORMATION AND HEALTH HISTORY

Welcome to our office. Please fill out both sides of this form.

TELL US ABOUT YOUR CHILD

Patient Name: _____ Age: _____ Birthdate: _____ Sex: _____
Home Address: _____ Nickname: _____
_____ Home phone: _____
         City   State   Zip Code   Fax / E-Mail: _____

Family History

Father's Name: _____ Living? No Yes Occupation: _____
Mother's Name: _____ Living? No Yes Occupation: _____
Siblings (name and age): _____
Marital status of parents: Married   Divorced   Separated   Not married
Patient living with: Mother _____   Father _____   Other _____

Person(s) Responsible for Financial Matters

Name(s): _____   _____
Address: _____   _____
_____   _____
Phone (Residence): _____   _____
Phone (Business): _____   _____
Place of Employment: _____   _____
Social Security Number: _____   _____

Is patient covered by insurance for orthodontic treatment?   No   Yes   Company? _____
PLEASE SUPPLY INSURANCE FORMS IF YOU WOULD LIKE US TO FILE FOR YOUR REIMBURSEMENT.

	FAMILY DENTIST	FAMILY PHYSICIAN	REFERRED BY
NAME:	_____	_____	_____
ADDRESS:	_____	_____	_____
CITY, STATE:	_____	_____	_____

Medical History

Has the patient ever had:

Allergy	Cold Sores	Heart Condition/Murmur	Oral Ulcer
Anemia	Diabetes	Head or Face Injury	Previous Surgery
Arthritis	Endocrine Problems	Hepatitis	Rheumatic Fever
Asthma	Emotional Problems	Herpes	Thyroid Problems
Bleeding	Epilepsy Seizures	HIV Positive	Tuberculosis
Cancer	Headache/Migraine	Kidney Disease	Other (Describe below)

Comments: _____

Has the patient been under the care of a physician during the past two years, other than for routine examination?
                                            No   Yes
Condition: _____

Does the patient require premedication for dental procedures?   No   Yes
Present drugs or medication: _____

Figure 2-5. Health history for child. A modified version of this form is used for adult patients.

Birth defects, congenital problems: _____

Has the patient reached puberty (menstruation, voice change, hair)   No   Yes   How long ago? _____

Respiratory History   Does the patient:

1. Have allergies to: Seasonal grasses: _____   Food: _____
   Drugs: _____   Other: _____
2. Breathe through mouth?   Seldom   Sometimes   Usually
3. Snore when sleeping?   No   Yes
4. Have frequent colds?   No   Yes
5. Have frequent "stuffy nose"?   No   Yes
6. Have frequent sore throat or tonsillitis?   No   Yes
7. Have chewing or swallowing difficulties?   No   Yes

Has the patient received medical treatment from allergist or ear, nose, and throat specialist?
   No   Yes   If Yes: When _____   By whom: _____
   Nasal Surgery: _____   Tonsils removed: _____   Adenoids removed: _____

Dental and Temporomandibular Joint History

Has the patient had any unusual dental experiences?   No   Yes
   Specify: _____
Date of last dental checkup: _____   Were patient's teeth cleaned?   No   Yes
Has the patient ever been treated for TMJ ("Jaw Joint") problems   No   Yes
Does the patient have:

1. difficulty in mouth opening?   No   Yes
2. pain or clicking in jaw joint?   No   Yes
3. pain on chewing, yawning or wide opening?   No   Yes
4. pain in or about the ears or cheeks?   No   Yes
5. a bite that feels "uncomfortable" or "unusual"?   No   Yes
6. a jaw that "locks", "gets stuck" or "goes out"?   No   Yes
7. noises in or from the jaw joints?   No   Yes

The following habits are of interest. List information as it pertains to this patient:

1. Thumb/finger/lip sucking until _____ (age)   No   Yes
2. Grinding or clenching of teeth   No   Yes
3. Tongue thrusting or other functional problem   No   Yes

Has the patient had a previous orthodontic consultation?   No   Yes   Or treatment?   No   Yes
   Date: _____   Dr: _____   City, State: _____
Why did patient seek this consultation? _____
What is the primary problem? _____
_____

What is expected from orthodontic treatment? _____
_____

Signature: _____   Relationship: _____   Date: _____

Figure 2-5. Health history for child (cont.)

The office staff tells the patient about the availability of the toothbrushing area, located in the main operatory. If brushing is not needed, the patient and parent then are directed to seats in the reception area.

The information typed into the workstation in the foyer is relayed through the computer network to a workstation in the main operatory. Information on the display screen in the operatory includes the patient's

CLINICAL EXAMINATION

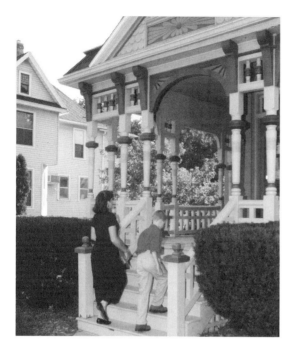

Figure 2-6. Patient and parent enter the office. The exterior decor adds to the ambiance of the visit.

first and last name, the type of procedure to be performed, the number of minutes that the patient has been in the office, and whether the patient is early or late regarding the scheduled appointment time.

Each day, one clinical staff person is designated as the "On-Deck coordinator." This person is responsible for making sure that clinical care functions on schedule. She is consulted if there is a desire on the part of the orthodontist to perform unschuled clinical procedures It also is her responsibility to determine the priority of the procedures being carried out simultaneously in the operatory area. She directs the orthodontists as to which chair she or he should attend to next.

Initial Interaction with the Treatment Coordinator

The On-Deck coordinator sees that the new patient is in the reception area and notifies the treatment coordinator. The treatment coordinator first will check the health history to familiarize herself with the patient. She then will walk to the reception area and greet the patient (Fig. 2-9).

Our treatment coordinator has found that it is better if her introduction of herself by name is delayed for a minute or two in order to allow the patient and parents to become accustomed to this new interaction. As she is accompanying the patient to the examination room, she talks with the patient and parent concerning a variety of general topics. When they are seated around the examination table (Fig. 2-10), she extends her hand to the patient and says, "We want to welcome you to the office. It is a pleasure to have you here. My name is Cherie." Then shaking the parent's hand, she says, "Thank you for letting us examine your child today." This initial interaction puts the patient at ease and lets the parents know that we appreciate their decision to bring their child to us for an orthodontic examination.

Radiograph Examination

Obtaining a panoramic radiograph (Fig. 2-11) at the initial examination appointment is extremely helpful in many ways. First, the radiograph reveals whether there are any missing or extra teeth present. The stage of den-

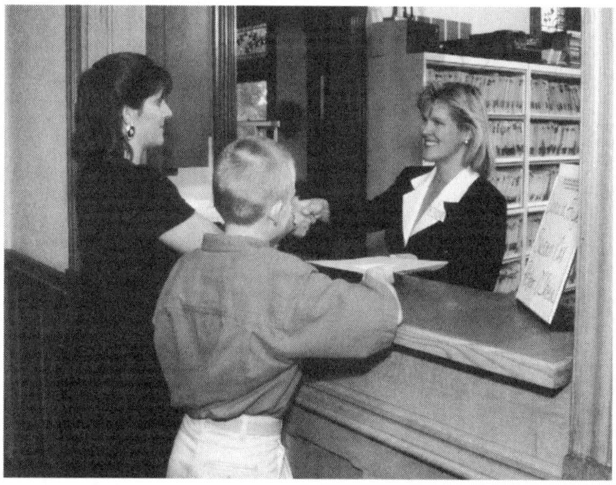

Figure 2-7. Patient and parent are greeted by the office manager. The family usually is carrying the new patient packet, so they are easily identifiable.

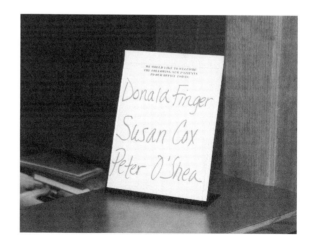

Figure 2-8. A framed sign is placed at the corner of the reception counter that lists the names of patients scheduled for initial examinations each day.

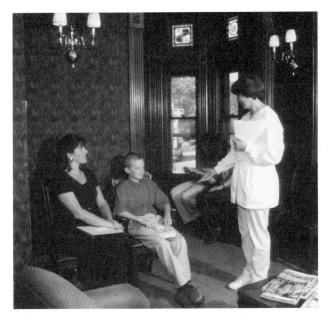

Figure 2-9. The treatment coordinator (CRL) greets the patient and parent in the reception area.

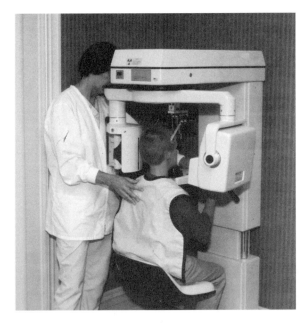

Figure 2-11. A panoramic radiograph is taken at the beginning of the initial examination.

tal development, critical in mixed dentition treatment, also can be evaluated. In addition, a cursory examination can be made of the contours of the mandibular condyles bilaterally. The panoramic radiograph also serves as an excellent teaching aid later in the examination.

Digital Imaging

At the initial examination appointment, various digital images can be obtained as well (Fig. 2-12). There are two excellent digital imaging programs that can be used routinely for manipulating digital images obtained photographically (Dolphin™, Dolphin Imaging, Woodland Hills CA; Showcase™, Dentofacial Software, Toronto, Ontario, Canada). A complete series of intra-oral or extraoral digital photographs can be taken (Fig. 2-13), or single images can be obtained for inclusion in correspondence to the referring practitioner.

We strongly suggest that careful attention is paid to the position of the head of the patient whenever radiographic or digital images are obtained. In order to provide guidelines for extraoral photography, a modified soft tissue Frankfort horizontal plane[3] is used. The top of the patient's ear is oriented along the same horizontal plane as is the midpoint between the eyebrow and the eyelash (Fig. 2-14) bilaterally. This head orientation can be visualized in both frontal and lateral views, min-

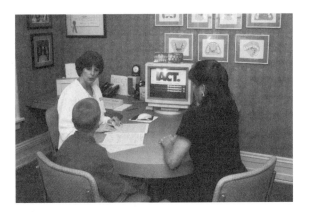

Figure 2-10. The treatment coordinator will initiate conversation on general topics and then will discuss the chief concerns of the patient and parent while reviewing the health history form.

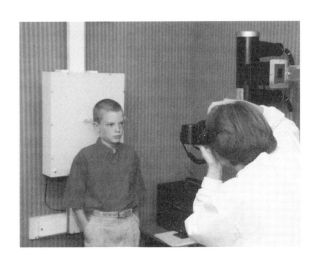

Figure 2-12. Extraoral (shown here) and intraoral digital photographs are obtained

CLINICAL EXAMINATION

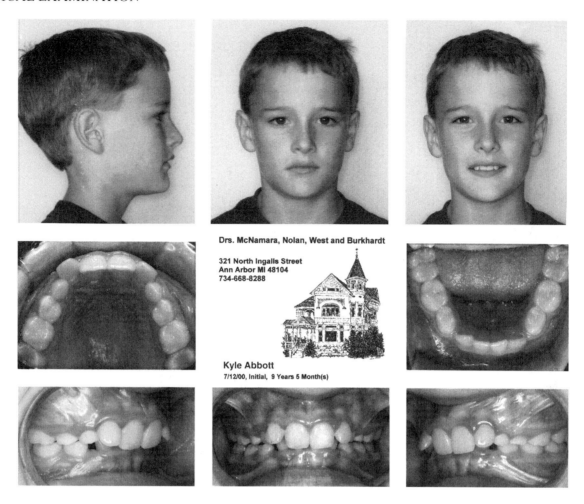

Figure 2-13. Composite digital photographs obtained with the Dolphin™ digital imaging system (Dolphin, Woodland Hills CA)

imizing variations in head position among patients and in serial headfilms and photographs of the same patient.

Personal History

After the radiographic and digital data have been obtained and processed, the treatment coordinator continues to interact with the patient and the parent while seated at a table in the examination room. The treatment coordinator inquires about the personal history of the patient and family (*e.g.*, nickname, grade in school, name of school, other patients being treated in our practice who are friends).

The treatment coordinator also will ask the patient and/or the parent to describe their chief concerns. These responses typically are recorded in the patient's or parent's own words (Table 2-4).

Family History

The treatment coordinator will ask about the general health and dental health status of the patient. This discussion covers family history, especially the occurrence of orthodontic problems linked to heredity (*e.g.*, Class III malocclusion, anterior open bite, deep bite). She also will discuss any history of previous orthodontic treatment of parents or siblings.

Medical History

The treatment coordinator then will evaluate the medical history, exploring any of the items that have been checked by the patient or parent. Of particular interest is any injury of the head or face region, especially if the patient has any signs or symptoms of temporomandibu-

Table 2-4. Typical responses of parents to inquiries about their chief concerns.

- "His teeth are too big and his jaws are too small."
- "Peter's lower teeth are crowded."
- "My child's overbite is too big."
- "Gayle (hygienist) said that Felipe has an overbite."
- "My dentist thought that it was time for Rachel to be seen in your office."

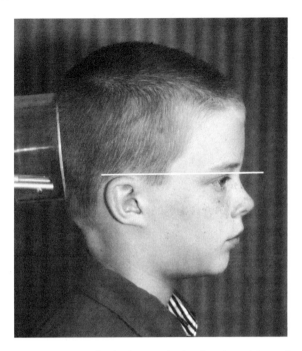

Figure 2-14. A method of reproducing head position when taking frontal and lateral photographs and radiographs. The head is oriented horizontally so that a line or plane is drawn between the top of the external ear and the midpoint between the eyebrow and the eyelash.

lar disorders. She also will identify the nature of any previous surgery, as well as any report of cold sores (differentiating between herpetic outbreaks and canker sores), hepatitis, rheumatic fever, or tuberculosis.

We have found it useful to ask a question defined in general terms as "emotional problems." Psychological and psychiatric conditions have been reported by many adult patients and have been noted in children as well. A general understanding of the nature of such problems is helpful to the orthodontist in defining future treatment options.

Respiratory History

The treatment coordinator then evaluates the responses to specific questions concerning respiratory history, including allergy, mouth breathing, snoring, sore throat, and tonsillitis. We also would like to know about the surgical treatments that have been performed by an otorhinolaryngologist, including intranasal surgery, adenoidectomy, or tonsillectomy (See Chapter 8 on the Vertical Dimension for a discussion of the relationship between altered respiratory function and craniofacial growth).

Dental and Temporomandibular Joint History

In the health history, seven questions that were defined in the 1983 ADA President's Conference on Temporo-

Table 2-5. Recommended questions about temporomandibular disorders. This series of questions originated at the 1983 ADA President's conference on the examination, diagnosis and management of temporomandibular disorders.[4]

Does the patient have:
- difficulty in mouth opening?
- pain or clicking in the jaw joint?
- pain on chewing, yawning or wide opening?
- pain in or about the ears or cheeks?
- a bite that feels "uncomfortable" or "unusual"?
- a jaw that "locks," "gets stuck" or "goes out"?
- noises in or from the jaw joints?

mandibular Disorders are asked.[4] These questions (Table 2-5) cover most of the signs and symptoms of temporomandibular disorders. Any positive responses are noted for later discussion with the orthodontist.

The treatment coordinator also notes any reports of habits or abnormal orofacial functions, including digital sucking, grinding or clenching of teeth, and tongue thrusting or other related problems for further discussion.

Oral Questions

The treatment coordinator will ask some specific oral questions that may or may not have been addressed in the review of the health history. She inquires about a history of facial trauma, and about the presence of facial scars other than those associated with chickenpox. She also asks about a history of bruxism and clenching and specifically about current or past temporomandibular joint symptoms, as well as whether there is a family history of temporomandibular disorders. She also inquires whether there is a history of arthritis either in the patient or in his or her parents.

Finally, the patient and parent are asked if there is any other information relevant to orthodontic treatment that has not been covered, including any unusual medical or dental occurrences.

CLINICAL EXAMINATION

The treatment coordinator has been trained to examine the patient and to obtain all objective measurements prior to the orthodontist's participation in the examination. These findings are recorded on the clinical examination form (Fig. 2-15).

Examination of the Temporomandibular Joints

The patient is examined for clicking in the joints, both by palpation and by auscultation by way of a stetho-

CLINICAL EXAMINATION

CLINICAL EVALUATION

DATE _____

NAME _____ AGE _____ SEX _____ EXAMINER _____

CHIEF COMPLAINT _____

_____

_____

_____

_____

_____

_____

_____

TMJ EXAMINATION

History of Facial Trauma	☐ Yes	☐ No	Facial Scars	☐ Yes	☐ No	
History of Bruxism	☐ Yes	☐ No	Clenching	☐ Yes	☐ No	LB — INT
History of TMJ symptoms	☐ Yes	☐ No	TM Disorders	☐ Mother	☐ Father	☐ None
Ortho Treatment	☐ Mother	☐ Father	Arthritis	☐ Mother	☐ Father	☐ Self ☐ None

Comments _____

CLICKING	LEFT	☐ None	☐ Opening ____ mm	☐ Closing ____ mm	☐ Protrusive ____
	RIGHT	☐ None	☐ Opening ____ mm	☐ Closing ____ mm	☐ Protrusive ____
CREPITUS		☐ None	☐ Left _____	☐ Right _____	
PAIN	LEFT	☐ None	☐ Within joint	☐ Muscular _____	
	RIGHT	☐ None	☐ Within joint	☐ Muscular _____	
OPENING/CLOSURE		☐ Straight	☐ Deviation Left	☐ Deviation Right	
CR/CO		☐ Straight	☐ Deviation Anterior	☐ Deviation Posterior	

Maximum Opening ____ mm   Lateral: Left: ____ mm   Right: ____ mm   Prot: ____ mm

Transpalatal Width ____ mm   Overjet ____ mm   Overbite ____ mm

SOFT TISSUE   ☐ Normal   ☐ Abnormal _____

   Incisor/lip ____ mm   Smile ____ mm   _____

MIDLINES   ☐ Coincident   ☐ Maxilla _____   ☐ Mandible _____

TOOTH SIZE   ☐ Normal   ☐ Large   ☐ Small   Diastema _____ ____ mm

OCCLUSAL WEAR   ☐ Mild   ☐ Moderate   ☐ Severe   Abnormalities _____

PERIODONTAL STATUS _____ Bleeding _____

PROVISIONAL DIAGNOSIS _____

_____

_____

PROVISIONAL TREATMENT PLAN _____

_____

_____

ESTIMATED DEGREE OF DIFFICULTY (0–100) _____   Initial Exam _____

TREATMENT TIME _____   Records _____

REFERRAL LETTERS NEEDED _____   PHASE I _____   COMPREHENSIVE _____

_____   Initial fee _____   Initial fee _____

COMMENTS _____   Monthly fee ____ x ____   Monthly fee ____ x ____

_____   Est. Ph II _____   PER VISIT _____

PARENT/SPOUSE _____   Initial _____   Retention _____

   Monthly fee ____ x ____

Figure 2-15. Clinical examination form.

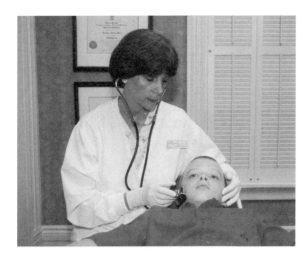

Figure 2-16. The treatment coordinator begins her evaluation of the temporomandibular joints with a stethoscopic examination.

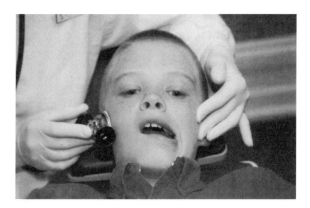

Figure 2-18. The patient is asked to move their jaw from side to side.

scope (Fig. 2-16). The patient is asked to open as wide as possible and then close, repeating this cycle several times (Fig. 2-17). The patient also is asked to move the jaw to the right and left in order to evaluate the range of motion (Fig. 2-18).

The stethoscope can be used to identify clicking in either or both joints, as well as crepitus, the "grinding" noise that occurs in some joints with soft tissue or hard tissue irregularities. We have developed a relatively simple scale in 0.5 units that indicates the severity of the crepitus. In a young patient with smooth sounding and feeling articular surfaces, the score given is 0. In a slightly older patient with normal sounding joints, a score of 0.5 is awarded. If clinically significant crepitus is noted in either or both joints, scores from 1.0 to 3.0 are given, with the larger numbers indicating more severe conditions.

Maximum interincisal opening is measured using a Therabite™ disposable ruler (Therabite Corp., Newtown Square PA; Figure 2-19). The notch at 0 mm is

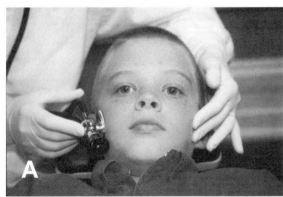

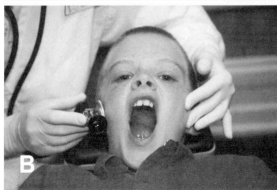

Figure 2-17. The patient is asked to A, close and B, open the mouth in order for the treatment coordinator to detect clicking or crepitus in either joint.

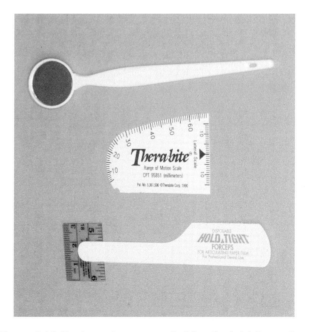

Figure 2-19. Basic equipment needed for the initial examination, including a disposable mouth mirror, a Therabite™ disposable ruler, a 30mm segment of a flexible plastic ruler held in a Hold Tight™ disposable forceps for articulating paper.

CLINICAL EXAMINATION

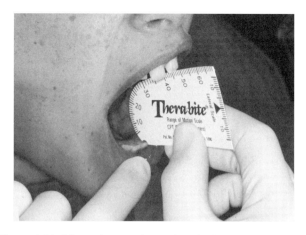

Figure 2-20. Measuring maximum interincisal opening with a Therabite™ disposable ruler.

placed on one of the lower incisors (Fig. 2-20). The patient then is instructed to open his or her mouth maximally, and a millimetric recording is obtained. A maximum interincisal opening of 40 mm or greater is considered within the normal range.

The flat end of the Therabite™ ruler can be used to measure the lateral movements of the mandible. Lateral excursions in both directions should be at least 10 mm. In fact, if a patient has unrestricted lateral movement, we do not make a specific measurement, but rather indicate that the range of movement was "10+ mm" in both directions. If there is any evidence of restricted movement, a specific millimeter measurement bilaterally is made and recorded on the clinical examination form. The flattened end of the Therabyte ruler can be used for this purpose (Fig. 2-19).

The treatment coordinator measures protrusion as the distance from the labial surface of the mandibular central incisors to the labial surface of the maxillary central incisors in maximum protrusion. Generally, this measurement should be at least 5 mm or greater.

The treatment coordinator completes her evaluation of the temporomandibular joint region by palpating the masticatory and facial musculature (Fig. 2-20) and the joints themselves. She also noted the path of opening and closure, as well as any discrepancy between centric occlusion and centric relation.

Other Oral Measurements

The treatment coordinator also measures transpalatal width, the shortest distance between the lingual surfaces of the maxillary first molars. This measurement can be obtained directly by using a flexible ruler or calipers. We have found it useful, however, to use a 30 mm section of plastic ruler attached to an articulation paper holder (Fig. 2-19). This ruler is placed intraorally between the maxillary first molars and the closest points between the upper molars are measured (Fig. 2-22). Typically, measurements of 2–5 mm on either side are estimated easily by the operator. Measurements of 30 mm or below are of clinical concern. Measurements of 36 mm or greater indicate that there is no significant transverse problem, given teeth of normal size.

The 30 mm ruler then is used to measure both overbite and overjet. Overjet is a direct measurement from the labial surface of the mandibular central incisors to the labial surface of the maxillary central incisors. Overbite can be measured by way of the millimeter ruler as well. More commonly, however, overbite is quantified as the percentage of vertical overlap of the upper incisor over the lower incisor (Figure 2-23). Ideally, overjet should be about 20% or 2 mm. The size of the di-

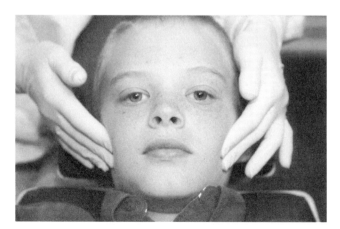

Figure 2-21. Muscle and joint tenderness is determined by palpation. Finger pressure of a consistent intensity should be applied to the masticatory musculature.

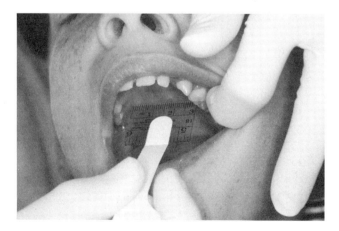

Figure 2-22. The intraoral determination of transpalatal width, as measured as the closest points between the permanent maxillary first molars.

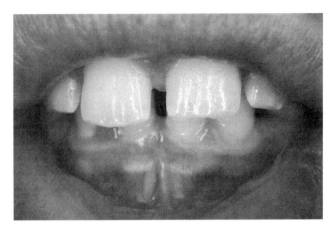

Figure 2-23. Overbite can be measured directly with a millimeter ruler (not shown) or it can be described as the percentage of overlap of the maxillary central incisors over the lower central incisors. In this example, the overbite is estimated to be 60%. The size of a midline diastema (if present) is measured as well.

astema between the maxillary central incisors (if present) is measured and noted as well.

At this time, a thorough evaluation of the soft tissue is made, including lifting the tongue with a piece of gauze. The cheeks, floor of the mouth and palatal area, as well as other regions of the mouth, are evaluated for both soft and hard tissue lesions.

The midlines are evaluated relative to the mid and upper face. The maxillary midline is measured relative to the maxilla. The lower midline is measured both to the mandible and to the maxillary midline. If a mandibular skeletal asymmetry is present, the lower midline may be centered relative to the mandible, but may be off to one side relative to upper facial structures.

Tooth size also is evaluated by way of a Boley gauge. We have found it useful to make a single measurement of the mesiodistal width of one maxillary central incisor. For European-Americans, a width of 8.9 mm (± 0.6) for males and 8.7 (± 0.6) mm for females is average, with a standard deviation of 0.6 mm.[5] The size of the central incisor serves as a guide as to whether the overall tooth size is within normal limits, is large, or is small. A central incisor width greater than 10 mm indicates that the upper central incisor is large. On the other hand, a mesiodistal diameter of 7.5 mm or less indicates that the central incisor is small relative to those of the general population. Although only an approximation of overall tooth size, this information about the relative size of the central incisors may be useful when deciding between orthopedic expansion and serial extraction in a mixed dentition patient.

The patient also is evaluated for the level of occlusal wear. Virtually all patients have some degree of wear. Generally, wear is marked as mild, moderate, or severe.

The treatment coordinator also will evaluate the periodontal status of the patient. At this point, she asks the patient: "Do your gums bleed when you brush your teeth or floss?" The answer to that question is written verbatim on the clinical examination form. The treatment coordinator also will measure the thickness of the attached gingiva in the lower anterior region, and will evaluate the patient for an abnormal frenum attachment in both arches.

After the treatment coordinator completes her evaluation, she will notify the orthodontist that the patient is ready for his or her examination.

Examination by the Orthodontist

Typically, the orthodontist is seeing patients concurrently in the main operatory, and so it may be several minutes before the orthodontist arrives at the initial examination. An experienced treatment coordinator can anticipate some of the general protocols that might be used for a specific patient, and she may begin some initial general discussion about these protocols, always saying that the orthodontist, of course, is the one to decide the specifics of the treatment protocol. She also uses this time to retrieve the panoramic radiograph and review the obvious anatomical features found on the film with the patient family.

The orthodontist enters the room, greets the patient and the parent, and then spends a few minutes in pleasant conversation. Questions are asked about the patient's school, sports or other activities, hobbies, etc. After the pleasantries are finished, the orthodontist will initiate a brief discussion with the patient and parent as to their chief concerns. He or she also may ask the treat-

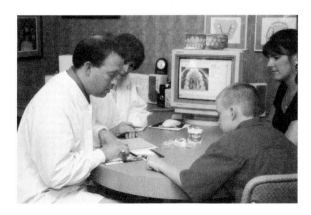

Figure 2-24. The orthodontist (PJN) reviews the findings of the panoramic radiograph with the patient and parent.

CLINICAL EXAMINATION

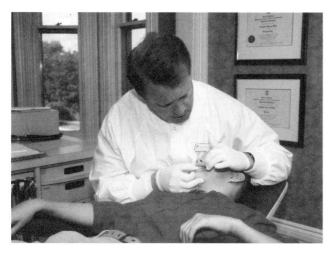

Figure 2-25. The orthodontist examines the patient, verifying the measurements and observations of the treatment coordinator.

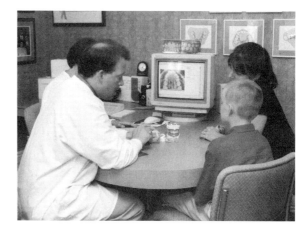

Figure 2-26. The orthodontist discusses the findings of the initial examination with the patient and parent, using examples of appliances as well as an interactive CD-Rom.

ment coordinator to reiterate the pertinent information gained thus far in the initial examination.

Review of the Panoramic Radiograph

The orthodontist will spend a minute or two discussing the findings of the panoramic radiograph (Fig. 2-23). He or she specifically will look for missing or extra teeth, cysts, tumors, or any other abnormal radiographic finding. It also is possible to obtain a general estimate regarding the size differential between the second deciduous molars and second premolars in this film. The presence or absence of third molars also is noted. Any abnormal findings are identified and discussed with the patient and parent.

At the completion of this phase of the examination, the orthodontist will ask the patient to stand, and the orthodontist will evaluate the soft tissue profile of the patient briefly. The patient then will be asked to sit again in the examination chair.

After appropriate hygienic and gloving procedures have been performed, the orthodontist will proceed with his or her clinical examination (Fig. 2-24). The orthodontist repeats the evaluation of the temporomandibular joint regions briefly. If any signs or symptoms of temporomandibular joint disorders are evident, however, the orthodontist will complete an in depth evaluation of these structures. An intraoral evaluation also is undertaken to verify the findings of the treatment coordinator.

The orthodontist will dictate to the treatment coordinator the findings of the intraoral orthodontic evaluation. This information either can be written on the clinical examination sheet by the treatment coordinator or can be entered directly into the clinical management system in the computer.

We have devised a sequence of information gathering shown in Table 2-6. This information is dictated to the treatment coordinator in sequence. The orthodontist then will dictate one or more treatment options.

After the clinical evaluation has been completed, specific demographic information about the patient's malocclusion is recorded on "Page 2" of the Ortho II™ management system. This information can be used later to retrieve data on patients with specific problems or certain types of malocclusions.

Treatment Options

After the orthodontist has completed the clinical examination, the patient and the orthodontist sit at the consultation table with the treatment coordinator and the parent (Fig. 2-26). The orthodontist then will summarize briefly the treatment options available.

We have found it effective to use a patient education

Table 2-6. The following information is gathered in sequence at the time of the orthodontist's examination:

- Angle classification
- Anteroposterior maxillary position
- Anteroposterior mandibular position
- Lower anterior facial height
- Transverse dimension
- Openbite or deepbite
- Dental crowding or spacing
- Presence of a diastema
- Abnormal tooth position
- Abnormal tooth shape
- Other relevant findings

CD-Rom program (Case Presenter™, Interactive Communication and Training (IACT), Birmingham AL) at this point. This interactive program provides illustrated and animated examples of the treatment protocols commonly used in our practice. Such protocols include routine fixed appliance therapy, orthopedic expansion, functional jaw orthopedics, and various types of orthognathic surgical procedures.

The orthodontist will explain the treatment options in general terms and then ask the patient and parent whether they have any questions about the proposed general course of treatment. Any questions are answered, and then the orthodontist thanks the family for coming to the office. He or she then departs to resume seeing patients in the main treatment operatory. Typically, the orthodontist will spend 7–10 minutes in the initial examination.

Explanation by Treatment Coordinator

The treatment coordinator describes the proposed treatment in detail (Fig. 2-27), once again using the interactive CD-Rom as a teaching aid in addition to actual models of sample appliances. She discusses the step-by-step procedures, beginning with the gathering of records. She explains that our routine records include extraoral and intraoral photographs, a panoramic radiograph and a lateral head film, as well as a set of study models. In some instances, another set of impressions is obtained for the fabrication of a diagnostic set up. Such a set up is used when an unusual extraction pattern is being considered by the orthodontist as a treatment option.

An explanation is given by the treatment coordinator about the day of appliance placement or delivery, which includes a risk management videotape. The consent form (Fig. 2-28) will be discussed in detail by the orthodontist during that visit, and the person responsible for treatment will be asked to sign this document.

In most instances, the general plan of treatment is established at the time of the initial examination. After the records are gathered at the next appointment, the records are reviewed in detail by one or more orthodontists, and the original treatment plan is verified or modified and then recorded on the treatment sheet for future reference. During the following appointment, after risk management issues have been handled, the records are reviewed again and discussed with the patient and parent. At this point, the patient will be given the appropriate appliance.

At the initial examination appointment, the typical financial arrangements are explained by the treatment

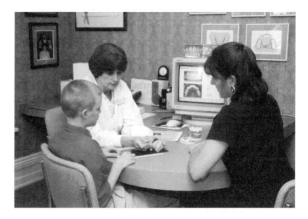

Figure 2-27. The treatment coordinator reviews the treatment options in detail, explaining the step-by-step process of the proposed treatment sequence.

coordinator, and the fees for the treatment are established. Typically, there are separate fees for the initial examination and for diagnostic records. Fees for active treatment may be included as one comprehensive phase or may be divided into two phases. The typical scheme of an initial payment followed by monthly payments for a specified number of months is used.

The final part of the initial examination involves reviewing practice policy. Once again, office hours are discussed, as is the necessity of scheduling longer appointments before 3:30 p.m.

The treatment coordinator will ask the family if they would like to schedule an appointment for records. This appointment can be scheduled on the management system computer in the initial examination room, or it can be scheduled by one of the front office staff. If the treatment coordinator escorts the patient to the front desk for scheduling, it is important that the treatment coordinator indicates by her verbal or non-verbal body language to the front desk staff whether the patient family wants to schedule another appointment.

"Care Call"

If a patient family has not scheduled a records appointment at the time of their departure from the office, it is the responsibility of the treatment coordinator to place a telephone call to the family within one week of the initial visit. The treatment coordinator will inquire as to whether the family has any questions or concerns that were not covered during the initial examination visit. She also will ask if they would like to schedule an appointment. Often, the follow-up call will result in the family scheduling a records appointment with us.

If the parent chooses not to schedule an appointment, the treatment coordinator will inquire about the

CLINICAL EXAMINATION

POTENTIAL RISKS AND LIMITATIONS OF ORTHODONTIC TREATMENT

(Patient Informed Consent)

Excellent orthodontic results can be achieved with informed and cooperative patients. You should be aware that orthodontic treatment, like treatment of any part of the body, has some inherent risks and limitations. These risks and limitations seldom are severe enough to offset the advantages of treatment, but they should be considered in making the final decision to undergo orthodontic treatment. Orthodontic treatment is usually elective, and no treatment always is an alternative.

Tooth decay, gum disease, and permanent markings (*decalcification*) on teeth can occur if patients do not brush their teeth frequently and properly and if they eat foods containing excessive sugar. Soft drinks containing sugar also should be avoided during orthodontic treatment. These same problems can occur in patients not wearing braces as well, but the risk is greater when wearing braces. Daily use of *Prevident 5000+* prescription toothpaste or rinsing with a fluoride mouthwash (for example, *Fluorigard* or *Act*) is recommended during orthodontic treatment. Decalcification also can occur under bonded acrylic appliances, such as a palatal expander.

A tooth that has been traumatized by an injury or a tooth that has a large filling may require root canal (*endodontic*) treatment when it is moved with an orthodontic appliance. Sometimes a tooth may have a non-vital or damaged nerve (*pulp*), which may not be apparent at the onset of orthodontic treatment. Orthodontics may make the need for root canal treatment apparent.

In some patients, the length of the roots of the teeth may be shortened (*root resorption*) during orthodontic treatment. Usually minor changes in root length are of no significant consequence, but on rare occasions it may become a serious threat to the longevity of the teeth involved. Rarely, root resorption may necessitate the early removal of orthodontic appliances.

After the braces are removed, patients are required to wear orthodontic retainers, as teeth have a tendency to change their position (*relapse*) after treatment. The wearing of retainers reduces this tendency. A common site for changes in tooth position to occur is in the region of the lower front teeth, where some changes in tooth position should be expected. The relationship of the maxillary to lower teeth can change adversely due to abnormal tongue position or other functional problems. Retainers usually are worn on a full time basis (except meals) for one year and then at night until the end of the active growth period.

Occasionally, unexpected or abnormal changes in the growth of the jaws may limit our ability to achieve the desired result. If growth becomes disproportionate, the relationship of the upper jaw to the lower jaw may change, requiring additional treatment or, in some instances, surgery. Severe growth disharmony is a biological process, which often is beyond the control of the orthodontist.

There is a risk that problems (*temporomandibular disorders*) may occur in the temporomandibular joint (TMJ), which is the joint in front of the ear, and/or the chewing muscles. In some patients, TMJ symptoms first may become evident during or after orthodontic treatment, especially during adolescence. If the patient experiences pain, clicking, or grinding sounds in the jaw joint region or cannot open or close the mouth, call the office immediately.

Patients wearing a face mask or headgear may become injured because of accidents, "horse play" and/or improper removal of the appliance. Do not wrestle or participate in competitive contact sports activities while wearing such an appliance. Do not wear it outside the house without the specific direction of the orthodontist and be sure to release the elastic force before removing the appliance from the teeth.

The total time required to complete treatment may exceed our estimate. Excessive or deficient growth of the jaw and bone, poor patient cooperation, broken appliances, poor oral hygiene, and missed appointments are all important factors which can lengthen treatment and affect the quality of the result.

It is our professional opinion that the potential benefits from orthodontic treatment in this patient outweigh the risks that reasonably may be anticipated. If you have any questions about treatment or if anything about this form is unclear, please ask for further explanation.

I grant permission for the use of clinical records for research, education, or professional publication. I understand that these clinical records will honor patient confidentiality.

I have read and understand the above and consented to treatment.

_____
Patient Name

_____   _____
Signature (of patient or parent, if minor)   Date

_____   _____   _____
Orthodontist   Staff member   Date

Figure 2-28. Patient consent form.

reason for not scheduling a return visit (we want to make sure that we have not offended them in any way). That reason is recorded in the chart, and the chart becomes inactive. If the decision to start is in the future, the treatment coordinator will mark down when the parent might be ready (usually 4–6 months), and she will contact the family at that time.

Some calls may result in leaving a message on an answering machine. After two calls, a letter is written to the parents. If no response is received, the patient is placed on inactive status.

CONCLUDING REMARKS

The sequence of events outlined in this chapter represent our current protocol regarding the initial experience of a patient and their family in our practice. We have found that the establishment of the treatment coordinator position (termed in other offices the "new patient coordinator") has been very beneficial in introducing a patient family to orthodontics in a relaxed and orderly fashion.

Typically, an orthodontic examination is scheduled for one hour. During this appointment, the panoramic radiograph is obtained, as are selected digital images. In addition, there is ample time within the initial examination to examine the patient in detail, obtaining many critical objective measurements including maximum interincisal opening and transpalatal width.

One of the advantages of using this examination protocol is that the patient family does not feel rushed when visiting our practice, even though the contact with the orthodontist is somewhat limited (typically less than 10 minutes). The patient family has the opportunity of having all of the their questions answered, with the possibility of follow-up contact with the orthodontist at the same appointment, if necessary. The need for a second contact with the orthodontist during the initial appointment arises infrequently.

In less than 10% of our patients is a formal consultation necessary. Typically, a consultation might be indicated in instances in which a patient has borderline crowding and additional documentation (*e.g.,* lateral cephalogram) is required. Also, most orthognathic surgical patients and patients with dentally compromised occlusions require a formal consultation appointment, as well as additional consultations with other dental specialists. These types of patients require added attention from the orthodontist, and the fees for these services are adjusted accordingly.

Throughout the rest of this text, the protocols used by us in the treatment of various types of malocclusions are described in detail. It is very important that the patient and his or her family have a thorough understanding of the established goals of treatment. They also must be informed of the risks associated with such treatments, as well as a reasonable expectation of the likelihood of a satisfactory treatment outcome and the approximate length of treatment. These goals can be met by a thorough initial examination appointment followed by diagnostic records and the verification or alteration of the provisional treatment plan.

REFERENCES CITED

1. Sondhi A. Personal communication, 2000.
2. White C. Personal communication, 1995.
3. Swain BF. Personal communication, 1982.
4. Laskin D, Greenfield W, Gale E, Rugh J, Neff P, Alling C, Ayer WA. The President's conference on the examination, diagnosis and management of temporomandibular disorders. Chicago: Am Dent Assoc, 1983.
5. Moyers RE, Van der Linden FPGM, Riolo ML, McNamara JA, Jr. Standards of human occlusal development. Ann Arbor: Monograph 5, Craniofacial Growth Series, Center for Human Growth and Development, The University of Michigan, 1976.

Chapter 3
DENTITIONAL DEVELOPMENT

A key element in successful orthodontic treatment of the growing patient is an understanding of the development of the dentition, particularly as it relates to the dynamics of dental arch maturation. Even though concepts of dental and occlusal development are taught in some detail to both undergraduate and graduate dental students, it is common that only the most basic concepts are retained by the practicing clinician (*e.g.*, the sequence of eruption and the timing of dental emergence).

As early treatment protocols have evolved, especially with an increasing trend toward more non-extraction treatment,[1] it has become obvious that an understanding of the size relationships between the deciduous and permanent dentitions is important in the clinical management of the transition of the dentition. In addition, many of the orthopedic expansion protocols described in this text are based in part on the relationship of dental crowding to aggregate tooth size and available arch size.

The literature on the development of the dentition is voluminous, as evidenced by the studies of Friel,[2] Cattell,[3] Clinch,[4] Sillman,[5] Schaur and Massler,[6] Diamond,[7] and Hurme.[8] The classic studies of Baume,[9–11] were followed by the articles and monographs of Lo and Moyers,[12] Nolla,[13] Vego,[14] Van der Linden,[15–18] McNamara,[19] and Nanda.[20]

Several studies of the development of the dentition have been published after analyzing changes in serial dental casts, including those of Clinch,[21] Moorrees,[22] Sillman,[5] Knott and Meredith,[23] Leighton,[24, 25] and Moyers and co-workers.[26] These studies have provided data on untreated individuals to which treated samples can be compared.

Other studies of the development of the dentition include the vast literature on genetics and inheritance,[27, 28] and the etiology of malocclusion.[29] In addition are monographs resulting from interdisciplinary conferences on the biological mechanisms underlying tooth eruption and tooth movement.[30, 31] Other publications have dealt with topics that have specific clinical relevance, including interarch tooth-size (Bolton) discrepancies[32, 33] as well as several mixed dentition analyses.[34–37]

This chapter considers several aspects of dental development that concern the dental arches. Specifically, deciduous/permanent tooth-size differences and the relationship between tooth size and arch size in individuals with dental crowding are discussed. Conclusions drawn from investigations on these topics serve as a basis for specific treatment strategies discussed later in this text.

DECIDUOUS AND PERMANENT TOOTH-SIZE RELATIONSHIPS

The first concept to be considered is the relationship between the size of the deciduous teeth and the size of the permanent teeth, given that one of the major goals of early treatment is to maintain or create enough space for the permanent teeth to erupt into an uncrowded position.

One indicator of future space requirements may be the presence or absence of interdental spacing in the deciduous dentition. The research of Leighton[24,25] has shown that interdental spacing of the primary dentition is an excellent indicator of the tooth-size/arch-size rela-

Table 3-1. Chances of crowding based on the available interdental spacing in the deciduous dentition according to Leighton.[24,25]

Deciduous Teeth	Chances of Crowding
Crowded	1 in 1
No spacing	2 in 3
<3 mm	1 in 2
3–5 mm	1 in 5
>6 mm	None

tionship in the permanent dentition. Studying a sample of 500 individuals monitored yearly from birth, Leighton reported that in every instance in which there was crowding of the deciduous incisors, crowding of the permanent incisors subsequently occurred (Table 3-1). When there was neither spacing nor crowding of the deciduous teeth, the chances were more than two in three that crowding would follow. When spacing existed that was less than 3 mm, there was a one in two chance of crowding, whereas with spacing between 3–6 mm there was a one in five chance of crowding. In instances of 6 mm of interdental spacing, however, there was little likelihood of crowding occurring at all (Fig. 3-1).

One explanation for the relationship of spacing in the deciduous dentition to crowding in the permanent dentition can be reached simply by comparing the size of the deciduous and permanent anterior teeth and the deciduous and permanent posterior teeth (Table 3-2). For this comparison, we used data gathered from children primarily of European-American ancestry who attended the University School on the University of Michigan campus. From 1935 to 1968, serial dental casts were obtained on all individuals enrolled in this "laboratory school" housed within the School of Education.[38] Annual radiographic, anthropometric, and psychometric data were obtained as well.

The dental cast data obtained from the *University of Michigan Elementary and Secondary School Growth Study*[26] indicate that in the maxilla the average width of the four deciduous incisors is 23.4 mm (Table 3-3). On average, an additional 8.2 mm of arch length is necessary to accommodate the four succeeding incisors. When significant spacing of the deciduous anterior teeth is not present, the reason underlying anterior crowding at the time of eruption of the maxillary central and lateral incisors is obvious. Similarly, there is an average discrepancy of 5.6 mm in the transition from the deciduous to the permanent mandibular incisors (Table 3-3).

During the later stage of the transition of the dentition, striking differences exist between the average values for the maxillary and mandibular posterior teeth. In the maxilla, there is an average reduction in tooth size of only 1.6 mm during the transition of the deciduous canines and molars to the permanent canines and premolars (Table 3-3). It should be noted, however, that if only the second premolar region is considered, slightly more than a 4 mm reduction in tooth size (*i.e.*, 2.2 mm per side; Table 3-2) occurs during the transition from

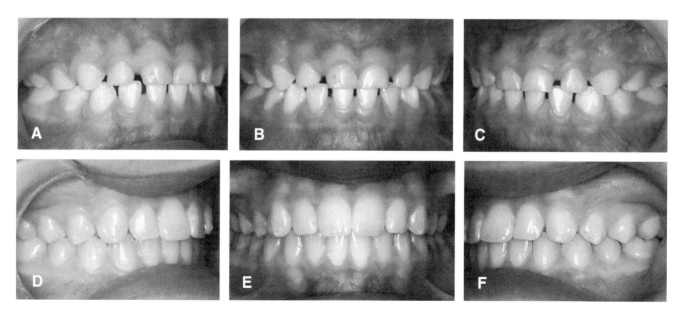

Figure 3-1. Interdental spacing. *A–C.* Intraoral views of a 5-year-old deciduous dentition subject with a normal occlusion and adequate (>5 mm) interdental spacing in both arches. *D–F.* Intraoral views of the same untreated subject at 13 years of age. A normal occlusion has been maintained with adequate space provided for the eruption of the permanent teeth.

Table 3-2. Mesiodistal diameters of deciduous and permanent teeth. Based on European-American data from the *University of Michigan Growth Study*.[26]

	Male			Female		
	Dec. Mean (mm)	Perm. Mean (mm)	Diff. (mm)	Dec. Mean (mm)	Perm. Mean (mm)	Diff. (mm)
Maxillary						
Central Incisor	6.4	8.9	2.5	6.5	8.7	2.2
Lateral Incisor	5.3	6.9	1.6	5.3	6.8	1.5
Canine	6.8	8.0	1.2	6.6	7.5	0.9
First DM/PM	6.7	6.8	0.1	6.6	6.6	0.0
Second DM/PM	8.8	6.7	−2.1	8.7	6.5	−2.2
Mandibular						
Central Incisor	4.1	5.5	1.4	4.1	5.5	1.4
Lateral Incisor	4.6	6.0	1.4	4.7	5.9	1.2
Canine	5.8	7.0	1.2	5.8	6.6	0.8
First DM/PM	7.8	6.9	−0.9	7.7	6.8	−0.9
Second DM/PM	9.9	7.2	−2.7	9.7	7.1	−2.6

the second deciduous molars to the second premolars. This latter observation will be discussed in detail elsewhere when the use of the transpalatal arch at the end of the transition period is considered.

The stage of dental arch development during which arch length can be manipulated most easily is the time of transition from the mandibular deciduous canine and molars to the mandibular permanent canine and premolars. Using the data of Moyers and co-workers,[26] the average mesiodistal size of the deciduous teeth in that region is 47.0 mm, a value that can be contrasted to the succeeding aggregate tooth dimension of 42.2 mm, indicating an average gain of 4.8 mm in available space (Table 3-3). Of particular importance is the transition from the second deciduous molar to the second premolar, when 2.6 mm of "leeway space" can be gained on either side of the arch (Table 3-2).

Table 3-3. Differences in tooth sizes of the deciduous and permanent dentition. Based on European-American data from the *University of Michigan Growth Study*.[26]

	Incisors	Canines/Premolars	Total
Maxillary			
Permanent	31.6 mm	43.0 mm	74.6 mm
Deciduous	23.4 mm	44.6 mm	68.0 mm
Difference	8.2 mm	−1.6 mm	6.6 mm
Mandibular			
Permanent	23.0 mm	42.2 mm	65.2 mm
Deciduous	17.4 mm	47.0 mm	64.4 mm
Difference	5.6 mm	−4.8 mm	0.8 mm

When all teeth are taken into consideration, the aggregate tooth size in the maxillary permanent dentition (anterior to the first molars) is 6.6 mm greater than in the deciduous dentition. This situation is in contrast to the mandible, where the aggregate permanent tooth size exceeds the deciduous tooth mass by only 0.8 mm.

The average maxillary and mandibular differences cited above, based on subjects in the *Michigan Growth Study*, are similar to those values published by Moorrees[22] and Leighton.[24] Leighton notes, however, that average values do not reflect the whole population, and that the range of variation of the population must be taken into consideration. Leighton reports an average difference in tooth size of 6 mm for the maxilla and 2 mm for mandible. These averages, however, represent ranges of 1.2 to 13.8 mm in the maxillary arch and −4.0 to 8.3 mm in the mandibular arch. This wide range of values illustrates the difficulty in predicting average space requirements based only on dental casts; it also demonstrates the value of using a radiographic comparison of the deciduous and permanent dentitions as viewed in periapical or panoramic radiographs.

Thus, a simple comparison of primary and permanent tooth size indicates an immediate need for additional space in both dental arches as soon as the deciduous incisors are lost, unless interdental spacing was present in the deciduous dentition. Due to the difference in the size of the posterior teeth, it is easier, on average, to maintain space in the mandibular arch than in the maxillary arch. The use of holding appliances, such as a transpalatal arch or a lingual arch, may be indicated to facilitate space maintenance during the transition of the dentition. If mandibular leeway space is used to resolve crowding, however, this same space cannot be used later to facilitate Class II correction.

TOOTH SIZE VS. ARCH SIZE

It is well known that crowding or protrusion of the dentition occurs when there is a discrepancy in the size of the available tooth mass and the size of the supporting bony bases. Logically, crowding can be due to teeth that are too large, bony bases that are too small, or some combination of these two factors. We have investigated the relationship between tooth size and arch size in both permanent and transitional dentitions.

Adult Dentition

Howe and co-workers[39] conducted a study on dental casts in which the dental arches of patients with severe crowding were compared to the dental arches of individuals who were classified as having ideal (or near-ideal) occlusions. The pretreatment study models of fifty patients with severe crowding were selected from a private practice sample. This group of dental casts was compared to sample casts of 54 individuals from the *University of Michigan Elementary and Secondary School Growth Study*[26] who had either ideal occlusions or occlusions with only minimal irregularities (*i.e.*, minor malocclusions that did not require treatment). Both dental and bony base dimensions were evaluated.

Evaluation of Tooth Size

The mesiodistal dimensions of each of the involved teeth were measured.

1. Individual Teeth. The first dimensions considered were individual tooth sizes (Table 3-4). There were no instances in which a statistically significant difference between the size of any given tooth was noted when the crowded and uncrowded dental arches were compared.

2. Aggregate Tooth Size. We then investigated whether

Table 3-4. Tooth size: Individual teeth. From Howe *et al.*[39]

Group	Tooth	Male				Female			
		N	Mean	S.D.	Sig	N	Mean	S.D.	Sig
Maxillary									
N	Central Incisor	24	8.7	0.5	ns	30	8.3	0.5	ns
C		18	8.6	0.7		32	8.3	0.4	
N	Lateral Incisor	24	6.7	0.5	ns	30	6.3	0.6	ns
C		18	6.8	0.5		32	6.4	0.6	
N	Canine	24	7.7	0.7	ns	30	7.4	0.5	ns
C		18	7.8	0.7		32	7.3	0.3	
N	First Premolar	24	6.8	0.4	ns	30	6.7	0.5	ns
C		18	6.8	0.5		32	6.7	0.4	
N	Second Premolar	24	6.6	0.5	ns	30	6.5	0.4	ns
C		18	6.7	0.4		32	6.4	0.4	
N	First Molar	24	10.7	0.5	ns	30	10.6	0.6	ns
C		18	10.8	0.5		32	10.4	0.6	
Mandibular									
N	Central Incisor	24	5.2	0.3	ns	30	5.1	0.3	ns
C		18	5.3	0.4		32	5.2	0.3	
N	Lateral Incisor	24	5.8	0.3	ns	30	5.5	0.4	ns
C		18	5.9	0.4		32	5.7	0.3	
N	Canine	24	6.7	0.3	ns	30	6.3	0.4	ns
C		18	6.8	0.5		32	6.3	0.3	
N	First Premolar	24	6.9	0.4	ns	30	6.8	0.4	ns
C		18	7.1	0.5		32	6.8	0.4	
N	Second Premolar	24	6.9	0.3	ns	30	6.8	0.4	ns
C		18	7.2	0.5		32	6.8	0.7	
N	First Molar	24	11.0	0.6	ns	30	10.6	0.6	ns
C		18	11.1	0.7		32	10.5	0.6	

N = Non-crowded   ns = not statistically significant
C = Crowded

the mesiodistal sums of the teeth in both arches were statistically different between the crowded and uncrowded samples. Measuring from the mesial aspect of the second molar, the average mesiodistal sum of teeth in the maxillary arch of the uncrowded cases was 94.3±3.9 mm as compared to 95.5±4.7 mm in the crowded subjects. Even though there was a slight tendency (~1 mm) toward larger teeth in the crowded cases, this observation was not significant statistically.

In the mandibular arch, the aggregate tooth size was 85.5±3.4 mm in the non-crowded cases and 86.6±4.1 mm in the crowded cases, a difference that again was not statistically significant. Although there did appear to be a tendency toward slightly larger teeth in crowded cases, tooth size did not appear to be a major contributor to crowding.

Evaluation of Arch Dimensions

In this aspect of the study, we evaluated various measures of arch width and perimeter. In both dimensions, there were statistically significant differences between the uncrowded and crowded cases, and there also was a greater variance in the crowded individuals. Similar, but slightly smaller, measures and differences were noted in the female sample (Table 3-5).

1. Arch Width. The average of the arch widths, as measured between the lingual points of antimeres, can be found in Table 3-5. Maxillary intermolar width was of particular interest. In the non-crowded males, the average distance between the maxillary first molars (Fig. 3-2), measured at the point of the intersection of the lingual groove with the gingival margin, was 37.4±1.7 mm, a value that can be compared to a similar measure in the crowded sample of 31.1±4.1 mm. Note that the intermolar width in the crowded sample was approximately 6 mm less than in the non-crowded group and that there also was a greater standard deviation in the crowded individuals. Similar, but slightly smaller, measures and differences are noted in the female sample (Table 3-5).

2. Arch Perimeter. Significant differences were found in dental arch perimeter measurements for both the maxilla and mandible, as measured from the mesial surface of one second molar around the arch to the mesial surface of the other second molar (Table 3-6). Maxillary arch perimeter for the 24 males in the non-crowded group averaged 99.3±4.3 mm, a value that was significantly larger than the average value of 94.7±7.7 mm for the 18 males in the crowded group, indicating an average 4.6 mm larger arch perimeter in the non-crowded subjects. The average difference in the female sample was 5.2 mm. There also was a 4.7 mm greater mandibular arch perimeter in the non-crowded group

Table 3-5. Differences in arch widths. From Howe et al.[39]

Group	Region	Male				Female			
		N	Mean	S.D.	Sig.	N	Mean	S.D	Sig.
Maxillary									
N	Canine	24	26.4	1.4	ns	30	25.1	2.1	*
C		18	24.6	3.8		32	23.5	3.3	
N	First Premolar	24	28.9	1.3	**	30	27.7	1.7	**
C		18	23.5	2.9		32	22.8	1.8	
N	Second Premolar	24	34.1	1.8	**	30	32.9	1.5	**
C		18	27.7	3.2		32	27.0	2.6	
N	First Molar	24	37.4	1.7	**	30	36.2	1.9	**
C		18	31.1	4.1		32	30.8	2.4	
Mandibular									
N	Canine	24	20.1	1.5	ns	30	19.3	1.4	**
C		18	19.4	2.2		32	18.2	1.9	
N	First Premolar	24	26.7	1.4	**	30	25.6	1.5	**
C		18	23.3	1.8		32	22.4	2.0	
N	Second Premolar	24	30.6	1.6	**	30	29.6	1.6	**
C		18	26.8	2.2		32	25.5	2.5	
N	First Molar	24	34.1	1.8	**	30	32.8	1.6	**
C		18	31.8	2.7		32	29.1	2.8	

N = Non-crowded   ns = not statistically significant
C = Crowded   ** = p <0.01   * = p <0.05

Table 3-6. Differences in arch perimeter (mm). From Howe and colleagues, 1983.[39]

	Male				Female			
Group	N	Mean	S.D.	Sig.	N	Mean	S.D.	Sig.
Maxillary								
Non-crowded	24	99.3	4.3	**	30	95.6	4.2	**
Crowded	18	94.7	7.7	(−4.6)	32	90.4	6.4	(−5.2)
Mandibular								
Non-crowded	24	88.1	5.9	**	30	84.6	3.7	**
Crowded	18	83.7	5.9	(−4.7)	30	79.9	5.1	(−4.7)

** = $p < 0.01$

when compared to the crowded group in both males and females.

Comparison with Other Studies

The results of the study of Howe and co-workers[39] are similar to those of several other investigators. For example, Moorrees and Reed,[40] Mills,[41] McKeown,[42] and Radnzic[43] all studied the relationships between tooth size, arch size, and crowding. These investigators found that arch size, particularly arch width, was strongly associated with the degree of crowding, whereas tooth size, in general, was not. Mills[41] found that the dental arches of those individuals with non-crowded dental arches were about 4 mm wider than were the crowded arches.

Lundström[44] and Doris and co-workers[45] have reported associations between tooth size and dental crowding. Radnzic[43] suggests that, although all parameters appear to be interrelated, arch size, particularly arch length and arch perimeter, seems to be more important than tooth size as a cause of dental crowding.

Transitional Dentition

In their study, Howe and co-workers[39] used the transpalatal width between the maxillary first molars (Fig. 3-2) as an indicator of arch dimension. A transpalatal width of 35–39 mm suggests a bony base of adequate size to accommodate a permanent dentition of *average size*. Of course, a larger total tooth size requires a larger bony base and *vice versa*.

Because the Howe study[39] dealt only with adults who had fully erupted second molars, that investigation did not address the issue of arch changes during the transition from the mixed to the permanent dentition, the time during which early treatment usually is initiated. The question considered in a second study[46] was the nature of normal changes in maxillary and mandibular transpalatal width from the early-mixed to the permanent dentition. We evaluated longitudinal changes in an untreated population from seven to fifteen years of age.

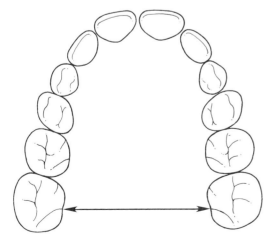

Figure 3-2. Maxillary transpalatal width, as measured at the intersection of the lingual groove with the gingival margin. For the purpose of routine clinical practice, however, the closest points between the maxillary first molars are measured.

Table 3-7. Transpalatal arch widths, genders combined (mm). Based on European-American data from the *University of Michigan Growth Study*.[26]

Age	N	Mean	S.D.
7	119	32.7	1.4
8	171	33.2	1.5
9	181	33.2	1.4
10	179	33.7	1.5
11	159	34.5	1.4
12	128	35.2	1.4
13	116	35.4	1.5
14	93	35.2	1.4
15	74	35.3	1.4

Mean change in arch width, age 7 to 15 = +2.6 mm

Table 3-8. Longitudinal changes in transpalatal arch width (mm). Based on European-American data from the *University of Michigan Growth Study*.[26]

	Initial AW <31 mm		Initial AW 31–35 mm		Initial AW >35 mm	
Age	Mean	S.D.	Mean	S.D.	Mean	S.D.
7	28.9	1.3	32.8	0.9	36.5	1.2
8	29.3	1.1	33.1	1.1	37.1	1.2
9	30.0	1.1	33.6	1.3	37.4	1.1
10	30.3	1.4	34.0	1.4	37.5	1.1
11	30.4	1.6	34.3	1.7	37.5	0.9
12	30.9	1.3	34.5	2.1	37.5	1.2
13	31.4	1.4	34.7	1.6	37.5	1.6
14	31.7	1.6	35.0	1.6	37.8	1.6
15	32.2	1.4	35.3	1.9	38.2	1.9

Mean change from age 7 to 15
+3.3 mm   +2.5 mm   +1.7 mm

Spillane and McNamara[46] examined data gathered previously by Moyers and associates.[26] Longitudinal records of 209 individuals were used in this evaluation. In one part of the study (Table 3-7), all patients who had records at a given age were evaluated, with the sample size ranging from 181 at age 9 to 74 at age 15. The average increase in transpalatal width between the maxillary first molars was 2.6 mm. A subsample of 40 individuals who had records taken at every age interval studied also was evaluated and demonstrated a similar change in transpalatal width (*i.e.*, a 2.7 mm increase from age 7 to 15).

We evaluated this sample further by dividing it into three subgroups on the basis of initial transpalatal width. The *narrow* group had an initial transpalatal width of less than 31 mm; the *neutral* group had a transpalatal width of between 31–35 mm; and the *wide* group had an initial transpalatal width of greater than 35 mm (Table 3-8). A similar subdivision was made of the true longitudinal sample of 40 subjects. Both of these subgroups demonstrated "good news/bad news" findings. For the total sample, the narrow group had an increase in transpalatal width of 3.3 mm. That increase was greater than the neutral (2.5 mm) or the wide (1.7 mm) subgroups. A favorable finding was that the narrow group expanded to a greater extent without treatment than did the wider group. The unfavorable finding was the observation that, even with this greater amount of expansion, the narrow group reached an average transpalatal width of 32.7 mm (32.2 mm in the true longitudinal group), dimensions that were very close to the transpalatal widths (31.1 mm in males and 30.8 mm in females) of the crowded individuals in the sample of Howe and co-workers[39] (see Table 3-5).

CONCLUDING REMARKS

This chapter covers basic information concerning the tooth-size/arch-size relationship during the development of the dentition. The results of our investigation that compared crowded and uncrowded adult dentitions indicated that there appeared to be a relationship between bony base dimensions, as indicated by maxillary transpalatal width, and dental crowding. Much less of a relationship existing between crowding and tooth size. Our second study indicated that about 2.5–3.0 mm of transpalatal width increase occurs in an untreated population from 7 to 15 years of age. The study also demonstrated that if a child had a very narrow dental arch (*e.g.*, transpalatal width less than 31 mm) early in the mixed dentition, it is unlikely that he/she would attain adequate arch dimensions through normal growth mechanisms alone.

One of the conclusions that can be drawn from the studies cited previously is that, by providing some mechanism of widening the bony bases and increasing arch width and perimeter, more space can be obtained for the alignment of the permanent dentition. Of course, the arches cannot be expanded *ad libitum*, as has been shown by many of the published studies of arch expansion. It seems logical, however, to consider increasing arch size at a young age so that skeletal, dentoalveolar, and muscular adaptations can occur prior to the eruption of the permanent dentition.

Arch expansion is only one option available in the treatment of tooth-size/arch-size problems, as will be discussed in the next chapter. No decision concerning the selection of treatment options should be reached until detailed clinical, cephalometric, and dental cast analyses are completed.

REFERENCES CITED

1. Proffit WR. Forty-year review of extraction frequencies at a university orthodontic clinic. Angle Orthod 1994;64: 407–414.
2. Friel S. Occlusion, observation on its development from infancy to old age. Inter J Orthod Oral Surg. 1927;13: 327-343.
3. Cattell P. The eruption and growth of the permanent teeth. J Dent Res 1928;8:279–287.
4. Clinch L. Variations in the mutual relationships of the upper and lower gum pads in the newborn child. Trans Brit Soc Study Orthod 1932:91–107.
5. Sillman JH. Dimensional changes of the dental arches: a longitudinal study from birth to 25 years. Am J Orthod 1964;50:824–842.
6. Schaur I, Massler M. The development of the human dentition. J Am Dent Assoc 1941;28:1153–1160.
7. Diamond M. The patterns of growth and development of human teeth and jaws. J Dent Res 1944;23:273–303.

8. Hurme VO. Ranges of normalcy in the eruption of permanent teeth. J Dent Child 1949;16:11–15.
9. Baume LJ. Physiological tooth migration and its significance for the development of occlusion. I. The biogenic course of the deciduous dentition. J Dent Res 1950;29:123–132.
10. Baume LJ. Physiological tooth migration and its significance for the development of occlusion. II. The biogenesis of accessional dentition. J Dent Res 1950;29:331–337.
11. Baume LJ. Physiological tooth migration and its significance for the development of occlusion. III. The biogenesis of the successional dentition. J Dent Res 1950;29:338–348.
12. Lo RT, Moyers RE. Studies in the etiology and prevention of malocclusion. I. The sequence of eruption of the permanent dentition. Am J Orthod 1953;39:460–467.
13. Nolla CM. The development of the permanent teeth. J Dent Child 1960;27:254–266.
14. Vego L. A longitudinal study of mandibular arch perimeter. Angle Orthod 1962;32:187-192.
15. Van der Linden FPGM, McNamara JA, Jr, Burdi AR. Tooth size and position before birth. J Dent Res 1972;51:71–74.
16. Van der Linden FPGM, Duterloo H. The development of the human dentition: An atlas. Haggerstown: Harper and Row Publishers, 1976.
17. Van der Linden FPGM. Transition of the human dentition. Ann Arbor: Monograph 13, Craniofacial Growth Series, Center for Human Growth and Development, The University of Michigan, 1982.
18. Van der Linden FPGM. Development of the dentition. Chicago: Quintessence Publishing Co, 1983.
19. McNamara JA, Jr, ed. The biology of occlusal development. Ann Arbor: Monograph 7, Craniofacial Growth Series, Center for Human Growth and Development, The University of Michigan, 1977.
20. Nanda SK. The developmental basis of occlusion and malocclusion. Chicago: Quintessence, 1983.
21. Clinch L. An analysis of serial models between 3 and 8 years of age. Dent Rec 1951;71:61–72.
22. Moorrees CFA. Dentition of the growing child: A longitudinal study of dental development between 3 and 18 years of age. Cambridge: Harvard University Press, 1959.
23. Knott VB, Meredith HV. Statistics on eruption of the permanent dentition from serial data for North American white children. Angle Orthod 1966;36:68–79.
24. Leighton BC. The early signs of malocclusion. Trans Europ Orthod Soc 1969;45:353–368.
25. Leighton BC. Early recognition of normal occlusion. In: McNamara JA, Jr, ed. The biology of occlusal development. Ann Arbor: Monograph 7, Craniofacial Growth Series, Center for Human Growth and Development, The University of Michigan, 1977.
26. Moyers RE, Van der Linden FPGM, Riolo ML, McNamara JA, Jr. Standards of human occlusal development. Ann Arbor: Monograph 5, Craniofacial Growth Series, Center for Human Growth and Development, The University of Michigan, 1976.
27. Garn SN. Genetics of dental development. In: McNamara JA, Jr, ed. The biology of occlusal development. Ann Arbor: Monograph 7, Craniofacial Growth Series, Center for Human Growth and Development, The University of Michigan, 1977.
28. Graber LW. Congenital absence of teeth: a review with emphasis on inheritance patterns. J Am Dent Assoc 1978;96:266–75.
29. Brash JC. The aetiology of irregularity and malocclusion of the teeth. London: Dental Board of the United Kingdom, 1956.
30. Norton LA, Burstone CJ. The biology of tooth movement. Boca Raton: CRC Press, 1986.
31. Davidovitch Z, ed. Biological mechanisms of tooth eruption and root resorption. Bethesda: The Ohio State University and National Institute of Dental Research, 1988.
32. Bolton WA. Disharmony in tooth size and its relation to the analysis and treatment of malocclusion. Angle Orthod 1958;28:113–130.
33. Bolton WA. The clinical application of a tooth-size analysis. Am J Orthod 1962;48:504–529.
34. Hixon EH, Oldfather RE. Estimation of the sizes of unerupted cuspid and bicuspid teeth. Angle Orthod 1958;28:236–240.
35. Moyers RE. Handbook of orthodontics for the student and general practitioner. Chicago: Yearbook Medical Publishers, 1958.
36. Moyers RE. Handbook of orthodontics. Chicago: Yearbook Medical Publishers, 1988.
37. Tanaka MM, Johnston LE, Jr. The prediction of the size of unerupted canines and premolars in a contemporary orthodontic population. J Am Dent Assoc 1974;88:798–801.
38. Hunter WS, Baumrind S, Moyers RE. An inventory of United States and Canadian growth record sets: preliminary report. Am J Orthod Dentofac Orthop 1993;103:545–555.
39. Howe RP, McNamara JA, Jr, O'Connor KA. An examination of dental crowding and its relationship to tooth size and arch dimension. Am J Orthod 1983;83:363–73.
40. Moorrees CFA, Reed RB. Biometrics of crowding and spacing of the teeth in the mandible. Am J Phys Anthrop 1954;12:77–88.
41. Mills LF. Arch width, arch length, and tooth size in young adult males. Angle Orthod 1964;34:124–129.
42. McKeown M. The diagnosis of incipient arch crowding in children. New Zeal Dent J 1981;77:94–96.
43. Radnzic D. Dental crowding and its relationship to mesiodistal crown diameters and arch dimensions. Am J Orthod Dentofac Orthop 1988;94:50–56.
44. Lundström A. The aetiology of crowding of the teeth (based on studies of twins and on morphological investigations) and orthodontic treatment (expansion or extraction). Trans Eur Orthod Soc 1951;27:176–189.
45. Doris JM, Bernard BW, Kuftinec MM, Stom D. A biometric study of tooth size and dental crowding. Am J Orthod 1981;79:326–36.
46. Spillane LM, McNamara JA, Jr. Arch width development relative to initial transpalatal width. J Dent Res, IADR Abstracts, p 374, 1989.

Chapter 4

TOOTH-SIZE/ARCH-SIZE DISCREPANCIES

The most common type of malocclusion observed in both mixed dentition and permanent dentition patients is "crowding." These patients usually are referred to the orthodontist by the family dentist or by the patient's parents because of obvious dental irregularities or lack of sufficient space for tooth eruption. Such patients usually present with a Class I molar relationship or a tendency toward either Class II or Class III malocclusion. Not only will the treatment of crowding problems be addressed in this chapter, but the issue of the "spontaneous" sagittal correction of Class II tendency and Class III tendency patients also will be discussed.

TREATMENT STRATEGIES IN THE PERMANENT DENTITION

If crowding and/or protrusion occur in the permanent dentition, three basic treatment strategies are used to solve this problem: extraction, interproximal reduction, and expansion. Each of these techniques is summarized briefly below.

Extraction

One approach to the treatment of tooth/arch discrepancy problems is the extraction of permanent teeth (Fig. 4-1). By removing one or more teeth within an arch, total tooth mass is reduced, and the relationship between the dentition and the bony bases can be corrected. The primary advocates of this technique during the last century include Case,[1] Tweed,[2,3] Strang,[4] Begg,[5,6] and Merrifield.[7,8]

A major goal of extraction treatment is to make tooth mass compatible with existing arch dimensions, thereby enhancing the stability of the occlusion. Intentional widening or expansion of the dental arches often is avoided, especially when standard edgewise appliances are used, because of the known tendency to relapse.[2,3]

The results of extraction therapy have proven reasonably stable over the long-term. As with untreated individuals,[9,10] however, incisor irregularity has been observed during the post-retention period.[11–13]

Interproximal Reduction

A second method of eliminating discrepancies between aggregate tooth size and existing basal arch perimeter is interproximal reduction or, as termed by Peck and Peck,[14] "reproximation." This technique involves the removal of enamel interproximally, especially in areas in which there are rounded tooth contacts. Depending on tooth shape and the degree of crowding, interproximal reduction can be used in the anterior and/or posterior regions. Interproximal reduction is indicated in patients exhibiting mild to moderate crowding (*e.g.*, 2–5 mm per arch), although Sheridan[15,16] states that 6–8 mm in arch length can be gained in both the maxillary and mandibular dentitions using his procedure (Fig. 4-2). This technique also is used in patients with tooth-size discrepancies.[17–19]

Interproximal reduction has been recommended to

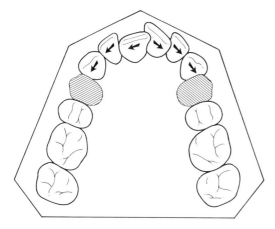

Figure 4-1. Extraction of permanent teeth. In this Class II, division 2 patient, the maxillary first premolars have been removed to solve both crowding and interarch problems.

flatten contact points between adjacent teeth. Through "locking" teeth into position by making contact areas broader, there is said to be less potential for relapse.[14] This procedure also is recommended near the end of active treatment to facilitate final settling of the occlusion.

A number of techniques for interproximal reduction have been recommended, including abrasive strips,[14,20] mounted rotary discs in a low-speed handpiece,[19] and tapered burs in a high-speed handpiece.[15,16] Using the air-rotor stripping technique, Sheridan recommends sequential stripping, beginning in the posterior interproximal regions (Fig. 4-2). Each patient must be evaluated individually, taking into account relative tooth size, the contour of the specific teeth involved, and the health of the supporting hard and soft tissue.

The clinical studies of interproximal reduction to date reveal no long-term unfavorable changes (*e.g.*, caries). Crain and Sheridan[21] maintain that there is no increase in caries susceptibility and periodontal disease following judicious interproximal reduction of enamel. Care must be taken to make sure that the enamel surfaces are smooth at the end of the procedure.[22] Remineralization of enamel occurs within a nine-month period.[23]

Expansion

A third approach to the treatment of discrepancy problems in the permanent dentition is expansion. Expansion can be divided into various arbitrary categories including orthodontic, passive, and orthopedic.

Orthodontic Expansion

It is well known that expansion of the dental arches can be produced by a variety of orthodontic treatments, including those that employ fixed appliances. Similar types of movement are produced by removable finger spring appliances (Fig. 4-3A), removable expansion plate appliances (Fig. 4-3B), or the quadhelix appliance (see Fig. 4-37). Orthodontic expansion of the dental arches produces lateral movement of the posterior buccal segments, with a tendency toward a lateral tipping of the crown and a resultant lingual tipping of the root. The forces of the cheek musculature remain, providing a force that may lead to a relapse or rebound of the achieved orthodontic expansion (Fig. 4-3).

Expansion of the dental arches also occurs in the anteroposterior dimension, typically in the maxilla.[24] Additional arch space can be gained with facebows and headgears (see Chapter 21 for a review of the literature on this subject), distalizing magnets,[25,26] NiTi coils,[27-31] and Pendulum appliances.[32] The compression or distortion of straight wires also has been used to produce distal molar movement.[33,34]

Many investigators in the past have warned that orthodontic expansion rarely is stable,[1,2,4,12,35-37] and that sagittal expansion of the mandibular dental arch is very difficult to maintain over the long-term. Most follow-up studies of fixed appliance treatment have shown that mandibular incisors that are proclined during treatment typically return to their pretreatment angulation relative to the mandibular bony base.[38-40] In most instances mandibular arch perimeter diminishes slightly over time, regardless of whether an individual receives conventional orthodontic treatment or no treatment at all.[10,12,41]

Passive Expansion

When the occlusion is shielded from the forces of the buccal and labial musculature, a widening of the dental

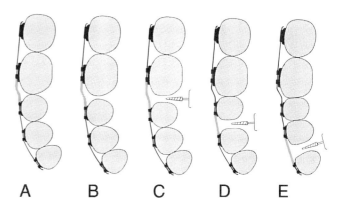

Figure 4-2. Air rotor stripping (ARS) technique of Sheridan. *A*, A compressed coil spring is used to open a space distal to the second premolar. *B*, The interproximal area now is open for ARS procedure. *C*, ARS in open embrasure. *D*, ARS of interproximal space distal to first premolar after distalization of second premolar. *E*, ARS of interproximal space distal to canine following distalization of first premolar (after Sheridan[15]).

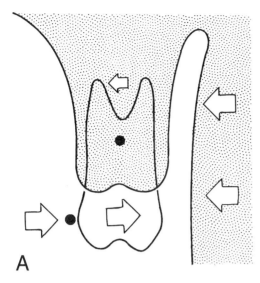 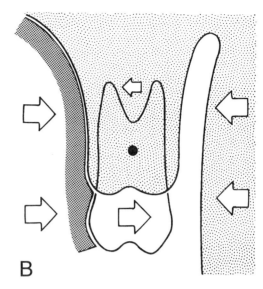

Figure 4-3. Orthodontic expansion. *A*, A finger spring appliance places lateral forces against the premolar, producing slight lingual movement of the root apices. The expansion is counterbalanced by the cheek musculature. *B*, Similar forces are produced by removable plate appliances. (After Fränkel.[42])

arches often occurs. This expansion is not produced through the application of extrinsic biomechanical forces, but rather by intrinsic forces such as those produced by the tongue (Fig. 4-4). Examples of passive expansion are the dimensional changes in the dental arches produced by such vestibular shield appliances as the FR-2 of Fränkel.[42–44] By changing the balances of forces within the orofacial region, 4–5 mm of spontaneous arch expansion has been reported.[45–47]

An implant study in Fränkel patients, conducted by Brieden and co-workers,[48] has demonstrated that bone deposition occurs primarily along the lateral aspect of the alveolus, rather than in the midpalatal suture. A related type of spontaneous arch expansion also has been observed following lip-bumper therapy.[49,50]

Orthopedic Expansion

Rapid maxillary expansion (RME) appliances (Figs. 4-5 and 4-6) are the best examples of true orthopedic expansion in that changes are produced primarily in the underlying skeletal structures rather than by the movement of teeth through alveolar bone.[51–57] RME not only separates the midpalatal suture but also affects the circumzygomatic and circummaxillary sutural systems.[58–60]

Inoue and co-workers[61] obtained occlusal radiographs of the midpalatal suture in patients who underwent rapid palatal expansion. Signs of bony filling (*e.g.*, spicule formation) were evident four to seven days after expansion, and complete ossification of the midpalatal suture was observed by two months post-expansion. Therefore, normal suture morphology is reestablished radiographically within 2–3 months when radiographic analysis indicates a general mineralization. Ekstrom and associates[62] used radioisotope labeling to measure the degree of mineralization that occurred in the midpalatal suture after it had been opened. Their findings also indicated that mineralization essentially was completed by three months post-expansion.

In contrast to passive expansion appliances that shield the teeth from the forces produced by the surrounding

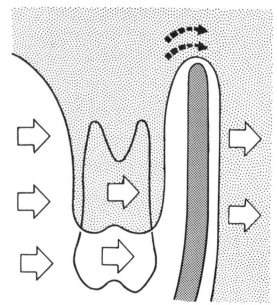

Figure 4-4. Passive expansion of the dental arch. The vestibular shield of the FR-2 appliance shields the dentition from the forces of the cheek musculature. Deposition of new bone may be observed along the lateral aspect of the alveolus. The tongue also influences lateral dental movement. (After Fränkel.[42])

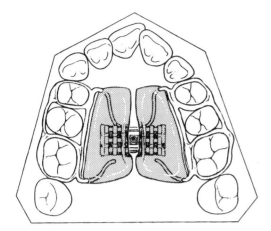

Figure 4-5. The Haas-type rapid maxillary expansion appliance. Bands are placed on the first premolar and first molars. The midline expansion screw is anchored in palatal acrylic.

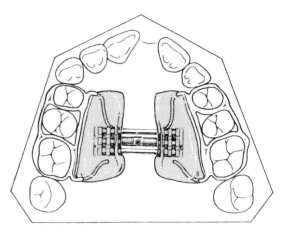

Figure 4-6. Separation of the two halves of the maxilla using the Haas-type RME appliance. Note the diastema created between the maxillary central incisors. Additional arch space is created to facilitate the eruption of the maxillary left canine. Interproximal reduction also is indicated following RME removal in this example to gain additional arch space.

soft tissues, RME appliances do not influence the adjacent soft tissues directly. As occurs in orthodontic expansion, the soft tissues usually produce forces that counteract expansion (Fig. 4-7). Thus, most rapid palatal expansion procedures are aimed at over-expansion of the maxilla. Haas[63] advocates opening the midline expansion screw so that the maxillary occlusion often is in a complete buccal crossbite relative to the mandibular dentition at the end of the expansion procedure.

Whereas some limited orthodontic and passive expansion is possible in patients virtually of any age, the ability to use RME decreases with the increasing age of the patient.[64,65] RME is accomplished most easily during the mixed-dentition period and can be performed routinely in young adolescent patients. Surgically assisted expansion procedures, however, are recommended in older adolescent patients and adult patients with severe maxillary constriction and in whom lateral tipping of posterior teeth is not desirable.

One obvious indication for the use of RME appliances is the existence of a posterior crossbite. Orthopedic expansion also is used much more frequently by us for other purposes, including increasing available arch length as well as correcting the axial inclinations of the maxillary posterior teeth (see Chapter 7 for discussion). RME also can be used in the initial preparation of a patient for functional jaw orthopedics, facial mask therapy, or orthognathic surgery.

TREATMENT STRATEGIES IN THE MIXED DENTITION

The treatment strategies outlined above for the adolescent and adult patient have applications in the mixed dentition. Serial extraction and orthopedic expansion can be initiated as part of a mixed dentition treatment protocol, whereas interproximal reduction is used infrequently in the mixed dentition, usually to facilitate the eruption of specific permanent teeth.

Serial Extraction

Serial extraction refers to the sequential removal of deciduous teeth to facilitate the unimpeded eruption of the permanent teeth. Such a procedure often, but not always, results in the extraction of four first premolar

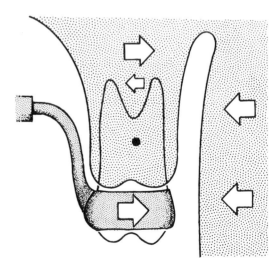

Figure 4-7. Lateral movement of the buccal dentition produced by a Hyrax-type expander. Note the rebound effect produced by the cheek musculature and also the tendency toward lingual movement of the root apices that results in tipping as well as bodily movement.

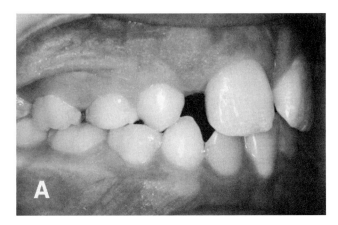
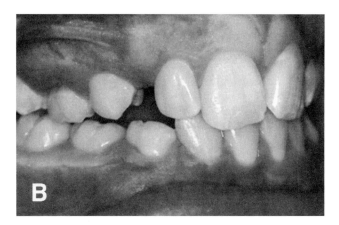

Figure 4-8. *A*, Intraoral view of the dentition of a patient who will undergo a serial extraction protocol. The need for additional arch space in the maxilla is obvious, especially given the large size of the maxillary central incisors. The need for extraction in the mandible is not so obvious, in that space is available for only three permanent mandibular incisors to erupt. *B*, Two and one half years later, following the removal of all deciduous canines and the maxillary deciduous first molars. Note the lingual tipping of the mandibular anterior teeth. There is insufficient space for the eruption of the maxillary and mandibular permanent canines.

teeth. This procedure began in Europe in the 1930s and has been advocated by a number of individuals, including Hotz,[66,67] Kjellgren,[68] Terwilliger,[69] Lloyd,[70] and Palsson.[71] The sequence of serial extraction has been clarified further in a series of articles by Dewel[72-74] and Ringenberg[75] as well as in chapters on this topic by Graber,[76] Dale,[77,78] Proffit,[79] and Moyers.[80]

The typical serial extraction protocol is initiated about the time of the appearance of the permanent lateral incisors, which erupt in rotated positions or initially are prevented from eruption by the deciduous canines (Fig. 4-8*A*). In the most commonly used protocol, the first teeth to be removed are the deciduous canines (Fig. 4-9). The removal of these teeth allows for the eruption, posterior movement, and spontaneous improvement in the alignment of the permanent lateral incisors.

In six to twelve months, the removal of the four deciduous first molars is undertaken (Fig. 4-10). Ideally, the root development of the four first premolars is ahead of that of the permanent canines, so that the first premolars will erupt before the canines. At this stage, some clinicians prefer to extract the first premolars at the same time that the first deciduous molars are removed, under the assumption that changes that are even more favorable are obtained when the first premolars are removed before they emerge.[81] Before emergence, the permanent canines can move within the jaws to the space where the first premolar crowns were located.

The next step in this protocol is the extraction of the first premolars (Fig. 4-11), if the teeth have been allowed to erupt into occlusion. It is common to observe that the adjacent teeth erupt toward the extraction sites, as is shown in Figure 4-12. The mandibular incisors often upright as well (Fig. 4-8*B*), sometimes too much so. As soon as the second molars near emergence, fixed appliances can be used to align and detail the dentition (Fig. 4-13).

Graber[76] states that serial extraction may be indicated when it is determined "with a fair degree of certainty that there will not be enough space in the jaws to accommodate all the permanent teeth in their proper alignment." Proffit[79] cites a predicted tooth-size/arch-size discrepancy of 10 mm or more as an indication for serial extraction, whereas Ringenberg[75] cites a discrepancy of 7 mm or greater. In addition, Graber[76] notes that the presence of gingival recession and alveolar destruction on the labial surface of one or both mandibular central incisors can indicate the need for this type of treatment regimen. Another indication is the early loss of one or both mandibular canines and a resultant midline discrepancy.

In addition, Graber[76] has stressed that the success of any program of serial extraction is dependent on the existing craniofacial morphology of the patient. If the sagittal relationship of the dentition is normal (Class I malocclusion), he states that the chances of success with this treatment are relatively good, with proper guidance and patient cooperation. If serial extraction procedures are undertaken in Class II and Class III malocclusion, however, great caution must be taken not only in solving the emerging intra-arch problem, but also the existing inter-arch relationship. Routine serial extraction protocols usually are not indicated in situations of extreme skeletal imbalance.

In our opinion, the primary factor to be evaluated

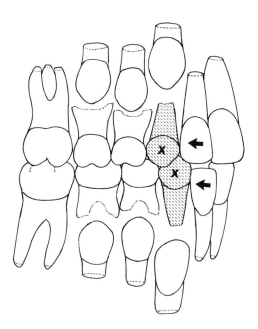

Figure 4-9. Serial extraction protocol. The removal of the maxillary and mandibular deciduous canines (**x**) allows for an improvement in the alignment of the maxillary and mandibular incisors.

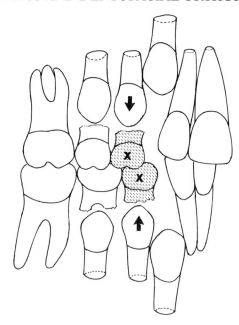

Figure 4-10. Serial extraction protocol (continued). The removal of the deciduous first molars encourages the eruption of the first premolars. Some clinicians choose to remove the first premolars at the same time to allow the mandibular canines to migrate posteriorly before emergence.

when making a treatment decision concerning serial extraction is the *size of the individual teeth*. In instances in which tooth sizes are abnormally large, as is indicated by the width of the erupted central incisors, serial extraction protocols may be appropriate. For example, the mean mesiodistal diameter of the maxillary central incisor in males and females is 8.9±0.6 mm and 8.7±0.6 mm, respectively.[82] A central incisor with a mesiodistal diameter of 10 mm or greater indicates that the patient may have larger than average teeth. Of course, more sophisticated mixed dentition analyses[80,83,84] can be used to estimate future arch-perimeter requirements, as can the panoramic radiograph taken at the initial examination

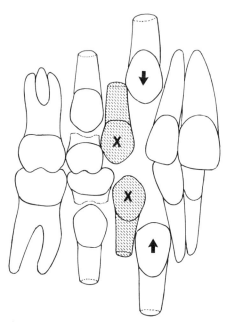

Figure 4-11. Serial extraction protocol (continued). The removal of the first premolars encourages the eruption and posterior movement of the permanent canines into the first premolar region.

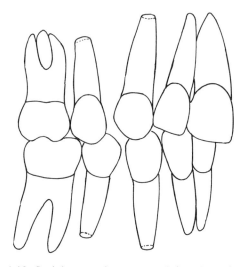

Figure 4-12. Serial extraction protocol (continued). The remaining teeth tend to tip toward the extraction sites. The mandibular incisors often tip lingually as well. Fixed appliance therapy follows as soon as the necessary permanent teeth erupt into occlusion.

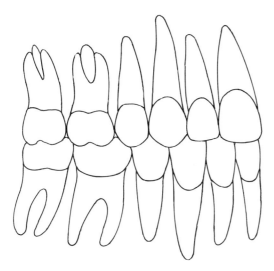

Figure 4-13. Serial extraction protocol (continued). After the mandibular second premolars near emergence, fixed appliances are used to align the teeth and level the occlusal plane.

appointment. Regardless of the method used, however, it is important to evaluate thoroughly the future arch-perimeter requirements of the mixed dentition patient.

Another factor that must be considered in the treatment planning of serial extraction regimens is the anteroposterior positioning of the mandibular incisors relative both to the associated skeletal elements as well as to the soft tissue, especially the lip musculature. Serial extraction in patients with extreme retrusion of the maxillary and mandibular anterior teeth obviously is not recommended due to unfavorable facial contour changes. In fact, mild residual crowding of the mandibular incisors is far preferable to creating a concave or "dished-in" facial appearance. Similarly, a serial extraction protocol in patients with bialveolar protrusion also is not indicated, because maximum retraction of the incisors is desirable, and maximum anchorage mechanics using fixed appliance therapy usually is the treatment of choice.

It is well known that serial extraction is not a panacea in all instances of tooth-size/arch-size discrepancy problems.[75] Care must be taken to avoid lingual tipping of the mandibular incisors as well as unfavorable changes in the sagittal position of the maxillary and mandibular dentitions. In addition, the initiation of serial extraction procedures may result in unwanted spacing in the dental arches.

Serial extraction may be combined with RME in certain patients with significant tooth-size/arch-size problems who also present with a narrow tapered maxilla and "negative space"[85] in the corners of the mouth during smiling. The arches can be expanded first to "broaden the smile," and serial extraction procedures are initiated subsequently to reduce or eliminate emerging tooth/arch imbalances.

In conclusion, not every orthodontic patient can be treated without the removal of permanent teeth, even given the possibility of orthodontic and orthopedic expansion of the dental arches. In patients who have large dental dimensions, the treatment plan often includes extraction.

Interproximal Reduction

As mentioned earlier, interproximal reduction, whether accomplished using burs, disks, or abrasive strips, can be incorporated into the overall treatment plan of the patient. It is uncommon for us to initiate this procedure in the mixed dentition. Many patients who undergo early treatment achieve a partial, rather than a complete, elimination of the pre-treatment tooth-size/arch-size discrepancy. In instances in which there is residual crowding of 2–4 mm at the time of the eruption of the permanent dentition, judicious interproximal stripping can be used to reduce tooth mass, thus enabling a proper alignment of the permanent dentition.

Mild crowding of the mandibular anterior teeth can be improved by removing mesial parts of deciduous teeth at strategic moments.[86] Slicing of the deciduous teeth is facilitated by way of a single-sided diamond strip whose abrasive side is placed against the permanent tooth.[81] The strip protects the permanent tooth against damage, and the rough texture of the strip prevents slippage. The smooth side allows controlled removal of deciduous tooth structure as a long thin diamond bur is guided against its surface.

Space for the alignment of the incisors is gained by removing a portion of the mesial surface of the adjacent deciduous canine. Similarly, stripping the mesial surface of the deciduous first molar can attain space for an erupting permanent mandibular canine. Further, reducing the mesial surface of the mandibular second deciduous molar allows the first premolar to erupt unimpeded, and the second premolar erupts without the mesial migration of the permanent first molar. A similar pattern of space maintenance, however, also can be achieved by way of a mandibular lingual holding arch.[87,88]

Orthopedic Expansion

In recent years, there has been an increasing interest among many members of both the professional and lay populations in avoiding the extraction of permanent teeth, an interest that is based on many concerns both real and perceived (*e.g.*, elimination of unfavorable facial changes, fear of litigation). This current trend once again

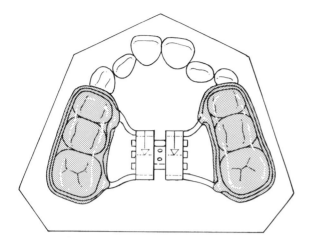

Figure 4-14. The acrylic splint RME appliance that is bonded to the primary molars and permanent first molars.

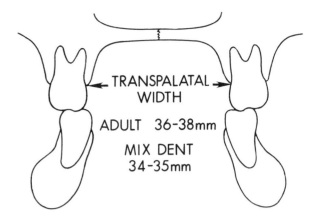

Figure 4-15. Ideal transpalatal width of the adult patient and mixed dentition patient, as measured from the closest points between the lingual surfaces of the maxillary first molars (frontal cross-sectional view.)

illustrates the ebb and flow of interest in non-extraction therapy that has existed since the days of Angle[89,90] and Case.[1] The move toward non-extraction treatment also has increased with the advent of bonded brackets and interproximal reduction procedures.

The cornerstone of early expansion treatment in patients with arch-length discrepancy problems is rapid maxillary expansion. Even though there will be a discussion of adjunctive treatments that produce tooth movement (e.g., Schwarz appliance, lip bumper, utility arch) as part of various mixed dentition protocols, rapid maxillary expansion is the most essential component of this treatment approach.

The appliance of choice is the acrylic splint rapid maxillary expansion appliance (Fig. 4-14). This appliance, which incorporates a Hyrax-type screw (Leone Co., Florence, Italy) into a framework made of wire and acrylic, is used to separate the halves of the maxilla. As mentioned earlier, it is widely recognized that maxillary expansion is achieved easily in a growing individual, particularly in an individual in the mixed dentition.[64,65,91]

The acrylic-splint type of appliance that is made from 3 mm thick, heat-formed acrylic (splint Biocryl™) has the additional advantage of acting as a posterior bite block, due to the thickness of the acrylic that covers the occlusal surfaces of the posterior dentition. The posterior bite block effect of the bonded acrylic splint expander prevents the extrusion of posterior teeth, a finding often associated with banded rapid maxillary appliances.[57] Thus, this type of expander can be used in patients with steep mandibular plane angles.

Much of the theoretical basis for this orthopedic treatment approach in the mixed dentition has been presented in the previous chapter. As mentioned in Chapter 3, an ideal transpalatal width in the adult patient with a Class I normal occlusion and average sized teeth is 35–39 mm.[92] Similarly, a transpalatal width of 33–35 mm can be considered ideal for a patient during the mixed dentition period,[93] of course depending on the relative size of the permanent teeth.

This treatment sequence is illustrated by the following example. The morphology of a patient in the mixed dentition with an idealized (e.g., 34 mm) transpalatal relationship (Fig. 4-15) can be compared to a patient with a narrow (e.g., 29 mm) transpalatal width (Fig. 4-16). A goal of orthopedic treatment initiated in the mixed dentition is to reduce the need for extractions in the permanent dentition through the elimination of arch length discrepancies as well as the correction of bony base imbalances.

In instances of constricted transverse dimensions, a bonded rapid maxillary expansion appliance is used (Fig. 4-17). The screw of the expander is activated a

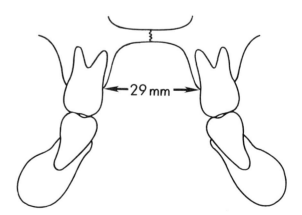

Figure 4-16. Frontal cross-sectional view of patient with a constricted maxilla, as indicated by an intermolar width of 29 mm. There also is a tendency toward a posterior crossbite due to the maxillary constriction.

TOOTH-SIZE/ARCH-SIZE DISCREPANCIES

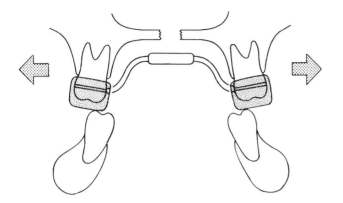

Figure 4-17. The effect of a bonded acrylic splint RME appliance. Note that the lingual cusps of the maxillary posterior teeth approximate the buccal cusp of the mandibular posterior teeth.

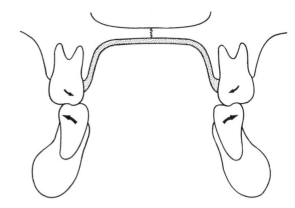

Figure 4-18. Frontal cross-sectional view of same patient during the post-RME period. A removable palatal plate has been added to stabilize the intra-arch relationship. Note slight spontaneous uprighting of the mandibular dentition.

quarter turn (90°) per day (~0.2 mm) until the lingual cusps of the maxillary posterior teeth approximate the buccal cusps of the mandibular posterior teeth. In contrast to Haas[63] who recommends full opening (e.g., 10–11 mm) of the expansion screw, an action that produces a buccal crossbite in many instances, we advocate only as much expansion as is possible while still maintaining contact between the maxillary and mandibular posterior teeth.

After the active phase of expansion is completed, the appliance is left in place for an additional five months to allow for the remodeling of the midpalatal suture. At the end of the treatment time, the RME appliance is removed, and the patient is given a removable palatal plate to sustain the achieved result (Fig. 4-18). Our studies of patients treated with this type of expander indicate that there may be some slight uprighting of the mandibular posterior teeth during the post-expansion period.[94,95] Little change in maxillary molar angulation is observed if a removable palatal plate is used for at least one year following RME treatment.

It has been well documented[59,60,96] that rapid maxillary expansion affects not only the midpalatal suture, but also the circumzygomatic and circummaxillary sutural systems. Figure 4-19A represents the skeletal and dental structures of an individual who has a Class I malocclusion characterized by narrow dental arches and a Class II, division 2 configuration of the maxillary in-

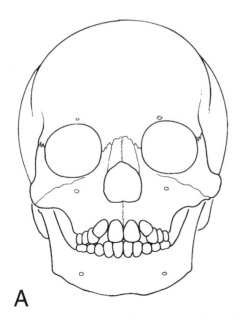
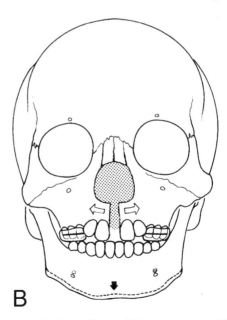

Figure 4-19. Frontal view of the skeletal structures of a patient with a constricted maxilla. A, Before treatment. Note the flared position of the maxillary lateral incisors. B, The effect of rapid maxillary expansion on the midpalatal suture as well as on adjacent sutural systems. Note the midline diastema.

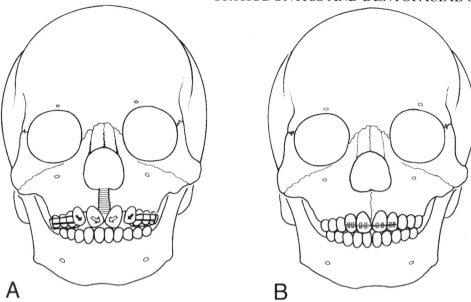

Figure 4-20. *A*, Frontal view of skeletal structures of patient originally with maxillary constriction during the post-activation period. Note the beginning reorganization of the midpalatal suture and the spontaneous drifting and tipping of the incisors toward the midline. *B*, After the RME appliance has been removed. "Temporary" brackets[97] have been placed on the maxillary incisors to align these teeth. Note that the sutural systems have become reorganized.

cisors. The bonded rapid maxillary expansion appliance is attached to the posterior dentition and, following activation once-per-day for 30 to 40 days, produces obvious changes in the midpalatal suture as well as in other sutural areas (Fig. 4-19*B*). After activation of the appliance has been discontinued, the maxillary teeth appear to be in an overexpanded position (Fig. 4-19*B*).

The active expansion of the two halves of the maxilla produces a midline diastema between the maxillary central incisors (Figure 4-19*B*). During the period following the active expansion of the appliance, a mesial tipping of the maxillary central and lateral incisors usually is observed (Fig. 4-20*A*). Such spontaneous tooth movement is typical following rapid maxillary expansion, and this movement often is interpreted as being evidence of "relapse" by patients or their parents. The clinician should advise the family about the probability of such tooth migration.

An adjunctive part of this type of treatment is the placement of brackets on the maxillary incisors (Figs. 4-20*B* and 4-21) and occasionally on the mandibular anterior teeth in instances of mandibular incisor irregularity. The placement of brackets not only will facilitate closure of an existing diastema, but also will correct any abnormalities in torque or angulation of these teeth. Auxiliary archwires (Fig. 4-22) can be used subsequently to intrude, extrude, retract, or procline the maxillary incisors if buccal tubes have been incorporated into the RME appliance posteriorly.

Mandibular Dental Decompensation

Although we had used a number of banded RME appliances in the mixed dentition in the 1970s, our experience with bonded acrylic splint expanders began about 1980. Little difficulty was encountered in producing the expected maxillary changes observed with RME, but no effort was made by us to produce active tooth movement in the mandible. After evaluating rapid maxillary

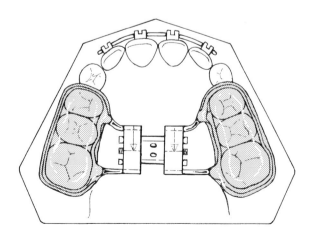

Figure 4-21. Occlusal view of the acrylic splint RME after expansion had been completed. Brackets are place on the maxillary anterior teeth for approximately six months to facilitate incisal alignment.

TOOTH-SIZE/ARCH-SIZE DISCREPANCIES

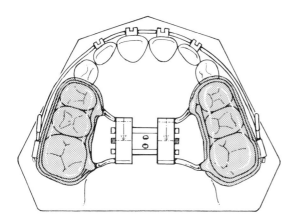

Figure 4-22. Intrusion of the maxillary anterior teeth by way of a continuous wire extending from optional buccal tubes places opposite the first molars and embedded in the acrylic splint expander.

expansion over a five-year period, we discovered that a spontaneous uprighting and "decrowding" of the mandibular teeth occurred in some patients, yet in others there was no clinically significant change in the alignment of the mandibular teeth.

Because one of the "cardinal rules" of orthodontics traditionally has been to avoid expanding the mandibular arch, we were reluctant to do so. Yet, because expansion in the mandibular arch was observed on a sporadic basis following RME, and also because expansion was observed following treatment with the FR-2 appliance of Fränkel (discussed in detail in Chapter 16), two types of appliances were used to produce additional arch length in the mandibular dentition intentionally: the Schwarz expansion appliance and the lip bumper.

The Schwarz Appliance

The Schwarz appliance is a horseshoe-shaped removable appliance that fits along the lingual border of the mandibular dentition (Fig. 4-23). The inferior border of the appliance extends below the gingival margin and contacts the lingual gingival tissue.

A midline expansion screw is incorporated into the acrylic; in addition, ball clasps lie in the interproximal spaces on either side of the second deciduous molars. Patients often use the ball clasps as handles when removing the appliance from the mouth.

The Schwarz appliance is indicated in patients with mild to moderate crowding in the mandibular anterior region or in instances in which there is significant lingual tipping of the mandibular posterior dentition. The appliance is activated once per week, producing about 0.2 mm of expansion in the midline of the appliance. Usually, the appliance is expanded for 3–5 months, depending on the degree of the incisor crowding, producing 3–5 mm of arch length anteriorly (Fig. 4-24).

Clinicians frequently have had difficulty understanding the rationale for using a Schwarz appliance *prior to* rapid maxillary expansion. The following example will illustrate our logic underlying this treatment decision. Figure 4-25 shows a bilateral posterior crossbite, a condition that easily is recognized clinically and for which rapid maxillary expansion is an appropriate treatment modality. In this example, the mandibular dental arch is of normal width and has normal posterior dental angulation, while the maxilla is constricted, with a transpalatal (TP) width of 29 mm.

In another patient with similar maxillary constriction, but in whom there also has been mandibular "dento-

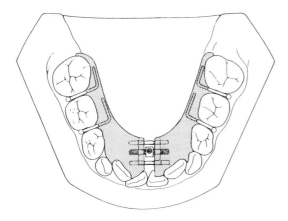

Figure 4-23. The removable mandibular Schwarz appliance is used for mandibular dental decompensation before orthopedic expansion of the maxilla. The Schwarz is activated once per week for 4-5 months. It is worn on a fulltime basis, including during meals and other activities, until the RME appliance is discontinued.

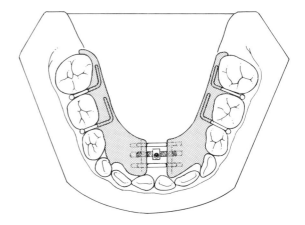

Figure 4-24. The removable mandibular Schwarz appliance after expansion. Orthodontic tooth tipping results in an uprighting of the mandibular posterior teeth and the gain of a modest amount of arch perimeter increase anteriorly. This movement is not orthopedic, in that separation of the fused mid-mandibular suture is not possible.

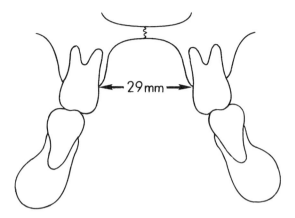

Figure 4-25. Frontal cross-sectional view of patient with a constricted maxilla and a bilateral posterior crossbite due to the upright orientation of the mandibular molars. A rapid maxillary expansion appliance is indicated in patients with this skeletal configuration.

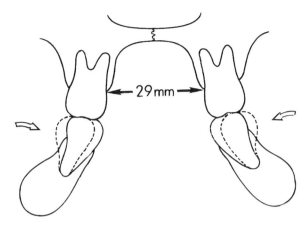

Figure 4-26. Frontal cross-sectional view of patient with a similar transpalatal width as in the previous figure and with the mandibular corpus in the same position. Note the mandibular teeth are more lingually inclined, camouflaging the maxillary constriction. The uprighting of the mandibular posterior teeth (mandibular dental decompensation) is indicated prior to RME.

alveolar compensation" (*i.e.*, the positions of the mandibular teeth have been influenced by the position and size of the narrow maxilla; Fig. 4-26), no obvious crossbite is present. Even though the width of the maxilla is the same as in the previous example, the mandibular posterior teeth have erupted with a lingual inclination. The palate is narrow (in this instance, a transpalatal width of 29 mm), and the arches are tapered in form. Mild to moderate mandibular incisor crowding also may be present. In such a patient, mandibular dental decompensation using a Schwarz appliance often is undertaken. The width and form of the mandibular dental arch is made as ideal as possible before rapid maxillary expansion. It has been our experience that by decompensating the mandibular dental arch, greater arch expansion of the maxilla can be achieved.[95] Also, the need for a second RME treatment due to a lack of adequate maxillary width is reduced.

Simply stated, the purpose of the Schwarz appliance is to produce *orthodontic tipping* of the mandibular posterior teeth, uprighting these teeth into a more normal inclination (Fig. 4-27). This movement would be unstable if no further treatment were provided to the patient, because a tendency toward a posterior crossbite is produced that is similar in many respects to the posterior crossbite shown in Fig. 4-25.

After adequate mandibular dental decompensation has been achieved, the Schwarz appliance is left in place as a passive retainer until the acrylic splint RME appliance treatment is completed. The maxillary arch is expanded so that the lingual cusps of the maxillary teeth barely contact the buccal cusps of the mandibular teeth (Fig. 4-28). After adequate expansion has been produced, the bonded expander is left in place for an additional five months. After that time, Schwarz appliance wear is discontinued, the bonded expander is removed,

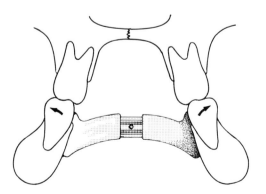

Figure 4-27. Mandibular dental decompensation using the Schwarz expander. Note the uprighting of the mandibular molars and the tendency to produce a posterior crossbite.

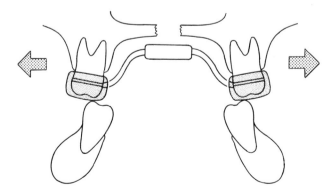

Figure 4-28. Frontal cross-sectional view of patient who has received a RME appliance following mandibular dental decompensation.

TOOTH-SIZE/ARCH-SIZE DISCREPANCIES

and a palatal plate is used to stabilize the dentition (see Fig. 4-33). During the subsequent retention period, there may be some further adjustment in the buccolingual relationship of the posterior teeth.

In many respects, the Schwarz appliance, when used as a mandibular decompensation appliance in the mixed dentition, can be viewed in a manner similar to the fixed appliance therapy performed in preparation for orthognathic surgery. In a surgery patient, the arches are idealized as much as possible to allow for unimpeded skeletal movement during surgery. In the instance of Schwarz appliance use, the mandibular arch is made as ideal as possible before midfacial orthopedics. If used alone, the Schwarz appliance produces only orthodontic tipping of teeth that is subject to the same soft tissue pressures as any other orthodontic expansion procedure (see Fig. 4-3B).

Lip Bumper

Another appliance that can be used effectively in both the mixed and permanent dentitions is the lip bumper (Figs. 4-29 and 4-30). The lip bumper is a removable appliance that attaches to buccal tubes located on mandibular first molar bands. The lip bumper is made from .036" stainless steel and is available in a variety of preformed sizes (GAC International, Central Islip NY).

The lip bumper is particularly useful in patients who have very tight or tense buccal and labial musculature. The lip bumper lies facially away from the dentition and shields the dentition from the forces of the labial and buccal musculature. The appliance usually is worn on a full-time basis and may be ligated in place. The lip bumper also should lie at the gingival margin of the mandibular central incisors (Fig. 4-30). The lip bumper not only increases arch length through passive lateral and anterior expansion but also serves to upright the mandibular molars distally, adding to the arch length increase.

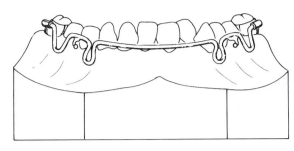

Figure 4-30. Removable lip bumper. The lip bumper should lie 2-3 mm away from the alveolus at the level of the gingival margin of the mandibular incisors.

From a neuromuscular perspective, the lip bumper, at least theoretically, appears to have a more desirable treatment effect than does the Schwarz appliance. The Schwarz appliance simply produces orthodontic tipping of the teeth through direct force application to the dentition and alveolus. On the other hand, the lip bumper shields the soft tissue from the dentition, allowing for spontaneous arch expansion.[49,50] We tend to favor the use of the Schwarz appliance over the lip bumper in most instances, however, because of the predictability of the treatment outcome. The Schwarz appliance is activated on a once-per-week basis; thus, the amount and rate of expansion is under the control of the orthodontist. In contrast, the rate of treatment response with the lip bumper varies widely among patients.

Anterior Bracket Placement

In a significant number of patients who present with tooth-size/arch-size discrepancy problems, irregularities exist in the alignment of the maxillary and mandibular anterior teeth. This condition occurs not only because of incisor irregularity subsequent to eruption but also as a consequence of rapid maxillary expansion used in the mixed dentition. Because usually only the maxillary and mandibular permanent incisors are erupted and the deciduous canines and deciduous molars remain, placement of brackets only on the incisors usually is indicated (Fig. 4-31).

Over the last few years, we have changed the terminology used when presenting the anterior brackets. Nolan[97] has suggested that such bonding of incisor brackets be presented to the patient and parents as "temporary braces" that will be in place for about six months. By using this phrasing, patients seem to realize the difference between the short period of limited fixed appliance treatment that occurs in Phase I and the longer comprehensive fixed appliance treatment that is

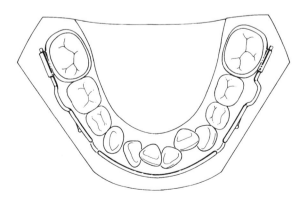

Figure 4-29. An occlusal view of a mandibular lip bumper that inserts into tubes on the mandibular first permanent molars and lies 2-3 mm labial to the anterior teeth.

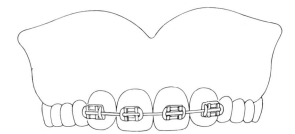

Figure 4-31. Placement of brackets on the maxillary anterior teeth to achieve incisal alignment. The ends of the wire are curved into the interproximal areas for patient comfort.

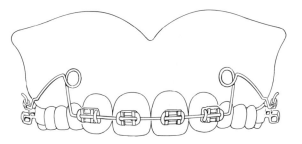

Figure 4-32. A retraction utility arch extends from the auxiliary tubes on the maxillary first molar to the incisors. This arch can be used to retract or intrude the maxillary anterior teeth.

characteristic of Phase II. We do not hear patients say as often, "but I already have had braces."

The alignment of the incisors can be achieved through a relatively simple sequence of archwires (*e.g.*, .0175″ co-axial archwire followed by a .016″ × .022″ chrome cobalt archwire). In other instances, more pronounced tooth movement is necessary. A variety of utility arches (Fig. 4-32; also see Chapter 11) can be used to intrude and/or retract maxillary or mandibular incisors, according to the needs of the individual patient. The management of a utility arch involves the placement of bands on the first molars. In the maxilla, a transpalatal arch (to be discussed later) can be used to anchor the utility arch posteriorly.

Maintenance Plates

Thus far we have discussed the use of a bonded rapid maxillary expansion appliance that may be preceded by a mandibular dental decompensation appliance and that may be followed by the placement of brackets on the maxillary and/or mandibular anterior teeth. In essence, this type of treatment represents the first phase of early corrective orthodontic therapy used in tooth-size/arch-size discrepancy patients. It is anticipated that this treatment will last 9–14 months.

The next stage in the treatment is stabilization of the expanded occlusion. We have found that it is efficient and effective to stabilize the maxilla using a removable palatal plate (Fig. 4-33). An impression for this plate is taken immediately following the removal of the rapid maxillary expander and the plate usually is delivered within 1–7 days, with the acrylic splint expander worn by the patient as a removable appliance until plate delivery. If there are any irregularities in the gingival contour due to transient gingival changes (*e.g.*, hypertrophy or irritation of the tissue immediately adjacent to the RME), these irregularities are filled with wax before the appliance is fabricated. A "salt-and-pepper" technique is used for the placement of the acrylic.

For patients who have had anterior brackets, we only occasionally use a retainer with a labial wire added to the anterior part of the maintenance plate (Fig. 4-34). This wire lies passively against the labial surface of the

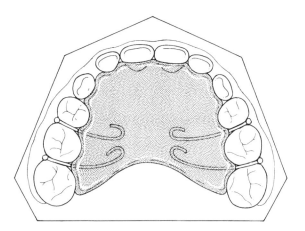

Figure 4-33. Removable maintenance plate. Clasps extend to the interproximal region between the first and second deciduous molars and the first permanent molar.

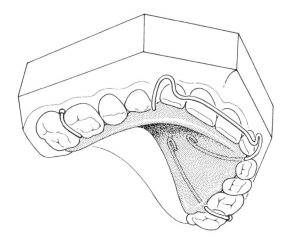

Figure 4-34. Removable maintenance plate (modified Hawley design). A maxillary labial wire is incorporated into the appliance when anterior brackets have been used.

anterior teeth and holds them in their corrected position. In most instances, however, we prefer to use the simple maintenance shown in Figure 4-33. We prefer to have the patient wear an appliance that is not obvious, as is a retainer without a labial wire. The parents are informed that some drifting of the maxillary anterior teeth may occur when the retainer without the labial wire is being worn. Such minor drifting of teeth is to be expected and will provide us with an early glimpse of the tendency of the maxillary anterior teeth to relapse, possibly indicating the need for soft tissue surgery (e.g., fiberotomy[98] or frenectomy[99]) after Phase II treatment is completed.

After the maintenance plate has been delivered, the patient usually is seen two months later and subsequently is placed on a four- to six-month recall schedule. The plate is worn for at least one year on a full-time basis. After one year, several options exist, including continuing full-time wear, switching to nighttime wear, or discontinuing the appliance altogether. This decision is made on the basis of patient compliance as well as retention need. Obviously, the larger the original tooth-size/arch-size discrepancy, the greater the necessity for long-term retention. The patient is monitored on an intermittent basis until the end of the transition to the permanent dentition.

Normally, no retention appliance is used in the mandibular dental arch unless there has been significant expansion of the mandibular arch or if severe rotations in the mandibular incisor region existed pre-treatment. In these instances, a simple Hawley-type retainer can be used to stabilize the mandibular dentition.

Transitional Appliances

As mentioned in the previous chapter concerning the development of the dental arches, some significant differences usually exist between the sizes of the second deciduous molars and the succeeding second premolars. On average, 2.5 mm per side can be gained in the mandibular arch and about 2 mm per side can be gained in the maxillary arch.[82] Wide variation in tooth size exists among patients, however. Thus, each patient must be evaluated radiographically (e.g., panoramic film) to determine the relative size of the second deciduous molars and their successors.

Two main appliances are used late in the transition of the dentition as holding appliances: the transpalatal arch and the lingual arch. In addition, the quadhelix appliance can be used after rapid palatal expansion has been completed to achieve additional arch expansion without having the patient undergo rapid maxillary ex-

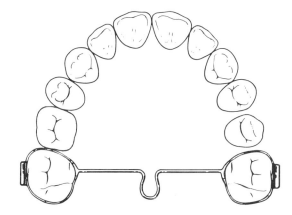

Figure 4-35. Transpalatal arch. This arch is used both as an active appliance and as a stabilization appliance during the transition from the deciduous to the permanent dentition.

pansion again. Each one of these appliances is discussed briefly below.

Transpalatal Arch

The transpalatal arch (described in detail in Chapter 12) is an .036″ stainless steel archwire that extends from one maxillary first molar along the contour of the palate to the molar on the opposite side (Fig. 4-35). The major role of the transpalatal arch in the late mixed dentition is to prevent the mesial migration of the maxillary first molars during the transition from the second deciduous molars to the second premolars. This appliance also is capable of producing molar rotation and changes in root torque. The transpalatal arch is placed at the time that the second deciduous molars have become loosened and usually remains in place until the completion of the final comprehensive phase of orthodontic therapy.

Lingual Arch

The lingual arch, typically used in the mandible, has a similar function to the transpalatal arch in the maxilla, that being as an anchorage appliance. The lingual arch, usually made out of .036″ stainless steel, extends along the lingual contour of the mandibular dentition from first molar to first molar (Fig. 4-36). An adjustment loop can be placed in the lingual arch in the region of the deciduous second molar.

The mandibular lingual arch is used less frequently than the transpalatal arch because there are many patients undergoing early orthodontic treatment who do not require the maintenance of the space in the second premolar region. Thus, the lower lingual arch only is used in patients in whom maximum anchorage is to be maintained. In contrast to the transpalatal arch, the

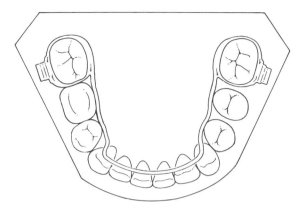

Figure 4-36. A soldered mandibular lingual arch. Note the maintenance of arch space following the loss of the second deciduous molar and the eruption of the second premolar on the left side. An adjustment loop is not shown.

lower lingual arch is removed as soon as the second premolars erupt fully into occlusion.

Quadhelix Appliance

The quadhelix appliance (Fig. 4-37) is a variation of the lingual arch in that loops have been incorporated into the arch to facilitate an active expansion movement of posterior teeth. Originally developed by Herbst,[100] and popularized by Ricketts[101] among others, the quadhelix can be adjusted in many regions to produce differential tooth movement as well as molar rotation. It also is made from .036″ stainless steel wire.

The quadhelix appliance usually is indicated when there is some residual narrowness in the maxilla, although a quadhelix (or bi-helix) appliance also can be used in the mandibular dental arch in patients who routinely lose removable expansion appliances.

The quadhelix appliance can be used to produce additional arch expansion, although a significant component of this expansion includes the buccal tipping of the posterior teeth. The appliance is not recommended for patients in whom pronounced arch expansion is indicated. The quadhelix is useful in instances in which a mild amount of expansion may be desirable after rapid maxillary expansion has been completed.

SPONTANEOUS CORRECTION OF SAGITTAL MALOCCLUSIONS

The major focus of the discussion thus far has been the resolution of tooth-size/arch-size discrepancy problems with regard to the resolution of crowding in the dental arches. Interestingly, there is another phenomenon that has been a serendipitous finding, that being the "spontaneous" correction of mild Class II and Class III malocclusions in patients with maxillary constriction, perhaps as a manifestation of "maxillary deficiency syndrome."[102]

It is not surprising that certain types of sagittal malocclusions also are associated with maxillary deficiency. One of the major components of Class III malocclusion is maxillary skeletal retrusion, a condition that occurs in nearly half of all Class III patients.[103] As will be discussed later, in our opinion the most efficient and effective treatment for Class III problems in the early mixed dentition is RME combined with the orthopedic facial mask. In some mixed dentition patients with only mild skeletal imbalances, however, simply widening the maxilla without initiating facial mask treatment may lead to a spontaneous correction of an anterior crossbite and the resolution of the Class III molar relationship.[104] In those patients with more severe problems, modest maxillary skeletal advancement combined with a similar amount of maxillary dentoalveolar advancement can be induced by RME combined with facial mask therapy.[105]

The most common surgical treatment for this condition in the mature patient today is the LeFort I osteotomy, a procedure during which the maxilla can be both advanced and widened, instead of reliance on surgical procedures that involve the mandible.

Counterintuitively, certain Class II malocclusions also may be associated with maxillary deficiency. From a sagittal perspective, maxillary skeletal protrusion occurs only in about 10–15% of Class II patients, whereas as many as 30% of Class II patients may have maxillary skeletal retrusion, often associated with an obtuse nasolabial angle and a steep mandibular plane angle.[106] Further, many Class II malocclusions, when evaluated clinically, have no obvious maxillary transverse con-

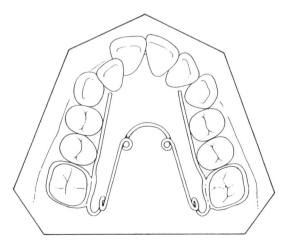

Figure 4-37. A quadhelix appliance soldered to the lingual surfaces of the maxillary first molar bands. This appliance can widen the maxilla, but also produces lateral tooth tipping.

TOOTH-SIZE/ARCH-SIZE DISCREPANCIES

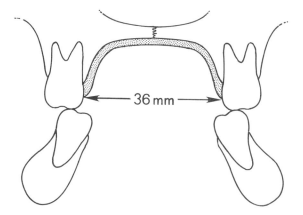

Figure 4-38. Frontal cross-sectional view of patient during the post-RME period. The maxilla has been expanded so that the intermaxillary width is 36 mm. Note the tendency toward a buccal crossbite bilaterally.

striction. When the study models of the patient are "hand-articulated" into a Class I canine relationship, however, a unilateral or bilateral crossbite is produced. In fact, Tollaro and co-workers[107] have shown that a Class II patient with what appears to be a normal buccolingual relationship of the posterior dentition usually has a 3–5 mm transverse discrepancy between the maxilla and mandible.

Spontaneous Correction of Class II Malocclusion

Most Class II malocclusions in mixed dentition patients are associated with maxillary constriction. Therefore, a reasonable first step in the treatment of mild-to-moderate Class II malocclusions, characterized, at least in part, by mild mandibular skeletal retrusion and maxillary constriction (*e.g.*, intermolar width <30 mm; see Chapters 7 and 13), should be orthopedic expansion of the maxilla. The maxillary posterior teeth can be left in an overexpanded position (Fig. 4-38), with contact still maintained between the maxillary lingual cusps and the buccal cusps of the mandibular posterior teeth. The occlusion subsequently is stabilized using a removable palatal plate in the mixed dentition or alternatively full orthodontic appliances combined with a transpalatal arch in the permanent dentition.

A most interesting (and somewhat surprising) observation following our initial efforts to expand Class II patients in the early mixed dentition was the occurrence of a spontaneous correction of the Class II malocclusion during the retention period (Fig. 4-39). Such patients had either an end-to-end or full cusp Class II molar relationship. Generally, these patients did not have severe skeletal imbalances but typically were characterized clinically as having either mild-to-moderate mandibular skeletal retrusion or an orthognathic facial profile.

At the time of expander removal, these patients had a buccal crossbite with only the lingual cusps of the maxillary posterior teeth contacting the buccal cusps of the mandibular posterior teeth. Following expander removal, a maxillary maintenance plate was used for stabilization (Fig. 4-38). Several appointments later, the tendency toward a buccal crossbite often disappeared, and some of the patient now had a solid Class I occlusal relationship (Fig. 4-39*B*).

It should be noted that the shift in molar relationship in these patients occurred before the transition from the mandibular deciduous second molars to the mandibular second premolars, the point at which an improvement

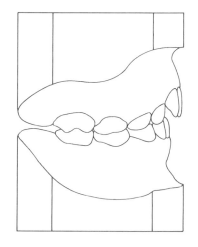
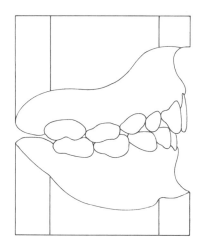

Figure 4-39. The spontaneous correction of Class II malocclusion. *A*, Before RME. Note the end-to-end molar relationship. *B*, One year following the removal of the RME appliance. Note Class I molar relationship.

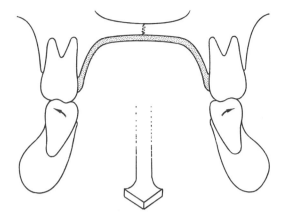

Figure 4-40. Frontal cross-sectional view of patient one year into the retention period. Note that the mandibular dentition has uprighted slightly and that there has been a forward sagittal movement of the mandible as the patient seeks to find a more stable position in which to occlude.

in Angle classification sometimes occurs in untreated subjects due to the forward movement of the mandibular first molar into the leeway space.[108]

This phenomenon has forced us to rethink our concept of Class II molar correction. Traditionally, clinicians have viewed a Class II malocclusion as primarily a sagittal and vertical problem.[109–112] Our experience with the post-RME correction of the Class II problem in growing patients indicates that many Class II malocclusions have a strong transverse component. The overexpansion of the maxilla, which subsequently is stabilized with a removable palatal plate, disrupts the occlusion. It appears that the patient becomes more inclined to posture his or her jaw slightly forward, thus eliminating the tendency toward a buccal crossbite and at the same time improving the sagittal occlusal relationship. Presumably, subsequent mandibular growth makes this initial postural change permanent.

The correction of a Class II tendency patient is illustrated in Figure 4-41, which shows the sagittal view of the skeletal and dentoalveolar structures of a Class II tendency patient who has excessive overjet and a narrow maxilla. The placement of a bonded maxillary expansion appliance immediately causes an increase in the vertical dimension of the face, because of the posterior occlusal coverage. The immediate change is not beneficial in Class II malocclusion (see Fig. 4-41B), because appliance placement initially may result in an upward slightly forward displacement (Fig. 4-41B) of the maxilla. (This phenomenon will be considered subsequently in the discussion of the spontaneous correction of Class III). The increase in the vertical dimension, however, prevents extrusion of the posterior teeth during the expansion process, a change favorable to Class II correction.

During the post-RME period, during which a removable palatal plate and anterior brackets may be worn (Fig. 4-41C), the mandible may be postured forward by the patient because of the overexpansion of the maxilla.[113] Thus, the spontaneous correction of patients with a tendency toward a Class II malocclusion does not occur during the active expansion period but rather during the time that the maintenance plate is being worn.

Spontaneous Class II correction, if it is going to occur, usually happens during the first 6–12 months of the post-RME period. The Class II correction can be enhanced further at the end of the mixed dentition pe-

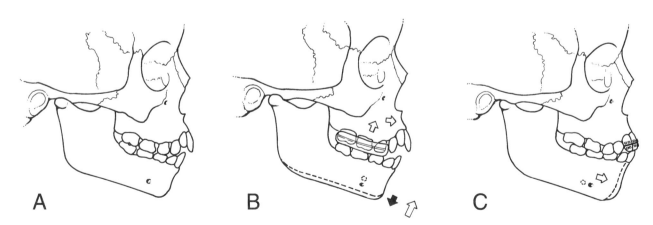

Figure 4-41. Sequence of events leading to a spontaneous correction of a sagittal malocclusion. A, Pre-treatment. The patient has excessive overjet and an end-to-end molar relationship. B, The placement of the appliance immediately creates a downward rotation of the position of the mandible due to the posterior occlusal acrylic. During treatment, an intrusive (and slightly protrusive) force is produced on the skeletal and dental structures of the maxilla. C, During the post-expansion period, the maxillary dental arch has been widened. The lower jaw often is postured forward to achieve a more stable occlusal relationship. In this illustration, brackets have been placed on the maxillary anterior teeth to facilitate incisal alignment.

riod by way of a transpalatal arch (Fig. 4-35) that not only maintains the maxillary leeway space but also can be activated sequentially to produce molar rotation and uprighting. At this point, if the occlusion still has a Class II component, additional treatment approaches (*e.g.*, extraoral traction, functional jaw orthopedics) may be indicated. The phenomenon of the spontaneous correction following RME treatment combined with the routine use of a transpalatal arch are now components of our mixed dentition treatment protocol. We have found that the frequency of subsequent functional jaw orthopedics has dropped substantially in our practice during the last ten years.

The relationship between the transverse dimension and the correction of Class II malocclusion has been recognized in the German literature. Reichenbach and Taatz [114] used the example of a foot and a shoe, with the foot representing the mandible and the shoe representing the maxilla. We have adapted this concept, as shown in Figure 4-42. If the shoe is too narrow, it is impossible for the foot to slide fully into the shoe. By widening the shoe, the foot slides forward into its usual position. From an orthopedic standpoint, the widening of the maxilla allows for the spontaneous repositioning of the lower jaw into a more forward position.

In fact, Kingsley[115] recognized the relationship between maxillary width and mandibular sagittal position as far back as 1880. In the part of his text dealing with the correction of Class II molar relationship, he wrote the following:

"The remedy evidently lay in the widening of the upper jaw until the lower would be received in its forward and natural place; and resolved itself, therefore, into three elements, viz: widening the upper arch so that the lower teeth could not articulate as they had been accustomed to; secondly compelling a new articulation in an advanced position (this action I have called in other places "*jumping the bite*"); and, thirdly, flattening the pointed and projected appearance of the incisors."

The phenomenon of the spontaneous correction following RME treatment occurs with sufficient frequency to become incorporated into our mixed dentition treatment plan. In patients with a Class II malocclusion and a reduced transpalatal width (*e.g.*, <31 mm measured between the maxillary first molars), we will widen the maxilla using RME and then stabilize the patient with a maintenance plate. The patient then will be monitored on a routine basis (*e.g.*, every 4–6 months), with the decision concerning functional jaw orthopedics or extraoral traction being deferred until toward the end of the mixed dentition period.

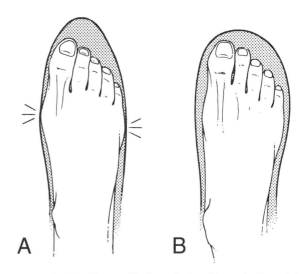

Figure 4-42. Maxillomandibular relationship as indicated by the foot and shoe example. *A*, The foot (mandible) is unable to be moved forward in the shoe (maxilla) due to transverse constriction. *B*, A wider shoe will allow the foot to assume its normal relationship. After Reichenbach and Taatz.[114]

Spontaneous Correction of Class III Malocclusion

The use of a bonded rapid maxillary expansion appliance also can lead to a spontaneous occlusal correction in a patient with a tendency toward a Class III malocclusion. At first glance, this phenomenon seems paradoxical, given the previous discussion concerning the spontaneous correction of Class II tendency problems. The mechanism of Class III correction, however, is distinctly different than that described previously.

An examination of Figure 4-41*B* provides some explanation for this phenomenon. The placement of an acrylic splint expander that opens the bite vertically 3 mm not only provides an intrusive force against the maxilla,[113] presumably due to the stretch of the masticatory musculature, but also may produce a slight forward repositioning of the maxilla. A slight forward movement of the maxilla following rapid maxillary expansion has been documented in both clinical[52,57] and experimental[116,117] studies. In addition, the placement of a bonded expander with acrylic coverage of the occlusion helps eliminate a tendency toward a pseudo-Class III malocclusion.

As with the Class II tendency patients described previously, patients in whom a borderline Class III malocclusion exists usually have a reasonably balanced facial pattern, often with only a slight tendency toward maxillary skeletal retrusion. Obviously, in patients in whom Class III malocclusion persists after expansion, aggressive types of therapy are indicated, as will be discussed in later chapters.

When contrasting the spontaneous correction of both Class II and Class III tendency patients, it must be emphasized that any spontaneous correction of a Class III malocclusion usually occurs (if it does occur) during the *active* phase of treatment (within the first 30 or 40 days). The spontaneous correction of Class II malocclusion usually is noted during the *retention* phase, after the bonded expander has removed and the maintenance plate has been worn for 6–12 months. When planning the treatment for a Class III tendency patient, facial mask hooks may be attached to the expansion appliance to facilitate the use of a facial mask if that treatment is deemed necessary later.

CONCLUDING REMARKS

This chapter has discussed a number of treatment options for dealing with patients who have tooth-size/arch-size discrepancies, either evidenced by crowding or dentoalveolar protrusion. Both serial extraction and orthopedic expansion of the dental arches were discussed, with the primary indication for serial extraction being large tooth size, and narrow arch dimensions for orthopedic expansion.

The bonded acrylic-splint expander can be used alone or following mandibular dental decompensation, either with a Schwarz appliance or a lip bumper. Brackets on the maxillary and mandibular anterior teeth are used to achieve incisal alignment. Various types of auxiliary archwires including utility arches are used to position the incisors in three dimensions.

The importance of monitoring early treatment patients during the transition from the deciduous to the permanent dentition cannot be overemphasized. The use of transpalatal arches and lingual arches to hold the position of the molars during the eruption of the premolars is an essential component of this treatment and may be as important as the active treatment procedures.

A final comment is made regarding the observation that some Class II and Class III malocclusions will correct spontaneously following rapid maxillary expansion. Although no specific clinical study has been conducted that has considered the actual percentage of patients exhibiting spontaneous correction, this phenomenon happens with sufficient frequency that we now incorporate this treatment effect routinely into the patient's overall treatment plan. The net result of this change in outlook has been a reduction in the number of functional jaw orthopedic appliances that now are used in the treatment of mild to moderate Class II malocclusions.

This chapter has discussed the two extremes in dealing with tooth-size/arch-size discrepancy problems: serial extraction and orthopedic expansion. Obviously, neither of these techniques is applicable in every mixed dentition patient who shows either a crowding of the dental arches or dentoalveolar protrusion. A careful analysis of the skeletal and dental relationships in all three planes of space is necessary before a specific treatment plan for a given patient can be established.

REFERENCES CITED

1. Case CS. Principles of occlusion and dento-facial relations. Dent Items Int 1905;27:489–527.
2. Tweed CH. A philosophy of orthodontic treatment. Am J Orthod Oral Surg 1945;31:74–103.
3. Tweed CH. Clinical orthodontics. St Louis: CV Mosby, 1966.
4. Strang RHW. The fallacy of denture expansion as a treatment procedure. Angle Orthod 1949;19:12–17.
5. Begg PR. Light-wire technique: Employing the principles of differential force. Am J Orthod 1961;47:30–48.
6. Begg PR. Begg orthodontic theory and technique. Philadelphia: WB Saunders, 1965.
7. Merrifield LL, Cross JJ. Directional forces. Am J Orthod 1970;57:435–464.
8. Merrifield LL. Dimensions of the denture: back to basics. Am J Orthod Dentofac Orthop 1994;106:535–542.
9. Sinclair PM, Little RM. Maturation of untreated normal occlusions. Am J Orthod 1983;83:114–123.
10. Carter GA, McNamara JA, Jr. Longitudinal dental arch changes in adults. Am J Orthod Dentofac Orthoped 1998;114:88–99.
11. Little RM, Wallen TR, Riedel RA. Stability and relapse of mandibular anterior alignment-first premolar extraction cases treated by traditional edgewise orthodontics. Am J Orthod 1981;80:349–365.
12. Little RM. Stability and relapse of dental arch alignment. Br J Orthod 1990;17:235–241.
13. McReynolds DC, Little RM. Mandibular second premolar extraction—postretention evaluation of stability and relapse. Angle Orthod 1991;61:133–144.
14. Peck H, Peck S. An index for assessing tooth shape deviations as applied to the mandibular incisors. Am J Orthod 1972;61:384–401.
15. Sheridan JJ. Air-rotor stripping. J Clin Orthod 1985;19:43–59.
16. Sheridan JJ. Air-rotor stripping update. J Clin Orthod 1987;21:781–788.
17. Bolton WA. Disharmony in tooth size and its relation to the analysis and treatment of malocclusion. Angle Orthod 1958;28:113–130.
18. Bolton WA. The clinical application of a tooth-size analysis. Am J Orthod 1962;48:504–529.
19. Tuverson DL. Anterior interocclusal relations. Part I. Am J Orthod 1980;78:361–370.
20. Hudson A. A study of the effects of mesiodistal reduction of mandibular anterior teeth. Am J Orthod 1956;42:615–624.
21. Crain G, Sheridan JJ. Susceptibility to caries and periodontal disease after posterior air-rotor stripping. J Clin Orthod 1990;24:84–85.

22. Radlanski RJ, Jager A, Zimmer B. Morphology of interdentally stripped enamel one year after treatment. J Clin Orthod 1989;23:748–750.
23. El-Mangoury NH, Moussa MM, Mostafa YA, Girgis AS. In-vivo remineralization after air-rotor stripping. J Clin Orthod 1991;25:75–78.
24. McNamara JA, Jr, Peterson JE, Jr, Alexander RG. Three-dimensional diagnosis and management of Class II malocclusion in the mixed dentition. Semin Orthod 1996;2:114–137.
25. Blechman AM, Smiley H. Magnetic force in orthodontics. Am J Orthod 1978;74:435–443.
26. Blechman AM. Magnetic force systems in orthodontics. Clinical results of a pilot study. Am J Orthod 1985;87:201–210.
27. Gianelly AA, Viatas AS, Thomas WM, Berger DG. Distalization of molars with repelling magnets. J Clin Orthod 1988;22:40–4.
28. Gianelly AA, Viatas AS, Thomas WM. The use of magnets to move molars distally. Am J Orthod Dentofac Orthop 1989;96:161–167.
29. Itoh T, Tokuda T, Kiyosue S, Hirose T, Matsumoto M, Chaconas SJ. Molar distalization with repelling magnets. J Clin Orthod 1991;25:611–617.
30. Bondemark L, Kurol J. Distalization of maxillary first and second molars simultaneously with repelling magnets. Eur J Orthod 1992;14:264–272.
31. Steger ER, Blechman AM. Case reports: molar distalization with static repelling magnets. Part II. Am J Orthod Dentofac Orthop 1995;108:547–555.
32. Hilgers JJ. The pendulum appliance for Class II noncompliance therapy. J Clin Orthod 1992;26:706–714.
33. Gianelly AA, Bednar J, Dietz VS, Locatelli R. Molar distalization with superelastic NiTi wire. J Clin Orthod 1992;26:277–279.
34. Kalra V. The K-loop molar distalizing appliance. J Clin Orthod 1995;29:298–301.
35. Lombardi AR. Mandibular incisor crowding in completed cases. Am J Orthod 1972;61:374–383.
36. Bishara SE, Chadha JM, Potter RB. Stability of intercanine width, overbite, and overjet correction. Am J Orthod 1973;63:588–595.
37. Little RM, Riedel RA, Årtun J. An evaluation of changes in mandibular anterior alignment from 10 to 20 years postretention. Am J Orthod Dentofac Orthop 1988;93:423–428.
38. Grieve GW. The stability of the treated denture. Am J Orthod Oral Surg 1944;30:171–195.
39. Tweed CH. Indications for extraction of teeth in orthodontic procedure. Am J Orthod 1944;30:405–428.
40. Mills JRE. The long term results of proclination of the lower incisors. Br Dent J 1966;120:355–363.
41. Sinclair PM, Little RM. Dentofacial maturation of untreated normals. Am J Orthod 1985;88:146–156.
42. Fränkel R. Technik und Handhabung der Funktionsregler. Berlin: VEB Verlag Volk and Gesundheit, 1976.
43. Fränkel R, Fränkel C. Technik und Handhabung der Funktionsregler. Berlin: VEB Verlag Volk and Gesundheit, 1984.
44. Fränkel R, Fränkel C. Orofacial orthopedics with the function regulator. Munich: S Karger, 1989.
45. Fränkel R. Guidance of eruption without extraction. Trans Europ Orthod Soc 1971;47:303–315.
46. Fränkel R. Decrowding during eruption under the screening influence of vestibular shields. Am J Orthod 1974;65:372–406.
47. McDougall PD, McNamara JA, Jr, Dierkes JM. Arch width development in Class II patients treated with the Fränkel appliance. Am J Orthod 1982;82:10–22.
48. Breiden CM, Pangrazio-Kulbersh V, Kulbersh R. Maxillary skeletal and dental change with Fränkel appliance therapy—an implant study. Angle Orthod 1984;54:232–266.
49. Bjerregaard J, Bundgaard AM, Melsen B. The effect of the mandibular lip bumper and maxillary bite plate on tooth movement, occlusion, and space conditions in the lower dental arch. Eur J Orthod 1983;84:147–155.
50. Nevant CT. The effects of lip-bumper therapy on deficient mandibular arch length. Dallas: Unpublished Master's thesis, Department of Orthodontics, Baylor University, 1989.
51. Haas AJ. Rapid expansion of the maxillary dental arch and nasal cavity by opening the mid-palatal suture. 1961;31:73–90.
52. Haas AJ. The treatment of maxillary deficiency by opening the mid-palatal suture. Angle Orthod 1965;65:200–217.
53. Haas AJ. Palatal expansion: just the beginning of dentofacial orthopedics. Am J Orthod 1970;57:219–255.
54. Haas AJ. Long-term posttreatment evaluation of rapid palatal expansion. Angle Orthod 1980;50:189–217.
55. Timms DJ. An occlusal analysis of lateral maxillary expansion with mid-palatal suture opening. Dent Pract 1968;18:435–440.
56. Timms DJ. Long-term follow-up of cases treated by rapid maxillary expansion. Trans Europ Orthod Soc 1976;52:211–215.
57. Wertz RA. Skeletal and dental changes accompanying rapid midpalatal suture opening. Am J Orthod 1970;58:41–66.
58. Cleall JF, Bayne DI, Posen JM, Subtelny JD. Expansion of the midpalatal suture in the monkey. Angle Orthod 1965;35:23–35.
59. Starnbach H, Bayne D, Cleall J, Subtelny JD. Facioskeletal and dental changes resulting from rapid maxillary expansion. Angle Orthod 1966;36:152–164.
60. Murray J, Cleall, JF. Early tissue response to rapid maxillary expansion in the midpalatal suture of the rhesus monkey. J Dent Res 1971;50:1654–1660.
61. Inoue N, Oyama K, Ishiguro K, Azuma M, Osaki T. Radiographic observation of rapid palatal expansion of human maxilla. Bull Tokyo Med Dent Univ 1970;17:249-261.
62. Ekstrom C, Henrikson CO, Jensen R. Mineralization in the midpalatal suture after orthodontic expansion. Am J Orthod 1977;71:449–455.
63. Haas AJ. Personal communication, 1992.
64. Melsen B. A histological study of the influence of sutural morphology and skeletal maturation of rapid palatal expansion in children. Trans Europ Orthod Soc 1972;48:499–507.
65. Melsen B. Palatal growth studied on human autopsy material. A histologic microradiographic study. Am J Orthod 1975;68:42–54.
66. Hotz R. Active supervision of the eruption of teeth by extraction. Trans Europ Orthod Soc 1948;24:134–160.

67. Hotz R. Orthodontics in daily practice: Possibilities and limitations in the area of children's dentistry. Bern: Hans Huber Publishers, 1974.
68. Kjellgren B. Serial extraction as a corrective procedure in dental orthopedic therapy. Acta Odont Scand 1948;8:17–43.
69. Terwilliger KF. Treatment in the mixed dentition. Angle Orthod 1950;20:109–113.
70. Lloyd ZB. Serial extraction. Am J Orthod 1953;39:262–267.
71. Palsson F. Foregangare til den s k serieextraktionen. Odont Revy 1956;7:118–135.
72. Dewel BF. Serial extractions in orthodontics: indications, objections, and treatment procedures. Int J Orthod 1954;40:906–926.
73. Dewel BF. A critical analysis of serial extraction in orthodontic treatment. Am J Orthod 1959;45:424–455.
74. Dewel BF. Serial extraction: its limitations and contraindications in orthodontic treatment. Am J Orthod 1967;53:904–921.
75. Ringenberg QM. Serial extraction: stop, look, and be certain. Am J Orthod 1964;50:327–336.
76. Graber TM. Orthodontics: Principles and practices. Philadelphia: WB Saunders, 1966.
77. Dale JG. Guidance of occlusion: serial extraction. In: Graber TM, Swain BF, eds. Orthodontics: Current principles and techniques. St. Louis: CV Mosby, 1985.
78. Dale JG, Dale HC. Interceptive guidance of the occlusion with emphasis on diagnosis. In: Graber TM, Vanarsdall RL, Jr, eds. Orthodontics: Current principles and techniques. St. Louis: C.V. Mosby, 2000.
79. Proffit WR. Contemporary orthodontics. St Louis: CV Mosby, 1986.
80. Moyers RE. Handbook of orthodontics. Chicago: Yearbook Medical Publishers, 1988.
81. Van der Linden FPGM. Personal communication, 2000.
82. Moyers RE, Van der Linden FPGM, Riolo ML, McNamara JA, Jr. Standards of human occlusal development. Ann Arbor: Monograph 5, Craniofacial Growth Series, Center for Human Growth and Development, University of Michigan, 1976.
83. Hixon EH, Oldfather RE. Estimation of the sizes of unerupted cuspid and bicuspid teeth. Angle Orthod 1958;28:236–240.
84. Tanaka MM, Johnston LE, Jr. The prediction of the size of unerupted canines and premolars in a contemporary orthodontic population. J Am Dent Assoc 1974;88:798–801.
85. Vanarsdall RL, Jr. Personal communication, 1992.
86. Nanda SK. The developmental basis of occlusion and malocclusion. Chicago: Quintessence, 1983.
87. Singer J. The effect of the passive lingual archwire on the lower denture. Angle Orthod 1974;44:146–55.
88. Wright NS. A comparison of the treatment effects of the Schwarz appliance and the lower lingual holding arch. Unpublished Master's thesis, Department of Orthodontics and Pediatric Dentistry, The University of Michigan, 2000.
89. Angle EH. Treatment of malocclusion of the teeth and fractures of the maxillae. Philadelphia: SS White Dental Manufacturing, 1900.
90. Angle EH. Treatment of malocclusion of the teeth. Philadelphia: SS White Dental Manufacturing Company, 1907.
91. Melsen B, Melsen F. The postnatal development of the palatomaxillary region studied on human autopsy material. Am J Orthod 1982;82:329–342.
92. Howe RP, McNamara JA, Jr, O'Connor KA. An examination of dental crowding and its relationship to tooth size and arch dimension. Am J Orthod 1983;83:363–373.
93. Spillane LM, McNamara JA, Jr. Arch width development relative to initial transpalatal width. J Dent Res, IADR Abstracts 1989:374,#1538.
94. Brust EW. Arch dimensional changes concurrent with expansion in the mixed dentition. Ann Arbor: Unpublished Master's Thesis, Department of Orthodontics and Pediatric Dentistry, The University of Michigan, 1992.
95. Brust EW, McNamara JA, Jr. Arch dimensional changes concurrent with expansion in mixed dentition patients. In: Trotman CA, McNamara JA Jr, eds. Orthodontic treatment: Outcome and effectiveness. Ann Arbor: Monograph 30, Craniofacial Growth Series, Center for Human Growth and Development, The University of Michigan, 1995.
96. Gardner GE, Kronman JH. Cranioskeletal displacements caused by rapid palatal expansion in the rhesus monkey. Am J Orthod 1971;59:146–155.
97. Nolan PJ. Personal communication, 1998.
98. Edwards JG. A surgical procedure to eliminate rotational relapse. Am J Orthod 1970;57:35–46.
99. Edwards JG. The diastema, the frenum, the frenectomy: a clinical study. Am J Orthod 1977;71:489–508.
100. Bimler HP. Personal communication, 1992.
101. Ricketts RM, Bench RW, Gugino CF, Hilgers JJ, Schulhof RJ. Bioprogressive therapy. Denver: Rocky Mountain Orthodontics, 1979.
102. McNamara JA, Jr. Maxillary transverse deficiency. Amer J Orthod Dentofac Orthop 2000;117:567-570.
103. Guyer EC, Ellis E, McNamara JA, Jr, Behrents RG. Components of Class III malocclusion in juveniles and adolescents. Angle Orthod 1986;56:7–30.
104. McNamara JA, Jr. An orthopedic approach to the treatment of Class III malocclusion in young patients. J Clin Orthod 1987;21:598–608.
105. McGill JS, McNamara JA, Jr. Treatment and post-treatment effects of rapid maxillary expansion and facial mask therapy. In: McNamara JA, Jr., ed. Growth modification: What works, what doesn't and why. Ann Arbor: Monograph 36, Craniofacial Growth Series, Center for Human Growth and Development, University of Michigan, 1999.
106. McNamara JA, Jr. Components of Class II malocclusion in children 8–10 years of age. Angle Orthod 1981;51:177–202.
107. Tollaro I, Baccetti T, Franchi L, Tanasescu CD. Role of posterior transverse interarch discrepancy in Class II, Division 1 malocclusion during the mixed dentition phase. Am J Orthod Dentofac Orthop 1996;110:417–422.
108. Bishara SE, Khadivi P, Jakobsen JR. Changes in tooth size-arch length relationships from the deciduous to the permanent dentition: a longitudinal study. Am J Orthod Dentofac Orthop 1995;108:607–613.

109. Andresen V. The Norwegian system of gnatho-orthopedics. Acta Gnathol 1936;1:4–36.
110. Kloehn SJ. A new approach to the analysis and treatment of mixed dentition. Am J Orthod 1953;31:161–186.
111. Graber TM. Extra-oral force-facts and fallacies. Am J Orthod 1955;41:490–505.
112. Schudy F. Vertical growth versus anteroposterior growth as related to function and treatment. Angle Orthod 1964;34:75-93.
113. Wendling LK. Short-term skeletal and dental effects of the acrylic splint rapid maxillary expansion appliance. Ann Arbor: Unpublished Master's thesis, Department of Orthodontics and Pediatric Dentistry, The University of Michigan, 1997.
114. Reichenbach E, Taatz H. Kieferorthopädische Klinik und Therapie. Leipzig: Johan Ambrosius Barth, 1971.
115. Kingsley NW. A treatise on oral deformities as a branch of mechanical surgery. New York: D Appleton, 1880.
116. Dellinger EL. A preliminary study of anterior maxillary displacement. Am J Orthod 1973;63:509–516.
117. McNamara JA, Jr. An experimental study of increased vertical dimension in the growing face. Am J Orthod 1977;71:382–395.

Chapter 5
CLASS II MALOCCLUSION

With Lorenzo Franchi and Tiziano Baccetti

Class II malocclusion is a commonly observed clinical problem, occurring in about one third of the population of the United States.[1-4] According to data from the most recent federally-funded study of the US population (the third National Health and Nutrition Examination Survey or NHANES III[5,6]), about 15% have overjets greater than 4 mm, whereas an additional 38% have overjets in the 3–4 mm range (Table 5-1). Excessive overjet occurs at about the same frequency in Caucasians, African Americans, and Mexican Americans.

Because Class II malocclusion is recognized easily by health professionals as well as by patients and their families, especially in instances of excessive overjet (Fig. 5-1) or, less frequently, retroclined maxillary incisors (Fig. 5-2), the correction of Class II problems may constitute nearly half of the treatment protocols in a typical North American orthodontic practice.

Many treatment approaches currently are available to the orthodontist for altering the occlusal relationships typically found in Class II malocclusions. These treatments include a variety of extraoral traction appliances, arch expansion appliances, extraction procedures, and functional jaw orthopedic appliances. Often, only a few of these modalities are applied to all patients with Class II malocclusion in any given orthodontic practice, depending on the experience, personal preference, and success rate of the clinician. Each treatment approach, however, may differ in its effect on the skeletal structures of the craniofacial region, sometimes accelerating or limiting the growth of the various structures involved.

COMPONENTS OF CLASS II MALOCCLUSION

The simplicity of the Angle classification of malocclusion[7] belies the fact that Class II malocclusion is not a single diagnostic entity. Angle based his classification system solely on the position of the permanent maxillary first molars. Underlying this occlusal condition can be numerous skeletal and dentoalveolar combinations, some intuitively obvious, some not. Ideally, a given treatment modality should directly (or sometimes indirectly) affect the particular skeletal and dentoalveolar components of the specific Class II patient.

Much has been written in the orthodontic literature concerning the nature of Class II malocclusions. Many investigators[8-17] have pointed out that a Class II molar relationship occurs in a variety of skeletal and dental configurations. Cross-sectional studies usually have compared Class II individuals to either a group of Class I or normal subjects or to existing cephalometric standards. Comparison of mean values is the most commonly employed analytical procedure in those studies.

In this review of the literature, the measures of the craniofacial region have been divided into four sets based on different anteroposterior criteria: maxillary skeletal position, maxillary dentoalveolar position, mandibular dentoalveolar position, and mandibular skeletal position.[16] In addition, the vertical and transverse configurations of the Class II patient are considered. These arbitrary divisions allow a comparison of

Table 5-1. Percentage of the US population with Class II-type occlusal discrepancies. Data derived from NHANES III[5,6]

Overjet (mm)	All racial/ethnic groups (years)			All ages			
	8–11	12–17	18–50	White	Black	Mexican American	Total
3 to 4	45.2	39.3	37.7	38.0	39.8	49.0	38.8
5 to 6	18.9	11.9	9.1	10.1	11.8	6.5	10.6
7 to 10	3.4	3.5	3.9	3.8	4.3	2.2	3.8
>10	0.2	0.2	0.4	0.3	0.4	0.4	0.3

various cross-sectional studies of patients possessing Angle Class II malocclusion.

Maxillary Skeletal Position

One prime component of a Class II molar relationship presumably is the anterior positioning of maxillary structures relative to other craniofacial components. Drelich,[18] Altemus,[19] Rothstein,[20] and Mastorakos[17] report this to be the case. On the other hand, Riedel,[21] Hunter,[22] and Hitchcock[23] state that in their samples the maxilla was normally positioned in both sexes, and Hitchcock[23] found that only nine of 57 patients had a pretreatment SNA angle one standard deviation above 81°. Further, Renfroe,[24] Henry,[25] and Harris and coworkers[26] reported that, on average, the maxilla was in a slightly retrusive position, and Henry reports that the SNA angle of his Class II sample averaged 1.5° less than the Class I mean.

McNamara,[16] analyzing the components of Class II malocclusion in 277 children 8–10 years of age, found that maxillary skeletal position was variable. Relative to the cranial base, the maxilla most often was in a neutral position (47–65%), and protrusion of the maxilla was noted in only a small percentage (10–15%) of the patients studied. (If the nasolabial angle and the cant of the upper lip were taken into consideration, the prevalence of maxillary skeletal protrusion would be less.) On the other hand, 23–39% of the Class II sample had a retrusive position of the maxilla relative to cranial base structures, a skeletal relationship that often is reflected in an obtuse nasolabial angle.[27,28]

Maxillary Dentoalveolar Position

Another obvious component of Class II malocclusion is the position of the maxillary dentition relative to maxillary skeletal structures. Most studies usually have associated protrusion of the maxillary anterior teeth with the majority of Class II patients. For example, Riedel[21] noted that the maxillary incisor in his Class II, division 1 sample was twice as far anterior to the facial plane as that in patients having normal occlusions. Hitchcock[23] reported maxillary dental protrusion relative to the A-Po line. In contrast, Henry[25] noted that, relative to a line from nasion to Point A, only 11 of 103 patients exhibited maxillary dentoalveolar protrusion.

Although most previous studies have reported maxillary skeletal protrusion as a major component of Class II malocclusion, such findings may have been in error,

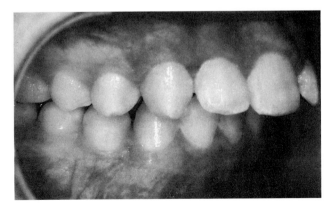

Figure 5-1. Intraoral view of patient with Class II, division 1 malocclusion characterized by flared maxillary incisors. At rest, the lower lip lies under the maxillary incisors.

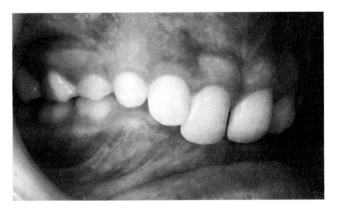

Figure 5-2. Intraoral view of patient with Class II, division 2 malocclusion and an impinging overbite. At rest, the retroclined maxillary incisors are trapped behind the lower lip.

due to the method of measurement. For example, the measurement maxillary incisor (U1) to the A-Po line[29] is influenced significantly by the position of the mandible, often retruded in Class II patients (see below). McNamara[16] compared findings for two measurements from the same group of mixed dentition patients, one method (U1 to A-Po) sensitive to mandibular position and a second method (U1 to Point A Vertical)[27] that is independent of mandibular position. The comparison of results was startling. With A-Po as the orientation line, maxillary incisors appeared protrusive 75% of the time; with Point A Vertical for orientation, the maxillary incisors were judged protruded only 20%, neutral 50%, and retruded 30% of the time. Thus, those findings derived from the method independent of mandibular position indicated that, in nearly one third of Class II patients, decompensation (e.g., forward movement) of the maxillary incisors at least should be considered as part of their overall treatment plan.

There also have been differences in the reported position of the maxillary first molar relative to maxillary skeletal structures. Altemus[19] stated that the posterior dentition was mesially located in the maxilla, whereas Baldridge[30,31] and Elsasser and Wylie[32] noted no difference in maxillary molar position between groups of Class II and Class I individuals. Renfroe[24] reported that the maxillary first molar in his Class II sample was located posterior relative to the Class I group.

Mandibular Dental Position

Less attention has been paid to the position of the mandibular dentition relative to the structures of the mandible. Generally, the investigators who considered the position of the mandibular dentition reported that, on average, the mandibular incisors were related normally to basal structures.[15,16] Disagreement exists, however, concerning the relative position of the mandibular first molars. Elman[33] reported no difference in the position of the mandibular molars relative to Class I individuals. On the other hand, Craig[34] and Altemus[19] reported that the mandibular molars in the Class II individual were located more posteriorly; Gilmore[35] found the anteroposterior position of the mandibular molars was variable.

Mandibular Skeletal Position

Much emphasis has been placed on the size and position of the mandible relative to other craniofacial structures. Adams[36] and Rothstein[20] stated that the absolute length of the mandibles in Class II patients did not differ from those of Class I subjects. Most other investigators, however, noted a mandibular deficiency in Class II individuals for both sexes. For example, Craig[34] noted that the mandibular body was shorter in Class II subjects. Most investigators did not differentiate between the absolute size and the position of the mandible, but Renfroe[24] and Henry[25] noted that, whereas certain Class II patients could be characterized as being deficient in mandibular size, other Class II patients had mandibles that were well formed but were retruded due to a posterior position of the glenoid fossa. All concluded that the mandibles of Class II individuals were retrognathic relative to other craniofacial structures.

McNamara[16] evaluated the variation in the position of the mixed dentition mandible relative to the cranial base and cranial structures by way of two cephalometric measures: pogonion to the nasion perpendicular[27] and the SNB angle.[21,37] These measures indicate that a deficiency in the anteroposterior position of the mandible is a common finding in Class II malocclusion, with about 60% of the patients demonstrating mandibular skeletal retrusion. Similar findings were noted in an adult Class II sample.[38]

Vertical Development

Although Class II malocclusion usually is perceived as a sagittal problem, the vertical dimension of the patient also must be considered. As has been shown by Schudy,[39,40] variations in facial height may conceal or intensify the clinical appearance of the malocclusion. Many other authors[10,13,14,41,42] have recognized the importance of excessive or deficient vertical development in the determination of occlusal relationships, yet few of the cephalometric studies of Class II malocclusion specifically mention anterior or posterior facial height.

Decreased Vertical Dimension

As is well known in prosthodontics and orthognathic surgery, a decrease in vertical dimension causes the mandible to rotate upward and forward. This same phenomenon occurs in the Class II orthodontic patient, in that a short lower anterior facial height can camouflage a mandible that is structurally small relative to the midface. These patients typically have a low mandibular plane angle, a deep overbite with a strong chin point, and either retruded (Fig. 5-3) or flared maxillary incisors. Mandibular dentoalveolar retrusion also occurs.

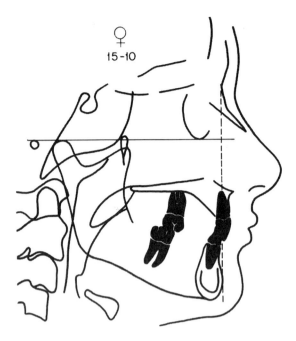

Figure 5-3. Cephalometric tracing of a patient with decreased vertical facial development and a low mandibular plane angle. The retrusion of the mandible is camouflaged by the short lower anterior facial height.

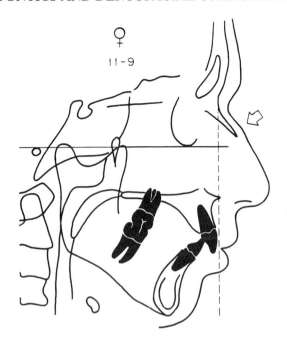

Figure 5-4. Cephalometric tracing of a patient with an increased vertical facial development, a steep mandibular plane angle, and maxillary and mandibular skeletal retrusion. The dorsal hump of the nose is indicated by the arrow.

Increased Vertical Dimension

A patient with an increased lower anterior facial height often is characterized by a retruded mandible (and occasionally the maxilla as well), a poorly defined chin point with a hyperactive mentalis muscle ("golf-ball chin"), and a tendency toward or an anterior openbite. A bump on the nasal contour ("dorsal hump") often is observed clinically in patients with both maxillary and mandibular skeletal retrusion and a Class II malocclusion (Fig. 5-4).

Drelich[18] noted that the Y-axis in Class II patients was directed more downward than in Class I individuals, and that the ratio of anterior to posterior face height was greater in Class II individuals than in Class I individuals. Henry[25] noted a larger mandibular plane angle in his Class II sample, Altemus[19] an increased vertical dysplasia, and Hunter[22] a slight increase in anterior face height.

To evaluate the frequency of occurrence of these conditions in a Class II mixed dentition sample, McNamara[16] examined two measures of vertical dimension. When the mandibular plane angle relative to the Frankfort horizontal was measured, approximately 40% of the sample had a neutral vertical dimension, whereas an increased mandibular plane angle (>26° relative to the Frankfort horizontal) was observed in nearly 50% of the children. A mandibular plane angle greater than 31° was seen in 17.5% of the sample. Only 10% of the sample had a short lower anterior facial height, and this decrease in facial height often is associated with Class II, division 2 malocclusion.

A direct measurement of lower anterior facial height (from anterior nasal spine to menton) indicated that over half of the individuals had a normal face height measurement, whereas 35% of the sample had an excessive lower anterior facial height.[16]

The results of this cephalometric evaluation[16] indicate that although Class II patients most frequently have a neutral or normal vertical dimension, at least one third have excessive vertical development. Decreased vertical development is less common, occurring only in about 10% of Class II subjects in the mixed dentition sample. As mentioned above, increases in lower anterior facial height often are associated with a chin point that is positioned downward and backward, whereas decreases in lower anterior facial height are associated with a forward and upward position of pogonion.

These changes are of critical importance when planning the treatment of a Class II patient, in that increasing the vertical dimension during Class II treatment will tend to camouflage positive changes in mandibular length. *Thus, if maximum advancement of the chin point is desired as a goal of treatment, increases in the vertical dimension of the patient during treatment should be minimized.*

Transverse Components

A dimension often overlooked in the evaluation of the Class II patient is the transverse relationship of the maxilla to the mandible. Most Class II patients appear to have a normal relationship of the buccal segments when the patient is in centric occlusion. Tollaro and colleagues,[43] however, have shown that an underlying transverse discrepancy of 3–5 mm exists in dental arches with Class II malocclusion and seemingly normal buccal relationships. This underlying transverse discrepancy can be unmasked clinically by having the patient posture the mandible in an anterior position so that the canines are positioned in a Class I relationship (Fig. 5-5). More pronounced transverse discrepancies are evidenced by unilateral or bilateral posterior crossbites in centric occlusion.

Baccetti and co-workers[44] evaluated two groups of untreated subjects (a Class II group and a normal occlusion group) during the transition from the deciduous to the mixed dentition. They noted that the transverse discrepancy that existed in the Class II group in the deciduous dentition persisted into the mixed dentition. These investigators also noted that all Class II subjects maintained full Class II molar and canine relationships, and mean overjet increased when compared to mean overjet in the deciduous dentition.

These observations are similar to those of Arya and co-workers[45] and Bishara and co-workers,[46] who have shown that in the absence of therapeutic intervention or a change in the orofacial environment (for example, the elimination of a habit or an airway obstruction), Class II malocclusion generally is not self-correcting. Only after the transition of the second deciduous molars to the second premolars is an improvement in molar relationship sometimes noted. Thus, Class II occlusal relationships tend to be self-perpetuating and continues to be associated with constricted transverse occlusal relationships.

The evaluation of the transverse dimension in Class II patients indicates that the goals of most Class II treatments should include the correction of obvious or camouflaged discrepancies between the maxilla and mandible. Whereas most clinicians recognize the need to eliminate unilateral or bilateral posterior crossbites as part of a treatment regimen, often the typical transverse discrepancy in the Class II patient with a seemingly normal buccal occlusal relationship is overlooked. Alteration of the transverse dimension by a variety of methods as described in the previous chapter, including rapid maxillary expansion, expanding the inner bow of a facebow, or widening as part of functional appliance

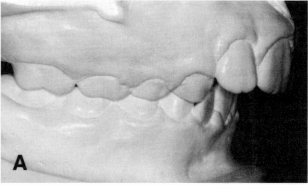
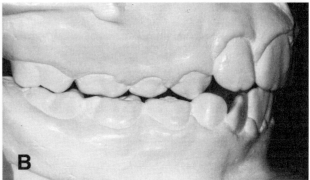

Figure 5-5. Study models of a patient with a Class II, division 1 malocclusion and excessive overjet. *A*, Normal buccolingual relationship with the models in centric occlusion. *B*, Maxillary constriction is evident when the dental casts are hand articulated anteriorly into a Class I canine relationship.

therapy, must be considered in addition to sagittal and vertical correction.

AVAILABLE TREATMENT STRATEGIES

My object all sublime
I shall achieve in time—
To make the punishment fit the crime.

The above quote from the second act of the 1885 Gilbert and Sullivan musical, *The Mikado*, in essence, should summarize the overall goal of treatment for a specific Class II patient, in that the treatment regimen selected should address the underlying needs of the given patient.

The first part of this chapter, as well as the detailed cephalometric analysis presented in Chapter 28, describes a method of determining the components of Class II malocclusion. Once the components have been identified, one or more specific treatment protocols can be used. Although there often is overlap of treatment effects produced by specific modalities, in that a given treatment may affect more than one component of malocclusion, the modalities available will be organized according to the skeletal and/or dentoalveolar effects that they have on craniofacial morphology.

Maxillary Skeletal Position

As mentioned previously, the best evaluation of maxillary skeletal (and dental) position is made at the time of the clinical examination through the evaluation of the nasolabial angle as well as the slope of the upper lip.[28] These observations can be verified through a routine cephalometric appraisal.

Protrusion

The most common treatment for true maxillary skeletal protrusion is extraoral traction. Extraoral traction appliances are divided arbitrarily into two types: facebows and headgears. Facebows attach to tubes on the maxillary first molar bands, whereas headgears attach directly to the archwire or to auxiliaries connected to the archwire.[47]

The cervical (low-pull) facebow (Fig. 5-6) is used most frequently in patients with decreased vertical dimensions. The inner bow of the facebow is anchored to tubes that are placed on the buccal surface of bands attached to the maxillary first molars. The outer bow is connected to a strap that extends to the cervical region and is anchored against the dorsal aspect of the neck. Usually, the outer bow of the facebow lies above the plane of occlusion to direct the force through the center of resistance and prevent distal tipping of the molars during treatment. Numerous clinical studies[48–53] have shown that the forward movement of the maxilla can be inhibited with this type of appliance. Cervical traction also can increase the vertical dimension through the extrusion of molars.[54,55]

The direction of force can be altered, depending on the place of attachment of the anchoring unit. For example, a high-pull facebow (Fig. 5-7) is used in individuals in whom increases in vertical dimension are to be minimized or avoided. The facebow is anchored to an occipital anchoring unit (headcap) to produce a more vertically directed force. As a growth guidance appliance, a high pull facebow can decrease the vertical development of the maxilla, thereby allowing for autorotation of the mandible and maximizing the horizontal expression of mandibular growth.[56] A facebow also can be anchored simultaneously to a cervical neckstrap and a headcap, a combination often termed a "straight-pull" facebow.

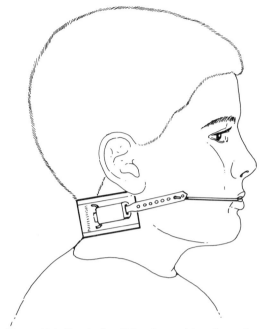

Figure 5-6. Cervical-pull facebow with safety release.

Retrusion

As mentioned earlier, there are a significant number of Class II patients whose malocclusions are characterized, in part, by maxillary skeletal retrusion (Fig. 5-4). This condition tends to be found in patients who have a long lower face height, a steep mandibular plane angle, and a retruded position of the chin point. Maxillary skeletal retrusion is extremely difficult to treat directly, except through orthognathic surgery, and usually no attempt is

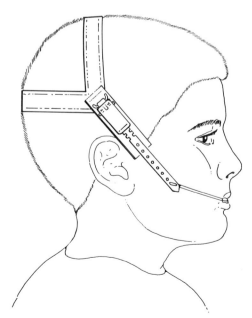

Figure 5-7. High-pull facebow with safety release.

TREATMENT OF CLASS II MALOCCLUSION

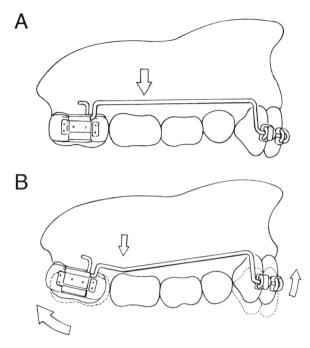

Figure 5-8. Intrusion utility arch. *A*, Before activation. *B*, After activation. The maxillary incisors are intruded and the maxillary first molars are tipped distally, sometimes leading to an improvement in the Class II molar relationship.

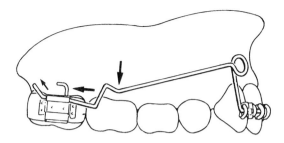

Figure 5-9. A retraction utility arch moves the maxillary incisors upward and backward. The retracting force is produced by activating the wire in the auxiliary tube on the maxillary first molar band.

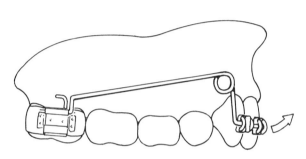

Figure 5-10. A protraction utility arch can be used to procline the maxillary incisors. Before the utility arch is tied into the anterior brackets, it typically lies passively 3-4 mm in front of the maxillary incisors.

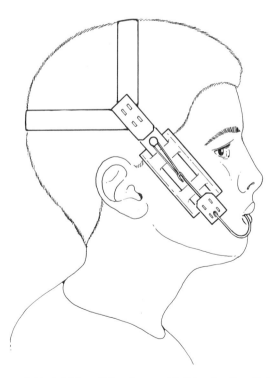

Figure 5-11. A high-pull headgear with J-hooks (Lee Laboratories, Ponco City OK).

made to correct maxillary skeletal retrusion in the mixed dentition. Occasionally, retrusion may be treated indirectly by using such appliances as the posterior biteblock or the vertical-pull chin cup that may produce a slight upward and forward movement of the maxilla and a counterclockwise rotation of the mandible.[57–59]

Maxillary Dentoalveolar Position

Problems with the position of the maxillary dentition can be divided into two types: simple and complex. Simple problems usually involve the anteroposterior position of the four incisors, with these teeth being either in a flared or a retruded position. In instances of flared maxillary incisors, the incisors can be intruded (Fig. 5-8) or retracted (Fig. 5-9) with a utility arch. In instances of retruded maxillary incisors, protraction utility arch treatment (Fig. 5-10) can be initiated. This latter archwire functions to normalize the position of the maxillary incisors prior to functional jaw orthopedic therapy in the mixed-dentition patient.

Flared maxillary incisors also can be retracted using a high-pull headgear with J-hooks (Fig. 5-11) or a straight-pull headgear (Fig. 5-12) combined with J-hooks that are attached to the archwire anteriorly or by using a closing arch supported by headgear. Headgears with J-hooks also are used to potentiate archwire me-

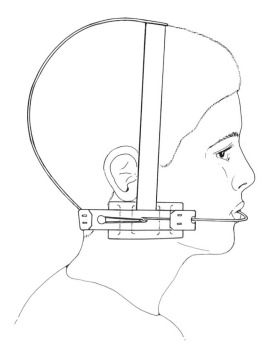

Figure 5-12. Straight-pull headgear with J-hooks.

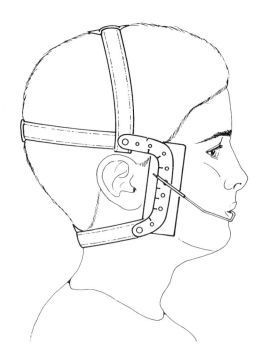

Figure 5-13. Interlandi-type headgear with J-hooks.

chanics by helping control forces incorporated into the archwire (*e.g.*, torque, intrusion).[47,60]

Complex problems involve more than simply correcting the flaring of the maxillary incisors. These conditions involve the protrusion of the entire maxillary dental arch relative to the skeletal portion of the maxilla. In this type of patient, the goal of treatment is either to retract the maxillary anterior teeth following the removal of two maxillary premolars or to move the maxillary dentition *en masse* in a distal direction. This latter goal can be achieved through a number of treatment options.

Extraoral Traction

As has been described previously, cervical, straight-pull, and high-pull facebows as well as low-pull, straight-pull, and high-pull headgear combined with J-hooks can be used to affect both maxillary skeletal and dentoalveolar structures.[61] These adjuncts are incorporated routinely into the treatment plan of patients with maxillary dentoalveolar protrusion.

The use of the Interlandi-type headgear[62,63] provides an additional treatment option with a variable direction of force. J hooks can be applied to the maxillary teeth in a variety of force vectors to retract and intrude the maxillary incisor teeth (Fig. 5-13). A similar type of retraction/stabilization of the mandibular dental arch also can be achieved. It also is possible to attach a high-pull headgear to the maxillary arch and a straight-pull headgear to the mandibular arch simultaneously.

Distalizing Plates

An adjunct to the extraoral traction procedure just described is the use of various distalizing plates, such as the ACCO (acronym of acrylic cervical occipital appliance).[64-67] The ACCO appliance consists of an acrylic palatal section, modified Adams clasps to the first premolars, and finger springs against the mesial surfaces of the maxillary first molars (Fig. 5-14). These plates fit against the maxillary dentition and create a force against the first molars, producing posterior molar movement of approximately one millimeter per month.[67] The plate is worn on a full-time basis except during meals and usually is used in conjunction with nighttime wear of a cervical or high-pull facebow. The finger springs on the plate tip the crowns distally; the facebow produces distal root torque to maintain an upright position of the molars. A 1-mm bite plate is added to disclude the posterior teeth slightly, facilitating posterior movement of the maxillary first molars.

Distalizing plates are useful not only in assisting in the production of additional space but also may serve to regain space that was lost due to the premature removal or loss of a second deciduous molar. In these instances, the plate sometimes may be used without ex-

TREATMENT OF CLASS II MALOCCLUSION

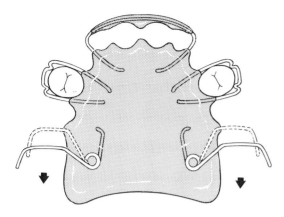

Figure 5-14. An ACCO appliance modified from the design of Cetlin[64,65] and Gianelly.[66,67] The springs anterior to the first molar produce the distalizing force. In this figure, the palatal surface of the appliance is shown. The wire is anchored in the acrylic, but the power arms and springs are free of acrylic, thus permitting activation of the appliance. (After Gianelly.[66])

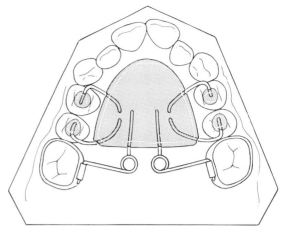

Figure 5-15. Typical design of the Pendulum appliance of Hilgers.[73,74] An acrylic palatal button is bonded to the occlusal surfaces of the maxillary first premolars. TMA springs extend from the acrylic to the sleeves on the first molar bands.

traoral traction. The ACCO also is effective in the correction of maxillary dental asymmetries.[67]

Pendulum Appliance

The Pendulum appliance is representative of a series of appliances that have been developed in recent years to facilitate efficient Class II correction by distalizing maxillary molars with relatively modest patient compliance requirements. Other related appliances include the Distal Jet,[68–70] the Jones Jig,[71] and the Lokar distalizing appliance.[72]

The Pendulum appliance, first described in 1992 by Hilgers,[73] consists of a large Nance-type acrylic button in the palate for anchorage, along with .032″ titanium molybdenum alloy (TMA™) springs that deliver a distal force to the maxillary first molars[73] (Fig. 5-15). The springs are activated 60° to 90° so that they lie nearly parallel to the midline of the palate when in a relaxed position,[74] delivering 200–250 grams per side to the maxillary molars when placed in the lingual sheaths on the maxillary first molar bands.[73] A swinging arc movement of the distalizing spring is produced; hence the name *Pendulum*.[75] The springs also may have adjustment loops that can be manipulated to increase molar expansion, molar rotation, or distal root tip.[76]

The Pendex version of the appliance (Fig. 5-16) incorporates a midpalatal jackscrew into the center of a Nance button that is activated in a manner similar to the Haas-type expander[77] when a transverse discrepancy is present. Because most Class II malocclusions have maxillary constriction as a component,[78] the Pendex typically is our version of choice.

We recommend expanding the pendex one turn per day until the lingual cusps of the maxillary posterior teeth approximate the mandibular buccal cusps. Then the wires connecting the molar bands to the acrylic palatal button are cut either unilaterally or bilaterally (see Chapter 20 for a discussion of the clinical management of the Pendex appliance), and the molars move posteriorly due to the action of the TMA™ springs (Fig. 5-17). Once the molars have been overcorrected into a super Class I molar relationship, Hilgers[73] recommends stabilization of the molar position for six to ten weeks in order to minimize mesial drift.

Achieving posterior movement of the remaining maxillary dentition has proved to be a challenge to the

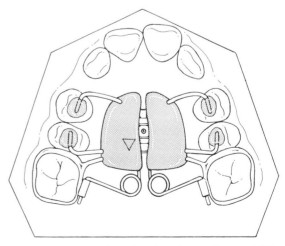

Figure 5-16. Typical design of the Pendex appliance of Hilgers. The midline expansion screw is activated in order to increase palatal width in patients with maxillary constriction.

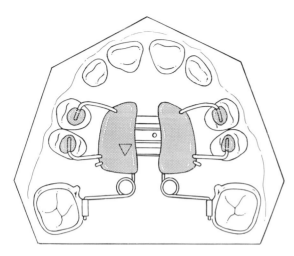

Figure 5-17. The Pendex appliance after expansion and molar distalization. The maxillary first molars also move slightly toward the midline and rotate posteriorly. An adjustment loop (not shown) can be used to minimize the distal tipping of the maxillary first molars.

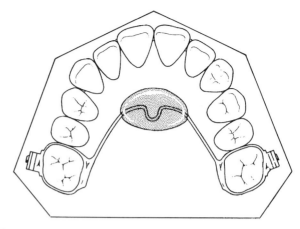

Figure 5-18. The Nance holding arch. An acrylic button is placed in the palate supported by a wire that extends from molar to molar. This appliance can be fabricated indirectly as a laboratory procedure (shown here) or directly in the mouth by means of light-cure acrylic and .036" stainless steel wire that fits into the lingual sheaths on the maxillary first molar bands.

clinician. After the molars have been distalized adequately into a slightly overcorrected (Class III) position, the occlusal rests on the maxillary second premolars are removed, and the second premolars are allowed to drift posteriorly, due to the pull of the transseptal fibers. One or two appointments later, the Pendex is removed and a "quick Nance" button,[79] fabricated intraorally from light-cure acrylic, is placed. A traditional Nance holding arch (Fig. 5-18), made from bands on a work model, also can be used to stabilize the position of the maxillary molars.

In addition to the Nance button, the placement of a passive utility arch (see Fig. 11-5 in Chapter 11) that extends from the auxiliary tube on the maxillary first molar to the brackets on the maxillary four incisors is recommended. The premolar teeth are not incorporated into the archwire but rather are allowed to drift posteriorly. After three or four months, brackets are placed on the premolars and canines, and retracting mechanics that incorporate elastomeric chain are used to complete the distalization of the premolars and canines. A retraction utility arch or a closing loop arch then is used to complete anterior space closure. The Class II correction can be supported by having the patient wear Class II elastics from the ball hooks on the maxillary canine brackets to the hooks on the bands of the mandibular first or second molars.

Other methods of molar stabilization have been suggested, including cementing the transpalatal arch that was used initially to rotate the molars into a proper orientation. A facebow can be used at this point in treatment to upright the molars if excessive distal tipping of the crowns of these teeth has occurred. A stopped maxillary continuous archwire also can be used to anchor the maxillary molars against the anterior teeth. In addition, Bowman[70] has suggested installing Jasper Jumper™ modules (see Chapter 19) as a method of stabilizing maxillary molar position.

Several clinical studies have been conducted concerning the treatment effects of the Pendulum/Pendex appliance.[75,76,80–82] The Pendulum appliance is effective in distalizing the maxillary molars by way of palatal anchorage in growing patients. Bussick and McNamara[82] reported that the average distalization of the maxillary first molar was 5.7 mm, with about 11° distal tipping of the maxillary molars. They estimated that about 25–30% of the total sagittal treatment effect was loss of anchorage anteriorly, a percentage that was less than reported by Ghosh and Nanda.[80] Bussick and McNamara[82] also noted a slight increase in lower anterior facial height and a slight opening of the mandibular plane angle during the Pendulum phase of treatment. Although this appliance can be used successfully in adults, no clinical studies have considered this age group.

NiTi Coils

Another source of distalizing force is the placement of NiTi coils into a fixed appliance system that incorporates palatal anchorage.[66,83] After derotating the molars by way of a transpalatal arch, a version of the Nance palatal button can be attached to the maxillary first or second premolars, depending on the anchorage requirements of the patient (Fig. 5-19). A continuous force of

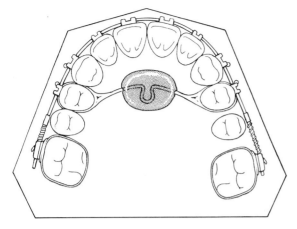

Figure 5-19. Occlusal view of NiTi coils activated to distalize maxillary first molars. A Nance button has been attached to the maxillary first premolars for anchorage.

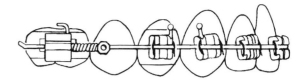

Figure 5-20. Sagittal view of fixed appliances and NiTi push-coil. A Gurin lock is used to activate the NiTi coil.

between 100 and 300 grams can be generated bilaterally with preformed NiTi coils (GAC International, Central Islip NY) that are threaded around the archwire (Fig. 5-20). Adjustable Gurin locks (3M Unitek, Monrovia CA) can be used to activate the NiTi coils intraorally.[66]

Mandibular Dentoalveolar Position

Many of the techniques described in the treatment of tooth-size/arch-length discrepancy patients also are applicable in the Class II individual. For example, a lip bumper can be used effectively in instances of mandibular dentoalveolar retrusion, especially in those individuals who have very tight cheek and lip musculature and a defined mentolabial sulcus.[65,84,85] Uprighting or distalizing the mandibular molars works against Class II correction but helps resolve existing tooth-size/arch-size discrepancies.

A passive utility arch also has proved to be effective in at least partially shielding the erupting dentition from the cheek musculature. Proclined mandibular incisors can be retracted (given sufficient interdental spacing) with a simple intrusion utility arch or a retraction utility arch. In a Class II patient with a mild-to-moderate deficiency (e.g., 2–5 mm) in mandibular arch length, a removable mandibular Schwarz appliance can be used to decompensate (e.g., expand, upright) the mandibular dental arch.

Of all the conditions relating to the position of the mandibular dentition in Class II malocclusion, the most challenging is the treatment of mandibular dentoalveolar retrusion. These patients often are characterized by a strong mentolabial band that may be part of the orbicularis oris muscle or, on the other hand, simply may be composed of fibroelastic connective tissue. Although many types of appliances have been used to address this problem, including the lip bumper and also the labial pads of the FR-2 of Fränkel, in many instances this tight soft tissue band prevents adequate correction of mandibular dentoalveolar retrusion despite orthodontic and even surgical intervention.

Mandibular Skeletal Position

As discussed earlier, the most consistent finding in Class II malocclusion is mandibular skeletal retrusion. If a patient has this problem as part of his or her overall craniofacial configuration, some type of functional jaw orthopedic (FJO) appliance may be indicated.

Over the last twenty-five years, there has been a gradual evolution regarding the way in which functional jaw orthopedics is used in a contemporary orthodontic practice, especially concerning appliance selection, the timing of intervention, and the need for "pre-orthopedic" orthodontic treatment. The majority of clinical studies to date seem to indicate that the length of the mandible can be increased over the short-term.[86–91] The long-term effects of orthopedic intervention, however, remain controversial and open to question. For example, long-term investigations of the Herbst appliance[92,93] demonstrate minimal skeletal increases over what would occur during normal growth, whereas long-term studies of the FR-2 of Fränkel[94] are more encouraging.

All functional jaw orthopedic appliances have one aspect in common: they induce a forward mandibular posturing (Fig. 5-21) as part of the treatment effect. Presumably, this alteration in the postural activity of the muscles of the craniofacial complex ultimately leads to changes in both skeletal and dental relationships.[94] Clinical studies of the treatment effects produced by specific FJO appliances will be discussed in detail in later chapters.

There are numerous FJO appliances that have been proposed for the treatment of Class II malocclusion. For the purpose of this discussion, however, only four will be considered: the FR-2 of Fränkel, the twin block appliance, the Herbst appliance, and the bionator. We use the first two appliances primarily in the mixed dentition, whereas the Herbst appliance is reserved for

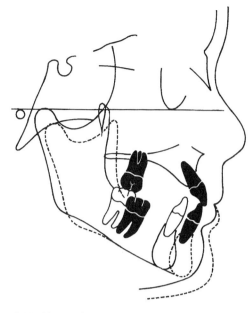

Figure 5-21. Change in mandibular posture produced by most functional jaw orthopedic appliances. No universal agreement exists as to the optimal amount of bite advancement (See Chapter 15 for discussion).

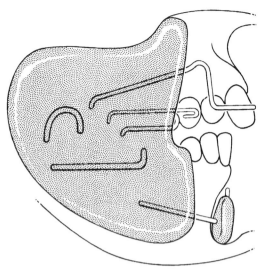

Figure 5-22. The FR-2 appliance of Fränkel. The base of operation is the maxillary and mandibular vestibule. The appliance has a direct effect on the postural activity of the masticatory and perioral musculature by producing a change in mandibular position. Spontaneous expansion of the dental arches also occurs due to the effect of the vestibular shields and lower labial pads on the soft tissue.

the early permanent dentition. We have not used the bionator at all since the early 1990s, but this appliance has been included in this discussion for the sake of completeness.

FR-2 of Fränkel

When treating the routine Class II malocclusion characterized in part by mandibular skeletal retrusion, the appliance that has the greatest effect on the skeletal, dentoalveolar and muscular components is the function regulator (FR-2) appliance (Fig. 5-22) of Fränkel.[94–97] Of all the so-called "functional appliances," the FR-2 appliance is unique in that it is essentially tissue-borne rather than tooth-borne. The base of operation is the maxillary and mandibular vestibule, and the appliance has a direct and primary effect on the neuromuscular system.

Fränkel designed the FR appliances according to the general orthopedic principles of Roux.[98] The appliance first is used as an exercise device in retraining the associated musculature and indirectly producing changes in skeletal and dentoalveolar relationships by retraining or reprogramming the central nervous system. In contrast to virtually every other type of functional appliance, the FR appliance interrupts abnormal patterns of muscle activity and ultimately produces an environment in which skeletal and dental arch changes occur. Not only have increases in mandibular length been noted following FR-2 treatment, but also changes in the transverse dimensions of the dental arches have been reported.

The FR-2 appliance is the appliance of choice in the treatment of patients with severe neuromuscular imbalances and skeletal discrepancies. For example, the lower labial pads help interrupt hyperactive mentalis activity, a clinical sign of lip incompetence. Fränkel and Fränkel[94] have stressed the importance of maintaining an adequate lip seal as a key element of successful orthopedic treatment. By balancing the neuromuscular environment, not only can severe malocclusions be treated successfully, but also the tendency toward relapse is minimized, because the neural and soft tissue factors associated with the skeletal malocclusion have been addressed as well. Because the appliance is tissue-borne rather than tooth-borne, maximum skeletal change can be achieved with minimal unwanted tooth movement.

Due to the protecting effect of the vestibular shields on the dentition, spontaneous expansion in both arches typically is observed during treatment.[94,96,99,100] Increases in mandibular length also have been noted.[88,89,94,97,101] The FR-2 appliance is an excellent appliance in patients with either a neutral or short lower anterior facial height, because this appliance may lead to an increase in lower facial height during treatment. The FR-2 also is used in patients with excessive vertical development, although care must be taken not to open the bite during treatment. A more extensive discussion

TREATMENT OF CLASS II MALOCCLUSION

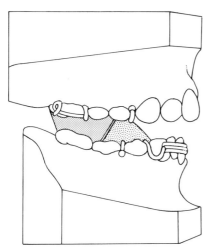

Figure 5-23. Modified twin block design. The anterior ball clasps of the original design of Clark[102] are replaced by a labial bow to which clear acrylic has been added, increasing anterior retention of the lower appliance, especially during the period of the transitional dentition.

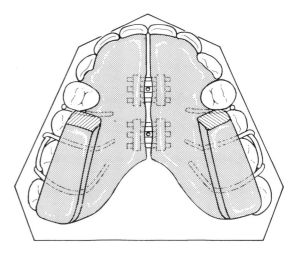

Figure 5-24. Maxillary occlusal view of the twin block appliance. Two expansion screws are placed in the midline. Delta clasps are used to secure the appliance to the molars posteriorly, and ball clasps are used to anchor the plate in the premolar/deciduous molar region.

of the biologic basis and clinical management of this appliance is found in Chapter 16.

Twin Block Appliance

Another functional appliance that has become more popular with orthodontists both in the United States and abroad is the twin block appliance (Fig. 5-23). This appliance, developed by Clark[102–104] in 1977, is perceived by most clinicians to be easier to manipulate than the FR-2 appliance of Fränkel, and thus has had a substantial rise in frequency of use during the 1990s. Although Class II correction can be achieved readily with this appliance within a 6–9 month period, the twin block does not have as direct an effect on the musculature as the FR-2.

The twin block appliance is composed of removable maxillary and mandibular plates that fit tightly against the teeth, alveolus, and adjacent supporting structures (Fig. 5-24). Delta clasps[105] are used bilaterally to anchor the maxillary appliance to the first permanent molars, and .030″ ball clasps are placed in the interproximal areas of the premolars or deciduous molars. The precise clasp configuration depends on the type (deciduous or permanent) and number of teeth present at the time of appliance construction. The use of two expansion screws in the midpalatal region is recommended.

In the mandibular arch, Clark[105] has recommended the use of a series of ball clasps that lie in the interproximal areas between the canines and mandibular incisors. We have modified this design by placing a labial bow covered with acrylic anterior to the mandibular incisors[106] (Fig. 5-25), similar to that of a mandibular spring retainer.[107] In contrast to the spring retainer, however, the positions of the mandibular incisors are not altered in the work model before appliance construction. The acrylic usually fills the interproximal areas below the contact points of the mandibular incisors.

The twin block appliance has the distinct advantage of being worn as a fulltime appliance, including during meals, although some clinicians have their patients remove their appliances while eating. In contrast to the bionator, which is a single acrylic and wire appliance and thus typically interrupts speech patterns, it is relatively easy for the patient to speak with the twin block appliance in place.

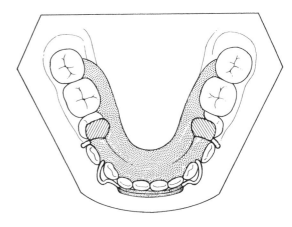

Figure 5-25. Modified design of the mandibular twin block appliance in which the lower lingual acrylic extends posteriorly into the permanent molar region. The lower labial bow with clear acrylic covering extends anteriorly to cover the labial surfaces of the mandibular anterior teeth.

The twin block appliance also provides the clinician with the ability to control the vertical dimension of the Class II patient. If a patient has a tendency toward an anterior openbite and excessive vertical development, the posterior bite blocks are not trimmed, allowing for differential eruption of the incisors while impeding the eruption of the posterior teeth. On the other hand, if a patient has a deep bite, an accentuated curve of Spee and a short lower anterior facial height, the posterior bite blocks can be trimmed to allow for eruption of the buccal segments as the curve of Spee is leveled.

Herbst Appliance

We use the first two appliances mentioned primarily in mixed dentition patients, although they can be used successfully in adolescents, given adequate patient compliance. Our choice of functional appliance in the permanent dentition generally is the Herbst appliance. Herbst developed this appliance system in 1910;[108] Pancherz,[86,87,109] reintroduced the Herbst appliance to the practicing orthodontist in the late 1970s.

The original design of the Herbst appliance involved gold castings on the maxillary and mandibular canines that were connected by the Herbst bite jumping mechanism,[108] a sliding rod and tube assembly. Pancherz originally advocated a banded design, although recently he has advocated a cast design as well.[110]

Today, we use two types of attachment mechanisms for the Herbst appliance: stainless steel crowns and the acrylic splints. The stainless steel crown Herbst[111-114] features crowns on the maxillary first molars (Fig. 5-26) and mandibular first premolars (Figs. 5-27 and 5-28). The pivots soldered to the crowns connect the tube and

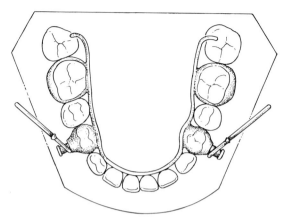

Figure 5-27. Mandibular view of the stainless steel crown Herbst appliance with a lingual arch and bands on the mandibular first molars.

plunger assembly, with the length of the maxillary tube determining the amount of bite advancement. A lower lingual arch connects the crowns on the mandibular first premolars to bands on the mandibular first molars (Fig. 5-27). Alternatively, the lingual arch extends posteriorly to the mandibular first molars. Occlusal rests formed from the ends of the lingual arch are bonded to the central grooves of the first molars (Fig. 5-28).

The second design of the Herbst appliance is the acrylic splint Herbst[115-118] (Fig. 5-29). This version is composed of a wire framework, over which has been adapted 2.5–3.0 mm thick splint Biocryl™. The posterior teeth are covered from the canines through the first molars in the maxillary arch; full occlusal coverage is provided for the mandibular dental arch. The axles of the Herbst bite-jumping mechanism are soldered adjacent to the mandibular first premolars and the maxillary

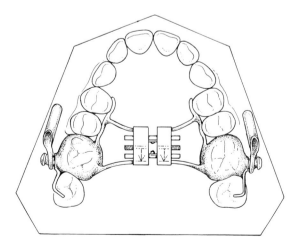

Figure 5-26. Maxillary view of the stainless steel crown Herbst appliance. A midline expansion screw routinely is incorporated into the appliance.

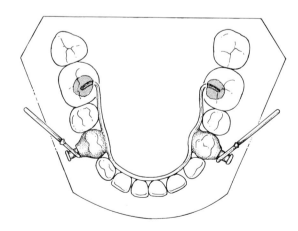

Figure 5-28. Mandibular view of the stainless steel crown Herbst appliance with a lingual arch, the ends of which have been bonded to the occlusal surfaces of the mandibular first molars.

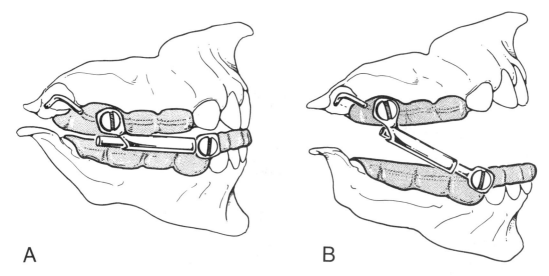

Figure 5-29. The acrylic splint Herbst appliance. *A.* In occlusion. *B,* During mandibular opening. The acrylic splints cover the mandibular dentition and the maxillary posterior teeth.

first molars (Fig. 5-27). A Hyrax-type screw can be utilized for expansion as the mandible is positioned forward. A step-by-step advancement also can be achieved easily by adding shims to the mandibular part of the bite-jumping mechanism.

In contrast to the crown Herbst that is cemented to the dentition, the mandibular part of the acrylic splint design always is removable. The maxillary portion of the acrylic splint type may be bonded in place in a manner similar to that used for the acrylic splint expander. On the other hand, both the maxillary and mandibular parts of the appliance can be removable, making the clinical management of this Herbst design relatively straightforward.

Both types of Herbst appliances are worn for 9–12 months, after which full fixed appliance therapy is initiated, usually for an additional 12–18 months. Class II elastics may be worn by the patient during Phase II treatment to sustain the Class II correction.

Although the Herbst appliance can be used in the mixed dentition,[119] it is not the appliance of choice for correction of mandibular skeletal retrusion, particularly in severe cases. Even though an adequate occlusal change can be produced, about 50% of this change tends to be due to tooth movement and 50% due to skeletal adaptation.[87,89] Significant tooth movement is not desirable in patients who require maximum skeletal change.

In mixed-dentition patients who have been followed for several years after Herbst therapy but before the placement of fixed appliances, we have noted a significant tendency toward a relapse to the original malocclusion. This observation with Herbst patients may be due, in part, to the lack of direct effect on the orofacial musculature produced by the appliance (in contrast to the FR-2 appliance). Also, the deciduous teeth tend to be relatively flat and thus do not provide the same type of occlusal interdigitation as does the permanent dentition. Thus, in our armamentarium today, the Herbst appliance is used primarily as an appliance in the permanent dentition.

Bionator

Another functional appliance that must be mentioned in this discussion of Class II correction is the bionator (Fig. 5-30), an appliance that has been available for over 40 years[120,121] and that has many devotees worldwide. Like the twin block, this appliance is much less technically demanding in its clinical management than the Fränkel appliance, but it does not affect directly the orofacial musculature like the FR-2 appliance.

With the availability of the twin block, and the ease with which patients function with the twin block in place, the argument could be made that the bionator may not be the appliance of choice in the 21st century. The bionator, however, still is used successfully by many clinicians today for the correction of Class II problems.[122–125]

A major indication for the use of the bionator or twin block instead of the FR-2 appliance is in patients with extremely short lower anterior facial heights. In these patients, there is not adequate vertical space for the positioning for the lower labial pads of the FR-2, and, thus, a bionator appliance is used, not only to bring the mandible in a more forward position but also to in-

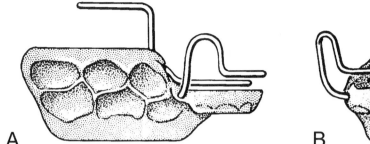 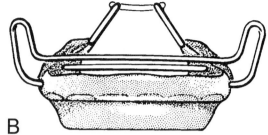

Figure 5-30. The Bionator. The "California Bionator" is an example of a bionator that can be used to correct Class II malocclusion. *A*, Lateral view. *B*, Frontal view.

crease vertical dimension through differential eruption of posterior teeth. In patients with excessive vertical facial height, the bionator also can be used if the posterior teeth are prevented from further eruption by way of an interocclusal acrylic bite block.

TREATMENT TIMING FOR FUNCTIONAL JAW ORTHOPEDICS

In the last two decades, several major changes have occurred within the field of functional jaw orthopedics. One of the most noted changes has been an alteration in the timing of treatment. One of the first investigations[88] to evaluate the role of age in the response to FJO treatment considered 100 patients with the FR-2 appliance of Fränkel, comparing them to longitudinal cephalometric data from 41 untreated Class II controls. The sample was divided almost equally into two groups, one with an average starting age of 8.5 years and the second 11.5 years. The older patients displayed a significantly greater growth response than did the younger patients. In 24 months, mandibular length increased 8.0 mm in the older group (4.4 mm in the older controls) and 6.4 mm in the younger group (4.0 mm in the younger controls).

McNamara and colleagues[88] hypothesized that the reason for this pronounced increase in growth response was due to the synergistic interaction between a change in function produced by a functional appliance and an increase in quantity of growth hormone during the circumpubertal growth period. The interaction between altered function and growth hormone has been demonstrated further in other experimental studies, including those of Petrovic and co-workers.[126] A corollary for this observation is that the effectiveness of therapy with functional appliances strongly depends on the responsiveness of the condylar cartilage, which in turn is dependent on the growth rate of the mandible.[127] Therefore, the evaluation of mandibular skeletal maturation and growth potential in the individual patient provides essential information for the anticipation of treatment results.

The growth rate of the human mandible is not constant throughout development. A peak in mandibular growth velocity (pubertal growth spurt) has been described in many cephalometric studies.[128–132] The intensity, onset, and duration of the pubertal peak in mandibular growth is characterized by significant individual variations.

Mandibular skeletal maturity can be assessed through a series of biological indicators that may include: increase in statural height,[128,133] skeletal maturation of the hand and wrist,[134–136] dental development and eruption,[135,137,138] menarche, breast, and voice changes,[139] and cervical vertebral maturation.[140,141]

This last method has proven to be effective and clinically reliable in detecting the peak in both statural height and mandibular growth in over 90% of subjects, including males and females.[142,143] One of the most practical advantages in using the cervical vertebral method when compared to other commonly used methods, such as the evaluation of hand and wrist x-rays, is that additional radiation exposure is avoided, as the vertebrae already are seen in the lateral cephalometric radiograph.

In the Cervical Vertebral Method (CVM), six stages corresponding to six different maturational phases in the cervical vertebrae can be identified during the pubertal period. The six stages (*Cervical vertebral stages, Cvs*) are characterized by definite morphological and dimensional changes of the bodies of the second through the sixth cervical vertebra (Fig. 5-31). *Stage 1 (Cvs 1)*: the inferior borders of the bodies of all cervical vertebrae are flat. The superior borders are tapered from posterior to anterior. *Stage 2 (Cvs 2)*: A concavity develops in the inferior border of the second vertebra. The anterior vertical height of the bodies increases. *Stage 3 (Cvs 3)*: A concavity develops in the inferior

TREATMENT OF CLASS II MALOCCLUSION

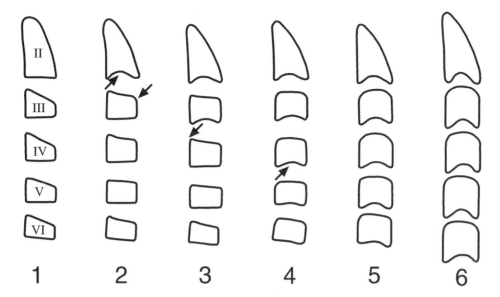

Figure 5-31. The six stages in cervical vertebral maturation. *Stage 1 (Cvs 1):* The inferior borders of the bodies of all cervical vertebrae are flat. The superior borders are tapered from posterior to anterior. *Stage 2 (Cvs 2):* A concavity develops in the inferior border of the second vertebra. The anterior vertical height of the bodies increases. *Stage 3 (Cvs 3):* A concavity develops in the inferior border of the third vertebra. *Stage 4 (Cvs 4):* A concavity develops in the inferior border of the fourth vertebra. Concavities in the lower borders of the fifth and sixth vertebrae are beginning to form. The bodies of all cervical vertebrae are rectangular in shape. *Stage 5 (Cvs 5):* Concavities are well defined in the lower borders of the bodies of all six cervical vertebrae. The bodies are nearly square and the spaces between the bodies are reduced. *Stage 6 (Cvs 6): All* concavities have deepened. The vertebral bodies are now higher than they are wide.

border of the third vertebra. *Stage 4 (Cvs 4)*: A concavity develops in the inferior border of the fourth vertebra. Concavities in the lower borders of the fifth and of the sixth vertebrae are beginning to form. The bodies of all cervical vertebrae are rectangular in shape. *Stage 5 (Cvs 5)*: Concavities are well defined in the lower borders of the bodies of all six cervical vertebrae. The bodies are nearly square in shape and the spaces between the bodies are reduced. *Stage 6 (Cvs 6)*: All concavities have deepened. The vertebral bodies are now taller than they are wide.

The six CVM stages include observations before the peak, *i.e.* during the accelerative growth phase (vertebral stages 1 to 3) and observations after the peak, *i.e.* during the decelerative phase of growth (vertebral stages 4 to 6). Pubertal growth peak occurs on average (93.5 % of the subjects) between vertebral stage 3 and 4.[143]

The CVM method has been used recently to define optimal timing for treatment of Class II malocclusion by means of a functional appliance (twin block).[143,144] In these studies, a comparison of both early and late treatment outcomes was performed. The subjects in the early-treated group started twin block therapy in Stage 1/Cvs 1 or Stage 2/Cvs 2 and they were compared with subjects treated either during or slightly after Stage 3/Cvs3 continuing on through Stage 5/Cvs 5. Untreated Class II subjects were used as controls for both of the treated groups.

More favorable mandibular skeletal modifications were induced with twin block therapy that started during or slightly after the onset of Stage 3/Cvs 3, which is concurrent with the onset of the peak in mandibular growth. The amount of supplementary elongation of the mandible in relation to controls measured along Co-Pg in the late-treated group (4.8 mm/year) was more than twice that of the early-treated group (1.9 mm/year). The pronounced increase in total mandibular length was associated with significant increases in the height of the mandibular ramus (Co-Go, 2.7 mm/year) and in the length of the mandibular body (Go-Pg, 1.7 mm/year) in the group treated at the peak when compared to the corresponding control group. The early-treated group (Stage 1/Cvs 1 and Stage 2/Cvs 2) showed no significant changes in these two measurements.

The increase in mandibular growth in the late-treated group was associated with significant changes in the direction of condylar growth. Individuals treated at the peak showed significantly more backward direction of growth in the mandibular condyle. This growth modification has been described previously as "posterior mandibular morphogenetic rotation,"[145] a biological mechanism leading to greater increments in total mandibular length and, thus, efficiently improving the skeletal sagittal relationships in Class II malocclusion.

The recent findings of Franchi and Baccetti on twin block therapy,[142,144] in association with previous data regarding other devices such as the FR-2[88,127] and the Herbst appliance[146] strongly suggest that optimum timing for functional/orthopedic treatment of Class II malocclusion is during or slightly after the pubertal growth spurt. From the point of view of occlusal development, this period correlates in most patients with the late mixed or early permanent dentition. The clinical consequence is that active treatment of the skeletal disharmony with the functional appliance can be followed almost immediately by a phase of fixed appliance therapy to refine occlusion and to give stability to the newly established intermaxillary relationship.

Long-term data for the Herbst appliance already exist indicating that a stable Class I intercuspation is an efficient factor in counteracting occlusal relapse.[147] Late functional/orthopedic therapy of Class II malocclusion just after the beginning of the peak in growth velocity (Stage 3/Cvs 3) is recommended to maximize the treatment effect and reduce the time of posttreatment retention.

Therefore, the onset of functional jaw orthopedic therapy in the mild-to-moderate Class II patient whenever possible should be delayed until the end of the mixed dentition period. These patients, however, often benefit from a "pre-orthopedic" phase of treatment in the early mixed dentition, as is described in detail below.

Need for Phase I Treatment

As we became more experienced in using various functional jaw orthopedic appliances, it became clear that some preparation of the dental arches was needed in a significant number of Class II patients. As mentioned earlier in this chapter, over 30% of the Class II patients evaluated[16] had maxillary incisors that were in a retroclined position. Thus, one of the initial treatments of a Class II patient may involve a flaring (and perhaps intrusion) of the maxillary incisors. The need for uprighting of the buccal segments, particularly in the lower arch, also was noted.

One of the other aspects of functional jaw orthopedic therapy was the realization that Class II malocclusion is not only an anteroposterior and vertical problem, but it also may have a strong transverse component. A deficiency in maxillary width, both at the occlusal and skeletal levels, is a main feature of developing Class II malocclusion.[44] A Class II patient in the mixed dentition usually presents with a 3–5 mm transverse discrepancy between the maxilla and mandible.[43] Thus, we advocate rapid maxillary expansion with a bonded acrylic splint appliance, as described in the preceding chapter. As has been discussed, the widening of the maxilla into a slightly overcorrected position often results in a spontaneous correction of a Class II relationship, occasionally even in a patient who has a full cusp Class II molar relationship. Therefore, the first major step in addressing a Class II problem may be intervention in the transverse dimension. Only in the late mixed dentition is a direct attempt made to correct the Class II problem in patients with mild to moderate discrepancies.

CONCLUDING REMARKS

There is no one ideal method of treating a Class II malocclusion in the mixed or early permanent dentition. Following a thorough clinical examination, a precise analysis of both the cephalometric radiographs and the dental casts should be undertaken to identify the components of the malocclusion that deviate from "normal." After a thorough diagnosis has been established, the clinician can select the appropriate treatment regimen from among a number of options.

A wide variety of treatment modalities have been considered in this chapter. Many of these modalities are discussed in detail in later chapters on the clinical management of various appliances. It should be noted, however, that not all of the treatment modalities discussed in this chapter are used with the same frequency. As true maxillary skeletal protrusion patients are observed relatively infrequently, extraoral traction is a less frequently used treatment option. On the other hand, mandibular skeletal retrusion is a relatively common problem in Class II malocclusion, and therefore our use of functional jaw orthopedics is a more frequently used treatment option. Subsequent to our initial experiences with rapid maxillary expansion and after observing spontaneous correction of some Class II problems, the frequency of use of FJO appliances has decreased significantly during the last decade.

The appliances mentioned in this chapter should be part of the routine armamentarium of the practicing clinician, so that he or she can deliver the appropriate treatment to a given patient. These mixed dentition treatment modalities are designed to alleviate skeletal and neuromuscular imbalances, but fixed appliances almost always are needed for final dental detailing in the permanent dentition.

REFERENCES CITED

1. Kelly JE, Sanchez M, Van Kirk LE. An assessment of the occlusion of the teeth of children. DHEW Publication No (HRA) 74-1612. Washington, DC: National Center for Health Statistics, 1973.
2. Kelly JE, Harvey C. An assessment of the teeth of youths 12–17 years, DHEW Publication No (HRA) 77–1644. Washington, DC: National Center for Health Statistics, 1977.
3. McLain JB, Steedle JR, Vig PS. Face height and dental relationships in 1600 children: A survey. J Dent Res 1983;62:308.
4. McLain JB, Proffit WR. Oral health status in the United States: Prevalence of malocclusion. J Dent Educ 1985;49:386–396.
5. Brunelle JA, Bhat M, Lipton JA. Prevalence and distribution of selected occlusal characteristics in the US population, 1988–91. J Dent Res 1996;75:706–713.
6. Proffit WR, Fields HW, Moray LJ. Prevalence of malocclusion and orthodontic treatment need in the United States: Estimates from the N-HANES III survey. Int J Adult Orthod Orthogn Surg 1998;13:97–106.
7. Angle EH. Treatment of malocclusion of the teeth. Philadelphia: SS White, 1907.
8. Case CS. Principles of occlusion and dento-facial relations. Dent Items Interest 1905;27:489–527.
9. Wylie WL. The assessment of anteroposterior dysplasia. Angle Orthod 1947;17:97–109.
10. Wylie WL, Johnson EL. Rapid evaluation of facial dysplasia in the vertical plane. Angle Orthod 1952;22:165–181.
11. Fisk GV, Culbert MR, Granger RM, Hemrend B, Moyers RE. The morphology and physiology of distocclusion. Am J Orthod 1953;39:3–12.
12. Woodside DG. The present role of the general practitioner in orthodontics. Dent Clin North Am 1968:483–508.
13. Sassouni V. A classification of skeletal facial types. Am J Orthod 1969;55:109–123.
14. Sassouni V. The Class II syndrome: differential diagnosis and treatment. Angle Orthod 1970;40:334–41.
15. Moyers RE, Riolo ML, Guire KE, Wainright RL, Bookstein FL. Differential diagnosis of Class II malocclusions. Part 1. Facial types associated with Class II malocclusions. Am J Orthod 1980;78:477–494.
16. McNamara JA, Jr. Components of Class II malocclusion in children 8–10 years of age. Angle Orthod 1981;51:177–202.
17. Mastorakos WL. Dental and skeletal relationships in children age 12–14 with Class II malocclusion: a comparative study. St Louis: Unpublished Master's thesis, Department of Orthodontics, St Louis University, 1984.
18. Drelich RC. A cephalometric study of untreated Class II, division 1 malocclusion. Angle Orthod 1948;21.
19. Altemus LA. Cephalometric studies on the form of the human mandible. Angle Orthod 1955;25:120–137.
20. Rothstein TL. Facial morphology and growth from 10 to 14 years of age in children presenting Class II, division 1 malocclusion: a comparative roentgenographic cephalometric study. Am J Orthod 1971;60:619–620.
21. Riedel RA. The relation of maxillary structures to cranium in malocclusion and normal occlusion. Angle Orthod 1952;22:142–145.
22. Hunter WS. The vertical dimensions of the face and skeletodental retrognathism. Am J Orthod 1967;53:586–595.
23. Hitchcock HP. A cephalometric description of Class II, division 1 malocclusion. Am J Orthod 1973;63:414–423.
24. Renfroe EW. A study of the facial patterns associated with Class I, Class II division 2 malocclusions. Angle Orthod 1948;19:12–15.
25. Henry R. A classification of Class II, division 1 malocclusion. Angle Orthod 1957;27:83–92.
26. Harris JE, Kowalski CJ, Walker SJ. Intrafamilial dentofacial associations for Class II, division 1 probands. Am J Orthod 1975;67:563–570.
27. McNamara JA, Jr. A method of cephalometric evaluation. Am J Orthod 1984;86:449–469.
28. McNamara JA, Jr., Brust EW, Riolo ML. Soft tissue evaluation of individuals with an ideal occlusion and a well-balanced face. In: McNamara JA, Jr, ed. Esthetics and the treatment of facial form. Ann Arbor: Monograph 28, Craniofacial Growth Series, Center for Human Growth and Development, University of Michigan, 1993.
29. Ricketts RM. The influence of orthodontic treatment on facial growth and development. Angle Orthod 1960;30:103–133.
30. Baldridge JP. A study of the relation of the maxillary first permanent molar to the face in Class I and Class II malocclusions. Angle Orthod 1941;11:100–109.
31. Baldridge JP. Further studies of the relation of the maxillary first permanent molars to the face in Class I and Class II malocclusions. Angle Orthod 1950;20:3–10.
32. Elsasser WA, Wylie WL. The craniofacial morphology of mandibular retrusion. Am J Phys Anthrop 1943;6:461–473.
33. Elman ES. Cephalometric studies on the positional changes of the teeth (The relation of the lower six year molar to the mandible). Angle Orthod 1948;18:9-10.
34. Craig CE. The skeletal patterns characteristic of Class I and Class II, division 1 malocclusions, in *normalateralis*. Angle Orthod 1951;21:44–56.
35. Gilmore WA. Morphology of the adult mandible in Class II, division 1 malocclusion and in excellent occlusion. Angle Orthod 1950;20:137–146.
36. Adams JW. Cephalometric studies on the form of the human mandible. Angle Orthod 1948;18:8.
37. Steiner CC. Cephalometrics for you and me. Am J Orthod 1953;39:729–755.
38. McNamara JA, Jr, Ellis E. Cephalometric analysis of untreated adults with ideal facial and occlusal relationships. Int J Adult Orthod Orthogn Surg 1988;3:221–231.
39. Schudy F. Vertical growth versus anteroposterior growth as related to function and treatment. Angle Orthod 1964;34:75-93.
40. Schudy FF. The rotation of the mandible resulting from growth: its implications in orthodontic treatment. Angle Orthod 1965;35:36–50.
41. Sassouni V, Nanda SK. Analysis of dentofacial vertical proportions. Am J Orthod 1964;50:801–823.
42. Harvold EP. The activator in interceptive orthodontics. St. Louis: CV Mosby, 1974.

43. Tollaro I, Baccetti T, Franchi L, Tanasescu CD. Role of posterior transverse interarch discrepancy in Class II, division 1 malocclusion during the mixed dentition phase. Am J Orthod Dentofac Orthop 1996;110:417–422.
44. Baccetti T, Franchi L, McNamara JA, Jr., Tollaro I. Early dentofacial features of Class II Malocclusion: A longitudinal study from the deciduous through the mixed dentition. Am J Orthod Dentofac Orthop 1997;111:502–509.
45. Arya BS, Savara BS, Thomas DR. Prediction of first molar occlusion. Am J Orthod 1973;63:610–621.
46. Bishara SE, Hoppens BJ, Jakobsen JR, Kohout FJ. Changes in the molar relationship between the deciduous and permanent dentitions: a longitudinal study. Am J Orthod Dentofac Orthop 1988;93:19–28.
47. Berger EV. Personal communication, 1992.
48. Kloehn SJ. Analysis and treatment in mixed dentitions, a new approach. Am J Orthod 1953;39:56-65.
49. Graber TM. Extra-oral force—facts and fallacies. Am J Orthod 1955;41:490–505.
50. Poulton DR. The influence of extraoral traction. Am J Orthod 1967;53:8–18.
51. Watson WG. A computerized appraisal of the high-pull face-bow. Am J Orthod 1972;62:561–579.
52. Wieslander L. Early or late cervical traction therapy of Class II malocclusion in the mixed dentition. Am J Orthod 1975;67:432–439.
53. McNamara JA, Jr, Peterson JE, Jr, Alexander RG. Three-dimensional diagnosis and management of Class II malocclusion in the mixed dentition. Semin Orthod 1996;2:114–137.
54. Boecler PR, Riolo ML, Keeling SD, TenHave TR. Skeletal changes associated with extraoral appliance therapy: an evaluation of 200 consecutively treated cases. Angle Orthod 1989;59:263–270.
55. Hubbard GW, Nanda RS, Currier GF. A cephalometric evaluation of nonextraction cervical headgear treatment in Class II malocclusions. Angle Orthod 1994;64:359–70.
56. Tweed CH. Clinical orthodontics. St Louis: CV Mosby, 1966.
57. Dellinger EL. A preliminary study of anterior maxillary displacement. Am J Orthod 1973;63:509–516.
58. Pearson LE. Vertical control in treatment of patients having backward-rotational growth tendencies. Angle Orthod 1978;48:132–40.
59. Pearson LE. The management of vertical problems in growing patients. In: McNamara JA, Jr, ed. The enigma of the vertical dimension. Ann Arbor: Monograph 36, Craniofacial Growth Series, Center for Human Growth and Development, The University of Michigan, 2000.
60. Vaden JL, Dale JG, Klontz HA. The Tweed-Merrifield edgewise appliance: Philosophy, diagnosis, and treatment. In: Graber TM, Vanarsdall RL, Jr, eds. Orthodontics: Current principles and practices, third edition. St Louis: CV Mosby, 2000.
61. Haas AJ. Headgear therapy: The most efficient way to distalize molars. Semin Orthod 2000;6:79–90.
62. Interlandi S. Ortodontia: Basespara a iniciação. Sao Paulo: Artes Medicas, 1994.
63. Mossey PA, Hodgkins JF, Williams P. A safety adaptation to Interlandi headgear. Brit J Orthod 1991;18:131–133.
64. Bernstein L. The ACCO appliance. J Clin Orthod 1969;3:461–468.
65. Cetlin NM, Ten Hoeve A. Nonextraction treatment. J Clin Orthod 1983;17:396–413.
66. Gianelly AA. Bidimensional technique theory and practice. Central Islip: GAC International, 2000.
67. Dietz VS, Gianelly AA. Molar distalization with the acrylic cervical occipital appliance. Semin Orthod 2000;6:91–97.
68. Carano A, Testa M. The distal jet for upper molar distalization. J Clin Orthod 1996;30:374–380.
69. Bowman SJ. Modifications of the distal jet. J Clin Orthod 1998;32:549–556.
70. Bowman SJ. Combination Class II therapy. J Clin Orthod 1998;32:611–620.
71. Jones RD, White JM. Rapid Class II molar correction with an open-coil jig. J Clin Orthod 1992;26:661–664.
72. Scott MW. Molar distalization: More ammunition for your operatory. Clin Impressions 1996;5:16–21, 26–27.
73. Hilgers JJ. The pendulum appliance for Class II non-compliance therapy. J Clin Orthod 1992;26:706–14.
74. Hilgers JJ. The pendulum appliance . . . An update. Clin Impressions 1993:15–17.
75. Joseph AA, Butchart CJ. An evaluation of the pendulum distalizing appliance. Semin Orthod 2000;6:129–135.
76. Byloff FK, Darendeliler MA, Clar E, Darendeliler A. Distal molar movement using the pendulum appliance. Part 2: The effects of maxillary molar root uprighting bends. Angle Orthodontist 1997;67:261–270.
77. Haas AJ. Rapid expansion of the maxillary dental arch and nasal cavity by opening the mid-palatal suture. Angle Orthod 1961;31:73–90.
78. Tollaro I, Baccetti T, Bassarelli V, Franchi L. Class III malocclusion in the deciduous dentition: a morphological and correlation study. Eur J Orthod 1994;16:401–408.
79. Burk S. The express-Nance: further streamlining an old favorite. Clin Impressions 1998;7:14–15.
80. Ghosh J, Nanda RS. Evaluation of an intraoral maxillary molar distalization technique. Am J Orthod Dentofac Orthop 1996;110:639–646.
81. Byloff FK, Darendeliler MA. Distal molar movement using the pendulum appliance. Part 1: Clinical and radiological evaluation. Angle Orthod 1997;67:249–260.
82. Bussick TJ, McNamara JA, Jr. Dentoalveolar and skeletal changes associated with the pendulum appliance. Am J Orthod Dentofac Orthop 2000;117:333-343.
83. Gianelly AA, Bednar J, Dietz VS. Japanese NiTi coils used to move molars distally. Am J Orthod Dentofac Orthop 1991;99:564–6.
84. Bjerregaard J, Bundgaard AM, Melsen B. The effect of the mandibular lip bumper and maxillary bite plate on tooth movement, occlusion, and space conditions in the lower dental arch. Eur J Orthod 1983;84:147–155.
85. Nevant CT. The effects of lip-bumper therapy on deficient mandibular arch length. Dallas: Unpublished Master's thesis, Department of Orthodontics, Baylor University, 1989.
86. Pancherz H. Treatment of Class II malocclusions by jumping the bite with the Herbst appliance. A cephalometric investigation. Am J Orthod 1979;76:423–442.
87. Pancherz H. The Herbst appliance—Its biologic effects and clinical use. Am J Orthod 1985;87:1–20.
88. McNamara JA, Jr, Bookstein FL, Shaughnessy TG. Skeletal and dental changes following functional regula-

tor therapy on Class II patients. Am J Orthod 1985;88: 91–110.
89. McNamara JA, Jr, Howe RP, Dischinger TG. A comparison of the Herbst and Fränkel appliances in the treatment of Class II malocclusion. Am J Orthod Dentofac Orthop 1990;98:134–144.
90. Mills C, McCulloch K. Treatment effects of the twin block appliance: A cephalometric study. Am J Orthod 1998;114: 15–24.
91. Toth LR, McNamara JA, Jr. Treatment effects produced by the twin block appliance and the FR-2 appliance of Fränkel compared to an untreated Class II sample. Am J Orthod Dentofac Orthop 1999;116:597–609.
92. Pancherz H. The Herbst appliance. Seville: Editorial Aguiram, 1995.
93. Wieslander L. Long-term effect of treatment with the headgear-Herbst appliance in the early mixed dentition. Stability or relapse? Am J Orthod Dentofac Orthop 1993;104:319–329.
94. Fränkel R, Fränkel C. Orofacial orthopedics with the function regulator. Munich: S Karger, 1989.
95. Fränkel R. The practical meaning of the functional matrix in orthodontics. Trans Eur Orthod Soc 1969;45:207–219.
96. Fränkel R. Technik und Handhabung der Funktionsregler. Berlin: VEB Verlag Volk and Gesundheit, 1976.
97. Fränkel R. Biomechanical aspects of the form/function relationship in craniofacial morphogenesis: a clinician's approach. In: McNamara JA, Jr, Ribbens KA, Howe RP, eds. Clinical alteration of the growing face. Ann Arbor: Monograph 14, Craniofacial Growth Series, Center for Human Growth and Development, The University of Michigan, 1983.
98. Roux W. Entwicklungsmechanik der Organismen, Bd. I und II. Leipzig: W. Engelmann Verlag W, 1895.
99. McDougall PD, McNamara JA, Jr, Dierkes JM. Arch width development in Class II patients treated with the Fränkel appliance. Am J Orthod 1982;82:10–22.
100. Fränkel R. Guidance of eruption without extraction. Trans Europ Orthod Soc 1971;47:303–315.
101. Falck F. Kephalometrische Längsschnittuntersuchung über Behandlungsergebnisse der mandibulären Retrognathie mit Funktionsreglen im Vergleich zu einer Lontrollgruppe. Berlin: Med Dissertation, 1985.
102. Clark WJ. The twin block traction technique. Eur J Orthod 1982;4:129–138.
103. Clark WJ. The twin block technique. A functional orthopedic appliance system. Am J Orthod Dentofac Orthop 1988;93:1–18.
104. Clark WJ. The twin block technique. In: Graber TM, Rakosi T, Petrovic AG, eds. Dentofacial orthopedics with functional appliances. St. Louis: Mosby-Yearbook, 1997.
105. Clark WJ. Twin block functional therapy. London: Mosby-Wolfe, 1995.
106. McNamara JA, Jr. Biological basis and clinical management of the twin block appliance. Rev d'Orthopéd Dento Faciale 1998;32:55–81.
107. Barrer HG. Protecting the integrity of mandibular incisor position through keystoning procedure and spring retainer appliance. J Clin Orthod 1975;9:486–494.
108. Herbst E. Atlas und Grundriss der Zahnärztlichen Orthopädie. Munich: JF Lehmann Verlag, 1910.
109. Pancherz H. The effect of continuous bite jumping on the dentofacial complex: a follow-up study after Herbst appliance treatment of Class II malocclusions. Eur J Orthod 1981;3:49–60.
110. Pancherz H. Personal communication, 1998.
111. Goodman P, McKenna P. Modified Herbst appliance for the mixed dentition. J Clin Orthod 1985;19:811–814.
112. Dischinger TG. Edgewise bioprogressive Herbst appliance. J Clin Orthod 1989;23:608–617.
113. Smith JR. Matching the Herbst to the malocclusion. Clin Impressions 1998;7:6–12, 20–23.
114. Smith JR. Matching the Herbst to the malocclusion: Part II. Clin Impressions 1999;8:14–23.
115. Howe RP. The bonded Herbst appliance. J Clin Orthod 1982;16:663–667.
116. Howe RP, McNamara JA, Jr. Clinical management of the bonded Herbst appliance. J Clin Orthod 1983;17: 456–463.
117. McNamara JA, Jr. Fabrication of the acrylic splint Herbst appliance. Am J Orthod Dentofac Orthop 1988;94:10–18.
118. McNamara JA, Jr., Howe RP. Clinical management of the acrylic splint Herbst appliance. Am J Orthod Dentofac Orthop 1988;94:142–149.
119. Dischinger TG. Full-face orthopedics with one multifunctional appliance—no cooperation required. Clin Impressions 1998;72-7, 23-25.
120. Balters W. Die Technik und Übung der allgemeinen und speziellen Bionator-therapie. Quintessenz 1964;1:77.
121. Balters W. Eine Einführung in die Bionatorheilmethode. Ausgewählte, Schriften und Vorträge. Heidelberg: Druckerei Hölzel, 1973.
122. Eirew HL. The bionator. Br J Orthod 1981;8:33–36.
123. Altuna G, Niegel S. Bionators in Class II treatment. J Clin Orthod 1985;19:185–191.
124. Janson I. Bionator-Modifikationen in der kieferorthopädischen Therapie. Munich: Karl Hanser, 1987.
125. Rudzki-Janson I, Noachtar R. Functional appliance therapy with the bionator. Semin Orthod 1998;4:33–45.
126. Petrovic A, Stutzmann JJ, Oudet C. Control process in the postnatal growth of the condylar cartilage. In: McNamara JA, Jr, ed. Determinants of mandibular form and growth. Ann Arbor: Monograph 4, Craniofacial Growth Series, Center for Human Growth and Development, The University of Michigan, 1975.
127. Petrovic A, Stutzmann J, Lavergne J. Mechanism of craniofacial growth and modus operandi of functional appliances: a cell-level and cybernetic approach to orthodontic decision making. In: Carlson DS, ed. Craniofacial growth theory and orthodontic treatment. Ann Arbor: Monograph 23, Craniofacial Growth Series, Center for Human Growth and Development, the University of Michigan, 1990.
128. Nanda RS. The rates of growth of several facial components measured from serial cephalometric roentgenograms. Am J Orthod 1955;41:658–673.
129. Björk A. Variations in the growth pattern of the human mandible: Longitudinal radiographic study by the implant method. J Dent Res 1963;42:400–411.
130. Ekström C. Facial growth rate and its relation to somatic maturation in healthy children. Swed Dent J (Suppl) 1982;11:1–99.
131. Lewis AB, Garn SM. The relationship between tooth formation and other maturation factors. Angle Orthod 1985;30:70–77.

132. Hägg U, Pancherz H, Taranger J. Pubertal growth and orthodontic treatment. In: Carlson DS, Ribbens KA, eds. Craniofacial growth during adolescence. Ann Arbor: Monograph 20, Craniofacial Growth Series, Center for Human Growth and Development, The University of Michigan, 1987.
133. Hunter CJ. The correlation of facial growth with body height and skeletal maturation at adolescence. Angle Orthod 1966;36:44–54.
134. Greulich WW, Pyle SI. Radiographic atlas of skeletal development of the hand and wrist. Stanford: Stanford University Press, 1959.
135. Björk A, Helm S. Prediction of the age of maximum pubertal growth in body height. Angle Orthod 1967;37:134–143.
136. Taranger J, Hägg U. Timing and duration of adolescent growth. Acta Odontol Scand 1980;38:57–67.
137. Hellman M. The process of dentition and its effects on occlusion. Dent Cosmos 1923;65:1329–1344.
138. Lewis AB, Garn SM. The relationship between tooth formation and other maturation factors. Angle Orthod 1960;30:70–77.
139. Tanner JM. Growth at adolescence. Oxford: Blackwell Scientific Publications, 1962.
140. Lamparski DG. Skeletal age assessment utilizing cervical vertebrae. Unpublished Master's thesis, Pittsburgh: Department of Orthodontics University of Pittsburgh, 1972.
141. O'Reilly M, Yanniello GJ. Mandibular growth changes and maturation of cervical vertebrae—a longitudinal cephalometric study. Angle Orthod 1988;58:179–184.
142. Franchi L, Baccetti T. New emphasis on the role of mandibular skeletal maturity in dentofacial orthopedics. In: McNamara JA, Jr, ed. The enigma of the vertical dimension. Ann Arbor: Monograph 36, Craniofacial Growth Series, Center for Human Growth and Development, The University of Michigan, 2000.
143. Franchi L, Baccetti T, McNamara JA, Jr. Mandibular growth as related to cervical vertebral maturation and body height. Am J Orthod Dentofac Orthop 2000;118:335–340.
144. Baccetti T, Franchi L, Toth LR, McNamara JA, Jr. Treatment timing for twin block therapy. Am J Orthod Dentofac Orthop 2000;118:159-170.
145. Lavergne J, Gasson N. Operational definitions of mandibular morphogenetic and positional rotations. Scand J Dent Res 1977;85:185–192.
146. Hägg U, Pancherz H. Dentofacial orthopaedics in relation to chronological age, growth period and skeletal development. An analysis of 72 male patients with Class II division 1 malocclusion treated with the Herbst appliance. Eur J Orthod 1988;10:169–176.
147. Pancherz H. The nature of Class II relapse after Herbst appliance treatment: a cephalometric long-term investigation. Am J Orthod Dentofac Orthop 1991;100:220–233.

Chapter 6
CLASS III MALOCCLUSION

With Tiziano Baccetti and Lorenzo Franchi

One of the most perplexing malocclusions to diagnose and treat is Class III malocclusion, particularly in the mixed and late deciduous dentitions. This occlusal problem is identified easily, not only by dental specialists and generalists but also by the lay public. The appearance of a negative horizontal overlap of the incisors (Fig. 6-1) often stimulates a parent to seek orthodontic treatment for his or her child.

Class III malocclusion and anterior crossbite are common clinical problems, especially in patients of Asian ancestry. For example, Lew and co-workers[1] report that the prevalence of Class III malocclusion to be about 12% in a Chinese population. Although the prevalence of Angle Class III molar relationship in individuals of Japanese ancestry has not been studied in detail, estimates of the frequencies of anterior crossbite and edge-to-edge incisal relationships in Japanese populations range from 2.3% to 13% and 2.7% to 7.4% respectively.[2–4] If the frequency of occurrence of these two manifestations of Class III malocclusion are combined, a substantial percentage of the Japanese population have characteristics of Class III malocclusion.

A relatively high prevalence of Class III malocclusion has been observed in other ethnic groups as well (*e.g.*, 9.4% in Saudi Arabian orthodontic patients[5]). In comparison, Class III malocclusion is seen less frequently in persons of European ancestry, with estimates ranging from 0.8% and 4.2%.[6–16] Slightly higher prevalence (6%) has been noted in Swedish men by Ingervall and colleagues.[17]

The occurrence of anterior crossbite and edge-to-edge incisal relationship also has been evaluated in non-Asian populations. Kelly and colleagues[18,19] reported that the prevalence of anterior crossbite in samples of European-Americans and African-Americans was 0.8% and 0.6–1.2% respectively. An earlier study of individuals of predominantly North-European ancestry by Mills[10] found slightly higher values. Based on an evaluation of incisor relationship regardless of Angle classification, Mills reported that 3.3% of males and 2.9% of females had an anterior crossbite, while an additional 5.0% of males and 3.8% of females were characterized as having an edge-to-edge incisal relationship.

The most recent data available from the third National Health and Nutrition Examination Survey (NHANES III)[20,21] conducted in the United States indicate that the prevalence of anterior crossbite is 0.8% in whites, 2.0% in blacks, and 1.6% in Mexican-Americans (Table 6-1). Additionally, edge-to-edge incisal occlusion occurs in 4.1% of whites, 6.1% of blacks, and 6.7% of Mexican-Americans, with a slight increase in frequency in older subjects. Molar relationship was not measured in this national survey of 7,000 individuals.[22]

COMPONENTS OF CLASS III MALOCCLUSION

Similar to the discussion of Class II malocclusion in the previous chapter, Class III malocclusion does not encompass a single diagnostic entity. Even though the terms "mandibular prognathism" and "Angle Class III malocclusion" often are regarded as similar, if not syn-

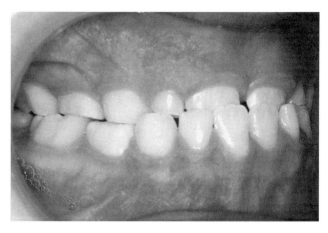

Figure 6-1. Intraoral view of a patient with a typical Class III malocclusion in the early mixed dentition.

onymous, in much of the dental literature, individuals possessing a Class III occlusal relationship may have various combinations of underlying skeletal and dental components.

We previously have described the components of Class III malocclusion in 144 Michigan children between the ages of 5 and 15 years.[23] Mandibular skeletal protrusion (commonly cited as a major skeletal aberration in individuals with Class III malocclusion) combined with a normal anteroposterior relationship of the maxilla was noted in less than 20% of the Michigan sample, a finding that was similar to the deciduous and mixed dentition samples of Dietrich[24] and the adult samples studied by Ellis and McNamara.[25] Maxillary skeletal retrusion and a normal sagittal relationship of the mandible was found in 25% of the individuals studied, an observation that agreed closely with similar investigations in adults by Sanborn,[26] Jacobson and co-workers,[12] and Ellis and McNamara[25] as well as the young patients studied by Dietrich.[24] A combination of maxillary skeletal retrusion and mandibular skeletal protrusion was found in approximately 22%. Thus, about 47% of the sample had a retrusive position of the maxilla and about 42% had some degree of mandibular prognathism. The remainder, about one-third of the Class III sample, had no anteroposterior skeletal imbalances.

Other areas within the faces of Class III individuals exhibited consistently significant differences from a comparison Class I sample,[27] including larger mandibular plane angles, larger gonial angles, longer mandibles, and compensations of the dentition, including maxillary dentoalveolar protrusion and mandibular dentoalveolar retrusion.[23] About 40% of the Michigan sample also had an increased lower anterior facial height compared to normal values.

Just as the prevalence of Class III malocclusion and anterior crossbite varies among racial and ethnic groups, so too do the components of these malocclusions. Masaki,[28] in a comparative study of native Japanese and of Americans of European ancestry, reported that maxillary skeletal retrusion occurred more often in Asians, whereas mandibular prognathism often is observed as a component of Class III malocclusion in individuals of European-American ancestry. Masaki reported that posterior cranial base length and facial height were significantly larger in Japanese children, whereas anterior cranial base length and facial depth were significantly larger in American children. The Japanese typically presented with a more retrusive facial profile and a longer lower anterior facial height than did the European-Americans. Masaki also noted that a backward rotation of the mandible in the Japanese appeared to be necessary to coordinate the occlusion relative to the small maxilla. He postulated further that maxillary skeletal retrusion with or without anterior crossbite may be more frequent in the Japanese; conversely, an orthognathic maxilla, combined with a larger cranial base, occurs more frequently in the European-American.

On average, a more retrusive profile and a relatively longer lower anterior facial height is observed even in Japanese with facial profiles and occlusions judged to be near-ideal by clinicians of the same ethnic group as the subjects selected. Miyajima and co-workers,[29] in a comparative study of Japanese and European-American individuals selected on the basis of having well-balanced faces and ideal occlusions, reported that the Japanese sample, in general, was smaller in anteroposterior facial

Table 6-1. Percentage of the US population with Class III-type occlusal discrepancies. Data derived from NHANES III.[21,22,87]

	All racial/ethnic groups (years)			All ages			
Overjet (mm)	8–11	12–17	18–50	White	Black	Mexican American	Total
0	2.2	4.6	4.8	4.1	6.1	6.7	4.5
−1 to −2	0.7	0.5	0.7	0.5	1.5	0.9	0.6
−3 to −4	0.0	0.6	0.2	0.2	0.4	0.4	0.3
>−4	0.0	0.0	0.1	0.1	0.1	0.3	0.2

dimensions and proportionately larger in vertical facial dimensions in comparison to the European-American sample. The facial axis angle was more vertical in Japanese subjects, indicating a more downward direction of facial development. Thus, it appears that diminished anteroposterior facial dimensions and elongated vertical facial dimensions in comparison to European-Americans is a common finding in Japanese subjects regardless of malocclusion type.

Thus, as with all malocclusions that are considered by Angle classification, the Class III malocclusion includes a variety of skeletal and dental components that may vary from our concept of normal or ideal. This observation is of significance when selecting from available treatment strategies.

GROWTH IN PATIENTS WITH CLASS III MALOCCLUSION

Because occlusal problems related to Class III malocclusion are recognized easily in the deciduous dentition, two major questions arise when approaching this type of malocclusion during early developmental stages. 1) Are Class III occlusal signs associated with a definite craniofacial skeletal disharmony? 2) How do subjects with Class III malocclusion grow? In other words, does Class III malocclusion worsen with growth? Both of these questions are extremely relevant to the issue of optimal treatment timing for Class III malocclusion.

The craniofacial skeletal pattern of children with Class III malocclusions is evident in the early deciduous dentition.[30] A sample of 69 Class III subjects was compared with 60 subjects exhibiting normal occlusion. The presence of both maxillary retrusion and mandibular protrusion was apparent as a result of the comparison. Additional skeletal characteristics in Class III subjects were represented by shorter anterior cranial base length and by larger mandibular ramus height and corpus length.

Information about the skeletal changes that occur in orthodontically untreated Class III subjects from childhood into adolescence is scarce. The longitudinal data that exist on untreated patients with Class III malocclusion or anterior crossbite or both[6,31–34] usually are very limited with regard to sample size and duration of longitudinal records, with most studies featuring few patients, short observation intervals, or a small number of cephalometric variables. All of the well-known "growth studies" of untreated individuals typically contain a preponderance of subjects with Class I and Class II malocclusion as well as normal occlusion.[27,35–37] Class III subjects are not well represented in these collections, even in proportion to their low occurrence in the general population. The few exceptions are represented by studies that analyze skeletal changes in subjects with mandibular prognathism of Asian ancestry.[38–40]

More recently, however, longitudinal data pertaining to growth changes in untreated Class III individuals of Caucasian ancestry have been gathered at the Department of Orthodontics of the University of Florence, Italy. The sample consists of two groups of untreated Class III subjects. The first group is comprised of 17 subjects observed longitudinally in the early mixed dentition (from 6.5 to 8.5 years of age) and the second group includes 15 subjects observed in the late mixed dentition (from 9.5 to 11.5 years of age). These samples of untreated Class III subjects have been used as control groups in investigations on the treatment effects of rapid maxillary expansion and facial mask therapy.[41,42]

The longitudinal analysis of skeletal modifications in these two groups of Class III subjects showed persistent evidence of both maxillary growth deficiency and mandibular growth excess throughout the mixed dentition. These changes were compared to samples of subjects with normal occlusion derived from *The University of Michigan Growth Study*.[35] The mean annualized growth increment for the maxilla (Ptm-A) was 0.8 mm in Class III subjects and 1.1 mm in normal subjects during the early mixed dentition. A similar deficiency in maxillary growth was found in the Class III group during the late mixed dentition (1.1 mm compared with 1.4 mm in normal subjects). The annual mandibular growth increments (Co-Gn) in Class III subjects were almost two times greater than those assessed in subjects with normal occlusion at both observation intervals (4.5 mm *vs.* 2.6 mm in the early mixed dentition, and 4.4 mm *vs.* 2.8 mm in the late mixed dentition).

In summary, the answers to the initial questions regarding growth in Class III malocclusion indicate that: 1) Class III skeletal imbalance concurrent with either an edge-to-edge incisor relationship or an anterior crossbite is established early (in the deciduous dentition); 2) the skeletal components of the malocclusion tend to worsen along with subsequent growth. Both these considerations significantly affect clinical decision-making in favor of early intervention.

THE SELECTION OF TREATMENT STRATEGIES

When a patient first is diagnosed as having a Class III malocclusion in the permanent dentition, treatment options are limited, particularly if there is a strong skeletal component to the Class III occlusal relationship. Such treatment usually includes comprehensive orthodontic therapy, either combined with extraction and/or orthognathic surgery. The orthognathic surgical procedure is designed to address the imbalance of the skeletal component (*e.g.*, mandibular setback in patients with mandibular prognathism, LeFort I advancement in instances of maxillary skeletal retrusion). In patients who are expected to have excessive skeletal growth in the future, the surgical procedure usually is deferred until the end of the active growth period.

In the diagnosis and treatment planning of patients who present with a Class III malocclusion in the late deciduous or the mixed dentition, several treatment options are available for use in specific types of Class III malocclusion. For example, the FR-3 appliance of Fränkel[43,44] has been recommended for the treatment of patients characterized by maxillary skeletal retrusion. On the other hand, the orthopedic chin cup[45-49] has been used in patients with mandibular prognathism. More recently, the orthopedic facial mask of Delaire[50-52] and Petit[53-55] has been used. Each of these treatments has been shown to produce favorable treatment effects in Class III patients, although there are substantial differences with regard to the speed of correction and in the regions of the craniofacial complex that are affected.

When selecting the appropriate regimen, a basic axiom of orthodontic treatment is that the treatment should address the specific nature of the skeletal and/or dentoalveolar imbalance. As discussed in the previous chapter on Class II malocclusion, extraoral traction is recommended for the treatment of maxillary prognathism, whereas the correction of mandibular skeletal retrusion may be approached using some type of functional jaw orthopedic appliance. An exception to this rule, however, may be the treatment of the developing Class III malocclusion.

Of the three treatment strategies mentioned above, the orthopedic facial mask may have the widest application and produces the most dramatic results in the shortest period. Thus, the orthopedic facial mask is our customary appliance of choice for most Class III patients seen in the early mixed dentition or late deciduous dentition, with the FR-3 appliance of Fränkel typically used effectively as a retention appliance in patients with initially severe skeletal and neuromuscular imbalances.

The Orthopedic Facial Mask

When we first heard Petit talk about his use of the orthopedic facial mask, we were critical of what appeared to be a lack of diagnostic criteria in selecting young patients for facial mask therapy. He was somewhat vague about the type of patients in whom this therapy was to be used, indicating that most young Class III patients were candidates for facial mask treatment.

After using this appliance for over two decades, we have found that, in fact, the facial mask is effective in most developing Class III patients, because the appliance system affects virtually all areas contributing to a Class III malocclusion (*e.g.*, maxillary skeletal retrusion, mandibular prognathism, decreased lower anterior facial height). Thus, this treatment protocol can be applied to most developing Class III patients regardless of the specific etiology.

The use of the facial mask in the mixed dentition is in marked contrast to the treatment of Class III malocclusion in surgical patients in whom surgical intervention must be targeted to the area of the craniofacial complex in which there is a deficiency or excess. In facial mask therapy, because the intervention is accomplished at an early age, the treatment effects produced by the facial mask ultimately are incorporated into the future craniofacial growth that occurs over a long period. Petit[54] describes such patients as having "prognathic syndrome" in which the underlying skeletal relationships may be out of balance in all three planes of space.

The orthopedic facial mask system has three basic components: the facial mask, a bonded maxillary splint, and elastics. The facial mask (Fig. 6-2) is an extraoral device that has been modified by Petit[54] and now is available commercially (Great Lakes Orthodontic Products, Tonawanda NY). In essence, the facial mask is composed of a forehead pad and a chin pad that are connected with a heavy steel support rod. To this support rod is connected a crossbow to which are attached elastics to produce a forward and downward traction on the maxilla. The position of the pads and the crossbow can be adjusted simply by loosening and tightening setscrews within each part of the appliance.

Although Petit[54] has recommended a number of different intraoral devices, both fixed and removable, to which the elastics can be anchored, it is our strong preference to use a bonded rapid maxillary palatal expansion appliance (Fig. 6-3) that is similar in design to the acrylic splint expander discussed previously in Chapter 4. The major modification in the appliance is the addition of facial mask hooks in the region of the maxillary deciduous first molars. In patients in whom treatment is started before the eruption of the maxillary first molars, the appliance is designed to incorporate the deciduous first and second molars as well as the deciduous canines.

The treatment effects produced by this type of appli-

TREATMENT OF CLASS III MALOCCLUSION

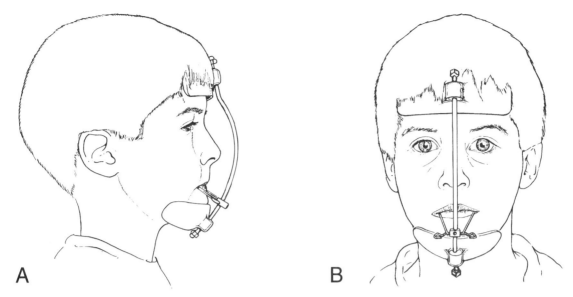

Figure 6-2. The orthopedic facial mask of Petit. *A*, Lateral view. *B*, Frontal view.

ance include a forward movement of the maxilla and maxillary dentition, a downward and backward rotation of the mandible, and a lingual tipping of the mandibular incisors.[54,56–58] In patients with a "pseudo-Class III" malocclusion, any discrepancy between centric occlusion and centric relation is eliminated as soon as the patient wears the appliance.

Once the decision has been made to use an orthopedic facial mask, the first step of the appliance therapy is the fabrication and bonding of the maxillary splint. The splint is activated once-per-day until the desired increase in transverse width has been achieved. In patients in whom no increase in transverse dimension is desired, the appliance still is activated for 8 to 10 days to disrupt the maxillary sutural system* and to promote maxillary protraction.[59]

As mentioned in detail in Chapter 4, spontaneous correction of Class III malocclusion occasionally occurs when the patient undergoes orthopedic expansion of the maxilla. This type of response usually is observed within the first few weeks or months of active expansion and may be due to a slight forward movement of the maxilla, a response that has been observed both clinically[66–68] and experimentally.[69] Thus, the clinician should monitor the sagittal relationship of the occlusion closely to determine if a spontaneous improvement occurs. This positive response typically occurs in patients with reasonably well-balanced faces and mild to moderate malocclusions. If such a response is observed, the facial mask may not be needed, or the hours per day of facial mask wear may be reduced (*e.g.*, nights only.)

If facial mask treatment is indicated, the facial mask is fitted to the requirements of the facial morphology of the patient (see Chapter 22 for the specifics of the clinical management of this appliance). Elastics of increasing force are used during the break-in period until a heavy orthopedic force is delivered to the maxillary complex. Normally, the facial mask is worn on a full-time basis (about 20 hours per day) for 4–6 months, and then it can be worn on a nighttime only basis for an additional period. Less than full-time wear (*e.g.*, 12–14 hours per day) by necessity results in a longer treatment time. It usually is unwise to have the splint remain bonded in position for more than 9–12 months due to the potential risk of leakage and subsequent decalcification.

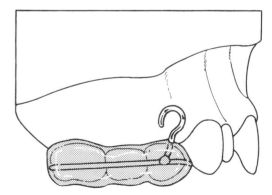

Figure 6-3. The bonded maxillary acrylic splint (lateral view). The hooks for the elastics usually are placed adjacent to the maxillary deciduous first molars.

---

*It should be noted, however, that in spite of intuitive logic, the clinical studies[58,60–65] conducted to date have not shown a superiority of this method of attachment over other methods of intraoral attachment, *e.g.*, fixed appliances, removable plates.

The ideal stage of dental development during which to begin facial mask therapy is at the time of eruption of the maxillary permanent central incisors. Usually the mandibular incisors already have erupted into occlusion. The achievement of a positive horizontal and vertical overlap of the incisors during treatment is essential in providing an environment that will help maintain the achieved anteroposterior correction of the original Class III malocclusion.

After the facial mask and rapid maxillary expansion appliance are removed, the patient can be retained using one of a number of appliances, including a simple maintenance plate, an FR-3 appliance of Fränkel, or a chin cup. Because facial mask treatment usually is begun in the early mixed dentition, a substantial period may elapse before the final phase of fixed appliance treatment can be initiated.

The selection of the orthopedic facial mask as the protocol of choice does not rule out the use of the FR-3 appliance of Fränkel or the orthopedic chin cup. The FR-3 can be used as a primary treatment appliance as well, especially in instances in which the patient declines to wear the facial mask as instructed (*e.g.*, to school). The FR-3 also can be selected as a retention appliance following initial correction of the Class III malocclusion.

The orthopedic chin cup can be used as an active appliance in patients with mandibular prognathism or with vertical excess or deficiencies, depending on the direction of pull of the appliance. The chin cup also can serve as a retention appliance following orthopedic facial mask wear.

The FR-3 Appliance of Fränkel

A removable appliance that has been used effectively in the treatment of Class III malocclusion is the FR-3 appliance of Fränkel.[43,44,70,71] Of all the Fränkel appliances, the FR-3 appliance (Figs. 6-4 and 6-5) is the easiest to manage clinically, because there is no change produced in the maxillomandibular relationship due to a forward positioning of the mandible, as occurs with the FR-2 appliance. Fränkel has stressed that the FR-3 appliance can be used in Class III patients of all levels of severity, including patients with severe skeletal and neuromuscular imbalances.[44,72]

As with all Fränkel appliances, the base of operation of the FR-3 appliance is the maxillary and mandibular vestibule. The appliance is designed to restrict the forces of the associated soft tissue on the maxillary complex (Fig. 6-5), transmitting these forces through the appliance to the mandible. Interestingly, the treatment effects produced by the FR-3 appliance have

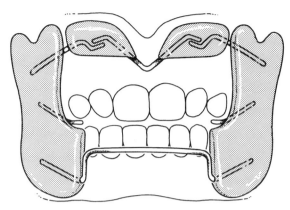

Figure 6-4. Frontal view of the FR-3 appliance of Fränkel. The vestibular shields and the upper labial pads shield the dentition from the forces of the associated musculature, producing mild expansion of the dental arches during treatment.

been shown to be similar to those produced by the orthopedic facial mask. These effects include the relative forward movement the maxilla as well as the maxillary dentition, a downward and backward redirection of mandibular growth, and some lingual tipping of the mandibular incisors.[44,57,70,73–75]

A major difference between the FR-3 appliance and the orthopedic facial mask is in the duration of treatment. In a routine Class III patient, the orthopedic facial mask may produce a correction of the malocclusion within a six-month period. Normally, 12–24 months are necessary to produce a similar response with the FR-3 appliance. It is obvious, however, that the FR-3 appliance has much more of an effect on the associated soft

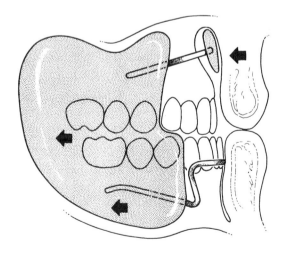

Figure 6-5. Mechanism of action of the FR-3 appliance of Fränkel (sagittal view). The vestibular shields and the maxillary labial pads shield the maxilla from the forces of the surrounding soft tissue. Because the lower portions of the vestibular shields contact mandibular hard and soft tissues, these forces are transmitted to the mandible.

tissue, particularly on any existing hyperactivity in the muscles associated with the maxilla, than does the facial mask. If a significant neuromuscular imbalance exists, the FR-3 is the appliance of choice.

The FR-3 appliance routinely is worn for about 20 hours per day, with the patient removing the appliance only for meals and contact sports. In contrast to the facial mask, which is obvious when it is worn, the FR-3 is less conspicuous, with the soft tissue of the patient's face adapting readily to the FR-3 appliance. In fact, in some instances in which significant maxillary skeletal retrusion exists, the overall soft tissue appearance of the patient actually may improve when wearing the appliance.

The Orthopedic Chin Cup

The chin cup (Fig. 6-6) is a relatively old orthopedic appliance that has been studied extensively in the orthodontic literature.[45–49,76–80] Much of the research has been conducted using Asian populations, due to the higher incidence of Class III malocclusion in those groups. Chin cups can be divided into two types, based on the direction of pull: occipital-pull and vertical-pull. The latter type of chin cup will be discussed in Chapter 8, when the treatment of the vertical dimension is considered.

The occipital-pull chin cup (Figs. 6-6 and 6-7) is the more frequently used type of chincup treatment for Class III malocclusion. This chin cup is indicated in instances of mild to moderate mandibular prognathism and is best initiated during the late deciduous or early mixed dentition.

Success is greatest in those patients who can bring their incisors close to an edge-to-edge position when in centric relation and in whom an increase in lower anterior facial height is not desired. The upward and backward pull of the chin cup (Fig. 6-7A) restricts both the forward and downward development of the mandibular face, at least in the short-term.

This treatment also can be used in patients with mandibular prognathism and a short lower face. If the pull of the chin cup is directed below the condyle (Fig. 6-7B), the force of the appliance may lead to a downward and backward rotation of the mandible.

The occipital-pull chin cup also is indicated in patients who have normally positioned or slightly protrusive mandibular incisors. Because the chin cup generates some force against the soft tissue in the chin region, some backward tipping of the mandibular incisors often is observed.

There have been a number of clinical studies that have evaluated the treatment effects produced by chin cup therapy.[45,47–49,76,77,80–85] These studies have shown

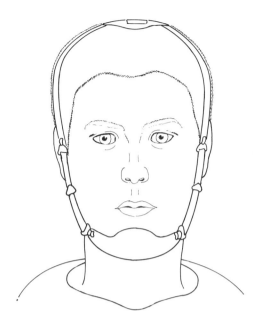

Figure 6-6. Frontal view of the occipital-pull chin cup made from soft fabric cup. The chin cup is connected to the headgear by an adjustable elastic strap.

treatment effects that are somewhat distinct from those discussed earlier regarding the orthopedic facial mask and the FR-3 of Fränkel.

One of the substantive concerns, particularly in the treatment of the patient with mandibular prognathism, is whether the growth of the mandible can be retarded during treatment. Sakamoto and co-workers[48] and Wendell and co-workers[82] have noted decreases in mandibular growth during treatment. Wendell and associates,[82] when examining a group of Class III patients treated in the mixed dentition, noted that mandibular length increases for the treated group were 60–68% of the control group. Mitani and Fukazawa[83] noted no differences in mandibular length in Class III patients who began treatment during the adolescent growth period. These findings support the observations of T.M. Graber,[86] Sakamoto,[81] and Sugawara and co-workers[49] who advocate the use of the occipital-pull chin cup as early as is practical. There is little evidence to date, however, that supports the concept that the ultimate length of the mandible is influenced significantly by chin cup therapy.

Another variation in treatment effect produced by the occipital-pull chin cup is the control of the vertical dimension. L.W. Graber[47] reported that, in his sample of young Class III patients, the predominantly horizontal mandibular growth pattern was redirected more vertically, indicating that the orthopedic chin cup can produce an increase in lower anterior facial height. On the other hand, Wendell and co-workers[82] report no in-

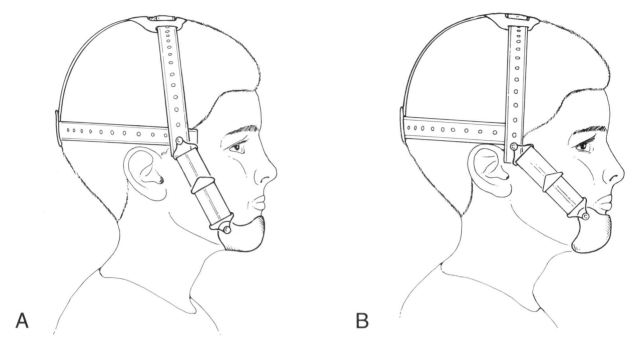

Figure 6-7. Lateral views of the occipital-pull chin cup. The chin cup is connected to the headgear by an adjustable elastic strap (Orthoband Corp., Barnhart MO). *A*, The direction of force is oriented vertically. *B*, The direction of force is oriented through the mandibular condyle.

crease in vertical vector of mandibular growth in comparison to controls.

Routine protocol for the use of the occipital-pull chin cup is as follows: The chin cup itself can be made from either a soft flexible material (Figs. 6-6 and 6-7) or from a hard acrylic material (Figs. 6-8) that either is available commercially or can be made from acrylic individually for each patient. The advantage of the soft cup is that it is relatively comfortable for the patient to wear. Soft chin cups, however, may cause more lingual tipping of the mandibular incisors than do hard cups.

The force on the chin cup is generated through traction placed against the headcap. An adjustable elastic strap (Fig. 6-6 and 6-7) can be used to connect the chin cup to the headcap. Elastics also can be used to connect the chin cup to an Interlandi-type headgear (Nola Orthodontic Specialties, Hilton Head SC). With the latter type of headgear, the direction of the elastics can be altered according to the desired direction of force application (Fig. 6-8).

At the time of appliance delivery, a force of 150–300 grams per side is used initially. Over the next two months, the force level is increased to 450–700 grams per side (16–24 ounces per side) if the force is directed through the condyle and slightly less if the force is directed below the condyle. The patient is instructed to wear the chin cup 14 hours per day (including sleep) with an acceptable range of wear being 10–16 hours per day. After the correction of a preexisting anterior cross-bite has been accomplished, the patient wears the appliance during the night only as a retention appliance.

Both occipital-pull and vertical-pull chin cups presumably create pressure on the temporomandibular joint region. Although this type of therapy has been used successfully for many decades, the increased sensitivity of the orthodontic specialist toward the diagnosis and treatment of temporomandibular joint problems should lead the clinician to monitor chin cup patients on an ongoing basis for signs and symptoms of TM disorders. If any are noted, the use of the chin cup should be discontinued immediately.

CONCLUDING REMARKS

This chapter has provided an overview of three different treatment modalities that can be used in the correction of Class III malocclusion. Both the facial mask and the FR-3 of Fränkel are described in detail in subsequent chapters.

It is our recommendation that the most useful of the three treatment modalities is the orthopedic facial mask worn with a bonded maxillary splint. This type of appliance produces treatment effects in both skeletal and dentoalveolar aspects of the craniofacial complex. In a young patient, the resolution of the underlying Class III relationship occurs relatively quickly (4–9 months). Then the mask can be worn for a few additional months

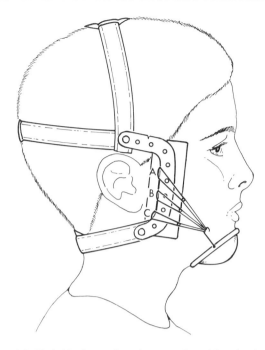

Figure 6-8. Variable force directions produced by elastics (A, B, C) attached from the Interlandi-type headgear to a hard chin cup.

as a retainer at night before the bonded maxillary splint is removed. Usually, a removable palatal plate to stabilize the correction is recommended, particularly if a positive horizontal and vertical overlap of the incisors has been created and is to be maintained.

The FR-3 appliance of Fränkel also is useful in mixed-dentition patients in the treatment of Class III malocclusion. This treatment regimen makes most biological sense, as the primary focus of this therapy is on the soft tissue, particularly the musculature, that may in part have been the etiology of the Class III relationship. The FR-3 is less intrusive to the everyday life of the patient but may take two or three times as much treatment time to complete the initial correction of the malocclusion. The FR-3 appliance also can be used effectively as a retention appliance following orthopedic facial mask or chin cup therapy, especially in those patients with persistent neuromuscular imbalances or who are expected to exhibit unfavorable subsequent patterns of craniofacial growth.

The orthopedic chin cup also can be used in patients with Class III malocclusion. In contrast to both the FR-3 appliance and the orthopedic facial mask, the chin cup is better suited to those patients in whom increases in lower facial height are not desirable and in patients who exhibit true mandibular prognathism. The correction of the malocclusion may be relatively rapid, depending on the force level used, but long-term chin cup wear usually is indicated.

Our experience in treating Class III malocclusion in the mixed dentition during the last thirty years has led to some interesting observations. Most importantly is that perhaps 50% of the patients who undergo any type of early Class III intervention will need another phase of treatment prior to the final phase of fixed appliance therapy. This may mean that chin cup wear is resumed or that another phase of rapid palatal expansion, with or without facial mask therapy, may be indicated.

The long-term stability of early Class III treatment is difficult to predict. In most instances, such intervention is successful, with a satisfactory occlusion attained. Since mandibular growth exceeds maxillary growth during adolescence, however, early Class III correction occasionally may be lost during the teenage years. The patient and parents should be advised of the possibility of surgical correction at the onset of interceptive treatment. The wise clinician never makes guarantees regarding the treatment of Class III malocclusion, because the outcome of the treatment of any individual Class III patient is very difficult to estimate.

REFERENCES CITED

1. Lew KKK, Foong WC, Loh E. Malocclusion status in Singapore school children. Cited in: Lew KKK, Foong WC. Horizontal skeletal typing in an ethnic Chinese population with true Class III malocclusion. Brit J Orthod 1993; 20:19–23.
2. Endo T. An epidemiological study of reversed occlusion in children 6-14 years old. J Jpn Orthod Soc 1971;30:73–77.
3. Susami R, Asai Y, Hirose K, Hosoi T, Hayashi I, Takimoto T. The prevalence of malocclusion in Japanese school children [in Japanese]. J Jpn Orthod Soc 1972;31:319–324.
4. Kitai N, Takada K, Yasada Y, Adachi S, Sakuda M. School health data base and its application [in Japanese]. J Kin-To Orthod Soc 1989;24:33–38.
5. Toms AP. Class III malocclusion: a cephalometric study of Saudi Arabians. Br J Orthod 1989;16:201–206.
6. Björk A. Some biological aspects of prognathism and occlusion of teeth. Acta Odontol Scand 1950;9:1–40.
7. Krogman W. The problem of timing of facial growth with special reference to the period of the changing dentition. Am J Orthod 1951;37:253–276.
8. Goose DH, Thompson DG, Winter FC. Malocclusion of the school children of the West Midlands (England). Brit Dent J 1957;102:174–178.
9. Ast DB, Carlos JP, Cons NC. The prevalence of malocclusion among senior high school students in upstate New York. Am J Orthod 1965;51:437–445.
10. Mills LF. Epidemiologic studies of occlusion. IV: The prevalence of malocclusion in a population of 1,455 school children. J Dent Res 1966;45:332–336.
11. Thilander B, Myrberg N. The prevalence of malocclusion in Swedish school children. Scand J Dent Res 1973;81: 12–20.

12. Jacobson A, Evans WG, Preston CB, Sadowsky PL. Mandibular prognathism. Am J Orthod 1974;66:140–171.
13. Foster TD, Day AJ. A survey of malocclusion and the need for orthodontic treatment in a Shropshire school population. Br J Orthod 1974;1:73–8.
14. Irie M, Nakamura S. Diagnosis and treatment to reversed occlusion cases [In Japanese]. Tokyo: Shorin, 1975.
15. Hannuksela A. The prevalence of malocclusion and the need for orthodontic treatment in 9-year-old Finnish schoolchildren. Proc Finn Dent Soc 1977;73:21–26.
16. Mohlin B. Need and demand for orthodontic treatment in a group of women in Sweden. Eur J Orthod 1982;4:231–242.
17. Ingervall B, Mohlin B, Thilander B. Prevalence and awareness of malocclusion in Swedish men. Comm Dent Oral Epid 1979;6:308–314.
18. Kelly JE, Sanchez M, Van Kirk LE. An assessment of the occlusion of the teeth of children. DHEW Publication No (HRA) 74-1612. Washington DC: National Center for Health Statistics, 1973.
19. Kelly JE, Harvey C. An assessment of the teeth of youths 12–17 years, DHEW Publication No (HRA) 77-1644. Washington DC: National Center for Health Statistics, 1977.
20. Brunelle JA, Bhat M, Lipton JA. Prevalence and distribution of selected occlusal characteristics in the US population, 1988–91. J Dent Res 1996;75:706–713.
21. Proffit WR, Fields HW, Moray LJ. Prevalence of malocclusion and orthodontic treatment need in the United States: Estimates from the N-HANES III survey. Int J Adult Orthod Orthogn Surg 1998;13:97–106.
22. Ezzati TM, Massey JT, Waksberg J, Chu A, Maurer KR. Sample design: Third National Health and Nutrition Examination Survey. Vital Health Stat 1992;2:1–35.
23. Guyer EC, Ellis E, McNamara JA, Jr, Behrents RG. Components of Class III malocclusion in juveniles and adolescents. Angle Orthod 1986;56:7–30.
24. Dietrich UC. Morphological variability of skeletal Class III relationships as revealed by cephalometric analysis. Trans Eur Ortho Soc 1970:131–140.
25. Ellis E, McNamara JA, Jr. Components of adult Class III malocclusion. J Oral Maxillofac Surg 1984;42:295–305.
26. Sanborn RT. Differences between the facial skeletal patterns of Class III malocclusion and normal occlusion. Angle Orthod. 1955;25:208–222.
27. Broadbent BH, Sr., Broadbent BH, Jr., Golden WH. Bolton standards of dentofacial developmental growth. St. Louis: CV Mosby, 1975.
28. Masaki F. Longitudinal study of morphological differences in the cranial base and facial structure between Japanese and American white [in Japanese]. J Jpn Orthod Soc 1980;39:436–456.
29. Miyajima K, McNamara JA, Jr, Kimura T, Murata S, Iizuka T. Craniofacial structure of Japanese and European-American adults with normal occlusions and well-balanced faces. Am J Orthod Dentofac Orthop 1996;110:431–438.
30. Tollaro I, Baccetti T, Bassarelli V, Franchi L. Class III malocclusion in the deciduous dentition: a morphological and correlation study. Eur J Orthod 1994;16:401–408.
31. Hopkins GB. A roentgenographic cephalometric analysis of treatment and growth changes in a series of cases of mesioclusion. Dent Pract 1963;13:394–410.
32. Love RJ, Murray JM, Mamandras AH. Facial growth in males 16 to 20 years of age. Am J Orthod Dentofac Orthop 1990;97:200–206.
33. Vasudevan SS. A cephalometric evaluation of maxillary changes during and after maxillary protraction therapy. Columbus: Unpublished Master's thesis, Department of Orthodontics, Ohio State Univ, 1994.
34. Ngan P, Hagg U, Yiu C, Merwin D, Wei SH. Treatment response to maxillary expansion and protraction. Eur J Orthod 1996;18:151–68.
35. Riolo ML, Moyers RE, McNamara JA, Jr, Hunter WS. An atlas of craniofacial growth: Cephalometric standards from The University School Growth Study, The University of Michigan. Ann Arbor: Monograph 2, Craniofacial Growth Series, Center for Human Growth and Development, The University of Michigan, 1974.
36. Prahl-Andersen BP, Kowalski CJ, Heydendael PHJM. A mixed-longitudinal interdisciplinary study of growth and development. New York: Academic Press, 1979.
37. Bishara SE, Jakobsen JR. Longitudinal changes in three normal facial types. Am J Orthod 1985;88:466–502.
38. Mitani H. Prepubertal growth of mandibular prognathism. Am J Orthod 1981;80:546–53.
39. Mitani H, Sato K, Sugawara J. Growth of mandibular prognathism after pubertal growth peak. Am J Orthod Dentofac Orthop 1993;104:330–6.
40. Miyajima K, McNamara JA, Jr, Kimura T, Murata S, Iizuka T. An estimation of craniofacial growth in the untreated Class III female with anterior crossbite. Am J Orthod Dentofac Orthop 1997;112:425–434.
41. Baccetti T, McGill JS, Franchi L, McNamara JA, Jr, Tollaro I. Skeletal effects of early treatment of Class III malocclusion with maxillary expansion and face-mask therapy. Am J Orthod Dentofac Orthop 1998;113:333–343.
42. Franchi L, Baccetti T, McNamara JA, Jr. Shape-coordinate analysis of skeletal changes induced by rapid maxillary expansion and facial mask therapy. Am J Orthod Dentofac Orthop 1998;114:418–442.
43. Fränkel R. Technik und Handhabung der Funktionsregler. Berlin: VEB Verlag Volk and Gesundheit, 1976.
44. Fränkel R, Fränkel C. Orofacial orthopedics with the function regulator. Munich: S Karger, 1989.
45. Thilander B. Treatment of Angle Class III malocclusion with chin cap. Trans Eur Orthod Soc 1963;39:384–398.
46. Graber TM, Chung DD, Aoba JT. Dentofacial orthopedics versus orthodontics. J Am Dent Assoc 1967;75: 1145–66.
47. Graber LW. Chin cup therapy for mandibular prognathism. Am J Orthod 1977;72:23–41.
48. Sakamoto T, Iwase I, Uka A, Nakamura S. A roentgenocephalometric study of skeletal changes during and after chin cup treatment. Am J Orthod 1984;85:341–350.
49. Sugawara J, Asano T, Endo N, Mitani H. Long-term effects of chincap therapy on skeletal profile in mandibular prognathism. Am J Orthod Dentofac Orthop 1990;98: 127–133.
50. Delaire J. Confection du masque orthopedique. Rev Stomat Paris 1971;72:579–584.
51. Delaire J. L'articulation fronto-maxillaire: Bases theoretiques et principes generaux d'application de forces

51. extra-orales postero-anterieures sur masque orthopedique. Rev Stomat Paris 1976;77:921–930.
52. Delaire J, Verson P, Lumineau JP, Ghega-Negrea A, Talmant J, Boisson M. Quelques resultats des tractions extra-orales a appui fronto-mentonnier dans le traitement orthopedique des maloformations maxillo mandibulaires de Class III et des sequelles osseuses des fente labio-maxillaires. Rev Stomat Paris 1972;73:633–642.
53. Petit HP. Syndromes prognathiques: schemas de traitement "global" autour de masques faciaux. Rev Orthop Dento Faciale 1982;16:381–411.
54. Petit HP. Adaptation following accelerated facial mask therapy. In: McNamara JA, Jr, Ribbens KA, Howe RP, eds. Clinical alterations of the growing face. Ann Arbor: Monograph 14, Craniofacial Growth Series, Center for Human Growth and Development, The University of Michigan, 1983.
55. Petit H. Normalisation morphogenetique, apport de l'orthopadie. Orthod Fr 1991;62:549–57.
56. McNamara JA, Jr. An orthopedic approach to the treatment of Class III malocclusion in young patients. J Clin Orthod 1987;21:598–608.
57. Ulgen M, Firatli S. The effects of Fränkel's function regulator on the Class III malocclusion. Am J Orthod Dentofac Orthop 1994;105:561–567.
58. McGill JS, McNamara JA, Jr. Treatment and post-treatment effects of rapid maxillary expansion and facial mask therapy. In: McNamara JA, Jr, ed. Growth modification: What works, what doesn't and why. Ann Arbor: Monograph 36, Craniofacial Growth Series, Center for Human Growth and Development, University of Michigan, 1999.
59. Haas AJ. The treatment of maxillary deficiency by opening the mid-palatal suture. Angle Orthod 1965;65:200–217.
60. Baik HS. Clinical results of the maxillary protraction in Korean children. Am J Orthod Dentofac Orthop 1995;108:583–592.
61. Shanker S, Ngan P, Wade D, Beck M, Yiu C, Hagg U, Wei SH. Cephalometric A point changes during and after maxillary protraction and expansion. Am J Orthod Dentofac Orthop 1996;110:423–430.
62. Ngan P, Hagg U, Yiu C, Wei H. Treatment response and long-term dentofacial adaptations to maxillary expansion and protraction. Sem Orthod 1997;3:255–264.
63. Williams MD, Sarver DM, Sadowsky PL, Bradley E. Combined rapid maxillary expansion and protraction facemask in the treatment of Class III malocclusion in growing children: a prospective study. Semin Orthod 1997;3:265–274.
64. Ngan P, Yiu C, Hu A, Hägg U, Wei SH, Gunel E. Cephalometric and occlusal changes following maxillary expansion and protraction. Eur J Orthod 1998;20:237–254.
65. Kapust AJ, Sinclair PM, Turley PK. Cephalometric effects of face mask/expansion therapy in Class III children: a comparison of three age groups. Am J Orthod Dentofac Orthop 1998;113:204–212.
66. Haas AJ. Rapid expansion of the maxillary dental arch and nasal cavity by opening the mid-palatal suture. 1961;31:73–90.
67. Haas AJ. Palatal expansion: just the beginning of dentofacial orthopedics. Am J Orthod 1970;57:219–255.
68. Haas AJ. Rapid palatal expansion: A recommended prerequisite to Class III treatment. Trans Eur Orthod Soc 1973:311–318.
69. Dellinger EL. A preliminary study of anterior maxillary displacement. Am J Orthod 1973;63:509–16.
70. Fränkel R. Maxillary retrusion in Class III and treatment with the function corrector III. Trans Eur Orthod Soc 1970;46:249–259.
71. Fränkel R. Biomechanical aspects of the form/function relationship in craniofacial morphogenesis: a clinician's approach. In: McNamara JA, Jr, Ribbens KA, Howe RP, eds. Clinical alterations of the growing face. Ann Arbor: Monograph 14, Craniofacial Growth Series, Center for Human Growth and Development, University of Michigan, 1983.
72. Fränkel R. Personal communication, 1999.
73. Loh MK, Kerr WJ. The function regulator III: effects and indications for use. Br J Orthod 1985;12:153–157.
74. McNamara JA, Jr, Huge SA. The functional regulator (FR-3) of Fränkel. Am J Orthod 1985;88:409–424.
75. Kerr WJ, TenHave TR, McNamara JA, Jr. A comparison of skeletal and dental changes produced by function regulators (FR-2 and FR-3). Eur J Orthod 1989;11:235–242.
76. Armstrong CJ. A clinical evaluation of the chin cup. Aust Dent J 1961;6:338–346.
77. Thilander B. Chin-cap treatment for Angle Class III malocclusion: a longitudinal study. Trans Eur Orthod Soc 1965;41:311–327.
78. Matsui Y. Effect of chin cap on the growing mandible. J Jpn Ortho Soc 1965;24:165–181.
79. Suzuki N. Cephalometric observation on the effect of the chin cap. J Jpn Orthod Soc 1972;31:64–74.
80. Irie M, Nakamura S. Orthopedic approach to severe skeletal Class III malocclusion. Am J Orthod 1975;67:377–392.
81. Sakamoto T. Effective timing for the application of orthopedic force in the skeletal Class III malocclusion. Am J Orthod 1981;80:411–416.
82. Wendell PD, Nanda R, Sakamoto T, Nakamura S. The effects of chin cup therapy on the mandible: a longitudinal study. Am J Orthod 1985;87:265–274.
83. Mitani H, Fukazawa H. Effects of chincap force on the timing and amount of mandibular growth associated with anterior reversed occlusion (Class III malocclusion) during puberty. Am J Orthod Dentofac Orthop 1986;90:454–463.
84. Deguchi T, Kitsugi A. Stability of changes associated with chin cup treatment. Angle Orthod 1996;66:139–145.
85. Deguchi T, McNamara JA, Jr. Craniofacial adaptations induced by chin cup therapy in Class III patients. Am J Orthod Dentofac Orthop 1999;115:175–182.
86. Graber TM. Extrinsic control factors influencing craniofacial growth. In: McNamara JA, Jr, ed. Determinants of mandibular form and growth. Ann Arbor: Monograph 4, Craniofacial Growth Series, Center for Human Growth and Development, The University of Michigan, 1976.

Chapter 7
THE TRANSVERSE DIMENSION

It is the purpose of this chapter to explore the possibilities of clinically altering the transverse dimension of the face, evaluating both short-term and long-term treatment effects produced by such intervention. The key to such adaptations in the transverse dimension is the use of rapid maxillary expansion (RME) as a routine treatment procedure. A number of somewhat non-traditional uses of RME also will be described, suggesting that this methodology may have a broader role in orthodontic treatment than has been recognized traditionally.

ROUTINE DIAGNOSIS AND TREATMENT PLANNING

Orthodontic diagnosis and treatment planning of patients with underlying skeletal malrelationships is a complex issue, one that incorporates not only fixed appliance therapy, but also may include growth modification or surgical intervention. Most clinicians recognize that the efficacy of conventional fixed appliances is limited and that both orthopedic and surgical options should be considered if significant skeletal and neuromuscular imbalances contribute to the clinical manifestation of the occlusal problem.

One example of such a situation is the adult patient with a Class II malocclusion and concomitant mandibular skeletal retrusion. When is surgical intervention indicated? On the one hand, most clinicians would agree that a maxillomandibular discrepancy of 10 mm typically warrants surgical intervention. Few would intervene surgically, however, if the anteroposterior skeletal discrepancy were only 2-3 mm. Similarly, surgical correction of vertical maxillary excess usually is indicated if the gingival display when smiling is 6–8 mm, but probably is not indicated if the vertical excess is only 1–2 mm. In fact, most surgical corrections of sagittal and vertical skeletal malrelationships are in the range of 5 mm or greater, with lesser discrepancies often handled by orthodontics-only camouflage mechanics.

A slightly less clear example is the treatment of a growing patient with Class II malocclusion and mandibular skeletal retrusion. Although controversy remains concerning the long-term effects of functional jaw orthopedic (FJO) therapy on the ultimate length of the mandible,[1-4] numerous clinical studies have shown that the growth of the mandible can be enhanced modestly over the short-term.[5-9] Once again, the question arises— When is functional appliance treatment indicated? Those clinicians who routinely use functional appliances might state that FJO treatment obviously is indicated in a patient with a maxillomandibular discrepancy of 8–10 mm, but these same clinicians probably would not initiated such treatment in a patient with skeletal discrepancy of only 2–3 mm.

In the examples cited above, the perceived magnitude of the structural and functional imbalances that triggers the use of a surgical or orthopedic option varies widely among clinicians, depending on their education and clinical experience. Some will embrace both adjunctive procedures with great enthusiasm, whereas others will use either procedure with very limited frequency or perhaps not at all. The important point in this discussion, however, is not that a clinician chooses to use adjunctive treatment in a given patient, but rather that the anteroposterior and vertical skeletal imbalances present in a given malocclusion typically are well recognized. It is the clinical judgment of each practitioner to determine the point at which the severity of the specific structural imbalance necessitates consideration of adjunctive surgical or orthopedic treatments. We will see later in this discussion that similar imbalances in the transverse dimension are not always recognized, let alone treated, by the average clinician.

The evolution of orthodontic diagnosis and treatment planning has been gradual. Initial emphasis was placed on sagittal relationships, as is indicated by the Angle classification of malocclusion. The Angle system of classification remains at the core of orthodontic diagnosis a century after its development, even though this classification scheme is not sensitive to imbalances in the vertical and transverse dimensions. In fact, it was not until the 1960s, in part due to the contributions of Schudy,[10] that the role of the vertical dimension finally was recognized.

Further, it only has been during the last two decades or so that the role of the transverse dimension has been a topic of interest to the typical practicing orthodontist. In fact, it is our opinion that skeletal imbalances in the transverse dimension often are ignored or simply not recognized. Thus, the treatment options for such patients by necessity are more limited than if these transverse skeletal problems were recognized. In contrast to the aggressive approaches often taken in treating skeletally-based anteroposterior and vertical problems, orthodontists traditionally have been reluctant to change arch dimensions transversely,[11,12] except in the instance of treating a unilateral or bilateral posterior crossbite.[13] Yet, it appears that the transverse dimension of the maxilla may be the most adaptable of all the regions of the craniofacial complex.

PROBLEMS IN THE TRANSVERSE DIMENSION

Most orthodontists cite crossbite (Fig. 7-1) as the primary reason to alter the transverse dimension clinically. It is very common for one or more of the maxillary posterior teeth to be in a lingual orientation relative to the mandibular dentition. Through the widening of the midpalatal suture, the correction of a posterior crossbite is accomplished readily in a patient in whom the maxillary sutural system still is patent. The research of Melsen[14-16] has indicated that the responses to orthopedic expansion of the maxilla are related to the age and maturation level of the patient (Fig. 7-2), with the sutural sys-

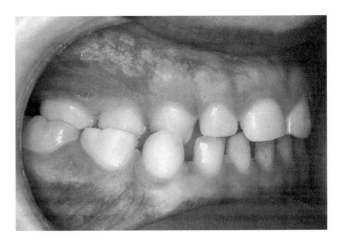

Figure 7-1. Intraoral view of a unilateral posterior crossbite in the deciduous dentition.

tems of younger patients very responsive to such orthopedic intervention.

The majority of (but not all) orthodontic practitioners use rapid maxillary expansion to correct such problems.[17] Applying a lateral force against the posterior maxillary dentition produces a separation of the midpalatal suture and results in orthopedic expansion (Fig. 7-3). Generally, RME appliances are fixed and generate 3–10 pounds of force.[18] After activation, RME produces a net increase in the transverse width of the maxillary basal bone, thereby leading to the correction of preexisting crossbites.

A less obvious but very common orthodontic problem, whose etiology in part is related to imbalances in the transverse dimension, is a discrepancy between tooth size and arch size (see Chapter 4). The most frequently observed type of malocclusion in routine orthodontic practice often is described as "crowding," an underlying imbalance between tooth size and available arch perimeter. As mentioned earlier, affected patients typically are referred to the orthodontist by the general or pediatric dentist or by the patient's parents because of obvious dental irregularities or lack of sufficient space for tooth eruption. In addition to crowding, tooth-size/arch-size discrepancies also can be manifested as protrusion and flaring of the teeth relative to underlying basal bone. Both conditions are highly visible and probably are responsible for much of the public's desire to have their "teeth straightened."

The transverse dimension of the maxilla can be widened, and this temporary defect in the midpalatal suture region remodels with osseous tissue. The transseptal fibers that connect the central incisors eventually cause a migration of the maxillary anterior teeth to close the midline diastema produced during expansion. The obvious clinical consequence of such a change is an

TRANSVERSE DIMENSION

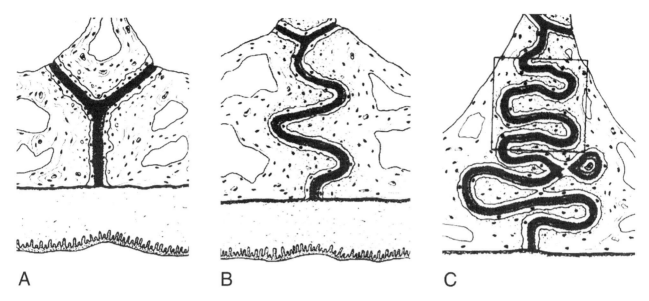

Figure 7-2. Maturational changes in the mid palatal suture based on human autopsy material. Drawings of histological sections in the frontal plane. The complexity of the suture increases with age. *A*, Two years of age. *B*, Nine years of age. *C*, Thirteen years of age (adapted from Melsen, 1975).

increase in total arch length that will allow the accommodation of rotated, displaced, or impacted permanent teeth into the dental arch (Fig. 7-4).

RME has been in common use for over thirty years. It is seen as an effective orthopedic means of correcting posterior crossbites, both unilateral and bilateral.[13,19–23] In addition, Adkins and colleagues[24] have examined the relationship between arch expansion and changes in arch perimeter and have shown that every millimeter of transpalatal width increase in the premolar region produces a 0.7 mm increase in available arch perimeter. By using RME in the early mixed dentition, it is hypothesized that an increase in transpalatal width ultimately should produce a net increase in the transverse width of maxillary basal bone, presumably leading to additional available arch length (Fig. 7-4). One obvious clinical consequence of such a change would be a reduction in the need for the extraction of permanent teeth.

CLINICAL STUDIES OF RAPID MAXILLARY EXPANSION

Short-term Studies

Numerous studies have considered the effects of RME on the craniofacial skeleton; however, most are limited to short-term outcomes.[13,19–21,25–34] Skeletal changes in-

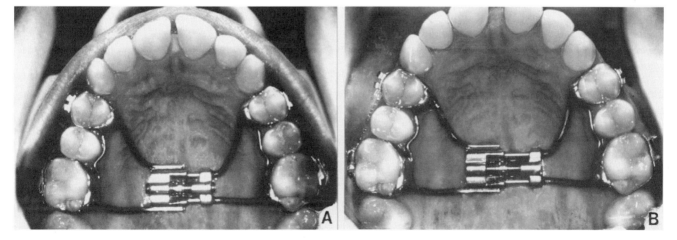

Figure 7-3. Typical maxillary response following once-per-day activation of the Hyrax-type expander. *A*) After 14 days. *B*) After 28 days. Note the midline diastema that becomes larger as the expansion continues.

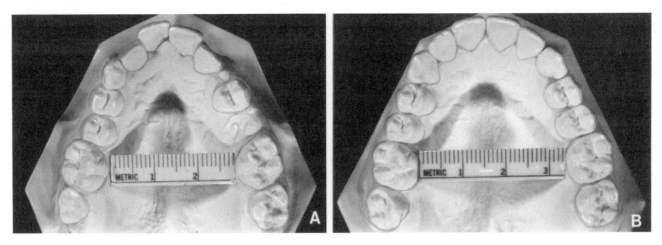

Figure 7-4. Arch perimeter changes associated with RME. *A)* The pretreatment transpalatal width is 28 mm, and the maxillary left canine is blocked out of the arch. *B)* After RME and fixed appliance treatment, the transpalatal width has increased to 33.5 mm.

duced by RME commonly are assessed from the time of appliance insertion to several weeks or months after initial RME activation. One of the first studies was by Thörne,[35] who examined 40 RME patients whose ages ranged from 8–15 years at the start of treatment. Thörne reported that bite opening occurred in about half the patients, but no statistical analysis was presented. Further, because there was a wide range of age at the start of treatment, he observed varying skeletal responses to RME, with greater orthopedic (rather than orthodontic) expansion in the younger patients. Studies by Haas,[13,36] Byrum,[37] and Wertz[19,28] also are compromised by variability in starting age, with patient age often extending to early adulthood.

Given the presumed importance of age in treatment response to RME, the findings from such studies are difficult to interpret.[26] The midpalatal suture becomes more interdigitated with increasing skeletal maturation,[15,16,38] thereby making skeletal expansion accomplished less easily.[14] Equally important, when RME therapy is attempted in skeletally mature patients, there is more dental tipping, a type of expansion—orthodontic, rather than orthopedic—that is prone to relapse.

Davis and Kronman[39] investigated the skeletal results of expanding the midpalatal suture in a sample of twenty-six patients. These patients had lateral and posteroanterior cephalograms as well as dental casts taken both before the cementation of the RME appliance and at the end of fixed retention (usually 3–6 months postexpansion). Forward displacement of Point A (measured in relation to the pterygomaxillary fissure) was observed in all but four patients. The exact amount of forward maxillary repositioning was not noted, however. Moreover, varying skeletal responses to RME were observed, but no statistical analysis was performed.

Wertz and Dreskin[28] also reported a varied response to RME that seemed to be age-related. The amount of bite opening (*i.e.,* change in mandibular plane angle) and the anteroposterior change in Point A depended on age at the start of treatment, with a tendency for greater anteroposterior and vertical change to occur in younger (less than 18-year-old) patients. Davis and Kronman[39] also observed a variable vertical change in response to RME, as did Thörne.[35] Haas,[36,40] on the other hand, asserted that in every one of his RME-treated patients the maxilla moved inferiorly with attendant opening of the mandibular plane angle. Thus, age at the start of treatment seems to be an important factor in determining the RME treatment outcome.

A study by da Silva Filho and co-workers[30] examined the skeletal alterations induced by RME in even younger age groups (*i.e.,* patients in the primary and mixed dentitions). They obtained lateral cephalograms from thirty patients before and immediately after the active phase of expansion. The two lateral cephalograms were taken 14–21 days apart, thereby eliminating the factor of growth. Da Silva Filho and co-workers reported that the maxilla did not move forward during the treatment period. In fact, the SNA angle decreased in 11 of 30 patients. The maxilla moved downward and backward and the mandible rotated downward and backward as well. The mandibular plane angle opened, the SNB angle decreased, and the palatal plane tipped down posteriorly.

Most previous studies of RME have involved patients treated with the Haas-type or hyrax-type banded expanders used in the late mixed or early permanent dentition. Relatively few studies deal with the treatment effects produced by the acrylic splint expander, a bonded appliance that has full posterior occlusal coverage. It has been hypothesized that this type of expander will prevent unfavorable bite opening due to the "posterior bite block effect" of the appliance.[41,42]

Sarver and Johnston[43] examined the effect of the acrylic splint expander in 20 patients who were on average 11 years of age at the beginning of treatment. The effects of treatment determined for these patients were compared to the findings from 60 patients who wore Haas-type expanders and who had been studied previously by Wertz.[19] A decrease in the displacement of the maxilla was noted in the bonded appliance group. Sarver and Johnston[43] suggested that the inferior displacement of the maxilla might be limited during treatment by the forces placed on the dentition by the elevator musculature and by the force associated with the stretch of other soft tissues. In the bonded-expander group, a slight superior movement of the posterior aspect of the palatal plane also was noted in comparison to the banded-appliance group. A downward and posterior movement of the anterior aspect of the maxilla also was observed at the anterior nasal spine.

One of the few prospective studies was conducted by Memikoglu and Iseri,[44] who set out to evaluate changes in the transverse plane following the use of an acrylic bonded rapid maxillary expansion appliance in growing individuals. The 14 consecutively treated orthodontic patients were 13 years old at the start of treatment, and the mean overall treatment time was three years. Frontal cephalograms and dental casts were used to assess treatment changes. Because of the expansion, lower nasal width, basal maxillary width, and maxillary molar width increased significantly. The greatest widening occurred in the dentoalveolar area, and the widening effect of the bonding device gradually decreased through the upper structures in a triangular pattern. At the end of active treatment, all measurements had remained constant. The results of this study suggest that dentoskeletal changes in the transverse dimension following the use of acrylic bonded RME are maintained satisfactorily at the end of fixed appliance therapy.

Despite numerous studies examining the effects of the rapid maxillary expander, however, its short-term skeletal effects remain somewhat controversial. For example, several studies have reported different responses in the maxilla and mandible. Short-term studies by Haas[36,40] revealed that the bite opens, the mandibular plane angle increases, and Point A is displaced anteriorly. Linder-Aronson[45] and da Silva Filho and co-workers,[30] however, observed no anterior movement of the maxilla. In fact, da Silva Filho and co-workers reported the antithesis of what Haas observed, namely that the maxilla displaces downward and backward with RME therapy.

Such disparities in findings, in part, are related to the nature of many previous short-term clinical studies of RME that are characterized by methodological problems, including limited sample size, lack of control data, large age range at start of treatment, lack of long-term data, and lack of statistical analysis. An alternative explanation to account for conflicting results, however, is that a varied response to RME truly exists. There may be certain categories of patients who can tolerate RME without increasing the vertical dimension significantly, whereas in others RME may produce a marked negative change, at least over the short-term.

Long-term Studies

There are few well-designed long-term studies of the effects of RME, and many of the earlier studies are based solely on case reports. For example, Haas[40] presented long-term data from 10 subjects. He reported that, immediately after expansion, the average initial increase was 9 mm in maxillary width and 4.5 mm in nasal cavity width. None of his subjects were said to have undergone a loss in either dimension at the time of re-evaluation 6–14 years post-retention. Slight loss of maxillary dental arch width was noted in two subjects following retention, and a slight increase in dental arch width was found in two other subjects.

Stockfish,[46] in one of the most extensive investigations of RME (150 patients), presented little in the way of statistical analysis, save for a summary graph presenting percentage relapse related to initial arch expansion. In contrast to the Stockfish study, the remaining long-term investigations of RME are compromised by small samples. Haas[13] examined only 10 patients; Krebs[26] and Linder-Aronson,[45] 23 patients; Timms,[47] 19 patients; and Wertz and Dreskin,[28] 56 patients, of whom only 27 were available for follow-up. Indeed, in the 1976 study of Timms,[48] 81 of 100 patients were excluded due to insufficient records.

Herberger[49] conducted one of the few long-term studies of RME involving a relatively large sample of patients. He evaluated 55 RME subjects with starting ages of 9 to 14 years who were treated with a Haas-design palatal expander. Nine years after RME, the residual dental expansion averaged 90% of that gained initially. The maxillary first molars on average uprighted almost 12° during the retention period to approximately pre-treatment values.

Moussa and co-workers[50] also investigated the long-term stability of rapid maxillary expander treatment and edgewise therapy. Their sample consisted of dental casts from 55 patients who had been out of retention for

8 to 10 years and who had a mean age of 30 years. Measurements were made directly on dental casts obtained at the three times: before treatment, after treatment, and after retention. Differences between post-treatment and post-retention measurements were statistically significant for all dimensions except mandibular intermolar width; only for mandibular and maxillary arch lengths and perimeters, however, were the differences greater than 2.0 mm. Treatment with the rapid maxillary expander presented good stability for maxillary intercanine width, maxillary and mandibular intermolar widths and incisor irregularity. Moussa and co-workers,[50] however, observed poorer stability in mandibular intercanine width, as well as mandibular arch length and arch perimeter.

It should be noted that the studies of Herberger[49] and Moussa and co-workers[50] are representative of most clinical studies of the long-term effects of RME, in that an untreated comparison group was not analyzed. In the absence of treatment, the dental arches typically become reduced in most dimensions during the late teen and early adult years. For example, it is a common clinical observation that mandibular incisor crowding increases with age in both males and females, regardless of whether orthodontic treatment was undertaken.[51-55] Such normally occurring decrements in arch dimensions must be taken into consideration in an analysis of the long-term changes in the dental arches of patients treated with RME. In fact, with the exception of the cephalometric study of Wertz and Dreskin,[28] no previous investigation has evaluated the change in arch dimensions relative to serial dental casts from a matched, untreated population. Thus, the long-term effect of RME on the dental arches must be evaluated in light of the so-called "developmental crowding" that often occurs in untreated individuals in the late teen and early adult years.

RECENT CLINICAL STUDIES

As part of an ongoing clinical trial, our group at The University of Michigan has been gathering data on all patients undergoing rapid maxillary expansion in the early mixed dentition, treated either in the Graduate Orthodontic Clinic or in a private group practice* in Ann Arbor. In addition, we have been assembling longitudinal dental cast and cephalometric records on samples treated elsewhere. The analysis of these samples already has resulted in multiple theses[56-61] and publications[62-65] concerning the treatment effects produced by rapid maxillary expansion.

*Drs. McNamara, Nolan, West and Burkhardt, Ann Arbor MI

Rapid Maxillary Expansion in the Late Mixed and Early Permanent Dentition

Dental Cast Analysis

The first RME sample studied in detail was obtained from the private practice of Drs. Robert and Thomas Herberger of Elyria, Ohio. An attempt was made to recall all patients treated during a specific time interval (1972–1985) who had undergone RME followed by standard edgewise orthodontics and who were five or more years post-treatment. Treatment outcome was not a selection criterion. Longitudinal dental casts from 70 patients who began treatment in the late mixed dentition and 41 patients in the early permanent dentition were obtained and analyzed by means of a digital imaging system.[57] A Haas-type rapid maxillary expansion device was used according to a common, uniform protocol.[13] Each patient then underwent comprehensive orthodontic treatment using a standard edgewise technique. On average, subjects were 11 years of age at the time of initial records (T_1), 14 years of age at the end of treatment (T_2), and 20 years of age at the time of long-term records (T_3). For controls, the longitudinal dental casts from 19 mixed dentition subjects and 24 permanent dentition subjects from the *University of Michigan Growth Study*[66] and the *University of Groningen (Netherlands) Growth Study* were matched according to age and analyzed at the time periods that corresponded to the three study ages of the treated subjects.

The most interesting findings concern changes in arch perimeter. The untreated controls demonstrated a net decrease in maxillary arch perimeter (−2.2 mm in early permanent dentition subjects; −3.4 mm in late mixed dentition subjects) from initial records to long-term follow-up. In contrast, the patient groups who had undergone rapid maxillary expansion had a net increase in maxillary arch perimeter (4.3 mm in the early permanent dentition and 2.1 mm in the late mixed dentition) when compared to untreated controls. An overall increase in maxillary arch perimeter (6.5 mm in the early permanent dentition and 5.5 mm in the late mixed dentition) was shown.

Similar changes were found in the mandibular dental arch. In the untreated sample, mandibular arch perimeter decreased (−5.7 mm in late mixed dentition subjects; −2.3 mm in early permanent dentition subjects), whereas the RME patients underwent a net increase in mandibular arch perimeter (0.4 mm in the late mixed dentition, 4.1 mm in the early permanent dentition). A comparison of changes in mandibular arch perimeter revealed that at age 20 years the group treated in the late mixed dentition had 6.1 mm more arch perimeter than did the controls, and the early permanent dentition group had an average advantage of 6.4 mm of arch perimeter relative to controls. Thus, when the decreases in arch perimeter seen in the control group are taken into consideration, the net treatment effect observed was an increase in maxillary arch perimeter of 5–6 mm and a 6 mm increase in mandibular arch perimeter. This long-term study indicates that, when RME is undertaken in the late mixed dentition or early permanent dentition, significant long-term treatment effects can be seen at least six years following fixed-appliance removal.

Another study that considered the long-term treatment effects of RME was conducted by Fenderson.[59] The purpose of the Fenderson study was to compare the long-term stability of maxillary expansion achieved by either RME or facebow expansion followed by fixed edgewise treatment. The original parent sample included 154 young adolescent patients that started their non-extraction orthodontic treatment between the years 1973 and 1981 in the private orthodontic practice of Dr. Charles Veith of Dover, Delaware. The exclusion criteria subsequently reduced the number of patients to 61 in the cervical pull facebow group (CFB) and 41 in the cervical pull facebow/rapid maxillary expansion group (CFB/RME). All subjects were in the late-mixed to early permanent dentition stage at the start of treatment. The maxillary and mandibular dental casts of these 102 patients were measured with the aid of our digital imaging system at four different times: Start of treatment (T_1), end of active treatment (T_2), end of retention (T_3), and post-retention follow up (T_4).

The results of the Fenderson[59] study indicated that the CFB/RME protocol produced a greater increase in maxillary arch width (6.1 mm) than did the CFB protocol (4.0 mm). The CFB/RME protocol also provided more net maxillary arch perimeter increase than did expansion with an inner bow of a cervical face bow. The CFB/RME group had 3.0 mm more arch perimeter 10 years after treatment completion than did the CFB group. The stability of expansion achieved with an inner bow of a facebow is equal to that achieved with a Haas-type rapid maxillary expansion appliance. Both expansion protocols retained 90% (5.5 mm group CFB/RME; 3.6 mm group CFB) of the initial intermolar expansion 15 years post-expansion therapy. Maxillary expansion by either method, however, had only a modest effect on mandibular arch perimeter. Neither method produced a net post-retention increase. Mandibular arch perimeters, however, were greater than they would have been had these patients not been treated. Thus, both methods of maxillary expansion evaluated in this study had sustained long-term effects on both the maxillary and mandibular dentitions, with the expansion produced appearing to be orthopedic rather than orthodontic in nature.

Cephalometric Analysis

Chang and co-workers[64] studied a randomly chosen subgroup of patients from the Herberger sample. The purpose of this investigation was to examine cephalometrically the long-term effects of RME on bite opening and on the anteroposterior position of the maxilla. The sample was composed of 25 patients who had undergone rapid maxillary expansion with the Haas-type expander followed by standard edgewise therapy. This RME sample was compared to a group of 25 patients who had undergone single-phase standard edgewise treatment and to an untreated control group of 23 subjects from the *University of Michigan Growth Study*.

Mean initial facial form and age at start of treatment were similar for all groups. Statistically significant among group differences were documented for only two of ten cephalometric variables that were assumed sensitive to anteroposterior and vertical skeletal changes. These differences, however, were small and of little clinical significance. This investigation implies, therefore, that RME therapy with the Haas-type expander has little long-term (*i.e.*, >6 years post-treatment) effect on either the vertical or anteroposterior dimensions of the face.

Rapid Maxillary Expansion in the Early Mixed Dentition

Dental Cast Analysis

The first investigation of patients in the longitudinal *Michigan Expansion Study* reported the effects seen in 162 subjects who had undergone rapid maxillary expansion during the mixed dentition before the eruption of the maxillary premolars and canines.[56,62] The expansion procedure was followed by a retention protocol that included the wearing of a removable palatal plate for at least one year, after which time a maintenance plate typically was worn on a full-time or part-time basis for at least one additional year. The average increase in intermolar width was about 6 mm.

During the post retention period, the expanded maxillary dental arches were stable. For example, more than 90% of the original expansion was maintained after the first year, and more than 80% remained at the end of the observation period at the time of Phase II records (records taken before the initiation of the final phase of comprehensive orthodontic treatment was begun) that were obtained 2.4 years post-expansion. Similar findings were observed during the transition from the primary molars to the premolars and from the primary canines to the permanent canines.

Brust[57,63] studied a larger sample that included 376 consecutively treated mixed-dentition patients who undergone rapid maxillary expansion, singly or in combination with prior mandibular expansion with a Schwarz appliance. Through the application of multiple exclusionary criteria, a subsample of 146 patients who received RME and 36 patients who received RME following Schwarz appliance therapy were studied. Serial dental casts of 50 untreated controls from *The University of Michigan Growth Study* were used as a matched control group. Longitudinal changes were analyzed with a digital imaging system (Bioscan Optimas, Seattle WA) specifically modified by our laboratory for the analysis of dental casts. Changes in arch width, arch perimeter, and molar angulation were evaluated pre-expansion, immediately post-expansion, and at the time of Phase II records.

At the end of the observation period, residual expansion was greatest in the RME/Schwarz group (7.2 mm), whereas in the RME group it was 4.9 mm; in the control group, it was 0.9 mm. This increase in width was mirrored by an increase in arch perimeter. Maxillary arch perimeter also increased following rapid maxillary expansion, with greater increases observed in mandibular expansion when a Schwarz appliance was used prior to RME. Indeed, clinically relevant increases in mandibular arch perimeter were noted only in the RME/Schwarz group. When the net arch length decrease in the control group was compared to the net arch length increase in the RME/Schwarz group, the net gain was about 3.3 mm. At first glance, this amount may seem like a small increase, but the gain is about half that seen with premolar extraction after anchorage loss from space closure is taken into consideration.

Cephalometric Analysis

Thus far, the primary focus of data analysis from this sample has been the development and implementation of the digital imaging system for dental cast analysis. In addition, Wendling[58] conducted a study of the short-term changes produced by an acrylic splint expander composed of a wire framework and 3 mm thick splint Biocryl™ during an initial six-months treatment interval. Pre- and post-treatment cephalograms on 25 patients treated solely with the acrylic splint expander and 19 patients treated with the removable mandibular Schwarz appliance followed by RME have been analyzed cephalometrically. The results of this analysis indicate that the acrylic splint expander appears to prevent the bite-opening effect of RME noted in previous short-term studies,[13,27,28,39] presumably due to the posterior bite block effect produced by the acrylic covering the maxillary posterior teeth. Some intrusion of the maxillary buccal segments was noted as well. The anteroposterior position of the maxilla and mandible remained unaffected by the expansion procedures, and an opening of the bite was not observed.

No significant between-group differences were observed with regard to vertical and horizontal changes during treatment. Further, the use of the Schwarz appliance to widen the mandibular dental arch did not produce proclination of the mandibular incisors, as might be expected with a removable expansion appliance. Thus, the mandibular incisors were not proclined by Schwarz treatment, a type of movement that has been shown to be unstable over the long-term.[54]

In summary, the results of clinical studies conducted both by our group and by others indicate that the maxillary complex appears to be responsive to orthopedic expansion not only over the short-term but over the long-term as well. It appears that the key to successful widening of the dental arches is the use of rapid maxillary expansion as in initial treatment modality. Mandibular expansion is not stable if attempted without concomitant orthopedic widening of the maxillary arch. The occlusal interdigitation of the teeth in the widened maxilla with the uprighted mandibular dentition may account for the stability of the treated results. Given the apparent stability of this type of treatment over the long-term, the efficacy of RME in a variety of clinical situations will be examined.

OTHER USES OF RAPID MAXILLARY EXPANSION

Over the last 20 years, we have seen the use of rapid maxillary expansion escalate greatly in routine clinical practice. Although this procedure was used initially to correct posterior crossbites and secondarily to increase available arch space, there now is a greater number of possible indications for this technique. Several other possible uses of RME are described below.

Correction of Axial Inclinations of the Posterior Teeth

One of the major goals of virtually all types of fixed appliance therapy is to idealize the positions of the teeth in all dimensions as much as possible. Of particular concern is the orientation of the lingual cusps of the maxillary posterior teeth that, in many instances, often lie

TRANSVERSE DIMENSION

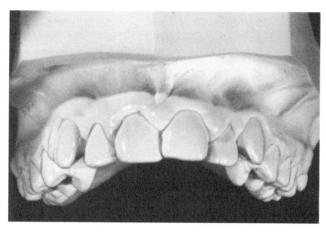

Figure 7-5. An example of a malocclusion characterized by a narrow transpalatal width (32 mm) and flared posterior teeth. The lingual cusps of the premolars and molars are inferior to the buccal cusps. RME is used to move the roots of the posterior teeth laterally as well as to increase available arch perimeter. Fixed appliances are used to tip the posterior teeth lingually, improving their axial inclinations and elimination balancing interferences during function.

below the occlusal plane (Fig. 7-5). This situation can lead to the production of balancing interferences during function. This common finding in patients with malocclusion often is due to maxillary constriction and subsequent dentoalveolar compensation in which the maxillary posterior teeth are in a slightly flared orientation.

One of the goals of our routine orthodontic treatment is not only to align the teeth properly, but also to level the curve of Wilson (Fig. 7-6). This transverse curvature of the dental arches is similar to the curve of Spee in the sagittal plane.

After identifying such a situation, the clinician has several choices of treatment protocols. Buccal root torque can be applied to the posterior teeth with conventional edgewise mechanics and rectangular archwires. While such an orthodontic technique is useful in patients who have mild-to-moderate flaring of the posterior teeth, it is contraindicated in instances of severe maxillary constriction because of the possibility that the roots of the maxillary teeth may erode through the buccal cortical plate (Fig. 7-7).

Another alternative, which we favor, is to approach such a problem in a two-step sequence of treatment. First, a rapid maxillary expansion appliance is used to widen the maxilla (Figs. 7-8 and 7-9), moving the roots of the maxillary posterior teeth into a near-ideal orientation. Of course, the application of RME will produce a tendency toward a buccal crossbite (an attempt normally is made to maintain contact between the lingual cusps of the maxillary posterior teeth and the buccal cusps of the mandibular posterior teeth; Fig. 7-8). After

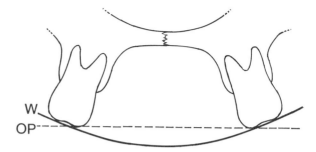

Figure 7-6. Diagrammatic representation of the curve of Wilson (W) in the molar region. Note that the lingual cusps are positioned below the buccal cusps. The goal of treatment is to flatten the occlusal plane (OP).

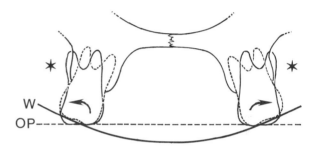

Figure 7-7. The application of buccal root torque to the posterior teeth with fixed appliances. In some instances, the buccal cortical plate can be perforated.

rapid maxillary expansion has been completed (Fig. 7-9) and the arch stabilized for three to five months, the expander is removed; fixed appliances then are placed. Subsequently, only tipping movements (Fig. 7-10), rather than the application of buccal root torque, are necessary to align the maxillary and mandibular dentitions and level the occlusal plane (Fig. 7-11). Some

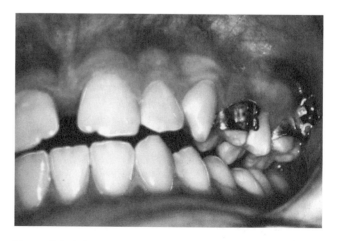

Figure 7-8. Adequate expansion is produced when the lingual cusps of the maxillary posterior teeth approximate the buccal cusps of the mandibular posterior teeth.

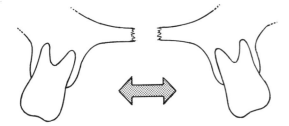

Figure 7-9. Correction of posterior tooth inclination. Rapid maxillary expansion separates the midpalatal suture, moving the apices of the posterior teeth laterally.

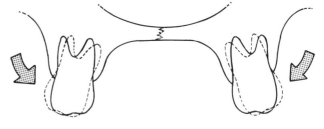

Figure 7-10. Correction of posterior tooth inclination (cont.) Fixed appliances are used to tip the teeth lingually, leveling the occlusal plane (OP).

spontaneous uprighting of the mandibular posterior teeth also may be observed in patients who have undergone RME.

Spontaneous Correction of Class II Malocclusion

As described in detail in Chapter 4, many Class II malocclusions, when evaluated clinically, have no obvious maxillary constriction. When the study models of the patient are "hand-articulated," however, it becomes obvious that when the dental casts are placed with the posterior dentition in a Class I relationship, a unilateral or bilateral crossbite is produced. This indicates the presence of maxillary constriction as a component of Class II malocclusion. In addition, transpalatal width usually is narrower than what is considered ideal.

Most Class II malocclusions in mixed dentition patients may be associated with maxillary constriction. When one is treating patients in the mixed dentition, the first step in the treatment of mild-to-moderate Class II malocclusions characterized, at least in part, by mild mandibular skeletal retrusion and maxillary constriction, may be expansion of the maxilla. The patient can be left in an "overexpanded" position (Fig. 7-8), with contacts still maintained between the maxillary lingual cusps and the mandibular buccal cusps of the posterior teeth. The occlusion is stabilized using a removable palatal plate in the mixed dentition or full orthodontic appliances in the permanent dentition. Widening the maxilla often leads to a spontaneous forward posturing of the mandible during the retention period. After six to twelve months, the spontaneous correction of Class II relationship can be seen in many mild and moderate Class II patients.

There is some indirect evidence from the previous described cephalometric study of Wendling[58] that treatment with an acrylic splint expander may create an environment conducive to spontaneous Class II correction. Fourteen of the original 63 patients in the sample gathered for use in this study were eliminated due to forward positioning of the mandible in the T_2 lateral cephalogram. No patients were excluded from consideration because of erroneous mandibular positioning before treatment (T_1). Because all headfilms were taken using a standardized protocol, and each patient was instructed to "move your tongue to the back of your mouth and bite on your back teeth," this forward posturing of the mandible may be a result of the disruption of the posterior occlusion, producing a tendency for the patient to bring their jaw into a forward position when closing. Following months of wear and significant alteration in the width of the maxilla, it is understandable that a child may experience a period of occlusal disorientation.

A final comment is made regarding the observation that some Class II malocclusions will correct spontaneously following rapid maxillary expansion. Although no specific clinical study has been conducted that has considered the actual percentage of patients exhibiting spontaneous correction, this phenomenon happens with sufficient frequency that we now incorporate this treatment effect routinely into the patient's overall treatment plan. The net result of this change in outlook has been a reduction in the number of functional jaw orthopedic appliances that now are used in the treatment of mild-to-moderate Class II malocclusions.

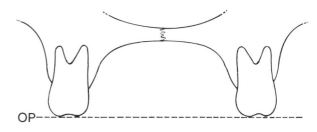

Figure 7-11. Correction of posterior tooth inclination (cont.) The occlusal plane (OP) is now level and the curve of Wilson has been flattened.

Preparation for Functional Jaw Orthopedics or Orthognathic Surgery

Many of the severe Class II malocclusions also benefit from rapid maxillary expansion. In instances in which a patient is being prepared for functional jaw orthopedics, an initial phase of rapid maxillary expansion may be indicated. Not only will the maxilla be widened, but also any intra-arch problems (*e.g.*, tooth-size/arch-size discrepancies) can be addressed. The transverse problem also may be treated at the same time Class II correction is attempted if expansion is produced by the functional appliance chosen (*e.g.*, FR-2 of Fränkel, twin block).

The use of rapid maxillary expansion as part of an orthognathic surgical protocol also must be evaluated thoroughly. In instances in which mandibular surgery alone is indicated to correct an anteroposterior problem, prior RME therapy during the presurgical phase of orthodontics may be necessary because the mandible will be advanced into a narrower part of the dental arch. In some non-growing patients, an initial phase of rapid maxillary expansion, even with a surgical assist, may be indicated because of preexisting arch length problems. In situations in which the patient is to undergo either maxillary surgery or maxillary surgery combined with a mandibular procedure, a two-piece LeFort I osteotomy may be used to widen the maxilla during the surgical phase of treatment.

Mobilization of the Maxillary Sutural System

Rapid maxillary expansion has become an integral part of the orthopedic correction of early Class III malocclusion.[41,42,67] The bonded rapid maxillary expansion appliance is used to anchor the elastic traction from the orthopedic facial mask to the maxillary dentition. Even in patients in whom no transverse expansion of the maxilla is indicated, the patient still is instructed to expand the appliance once-per-day for eight to ten days to disrupt the circummaxillary sutural system, presumably facilitating the response of the maxilla to the forward traction of the facial mask.

Although this approach to facial mask therapy seems to make sense from a clinical intuition perspective, no clinical studies have demonstrated that facial mask therapy combined with rapid maxillary expansion produces an orthopedic result that is superior to that produced by facial mask therapy combined with other types of intraoral anchorage systems.

It is our best guess, however, that RME does produce a positive effect during Class III treatment. As mentioned previously, we often have observed the spontaneous correction of mild-to-moderate anterior crossbites after rapid maxillary expansion without facial mask therapy. The clinical research of Haas[27,36,40] and Wertz[19] and the experimental investigation of Dellinger[68] have shown that 1–2 mm of anterior movement of Point A has been observed in some individuals treated with RME, although other investigators have shown the opposite results. In any event, it has been our clinical protocol to deliver an acrylic splint RME appliance (to which have been attached facial mask hooks) and to wait several appointments before delivering the facial mask in order to allow for the possible spontaneous correction of mild-to-moderate Class II problems to occur.

Reduction in Nasal Resistance

Although not a predictable part of RME treatment, a significant number of patients demonstrate a reduction in nasal resistance following rapid maxillary expansion. The study of Hartgerink[69] demonstrated that about two-thirds of the patients undergoing rapid maxillary expansion exhibited a decrease in nasal resistance. Clinically, these patients reported less difficulty breathing through the nose. Unfortunately, the reduction in nasal resistance is not predictable. It may be prudent for the clinician who is contemplating referral of a patient to an otolaryngologist for evaluation of possible nasal obstruction to defer such a referral until after RME therapy has been completed, if RME therapy is to be used for other reasons.

"Broadening the Smile"

Perhaps the use of RME least supported by clinical research and at this point is primarily the product of clinical intuition is widening the maxilla to make the smile of the patient more attractive. Vanarsdall[70] has used the term "negative space" to refer to the shadows that occur in the corners of the mouth during smiling in some patients with a narrow, tapered maxilla and a mesofacial or brachyfacial skeletal pattern (Fig. 7-12). Regardless of whether teeth are extracted, the maxilla is widened and the distance between the maxillary canines is increased, eliminating or reducing the dark spaces between the teeth and the inside surfaces of the cheeks. This type of orthopedic intervention results in what many consider a more pleasing facial appearance. It is our opinion that RME for esthetic purposes (*e.g.*, "broadening the smile") will become an increasingly

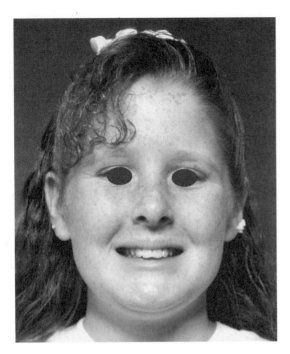

Figure 7-12. Patient with maxillary constriction and "dark spaces" at the corners of the mouth. RME can be used to broaden the smile and improve facial esthetics.

recognized indication for rapid maxillary expansion in patients with narrow dental arches in the future.

CONCLUDING REMARKS

A wide variety of orthodontic problems have been covered in this chapter, all linked to maxillary deficiency in the transverse or sagittal dimension or both. Signs of maxillary deficiency include far more than just anterior and posterior crossbite as well as crowding of the maxillary dentition. In fact, the signs of maxillary deficiency are such that they often appear together, as in what might be termed "maxillary deficiency syndrome."[65] We are fortunate to have at our disposal a proven orthopedic appliance, the rapid maxillary expander, that can be incorporated easily into treatment plans directed toward a variety of orthodontic conditions. In addition, other appliances including the quadhelix and the facebow also can have a positive effect on the transverse dimension.

Traditionally orthodontists have thought primarily in two dimensions, especially with the routine use of lateral headfilms as perhaps the principle quantifiable diagnostic tool. Although dental casts routinely are used in orthodontic diagnosis, the analysis of this type of patient record has been qualitative at best, with little in the way of quantification carried out routinely.

An attempt has been made to provide evidence that orthopedic expansion of the maxilla in a growing individual can be useful clinically over the long-term. Clinically significant increases in both maxillary and mandibular arch perimeters have been documented. In addition, RME can be used for other reasons, both functional and esthetic. RME typically is indicated as an initial treatment of Class II malocclusion because of the transverse discrepancy that usually occurs in such patients. It also can be used in patients who would benefit esthetically from so-called "broadening of the smile." Although the clinical situation of patients with relative bimaxillary transverse constriction generally has not been recognized as a specific clinical problem, RME has been shown to be useful in addressing this condition as well.

It is our opinion that during this century orthodontists will show an increased interest in rapid maxillary expansion as a method of orthopedically altering craniofacial growth in a variety of clinical situations. This type of orthopedic intervention ultimately may prove to be the most useful clinically and have the broadest application to routine clinical orthodontic treatment of all of the so-called "growth modifying" appliances currently available.

REFERENCES CITED

1. Pancherz H, Fackel U. The skeletofacial growth pattern pre- and post-dentofacial orthopaedics. A long-term study of Class II malocclusions treated with the Herbst appliance. Eur J Orthod 1990;12:209–218.
2. Wieslander L. Long-term effect of treatment with the headgear-Herbst appliance in the early mixed dentition. Stability or relapse? Am J Orthod Dentofac Orthop 1993; 104:319–329.
3. Johnston LE, Jr. Functional appliances: A mortgage on mandibular position. Austral Orthod J 1996;14:154–157.
4. Lai M, McNamara JA, Jr. An evaluation of two-phase treatment with the Herbst appliance and preadjusted edgewise therapy. Semin Orthod 1998;4:46–58.
5. Fränkel R. The treatment of Class II, division 1 malocclusion with functional correctors. Am J Orthod 1969;55: 265–275.
6. Pancherz H. Treatment of Class II malocclusions by jumping the bite with the Herbst appliance. A cephalometric investigation. Am J Orthod 1979;76:423–442.
7. McNamara JA, Jr., Howe RP, Dischinger TG. A comparison of the Herbst and Fränkel appliances in the treatment of Class II malocclusion. Am J Orthod Dentofac Orthop 1990;98:134–144.
8. Mills C, McCulloch K. Treatment effects of the twin block appliance: A cephalometric study. Am J Orthod 1998;114: 15–24.
9. Toth LR, McNamara JA, Jr. Treatment effects produced

by the twin block appliance and the FR-2 appliance of Fränkel compared to an untreated Class II sample. Am J Orthod Dentofac Orthop 1999;116:597–609.
10. Schudy F. Vertical growth versus anteroposterior growth as related to function and treatment. Angle Orthod 1964; 34 75-93.
11. Strang RHW. The fallacy of denture expansion as a treatment procedure. Angle Orthod 1949;19:12–17.
12. Tweed CH. Clinical orthodontics. St Louis: CV Mosby, 1966.
13. Haas AJ. Rapid expansion of the maxillary dental arch and nasal cavity by opening the mid-palatal suture. Angle Orthod 1961; 31:73–90.
14. Melsen B. A histological study of the influence of sutural morphology and skeletal maturation of rapid palatal expansion in children. Trans Europ Orthod Soc 1972;48: 499–507.
15. Melsen B. Palatal growth studied on human autopsy material. A histologic microradiographic study. Am J Orthod 1975;68:42–54.
16. Melsen B, Melsen F. The postnatal development of the palatomaxillary region studied on human autopsy material. Am J Orthod 1982;82:329–342.
17. Gottlieb E, Nelson A, Vogels D. 1996 JCO study of orthodontic diagnosis and treatment procedures. Part I. Results and trends. J Clin Orthod 1996;30:615–629.
18. Zimring JF, Isaacson RJ. Forces produced by rapid maxillary expansion. Angle Orthod 1965;35: 178–186.
19. Wertz RA. Skeletal and dental changes accompanying rapid midpalatal suture opening. Am J Orthod 1970;58: 41–66.
20. Hicks EP. Slow maxillary expansion. A clinical study of the skeletal versus dental response to low-magnitude force. Am J Orthod 1978;73:121–141.
21. Herold JS. Maxillary expansion: a retrospective study of three methods of expansion and their long-term sequelae. Br J Orthod 1989;16:195–200.
22. Vadiakas G, Roberts, MW. Primary posterior crossbite: diagnosis and treatment. J Clin Pediatr Dent 1991;16:1–4.
23. Ngan P, Wei, SH. Treatment of anterior and posterior crossbites in the primary and mixed dentitions. Update Pediatr Dent 1991;4:1-4,6–7.
24. Adkins MD, Nanda RS, Currier GF. Arch perimeter changes on rapid palatal expansion. Am J Orthod Dentofac Orthop 1990;97:194–199.
25. Krebs A. Expansion of the midpalatal suture studies by means of metallic implants. Trans Europ Orthod Soc 1958; 34:163–171.
26. Krebs A. Midpalatal suture expansion studies by the implant method over a seven year period. Trans Europ Orthod Soc 1964;40:131–142.
27. Haas AJ. The treatment of maxillary deficiency by opening the mid-palatal suture. Angle Orthod 1965;65: 200–217.
28. Wertz R, Dreskin M. Midpalatal suture opening: a normative study. Am J Orthod 1977;71:367–381.
29. Linder-Aronson S. Respiratory function in relation to facial morphology and the dentition. Br J Orthod 1979;6: 59–71.
30. da Silva Filho OG, Boas MC, Capelozza Filho L. Rapid maxillary expansion in the primary and mixed dentitions: a cephalometric evaluation. Am J Orthod Dentofac Orthop 1991;100:171–179.
31. da Silva Filho OG, Montes LA, Torelly LF. Rapid maxillary expansion in the deciduous and mixed dentition evaluated through posteroanterior cephalometric analysis. Am J Orthod Dentofac Orthop 1995;107:268–275.
32. Kurol J, Berglund L. Longitudinal study and cost-benefit analysis of the effect of early treatment of posterior crossbites in the primary dentition. Eur J Orthod 1992;14: 173–179.
33. Ladner PT, Muhl ZF. Changes concurrent with orthodontic treatment when maxillary expansion is a primary goal. Am J Orthod Dentofac Orthop 1995;108:184–193.
34. Velazquez P, Benito E, Bravo LA. Rapid maxillary expansion. A study of the long-term effects. Am J Orthod Dentofac Orthop 1996;109:361–367.
35. Thörne N. Experiences on widening the median maxillary suture. Trans Europ Orthod Soc 1956;32:279–290.
36. Haas AJ. Palatal expansion: just the beginning of dentofacial orthopedics. Am J Orthod 1970;57:219–55.
37. Byrum AG, Jr. Evaluation of anterior-posterior and vertical skeletal change vs. dental change in rapid palatal expansion cases as studied by lateral cephalograms. Am J Orthod 1971;60:419.
38. Persson M. Closure of facial sutures: A preliminary report. Trans Europ Orthod Soc 1976;52:249–253.
39. Davis WM, Kronman JH. Anatomical changes induced by splitting of the midpalatal suture. Angle Orthod 1969;39: 126–32.
40. Haas AJ. Long-term posttreatment evaluation of rapid palatal expansion. Angle Orthod 1980;50:189–217.
41. McNamara JA, Jr. An orthopedic approach to the treatment of Class III malocclusion in young patients. J Clin Orthod 1987;21:598–608.
42. McNamara JA, Jr, Brudon WL. Orthodontic and orthopedic treatment in the mixed dentition. Ann Arbor: Needham Press, 1993.
43. Sarver DM, Johnston MW. Skeletal changes in vertical and anterior displacement of the maxilla with bonded rapid palatal expansion appliances. Am J Orthod Dentofac Orthop 1989;95:462–466.
44. Memikoglu TUT, Iseri H. Effects of a bonded rapid maxillary expansion appliance during orthodontic treatment. Angle Orthod 1999;69:251–256.
45. Linder-Aronson S, Lindgren J. The skeletal and dental effects of rapid maxillary expansion. Br J Orthod 1979;6: 25–29.
46. Stockfish H. Rapid expansion of the maxilla-success and relapse. Trans Europ Orthod Soc 1969;45:469–481.
47. Timms DJ. An occlusal analysis of lateral maxillary expansion with mid-palatal suture opening. Dent Pract 1968; 18:435–440.
48. Timms DJ. Long-term follow-up of cases treated by rapid maxillary expansion. Trans Eur Orthod Soc 1976;52: 211–215.
49. Herberger TA. Rapid palatal expansion: long term stability and periodontal implications.: Unpublished Master's thesis, Department of Orthodontics, University of Pennsylvania, Philadelphia, 1987.
50. Moussa R, O' Reilly MT, Close JM. Long-term stability of rapid palatal expander treatment and edgewise mechanotherapy. Am J Orthod Dentofac Orthop 1995;108: 478–88.
51. Shapiro PA. Mandibular dental arch form and dimension.

Treatment and postretention changes. Am J Orthod 1974; 66:58–70.
52. Bishara SE, Jakobsen JR, Treder JE, Stasi MJ. Changes in the maxillary and mandibular tooth size-arch length relationship from early adolescence to early adulthood. A longitudinal study. Am J Orthod Dentofac Orthop 1989; 95:46–59.
53. Bishara SE, Treder JE, Jakobsen JR. Facial and dental changes in adulthood. Am J Orthod Dentofac Orthop 1994;106:175–186.
54. Little RM. Stability and relapse of dental arch alignment. Br J Orthod 1990;17:235–241.
55. Carter GA, McNamara JA, Jr. Longitudinal dental arch changes in adults. Am J Orthod Dentofac Orthoped 1998;114:88–99.
56. Spillane LM. Arch dimensional changes in patients treated with maxillary expansion during the mixed dentition. Unpublished Master's thesis, Department of Orthodontics and Pediatric Dentistry, The University of Michigan, Ann Arbor, 1990.
57. Brust EW. Arch dimensional changes concurrent with expansion in the mixed dentition. Ann Arbor: Unpublished Master's thesis, Department of Orthodontics and Pediatric Dentistry, The University of Michigan, 1992.
58. Wendling LK. Short-term skeletal and dental effects of the acrylic splint rapid maxillary expansion appliance. Ann Arbor: Unpublished Master's thesis, Department of Orthodontics and Pediatric Dentistry, The University of Michigan, 1997.
59. Fenderson FA. Long-term post-retention comparison of two methods of maxillary expansion. Ann Arbor: Unpublished Master's thesis, Department of Orthodontics and Pediatric Dentistry, The University of Michigan, 1998.
60. Wright NS. A comparison of the treatment effects of the Schwarz appliance and the lower lingual holding arch. Ann Arbor: Unpublished Master's Thesis, Department of Orthodontics and Pediatric Dentistry, The University of Michigan, 2000.
61. Cameron CG. Short-term and long-term effects of rapid maxillary expansion: A posteroanterior cephalometric and morphometric study. Ann Arbor: Unpublished Master's thesis, Department of Orthodontics and Pediatric Dentistry, The University of Michigan, 2000.
62. Spillane LM, McNamara JA, Jr. Maxillary adaptations following expansion in the mixed dentition. Sem Orthod 1995;1:176–187.
63. Brust EW, McNamara JA, Jr. Arch dimensional changes concurrent with expansion in mixed dentition patients. In: Trotman CA, McNamara JA, Jr, eds. Orthodontic treatment: Outcome and effectiveness. Ann Arbor: Monograph 30, Craniofacial Growth Series, Center for Human Growth and Development, The University of Michigan, 1995.
64. Chang JY, McNamara JA, Jr, Herberger TA. A longitudinal study of skeletal side-effects induced by rapid maxillary expansion. Am J Orthod Dentofac Orthop 1997;112: 330–337.
65. McNamara JA, Jr. Maxillary transverse deficiency. Amer J Orthod Dentofac Orthop 2000;117:567-570.
66. Moyers RE, Van der Linden FPGM, Riolo ML, McNamara JA, Jr. Standards of human occlusal development. Ann Arbor: Monograph 5, Craniofacial Growth Series, Center for Human Growth and Development, University of Michigan, 1976.
67. McGill JS, McNamara JA, Jr. Treatment and post-treatment effects of rapid maxillary expansion and facial mask therapy. In: McNamara JA, Jr, ed. Growth modification: What works, what doesn't and why. Ann Arbor: Monograph 36, Craniofacial Growth Series, Center for Human Growth and Development, University of Michigan, 1999.
68. Dellinger EL. A preliminary study of anterior maxillary displacement. Am J Orthod 1973;63:509–516.
69. Hartgerink DV. The effect of rapid maxillary expansion on nasal airway resistance: a one-year follow-up. Ann Arbor: Unpublished Master's thesis, Department of Orthodontics, The University of Michigan, 1986.
70. Vanarsdall RL, Jr. Personal communication, 1992.

Chapter 8
THE VERTICAL DIMENSION

With Frans P.G.M. van der Linden

The vertical dimension of the face has been the most difficult to modify clinically, with a multitude of orthodontic, orthopedic, and surgical interventions suggested over the years for the correction of associated skeletal, dentoalveolar, and neuromuscular abnormalities. Problems in the vertical dimension include open bite (Fig. 8-1) and deep bite (Fig. 8-2) malocclusions and also facial disfigurations.

Vertical malocclusions and disfigurations result from the interaction of many different etiological factors, some identified easily, others not. Studies of open bite have implicated many potential causes, including faulty postural performance of the associated musculature,[1-4] digit sucking habits,[5-10] tongue activity,[11-15] lymphatic tissue and obstructed nasorespiratory function,[7,9,16-18] unfavorable growth patterns,[6,19-21] imbalances between jaw posture, occlusal and eruptive forces and head position,[22] mental retardation,[9] and heredity.[10,23-25]

Similarly, a number of factors have been cited regarding the development of deep bite, including overeruption of the maxillary incisors,[26-28] incisor angulation,[28-32] width of the anterior teeth,[29,33] excessive overjet,[34] undereruption of the molars,[26,27,30,35] mandibular ramus height,[30] vertical facial type,[35,36] and failure of natural eruption.[37,38] The broad nature of the suggested etiologies, combined with the numerous proposed treatments, indicates the complexity of this subject area.

Dental and particularly skeletal vertical dysplasias are clinical problems for which there are many treatment options that have varying degrees of effectiveness, with certain types of problems occasionally defying conservative treatment, regardless of the efforts made by the clinician, as is illustrated by the unfavorable posttreatment growth changes shown in Figure 8-3.

TYPES OF VERTICAL MALOCCLUSION

Vertical malocclusions may be described according to the nature of the overlap of the maxillary and mandibular anterior teeth. Such problems can be divided into those that are limited to the dentoalveolar area and those that predominantly are of skeletal nature. Johnston[39] notes, however, that the division of these malocclusions into skeletal and dentoalveolar is arbitrary, in that virtually all so-called "skeletal" measures involve the existence and effects of the teeth.

If only dentoalveolar structures are involved, the terms *open bite* and *deep bite* are used. If skeletal structures are involved, the types of vertical facial patterns can be described as *hyperdivergent* and *hypodivergent*.[40] These vertical dysplasias clinically have been termed *long face syndrome*[41-43] and *short face syndrome*,[44] respectively. Generally, facial patterns with a mandibular plane angle* greater than 30° are considered hyperdivergent, and less than 20° hypodivergent.[45,46]

---

*For the purpose of this discussion, the mandibular plane angle is described relative to the Frankfort horizontal plane. If the MP-SN angle was measured, this angle is reduced by seven degrees to approximate the corresponding MP-FH value.

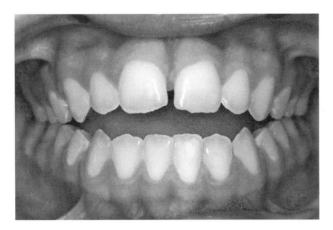

Figure 8-1. Intraoral view of patient with an anterior open bite that extends anteriorly from the maxillary premolars to the canines and the incisors.

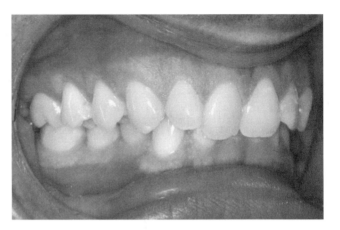

Figure 8-2. Intraoral view of a patient with an impinging overbite. The labial surfaces of the mandibular incisors are not visible. A posterior crossbite also is present in the premolar region.

The most current data[47,48] (Table 8-1) indicate that about half of the U.S. population has a normal vertical overlap of the incisors (0–2 mm). The overall prevalence of anterior open bite, defined as an absence of vertical overlap, is 3% in whites, 7% in blacks, and 2% in Mexican-Americans, with an average prevalence of 3%. There is no appreciable difference in the occurrence of open bite among the three age groups studied.

The prevalence of deep bite is greater in whites, *i.e.*, 52% in Caucasians as opposed to 41% in Mexican-Americans and 37% in Blacks (Table 8-1). Severe and extreme overbite is observed twice as frequently in European Americans than in African Americans or Mexican Americans.

Overview of Open Bite

Non-occlusion

Traditionally, the term open bite* has been used for conditions in which opposing teeth do not overlap.[49–52] Van der Linden, however, has indicated that the overlap criterion is arbitrary and is associated with the sagittal relation between the teeth involved. In essence, the absence of an occlusal stop between the teeth with their antagonists or opposing gingiva is of greater significance.[53] Absence of such a stop means that the eruption process has been arrested by one or more factors. The same view was expressed by Moyers,[54] who stated that it is most important to use the term "open bite" for all conditions characterized by the absence of an occlusal stop.

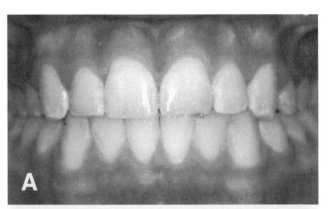

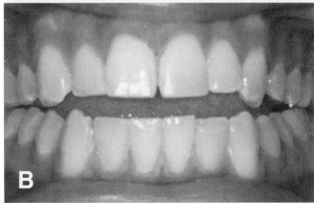

Figure 8-3. Intraoral views of a patient who exhibited an unexpected opening of the bite following routine two phase orthodontic treatment. *A*, Post-treatment. *B*, Two years post-treatment. The bite opened anteriorly during the retention period, while the posterior teeth erupted further. A posterior bite block then was used in an attempt to intrude the posterior teeth, but this treatment was unsuccessful. The patient ultimately underwent a LeFort I osteotomy, with the post-surgical occlusion essentially the same as shown in *A*.

*Just as there is confusion regarding the classification and etiology of open bite, so is there also about the spelling of the word. We have chosen to spell "open bite" as two words, although various other spellings have appeared in the literature (*i.e.*, openbite, open-bite)

VERTICAL DIMENSION

Table 8-1. Percent of US population with vertical occlusal discrepancies (data from NHANES III)[48]

Vertical Overlap (mm)	Age Groups			All Ages			
	All racial/ethnic groups			White	Black	Mexican American	Total
	8–11	12–17	18–50				
Openbite							
−4 (extreme)	0.3	0.2	0.1	0.1	0.7	0.0	0.1
−3 to −4 (severe)	0.6	0.5	0.5	0.4	1.3	0.0	0.5
0 to −2 (moderate)	2.7	2.8	2.7	2.4	4.6	2.1	2.7
Ideal							
0 to 2	40.2	45.0	49.0	45.5	56.4	56.5	47.5
Deepbite							
3 to 4 (moderate)	36.2	34.7	32.5	34.0	28.5	32.6	33.1
5 to 7 (severe)	18.8	15.5	13.4	15.7	7.5	8.7	14.2
>7 (extreme)	1.2	1.3	1.8	1.9	0.9	0.0	1.7

In the international literature, however, this recommendation has not been implemented, and the term "open bite" still is used only for conditions without vertical overlap. Generally, to avoid further confusion and misunderstanding, Van der Linden has suggested the term *non-occlusion* for situations with vertical overlap and yet the absence of an occlusal stop. Accordingly, the recently published *Glossary of Orthodontic Terms*[55] defines *non-occlusion* as any situation in which the teeth do not have maximum contact with their antagonists in habitual occlusion. *Anterior non-occlusion* (Fig. 8-4A) occurs in the incisor area and usually is associated with some degree of overlap of the incisors, as observed often in patients with Class II, division 1 malocclusion. *Posterior non-occlusion* (Fig. 8-4B) can occur in the premolar or molar region, with great variation occurring in the number of teeth and the occlusal surfaces involved. In *total non-occlusion*, the tongue is positioned between the opposing teeth most of the time.[55]

Non-occlusions are more common than open bites. That holds true for the anterior and posterior regions. Frequently, however, these relationships do not receive the attention they deserve in diagnosis and treatment planning. In the remaining part of this chapter, non-occlusions will not be mentioned separately, but are included in the concept of dental open bites.

Open Bite

The *Glossary of Orthodontic Terms*[55] defines open bite as a developmental or acquired malocclusion whereby no vertical overlap exists between maxillary and mandibular anterior teeth (*anterior open bite;* Fig. 8-5) or posterior teeth (*posterior open bite;* Fig. 8-6). The latter are caused by tongue interposition or by disturbances in eruption (*e.g.*, ankylosis). Posterior (lateral) open bites rarely are due to primary failure of eruption.[56] Defects in eruption often are associated with various craniofacial syndromes, including cleidocranial dysplasia and Carpenter's syndrome.

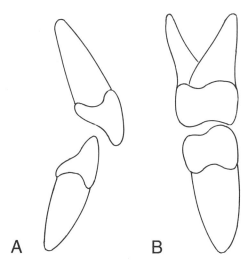

Figure 8-4. Non-occlusion. *A,* In anterior non-occlusion, the anterior teeth overlap vertically but do not contact. *B,* In posterior non-occlusion, the posterior teeth also overlap vertically but do not occlude. (After Daskalogiannakis.[55])

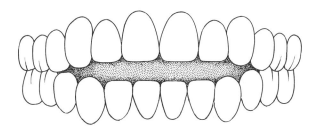

Figure 8-5. Anterior open bite. (After Daskalogiannakis.[55])

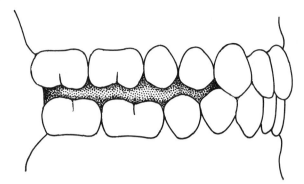

Figure 8-6. Posterior open bite. (After Daskalogiannakis.[55])

An open bite without facial disfiguration is classified as a *dental open bite*[55,57] (Fig. 8-7) and frequently is associated with a digital sucking habit and/or tongue interposition. The characteristics of a dental open bite include problems typically restricted to the anterior teeth and immediately associated hard and soft tissue structures without remarkable cephalometric findings (Fig. 8-8).[51]

In contrast, an open bite associated with a divergence of the skeletal planes is termed a *skeletal open bite* or *apertognathia*.[55,57,58] Such patients present significant vertical (and often anteroposterior and transverse) skeletal imbalances (Fig. 8-9). The latter type of malocclusion generally does not improve with growth and is difficult to treat, except by way of orthognathic surgery, or in some instances by use of posterior intrusive forces.[59]

The characteristics of a skeletal open bite occur throughout the craniofacial region. The major indicators of a skeletal relationship that predispose an individual to a skeletal open bite pattern are a short mandibular ramus and a downward rotation of the posterior part of the maxilla.[60] These relationships lead to a downward and backward rotation of the mandible, relative mandibular retrognathia, and anterior open bite (Fig. 8-9). Other characteristics of a skeletal open bite include increased lower anterior facial height, increased total anterior facial height, increased gonial, mandibular plane and occlusal plane angles, decreased palatal plane angle, occasional maxillary retrognathia, and increased vertical maxillary and mandibular dentoalveolar dimensions.[6,24,45,60–68]

Proffit and colleagues[69] note that, although increased lower anterior facial height exacerbates the problem by adding a skeletal element, about one-third of patients seeking surgical correction of long-face syndrome have a normal or excessive overbite, rather than an open bite. This type of occlusion is an indication of the compensatory dental eruption that can occur in these patients.

This observation by Proffit and colleagues[69] illustrates that the long face syndrome and the dental open bite are

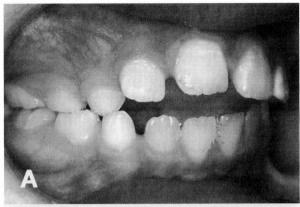
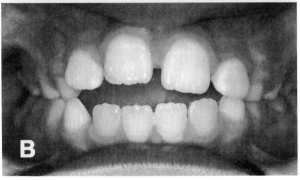

Figure 8-7. Intraoral view of a girl with a dental open bite due to a thumb sucking habit. The posterior teeth are not involved. She sucked her right thumb; note the slight asymmetry in arch form.

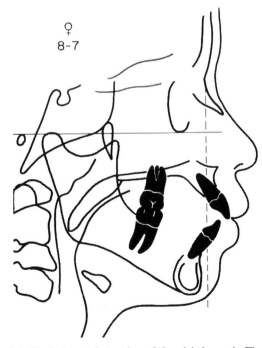

Figure 8-8. Cephalometric tracing of the girl shown in Fig. 8-7. Generally, she has a normal facial pattern, with a mandibular plane angle of 26° relative to the Frankfort horizontal plane. A tendency toward bialveolar protrusion also is present in this patient of European-American ancestry.

VERTICAL DIMENSION

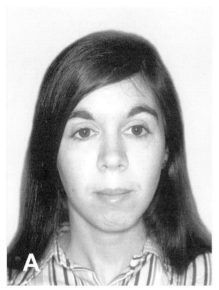 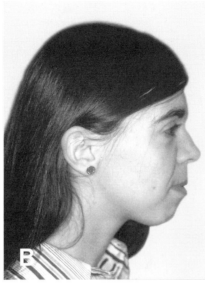 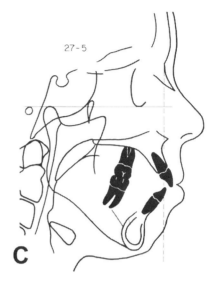

Figure 8-9. Twenty-seven year old female with skeletal open bite. *A*, Frontal view. *B*, Lateral view. *C*, Cephalometric tracing. She has a steep mandibular plane angle, an increased lower anterior facial height, and a hyperactive mentalis muscle when the lips are closed.

different entities. Indeed, the facial disfiguration seen in skeletal open bites can be found without the presence of dental open bites; however, in most instances, skeletal open bite is combined with dental open bite.

In studies examining the differences between faces with increased and normal vertical dimensions, the muscles of mastication have been analyzed. Magnetic resonance imaging (MRI) revealed that the size of the jaw muscles in long face subjects was up to 30% smaller than in normal individuals, whereas the position of the muscles was comparable in both groups.[70] Maximum bite force in long face subjects, however, was roughly half that in normal subjects.[71] The variation in long face and normal jaw geometry explained only half of the differences in their average maximum bite force.[71,72] Muscle fiber-type composition may account for the remaining differences.[73,74]

Extreme skeletal open bites often are associated with craniofacial malformations, such as the Crouzon's syndrome patient shown in Figure 8-10, in whom there are gross imbalances in skeletal structures in all three dimensions of the face. These types of problems are addressed only with aggressive craniofacial surgery, including distraction osteogenesis.[75–81]

Overview of Deep Bite

Patients with deep bite represent the other end of the spectrum, with vertical deficiencies that simply may be related to the overeruption of the anterior teeth or may be associated with skeletal and neuromuscular problems, such as short lower anterior facial height and overclosure. Some problems associated with a decreased vertical dimension may go unrecognized by the clinician, as mandibular skeletal retrusion often is camouflaged by a decreased lower anterior facial height,[82] resulting, for example, in an ANB angle that may fall within a clinically acceptable range.

In theory, patients with deep bites can be differentiated into *dental deep bites* and those with *short face syndrome*. Both features can occur together, but each can be present without the other.

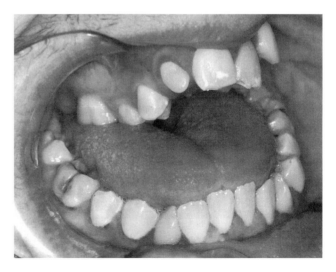

Figure 8-10. Extreme open bite in a patient with Crouzon's syndrome. The patient has occlusal contact only on the terminal molars.

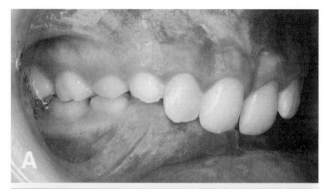

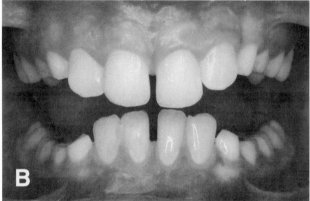

Figure 8-11. Intraoral views of a patient with excessive eruption of the maxillary and mandibular anterior teeth. *A*, The patient has an impinging overbite. *B*, The curve of Spee is accentuated.

A normal occlusion is characterized by a vertical and horizontal relationship of the anterior teeth of about 2 mm, as measured from the incisal edges.[49] If a patient has a normal vertical skeletal relationship, but excessive overlap of the teeth anteriorly (Fig. 8-2), a *dental* deep bite is present, as often is observed in Class II, division 2 malocclusion.

A deep bite can be characterized by an *impinging* overbite, a situation in which there is an overeruption of both the maxillary and mandibular anterior teeth (Fig. 8-11*A*) and an accentuated curve of Spee (Fig. 8-11*B*). In this type of deep bite, the mandibular incisors often contact the palatal tissue behind the maxillary anterior teeth, occasionally resulting in long-term periodontal breakdown. Such a condition can exist in a patient with a normal vertical skeletal configuration, but it also occurs in patients with vertical skeletal deficiencies.

Skeletal deep bite typically is characterized by a short lower anterior facial height and overclosure, as is illustrated by the 37-year-old male presenting with reduced vertical facial dimensions and mandibular skeletal retrusion shown in Figure 8-12. The cephalometric evaluation (Fig. 8-12*C*) reveals a short lower anterior facial height (−11 mm compared to ideal values), a low mandibular plane angle, and mandibular overclosure.

Overclosure occurs when the mandible closes from its rest position through an excessive interocclusal clearance or freeway space, resulting in a short lower anterior facial height relative to upper facial height.[83] A freeway space greater than 2–3 mm is considered an indication of overclosure.[84-86] A significant correlation between deep bite and diminished lower anterior facial height has been found in both children and adults.[67, 87, 88]

Linder-Aronson and Woodside[89] have proposed that this excessive freeway space seen in overclosure may represent a lack of vertical development in the posterior segments. A failure in posterior dentoalveolar development can occur if there is interference with the normal process of tooth eruption. For example, the habitual postural interposition of the tongue or cheeks between the occlusal surfaces of the posterior teeth can interfere with normal tooth eruption, leading to overclosure.[56,83,90,91]

Hypertonic muscles of mastication and hyperactive muscles of mastication also have been suggested as etiologic factors leading to overclosure.[83] Hypertonicity is a chronic low-grade activity, whereas hyperactivity is transient in nature. Ueda and co-workers[92] recorded the activity of the muscles of mastication for an extended period and found that the activities of the masseter, temporalis, and digastric muscles during the day consisted primarily of low-amplitude bursts that may be related to craniofacial morphology. They reported a negative correlation between masseter and digastric activities and the vertical dimension of the face, whereas temporal muscle activity was correlated positively with long lower anterior facial height.

A number of other investigators have examined the activity of the masticatory musculature relative to the reduced vertical dimension of the face.[85,93-95] These investigators report that, in overclosed subjects, strong activity occurs in the temporalis and masseter muscles during swallowing. Further, the activity recorded when biting in the intercuspal position and during chewing was correlated with the facial features of short-faced subjects. In addition, other studies have documented higher maximum bite force in subjects with reduced or normal vertical dimensions when compared to subjects with increased facial dimensions.[70,71,96]

PATTERNS OF GROWTH IN VERTICAL DYSPLASIA

A number of factors are related to the development of vertical skeletal dysplasias. Among the most obvious are the growth, remodeling, and rotation of the mandible and maxilla during growth. This discussion focuses on *how* the jaws rotate during growth in various

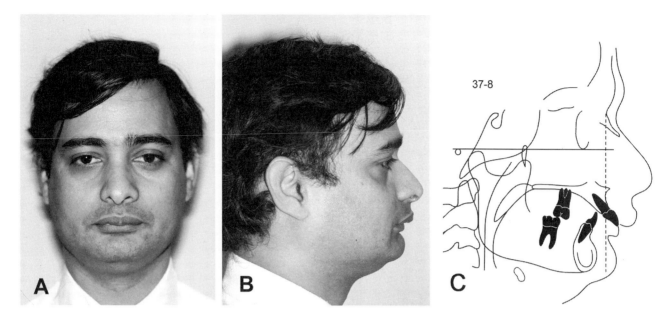

Figure 8-12. Patient with short face syndrome. *A*, Frontal view. *B*, Lateral view. *C*, Cephalometric tracing. This 37-year-old male has a Class II, division 1 malocclusion with an impinging overbite and flared maxillary incisors. His lower anterior facial height is 11 mm below normal values,[82] which helps camouflage significant mandibular skeletal retrusion.

vertical facial types; later, the issue of *why* specific types of growth rotations occur will be addressed.

Mandibular Development

One of the key factors associated with the development of open bite and deep bite malocclusions is the pattern of the growth of the mandible. The implant studies of Björk[97-102] have shown that the direction of mandibular growth varies greatly (Fig. 8-13). Mostly the direction of condylar growth is superior with some anterior component (Fig. 8-13*AB*). A posteriorly directed vector of growth (Fig. 8-13*C*) is observed less frequently.[57]

The implant studies of Björk provide a unique look at the complexity of the growth process in both open bite and deep bite individuals. For example, the subject from the Björk studies shown in Figure 8-14 can be characterized by maxillary and mandibular skeletal retrusion and an increased lower anterior facial height. The mandibular plane angle is steep and an anterior open bite is present. The direction of mandibular growth is vertical. Patients with this type of skeletal discrepancy typically have Class I or Class II, division 1 malocclusions and an open bite or open bite tendency.

Superimposition on metallic implants in the mandible allows for the evaluation of the direction and extent of condylar growth in this individual (Fig. 8-15). Instead of the typical vertical and slightly forward growth of the condyle, the direction of condylar growth is posterior and superior, leading primarily to vertical movement of the chin point during growth. The associated pattern of dental eruption generally is vertical, and in some individuals, the anterior teeth may become more retroclined during growth. Late mandibular anterior crowding often is seen in patients with this type of growth pattern.[57]

The opposite type of growth pattern is observed in another one of Björk's subjects (Fig. 8-16), a boy who had a Class II, division 2 type of malocclusion. He had a normal to slightly retruded position of the maxilla and slight mandibular skeletal retrusion that was camouflaged by a short lower anterior facial height. A marked mentolabial sulcus persisted during the six-year observation period. Patients with this type of skeletal pattern typically have a Class I deep bite or Class II, division 2 type of malocclusion.

Superimposition on the implants within the mandible of this subject (Fig. 8-17) indicated that mesial movement of the mandibular teeth occurred during eruption. In fact, patients with a deep bite skeletal configuration typically undergo a considerable amount of mesial migration of both the maxillary and mandibular dentition, along with proclination of the mandibular incisors.

Growth Rotation and Vertical Dysplasias

The vertical growth of the face is related closely to mandibular growth rotation. The differences between long face and short face individuals are not only the effect of differences in the pattern of mandibular growth,

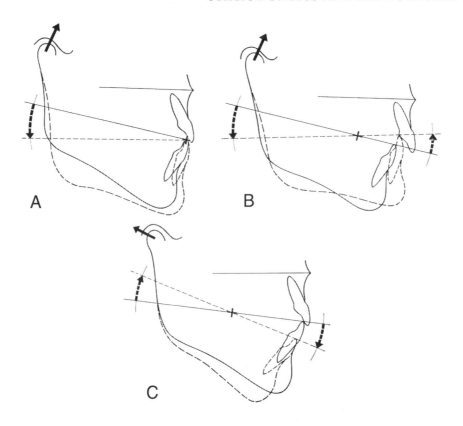

Figure 8-13. Three types of mandibular rotation during growth. *A*, forward mandibular rotation with the center of rotation at the incisal edges of the mandibular incisors. The direction of condylar growth is upward and forward. *B*, Forward rotation with the center at the premolars. *C*, backward rotation with the center at the occluding molars. The direction of condylar growth is backward and upward, and there is an backward and downward rotation of the mandible. (Modified from Björk and Skieller.[102])

but also are related to differential development of lower anterior and posterior facial heights.[45] These differences in facial heights are associated with rotational growth or positional changes of the mandible that affect chin position.

Factors that determine the increase in lower anterior facial height include the eruption of the maxillary and mandibular posterior teeth and the amount of sutural lowering of the maxilla.[57] Posterior facial height is determined by condylar growth as well as by a slight lowering of the temporal fossa.[45,57] Vertical condylar growth that exceeds the amount of vertical tooth eruption is associated with forward rotation of the mandible. On the other hand, tooth eruption that exceeds vertical condylar growth is associated with downward and backward mandibular rotation. Schudy[19] has suggested that the inclination of the mandibular plane is a good indicator of mandibular rotation. For example, a small mandibular plane angle (MPA) indicates that the mandible had rotated forward, whereas a large MPA is a sign of backward rotation.

Patients with an upward and forward direction of condylar growth often have a reduced lower anterior facial height. If this pattern is associated with a malocclusion, deep bite typically is a component, and rotation of the mandible occurs that results in a horizontal displacement of the chin anteriorly.

Maxillary Development

Although much emphasis is placed on mandibular rotation, rotation of the maxilla occurs as well. Basal rotation of the maxilla is concealed by surface remodeling that maintains the orientation of the palatal plane.[102–104] Unfortunately, the normal pattern of maxillary rotation does not always occur in patients with vertical growth problems.[105] Lavergne and Gasson[106] hypothesize that if the posterior part of the maxilla rotates downward posteriorly or upward anteriorly, space for the eruption of the posterior teeth is reduced, space for the eruption of the maxillary anterior teeth increases, and there is a tendency toward an anterior open bite. Conversely, if the anterior part of the maxilla rotates in a downward direction, a deep bite anteriorly may result.

VERTICAL DIMENSION

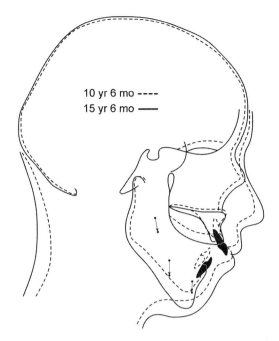

Figure 8-14. Subject from Björk's implant studies[98] with a characteristic vertical facial growth pattern. The arrows indicate the direction of implant movement. The maxilla and mandible rotated downward and backward during growth, resulting in an increase in the mandibular plane angle and lower anterior facial height. (Modified from Björk[98] and Nielsen.[57])

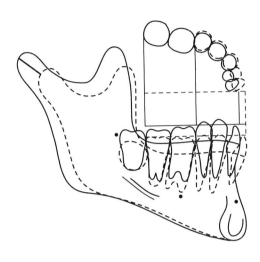

Figure 8-15. Mandibular growth and dentoalveolar development in the subject shown in Figure 8-14. The direction of condylar growth is mainly posterior, and the direction of tooth eruption is almost vertical. The mandibular incisors are erupting posteriorly, resulting in increased crowding with time. (Modified from Björk[98] and Nielsen.[57])

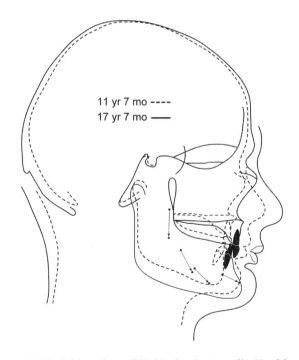

Figure 8-16. Subject from Björk's implant studies[98] with a characteristic skeletal deep bite pattern. The arrows indicate the direction of implant movement. Both the maxilla and the mandible rotated forward during growth. No change in the anterior occlusion occurred during this period. (Modified from Björk[98] and Nielsen.[57])

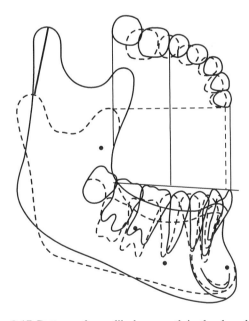

Figure 8-17. Pattern of mandibular growth in the deep bite patient shown in Figure 8-16. The condyle grows in an upward and slightly forward direction, and there is a pronounced mesial eruption of the mandibular teeth. Extensive remodeling of the lower border of the mandible masks about half of the actual mandibular rotation during growth. (Modified from Björk[98] and Nielsen.[57])

ROLE OF THE SOFT TISSUE

Interest in the role of soft tissue in the formation of malocclusion can be traced back to Angle.[107] Angle believed that certain types of malocclusion as well as relapse following treatment was caused by forces on the teeth resulting from an improper soft tissue environment, especially "mouthbreathing." Others also stressed the importance of the soft tissue, recognizing the relationship between tongue posture and anterior open bite.[5, 108–110]

During the 1950s and 1960s, some clinicians reincarnated and popularized the idea that open bite was caused by tongue thrusting and abnormal swallowing habits. Particular emphasis was placed on abnormal patterns of tongue behavior, with "tongue thrust," a deviant pattern of swallowing, considered a major factor in opening the bite.[111,112] Some treatment approaches to open bite were aimed at retraining or restricting the action of the tongue[11–13,111,113–115] and correcting speech patterns.[116,117] On the other hand, Proffit and Mason[118] reported that a poor correlation existed between tongue thrust and open bite malocclusion. Their recommendations concerning myofunctional therapy were more guarded and pessimistic, stating in general that myofunctional therapy was not effective. Other data have shown that so-called "tongue thrust" patterns are ten times as prevalent as are the malocclusions they are purported to cause.[119,120]

The research of Proffit[105,118] has demonstrated that such phasic activities as swallowing, chewing, and speaking have no impact on the morphology of the dentition. Conversely, postural alterations leading to changes in lip and tongue resting pressure and posture play a significant role. Both orthodontic clinical experience and laboratory studies indicate that there is a threshold for duration somewhere between 4–8 hours per day, below which force has no effect on tooth position. On the other hand, resting pressures apparently have an effect, even if the forces are light. Proffit[22] has stressed, however, that resting pressures rarely are perfectly balanced, and "active stabilization" from metabolic activity in the periodontal ligament probably plays a role in maintaining equilibrium of forces in the orofacial region, particularly regarding the positions of the anterior teeth.

Proffit[105] also described the forces contributing to vertical equilibrium. Teeth erupt until they reach occlusal contact or are stopped otherwise and continue to erupt as long as the face grows vertically. The teeth remain in the same vertical orientation after growth has ceased, but retain the potential for eruption if their antagonists are lost.

The findings of tooth eruption studies[121–123] indicate that the factors involved in vertical equilibrium are similar to those involved in anteroposterior and transverse equilibrium. Also regarding tooth eruption, short acting forces have no effect, but long lasting forces do. The studies of Proffit and Sellers[124] indicate that the force has to be active for at least 25% of the time, and that 50% time has about the same effect as a continuous force application.

The observations of Proffit and co-workers and their conclusions that short-lasting activities as speech, swallowing, and chewing have no impact on the morphology of the dentition, but that posture and resting pressure are predominant and of great clinical significance. Nevertheless, many clinicians do not seem to accept the consequences of these conclusions. Much emphasis still is placed on "tongue thrust." This deviant pattern of swallowing has to be considered as a secondary phenomenon that provides seal of the oral cavity, essential for the swallow in conditions of anterior open bite. Therefore, the "tongue thrust" is adaptive, not causal.

Tongue-inhibiting appliances were developed to counteract the forward movement of the tongue during function, including tongue-restraining devices[125] (Fig. 8-18). Graber[126] reported an initial 92% success rate with palatal crib treatment, but the occlusions of many patients relapsed following the removal of the "tongue-habit" appliance.[3]

Fränkel's experience with such appliances led him to examine patients who had relapsed following tongue crib treatment.[4] Fränkel first assumed that the relapse seen was due to too short of a treatment duration to "reeducate" tongue behavior, but he found that occlusal relapse occurred even after renewed treatment with the palatal crib appliance. In general, attempts to change the resting position of the tongue have met with little suc-

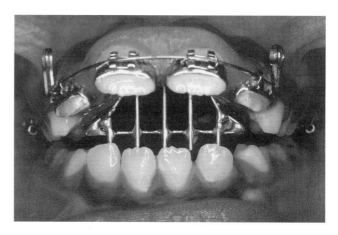

Figure 8-18. Intraoral view of a palatal tongue crib in a patient with an anterior open bite.

cess. That also applies to attempts to alter the activities of the tongue.[174]

Fränkel[4] discovered that some patients show a marked discrepancy between lower facial height and lip length. His observations were similar to those of Ballard,[127] who already in 1965 advocated paying more attention to the size and shape of the lips when evaluating habit behaviors. Ballard stated that too much emphasis was being placed on the role of tongue thrust in open bite malocclusions. Rather, he felt that the anterior postural position of the tongue appeared to compensate for the lack of an anterior oral seal formed by lip competency (Fig. 8-19), as indicated above. Indeed, if a proper lip seal is not maintained during normal functional activities, the tongue serves to seal the oral cavity through an adaptive change in postural position.

Fränkel's approach to the treatment of anterior open bite differs somewhat from that of Ballard, in that Ballard thought that lip incompetence was a consequence of a discrepancy between skeletal and soft tissue growth. Fränkel, on the other hand, concluded that a absence of competent oral seal was due to a lack of adequate postural activity of the lip-valve musculature[4] and advocated the initiation of a regimen of lip seal exercises to address such problems. (The use of lip seal exercises, as advocated by Fränkel[2,4] will be discussed later in this chapter.)

Fränkel[128-131] hypothesized that the deficiency of an oral seal was due, at least in part, to a "poor postural behavioral of the facial musculature, particularly in the lip area, even in cases of skeletal discrepancies associated with a steep mandibular plane." Thus, he instituted functional therapy with vestibular shields and lip seal training for anterior open bite patients. Fränkel observed that a normal overbite was obtained and remained stable, providing that a competent anterior oral seal also was established and maintained.

Fränkel and Fränkel[3] state that it seems reasonable to assume that, if a deviation in the postural activity of the orofacial musculature can result in skeletal open bite as well as other types of malocclusion, the improvement of faulty postural activity of the orofacial musculature might help correct the associated skeletal deformity. Thus, one of the Fränkel's underlying tenets when developing a therapeutic strategy was aimed at the establishment of a normal pattern of nasal breathing by correcting the lips-apart condition and faulty tongue posture.

To evaluate this hypothesis, Fränkel and Fränkel[3] evaluated the form-function relationship in patients with severe skeletal open bite. Serial lateral head films were taken of 30 patients and 11 untreated subjects, all of whom were characterized by what they termed "severe skeletal open bite." The patients were treated with lip-seal training and a function regulator appliance. During the 8-year interval, the values for the mandibular plane relative to sella-nasion on the palatal plane changed in the treated group and fell to within the normal range, as did the ratios of the anterior facial height to lower anterior facial height and anterior facial height to posterior facial height. In contrast, the same measurements for the untreated controls remained unchanged or became worse. In all patients treated with the FR appliance, ramus length increased more than did lower anterior facial height, if a competent oral seal was established.

Fränkel's emphasis on the postural activity of the

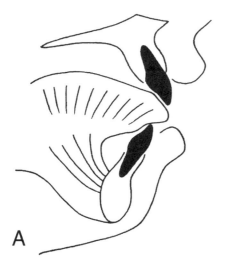 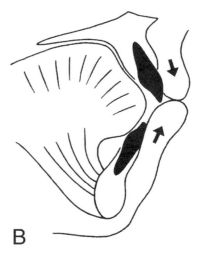

Figure 8-19. *A*, Incompetence of an anterior oral seal requires a compensatory interdental posture of the tongue. *B*, Lip seal training, as advocated by Fränkel,[2] is necessary to overcome an abnormal postural behavior of the tongue and to strengthen the lip musculature. (Modified from Fränkel and Fränkel.[4])

orofacial musculature has been supported by much of the research dealing with this issue. For example, as mentioned previously, Proffit[105] has shown that the influences of function on form are mediated almost entirely by the light but long-lasting pressures of soft tissues at rest, and posture is critically important in determining the pattern of resting pressures. In addition, the postural activity of the craniofacial musculature plays an integral part in maintaining the mandible in an adequate anteroposterior and vertical position, while stabilizing the tongue and posterior pharyngeal wall relationships. These postural activities are necessary for the maintenance of an adequate airway, as will be discussed in the next section of this chapter.

INFLUENCE OF NASORESPIRATORY FUNCTION

One proposed cause of vertical dysplasia is deviating neuromuscular function associated with an abnormal breathing pattern.[17,18,132–134] Physiologic adaptations to various types of upper respiratory obstruction (*e.g.*, constricted external nares, deviated septum, nasal polyps, enlarged adenoids, enlarged tonsils) initially may lead to altered functional activity of the muscles associated with respiration. It is hypothesized that this change in the level of postural activity of certain craniofacial muscles ultimately may lead to a change in craniofacial morphology, particularly in the vertical dimension.

Solow and Kreiborg[135] have proposed the *soft tissue stretching theory*, which postulates a relationship between airway obstruction and head posture relative to the cervical spine. Changes in the level of activity of certain craniofacial muscles leads to an extension of the head and airway maintenance. This alteration causes a stretching of the masticatory and facial muscles as well as the associated soft tissue. A prolonged obstruction of the airway can lead to skeletal remodeling and ultimately a change in craniofacial morphology.

The theory of Solow and Kreiborg[135] is representative of a discussion that has been ongoing for over a century, that being the relationship between an obstructed nasopharyngeal airway and craniofacial growth. This topic remains controversial, however, due in part to a lack of consensus regarding terminology (*e.g.*, "mouthbreathing") as well as conflicting evidence from clinical studies.

The classic clinical example of the possible relationship between airway obstruction and aberrant craniofacial growth is the type of patient described as having "adenoid facies"[107,136–140] (Fig. 8-20). These patients typically present a mouth-open posture, a small nose with button-like tip, nostrils that are small and poorly developed, a short upper lip, prominent maxillary incisors, a pouting lower lip, and a vacant facial expression. "Mouth-breathing" individuals classically have been described as possessing a narrow, V-shaped maxillary arch, a high palatal vault, proclined maxillary incisors, and a Class II occlusion. Proof is lacking, however, that the concept of adenoid facies is indeed valid. It also may be that one of the associated features of "adenoid facies" is the airway obstruction. A cause-effect relationship has not been demonstrated in humans.

Patients who have severe allergies often present with similar facial manifestations. In addition, they may have what are termed "allergic shiners" (Fig. 8-21), which represent a pooling of blood under the eyes, a sign of the allergic response.

Naso-Respiratory Physiology

The physiology of airway maintenance is well documented. When the nasal airway is obstructed, the respiratory system responds both behaviorally and physiologically, with compensations that tend to maintain an optimal level of air intake.[141,142] These responses follow the general rules of a homeostatic regulating system. Of particular relevance to this discussion is the response that deals with potential effects on craniofacial growth and development of postural compensations by oral structures whenever there is impairment of the nasal airway.[142]

Oral posture depends to a significant degree on the status of the nasal airway. Warren and co-workers[143] have shown that a nasal airway size of 18 mm^2 physically limits airflow (normal adult airway size is about 60–70 mm^2). Thus, when the cross-sectional area of the airway at its narrowest point is approximately 25% of the normal size, airflow is reduced significantly, and the nose can be considered severely obstructed.[142] Airways with a cross-sectional area above 40 mm^2 measured during relaxed breathing meet normal respiratory requirements without physical constraints.[144]

There is no direct correlation, however, between airway obstruction and mode of breathing. For example, an individual with an open mouth posture is not necessarily a mouth breather. If the tongue occludes the oral cavity or lingual palatal closure occurs, the oral cavity essentially is closed.[145] Warren[142] suggests an operational definition of breathing mode, with impairment occurring when the airway size is less than 40 mm^2.[143,146] Further, Warren[142] states that the term "mouthbreathing" should be used with some caution, because even

VERTICAL DIMENSION

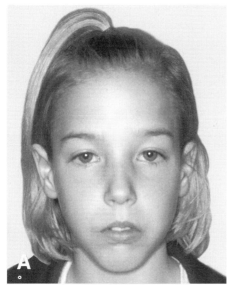

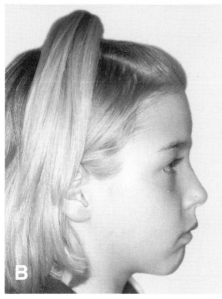

Figure 8-20. Girl with classic signs of "adenoid facies," including lips apart posture at rest, convex facial profile, and steep mandibular plane. *A*, Frontal view. *B*, Lateral view.

impaired nasal breathers demonstrate a wide range of nasal-oral volumes with each breath. Although some such individuals indeed may be oral breathers, others are predominantly oral, mixed, or even nasal breathers.

Johnston[147] and Rubin[148] have stated that mouthbreathing does not in itself cause altered facial growth. Rather, mouthbreathing may cause habitual mouth open posture, a proximal cause of long face syndrome. Posterior crossbite may occur because the tongue is lowered, leaving the constricting effect of the buccinator musculature unopposed. Dental eruption and vertical posterior alveolar growth are enhanced because the forces restraining these changes are reduced due to the chronic mouth open posture.

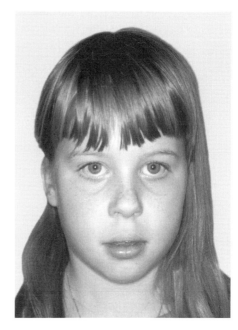

Figure 8-21. Girl with classic signs of allergy, including "allergic shiners" under the eyes.

Adenoid facies and a steep mandibular plane are frequent findings in patients with upper respiratory obstruction, but they are by no means the only types of adaptation that can occur. A low mandibular plane angle may result if the patient postures the tongue over the occlusal surfaces of the teeth in order to maintain an oral airway.[149] This type of patient may even exhibit a deep anterior overbite.

Experimental Studies of Respiratory Obstruction

As in many other areas of craniofacial biology, it often is difficult to detect basic biological relationships in clinical investigations. Thus, the relationship between airway obstruction and craniofacial growth has been addressed by experimental studies, the most definitive of which are those conducted by Harvold, Miller and associates[91,150–156] In these experiments, latex plugs were inserted into the nasal openings of young rhesus monkeys. The sudden change from nasal respiration to oral respiration (Fig. 8-22) involved the recruiting of some of the facial and masticatory musculature to serve as accessory muscles of respiration.

The first noticeable changes were functional in nature, in that the animals altered their patterns of neuromuscular activity in order to accomplish oral breathing. Individual monkeys met this challenge in different ways. Some of the animals learned to posture their mandible with a downward and backward (retrusive)

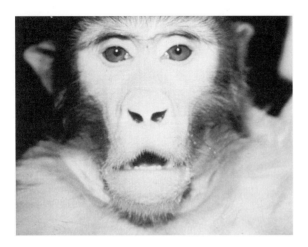

Figure 8-22. Harvold and co-workers[157] placed latex plugs in the nostrils of rhesus monkeys (*Macaca mulatta*). This type of airway obstruction changes the mode of breathing from nasal to oral respiration. The monkeys often assumed a facial expression that was similar to the "adenoid facies" appearance of humans. (Photograph courtesy of Egil Harvold.)

opening rotation. Some rhythmically lowered and raised their mandibles with each breath (Fig. 8-23). Still others postured their jaw in a downward and forward (protrusive) position, but each in its own way managed to breathe through its mouth.

Morphological changes gradually followed the postural changes, with soft tissue changes occurring first (Fig. 8-22). Notching of the upper lip and grooving of the tongue gradually develop in specific animals. Those animals augmenting the oral airway by pointing the tongue in a forward position also developed a moderate change in mandibular shape. The tongue itself became long and thin, and an anterior open bite developed. Moderate mandibular changes also were observed in those animals that lowered their mandible for each breath. Dramatic changes in mandibular morphology, particularly at the gonial region and at the chin, were produced in those animals that maintained a lowered mandibular postural position (Fig. 8-24).

Harvold[154] reported that the distance from nasion to the chin increased significantly in mouth-breathing animals, as did the distance from nasion to the hard palate. This change in the pattern of growth indicates that the lowering of the mandible was followed by a downward displacement of the maxilla. The lower border of the mandible became steeper and the gonial angle increased (Fig. 8-24). The most distinctive remodeling of the mandible occurred in the ramus, which maintained its normal relationship to the skull even when the chin assumed a lowered position. Harvold[157] speculated that the masticatory muscles attaching the ramus to the skull were relatively unaffected by the respiratory function and continued to maintain a normal

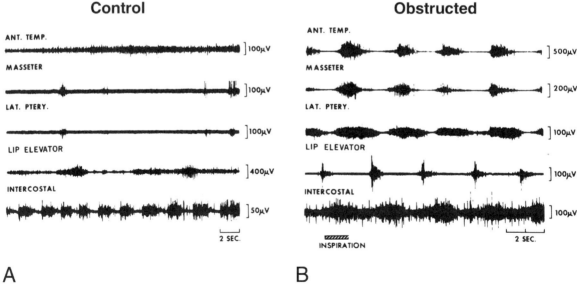

Figure 8-23. Electromyographic recordings of spontaneous activity in four craniofacial muscles and one primary respiratory muscle in the rhesus monkey.[152] *A*, Spontaneous activity with a few brief clenches and some upper lip movement in a control animal. The anterior temporalis muscle was tonically active. The lateral pterygoid was active during jaw closure and clenching. *B*, Spontaneous activity in a monkey adapted to mouth breathing that remained quiet except for periodic raising and lowering of the mandible. The jaw elevators were active during expiration as the mandible was raised. The lip elevator region demonstrated rhythmic activity in synchrony with the start of inspiration and while the upper lip was elevated rhythmically. The intercostals recording reflected the pattern of breathing. (Adapted from Miller and Vargervik.[152])

VERTICAL DIMENSION

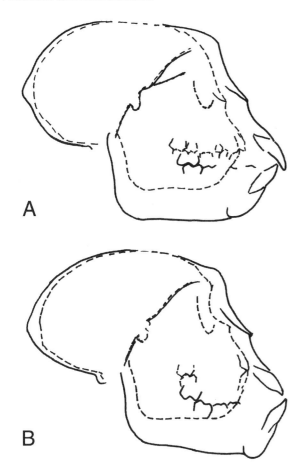

Figure 8-24. Superimposed cephalometric tracings of rhesus monkeys during a two-year interval. *A*, Control animal. *B*, Animal with nasal obstruction. (Adapted from Harvold.[157])

relationship to the ramus, whereas the mandible remodeled in response to the postural change.

What conclusions can be drawn from these experimental studies? First, every animal was subjected to essentially the same environmental insult, *i.e.,* the blockage of the nasal airway with nasal plugs; however, all animals did not adapt functionally in the same way. The nature of the structural changes produced by insertion of the nasal plugs depended on the unique neuromuscular adaptation of the individual animal.

Occlusal effects also varied. The animals that rotated their mandible in a posterior and inferior direction developed a Class I skeletal open bite or a Class II malocclusion. The animals that maintained an anterior position of the mandible developed a Class III malocclusion. Thus, a change in breathing pattern led to a variety of skeletal and dental deformities *in a species of animal that does not ordinarily develop malocclusions*. It was not the change in breathing pattern *per se* that caused the malocclusion. Rather, it appeared that the changes in related functional demands on the craniofacial muscles and their obligatory response were responsible for the altered craniofacial morphology.

If there is a relationship between nasal obstruction and the pattern of craniofacial growth, and if this interaction is an expression of the form-function relationship, it can be hypothesized that the removal of the causative obstruction might initiate a reversal of the change in function. Such a reversal then should be followed by a gradual corrective or positive change in the previously altered craniofacial configuration.

Miller and colleagues[158] measured changes cephalometrically and electromyographically (EMG) when the monkeys were forced to breathe orally, according to the Harvold protocol.[154] As discussed earlier, they reported an increase in lower anterior facial height, the mandibular plane angle, and the gonial angle, but the neuromuscular morphological changes were variable. The removal of the nasal obstructions two years later often reversed the morphological changes that had occurred during the oral respiration period, but Miller and co-workers[158] reported that the response was variable. The EMG recordings showed a non-uniform neuromuscular response to the removal of the nasal obstruction as well, with a number of animals not changing their new neuromuscular patterns at all.

From the investigations of the Harvold and Miller group, it is possible to derive a theoretical model of the influence of upper respiratory obstruction on craniofacial morphology, as is shown in Figure 8-25. Upper respiratory obstruction, whether following experimental placement of latex plugs in monkeys or from anatomical obstruction of the upper airway in humans, results in an alteration in the postural activity of the associated masticatory and facial musculature (Fig. 8-23), leading to long-term morphological changes (Fig. 8-24), the nature of which depends on the specific functional adaptations of the individual. If the obstruction subsequently is eliminated (*e.g.*, latex plugs removed, adenoidectomy, tonsillectomy), some subjects assume a more normal pattern of neuromuscular function, whereas others do not. In the latter, the habitual pattern of neuromuscular activity is continued in spite of the elimination of the obstruction. Further, superimposed on this relationship is the general level of postural activity, as regulated by the central nervous system (Fig. 8-25).

Clinical Studies of Respiratory Obstruction

From the beginning of the last century to the present, a number of prominent clinicians have given credence to the association between obstructed respiratory function and altered craniofacial growth,[107,139,148,159–163] whereas

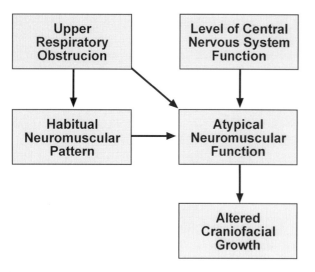

Figure 8-25. Flowchart of proposed relationship between obstructed respiratory function and altered craniofacial growth. A reduced nasal airway presumably leads to an altered pattern of muscle activity and subsequently altered craniofacial growth. Occasionally, the habitual pattern of muscle activity is maintained after surgery, resulting in little post-surgical skeletal change. In addition, the general level of neuromuscular activity mediated by the central nervous system is superimposed on this form-function relationship.

others have questioned this relationship.[164–167] Angle[107] included airway obstruction as an important etiological factor in Class II malocclusion, and Ketcham[168] recommended that patients see the rhinologist as well as the orthodontist.

The emphasis on the "adenoid facies" patient in the literature has been unfortunate in one sense, because it implies that all patients having these facial characteristics are mouth breathers and that all mouth breathers have these facial characteristics. This is not always the case.[169] Studies of clinical populations have indicated that obstructed respiratory function can be found in patients with a variety of facial types and occlusal configurations, a finding that is consistent with the animal studies discussed earlier.[170–172]

Retrospective studies of medical histories also have provided useful information on the relationship between airway problems and craniofacial morphology.[173] Analysis of data derived from a medical questionnaire given to patients with high mandibular plane angles and those with low mandibular plane angles showed that there was little difference in the incidence of allergic rhinitis, maxillary sinusitis, or deviated nasal septa between the two groups. Significant differences, however, were found in the incidence of enlarged adenoids or previous adenoidectomy. Nasopharyngeal impairment was noted in nearly two-thirds of the patients in the long-faced (high angle) group and in a quarter of the short-faced (low angle) group. The long-faced group also had a significantly higher incidence of symptoms of nasal obstruction due to undetermined causes. Cephalometric analysis of the two groups indicated that the nasopharyngeal cavity was smaller in the long-faced individuals, so that even moderate adenoid enlargement could cause marked symptoms of upper respiratory obstruction in these individuals.

Studies of the relationship of airway resistance to facial type also are relevant. Linder-Aronson and Backstrom[132] compared facial type and type of occlusion in nose breathers and habitual mouth breathers. They noted that children with long narrow faces have greater nasal resistance, on average, than those with short, wide faces; and that children with a high narrow palate tend to have a greater nasal resistance to air flow than those with a low, broad palate. No direct relationship between mouth breathing and type of occlusion could be found, particularly with regard to overbite and overjet.

In a follow-up study, Linder-Aronson[174] noted that the mouth-breathing individuals continued to have a significantly higher nasal resistance even after the use of nose drops. In both studies, variations in palatal height were notably greater in the mouth-breathing group than in the nose-breathing group.

These studies seem to indicate that there is a relationship between upper respiratory obstruction and the configuration of the craniofacial structures of a given individual, but that there is no one specific pattern that can be correlated directly with mouth breathing.

Airway Parameters and Facial Form

The relationship between airway parameters and facial form remains unclear. Some investigators[16,175,176] postulate a direct relationship between increased airway resistance and enlarged adenoid tissue. In these studies, airway resistance was estimated indirectly by the analysis of lateral cephalometric radiographs. Woodside and co-workers[177] assessed nasal obstruction in a sample of children by posterior rhinomanometry immediately post-adenoidectomy and five years post-adenoidectomy. They found that during the five-year post-treatment interval, there was a small but statistically significant increase in the amount of mandibular growth in children who had undergone adenoidectomy than in a control group; there was no difference in maxillary growth.

Conversely, studies comparing breathing pattern to dentofacial form demonstrate inconclusive results.[178–180] Ung and co-workers[180] found that, over a

VERTICAL DIMENSION

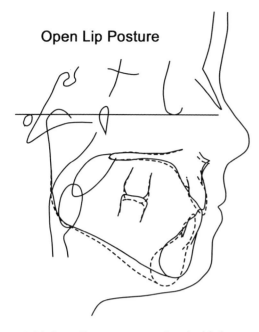

Figure 8-26. Open lip posture associated with features seen in the characteristic backward rotating growth pattern, a retrognathic face, and enlarged lower face height. This figure was constructed by incorporating the significant mean differences for lip posture in an arbitrarily chosen tracing and provides a general picture rather than a quantitative representation of the data. (From Trotman and co-workers.[18])

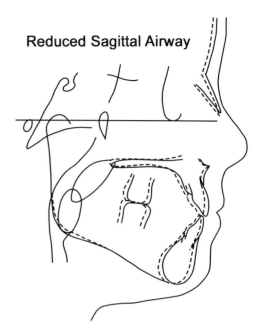

Figure 8-27. Skeletal pattern associated with a reduced sagittal airway—or larger adenoids—characterized by features of less horizontal growth of the face. This figure was constructed by incorporating the significant mean differences for the sagittal airway in an arbitrarily chosen tracing and provides a general picture rather than a quantitative representation of the data. (From Trotman and co-workers.[18])

24-hour period, subjects varied in their mode of breathing. They also found that nasal airway resistance was not correlated with either dental or skeletal variables.

Lip posture also has been used as a method of assessing airway resistance indirectly. It is hypothesized that individuals who have a more open lip posture also have increased nasal airway resistance.[18] Previous studies have demonstrated that children who have a more open lip posture also have larger mandibular and palatal plane angles,[181] decreased maxillary growth,[182] and increased lower anterior facial height.[183] Further, there have been reports of an association between head posture and airway size, but the results of these studies are inconclusive.[184,185]

Trotman and co-workers[18] assessed the separate associations of lip posture, sagittal airway size, and tonsil size with selected cephalometric measures. Clinical and cephalometric data from over 200 severely affected children who presented for evaluation of tonsil and/or adenoid problems were evaluated. Open lip posture, reduced sagittal airway, and large tonsils were associated statistically with a characteristic but different skeletal configuration. Specifically, a more open lip posture was associated with a more backward rotated face and larger lower face height (Fig. 8-26). Reduced sagittal airway size was associated with a *backward* relocation

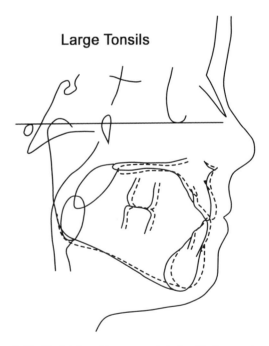

Figure 8-28. Skeletal pattern associated with larger tonsils characterized by increased posterior but decreased lower anterior facial height, and a prognathic face. All these are features of more horizontal growth. This figure was constructed by incorporating the significant mean differences for tonsils in an arbitrarily chosen tracing and provides a general picture rather than a quantitative representation of the data. (From Trotman and co-workers[18])

of the maxilla and mandible (Fig. 8-27). Because the sella-nasion dimension shortened proportionately, the SNA and SNB angles were not affected. Larger tonsils, on the other hand, were associated with a *forward* relocation and rotation of the maxilla and mandible and increased SNA and SNB angles (Fig. 8-28). Because each of the three parameters studied was associated proportionately with a different craniofacial morphology, Trotman and co-workers[18] concluded that lip posture, sagittal airway size, and tonsil size represent three different and unrelated phenomena with respect to their effects on craniofacial growth and form.

One of the most comprehensive clinical studies of the effects of removal of nasal obstructions is that carried out by Linder-Aronson.[186] He followed 41 children who had undergone adenoidectomies for a period of five years postoperatively. The thirty-four children who had switched post-operatively from oral breathing to nasal breathing were compared to 54 normal children. The significant group mean differences found initially between the dentitions and facial skeletons of the operated and control children tended to disappear during the postoperative years.

The greatest changes occurred in the dentition and in the sagittal depth of the nasopharynx during the first postoperative year. Linder-Aronson[16] noted at the beginning of the study that the mouth breathers had more retroclined maxillary and mandibular incisors than did the nose breathers. Other skeletal parameters also changed but more gradually than in the dentition and the nasopharynx. The amount of change, however, was of minor clinical relevance, as evidenced by the mandibular plane angle of the children who had undergone adenoidectomy diminished approximately 4°, twice the reduction found in the control children.

A Few Comments about Airway Obstruction

In spite of the relatively modest number of experimental studies and numerous clinical studies dealing with this issue that have been conducted to date, the relationship between upper respiratory obstruction and altered craniofacial growth remains controversial. In our opinion, there are reasonable biologic data to support a relationship between altered breathing pattern and subsequent adaptive craniofacial growth. As described previously, both experimental and clinical research has shown that a change in the postural activity of the orofacial musculature is a key factor in altering the direction and extent of craniofacial growth. Such a condition usually exists to varying extents in obstructed patients.

Why then the controversy? We take comfort in relatively straightforward clinical trials in medicine and dentistry in which patients undergoing "Treatment A" are compared to patients undergoing "Treatment B" or to an untreated group. In these studies, a single anticipated outcome (the recovery from an illness, the speed of retraction of a canine, etc.) is measured. When it comes to studies of airway obstruction, however, the difficulty in interpretation lies in categorizing or measuring the many functional and morphological reactions to the same environmental insult (*e.g.*, open bite, deep bite, Class II malocclusion, Class III malocclusion). The Harvold studies in non-human primates[91,152,154] and the Trotman study in humans,[18] for example, illustrate the variety of responses in severely affected respiratory obstruction subjects.

If we seek to differentiate between outcomes of clinical studies of upper airway obstruction to validate or refute a proposed relationship, the multiple responses observed both in experimental and clinical studies make an evaluation of mean values difficult, if not impossible. The situation is complicated further by the recognized maintenance of an altered breathing pattern* in some surgical patients in spite of airway obstruction removal. The definitive clinical study of the relationship between respiratory obstruction and altered craniofacial morphology that will satisfy clinicians on all sides of the issue may never exist, as evidenced by the debate that has been ongoing for over 100 years.

TREATMENT OF OPEN BITE

Suggested treatment for open bite malocclusions cover a broad spectrum that ranges from behavior modification to orthodontic, orthopedic, and surgical interventions. Each of the major treatments is reviewed below.

Lip Seal Exercises

One of the most useful treatments for patients with lip incompetence is a regimen of lip seal exercises, as advocated by Fränkel.[2,4] Lip seal exercises are an integral part of Fränkel therapy, but also can be incorporated successfully into routine orthodontic, orthopedic, and surgical treatments. Lip seal training also can be initiated without orthodontic intervention, in an attempt to improve facial balance and soft and hard tissue esthetics and function. An improvement in mandibular growth to a more hori-

---

*Many orthodontists term this pattern of respiration an "abnormal breathing pattern." Proffit[236] states that such a pattern is not abnormal but rather a necessary physiologic adaptation to that individual's circumstances.

VERTICAL DIMENSION

zontal direction with lip seal exercise alone is shown in Figure 8-29.

The underlying goal of this type of treatment is to establish normal neuromuscular function, particularly as it pertains to the perioral and masticatory musculature, as well as a pattern of nasal rather than oral breathing. The patient is instructed to keep the lips together at all times. By doing so, nasal respiration is encouraged. Patients often are given some type of reminder sticker that should be placed on the desk at school and in the study area at home. These types of reminders are useful in encouraging lip closure.

Fränkel and Fränkel[187] do not advocate a specific "minutes-per-day" regimen of lip seal exercises. They recommend, however, that while a child is watching television or reading, the child be given some type of small object to be kept between the lips. Such objects can include plastic disks, Popsicle™ sticks, and toothpicks (Fig. 8-30).

Patients who are candidates for this type of exercise regimen often have hyperactivity of the mentalis muscle as part of the abnormality. The patient can be instructed to press on the muscle with a finger (Fig. 8-31), This exercise can be performed inconspicuously, especially when watching television at home or listening to a teacher in a classroom setting. By pressing on the mentalis muscle posteriorly against the mandibular symph-

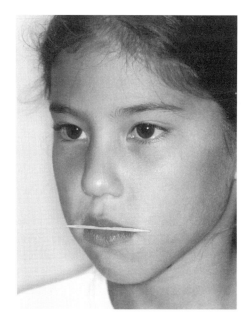

Figure 8-30. Lip seal training. A toothpick, plastic disk, or other object can be held between the lips to remind the patient to keep the lips together and to breathe through the nose.

ysis when the muscle is in a relaxed position (Fig. 8-31A) and then attempting to hold the lips together while maintaining pressure on the chin (Fig. 8-31B), the function of the mentalis muscle is inhibited and increased activity of the orbicularis oris muscle is encouraged. When such problems are identified, lip seal training can be initiated immediately, even at the time of the initial examination,

Elimination of Digital Habits

Digital habits (*i.e.*, thumb and finger sucking) have been associated with the formation and maintenance of anterior open bite.[9,10,22,188] Typically, we do not become too concerned about a digital sucking habit until about the time of the eruption of the permanent anterior teeth, and intervention usually is deferred until that developmental stage.

A wide range of therapeutic possibilities have been suggested in the literature,[113,125,189,190] including the use of digit inhibiting appliances similar in appearance to the tongue crib discussed previously (Fig. 8-18). Other treatment approaches include painting a foul-tasting or annoying substance (*e.g.*, hot pepper solution) on the offending digit as well as covering the hand with a sock during sleeping hours.

One of the simplest yet most effective behavior modification strategies is what we term the "thumb contract" (Fig. 8-32), although this technique is used regardless of whether a thumb or one or more fingers is

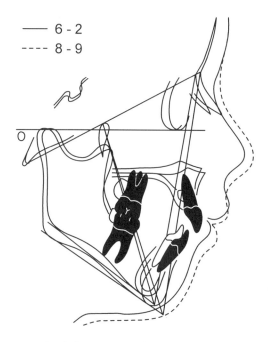

Figure 8-29. Cephalometric tracings of a patient of Rolf Fränkel who underwent only lip seal training without active orthodontic treatment. Note the closure of the mandibular plane angle. In an untreated subject, a further opening of the mandibular plane angle typically will occur during the same time interval. (Cephalograms courtesy of Rolf Fränkel.)

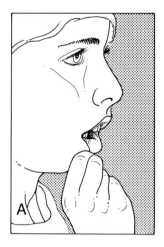
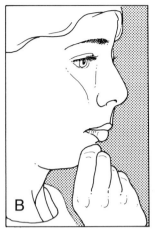

Figure 8-31. Muscle exercise used to strengthen the orbicularis oris muscle. *A*, With lips at rest, the patient pushes on the mentalis muscle, deactivating the muscle. *B*, The lips are closed. This exercise can be used alone or in conjunction with the function regulator of Fränkel.

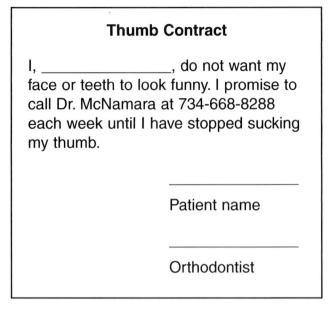

Figure 8-32. Thumb contract.

involved. Usually a digital sucking habit is identified during the initial examination through an evaluation of the written health history or in conversation between the parent and the treatment coordinator or orthodontist. If a sucking habit is denied by the patient, one especially clean digit with callous formation can betray the patient. Besides, intense digit sucking usually leads to a typical arrangement of the anterior teeth (Fig. 8-7).

Before proceeding with the formal examination, the orthodontist initiates a discussion with the young patient about the detrimental effects of the digital sucking habit, reinforcing the discussion with examples of the long-term effects of such a habit (Fig. 8-33). Usually such an example makes quite an impression on the young patient.

The patient is asked to sign a written contract with the orthodontist not to suck the thumb or finger(s) for one week. If the patient forgets and later realizes the error, even though the sucking has not stopped, the contract is not broken. Typically, if a patient wants to stop the habit, the thumb contract with the orthodontist provides enough incentive to terminate the habit (the patient can negotiate a separate reward arrangement with the parent, if indicated). The child is instructed to call the orthodontist personally each week until success is achieved. We have used this technique for over 20 years and estimate our rate of success at about 75%.

Conventional Orthodontic Treatment

In general, dental open bites respond reasonably well to conventional orthodontic treatment and to certain types of myofunctional therapy, although there is evidence that many such open bites disappear with maturation and without treatment. These treatments generally are not effective in improving skeletal open bite. Nahoum[63] states that the degree of success with conventional orthodontic procedures is inversely proportional to the extent of the skeletal dysplasia and to the number of teeth involved in the open bite. The rate of success diminishes as the open bite extends laterally and posteriorly into the canine, premolar, and molar regions.[50]

Proffit and co-workers[60] state that successful treatment of skeletal open bite in a growing patient requires control of the downward growth of the maxilla as well as control of the eruption of the posterior teeth, so that further mandibular rotation is prevented. Such effects are extremely difficult to achieve. Further, continued vertical growth in the late teen years (see Fig. 8-3 earlier in this chapter) can undo the outcome of what appears to be an otherwise successful routine orthodontic treatment and can lead to the need for a surgical correction of the problem.

Through the years, a number of non-surgical treatment approaches to open bite have been suggested, and clinicians have tended to use those therapeutic approaches popular at that time. For example, from the turn of the century to the 1930s, open bite was considered by some to be the result of inadequate development of the anterior alveolar processes.[191] The treatment approach required the use of vertical intermaxillary elastics in an effort to bring the anterior teeth together.[49,160,192] This mode of treatment has not always led to a sufficient correction (especially from an esthetic

VERTICAL DIMENSION

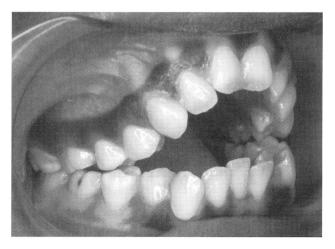

Figure 8-33. Intraoral photograph of 26-year-old female with chronic thumb sucking habit that continued into adulthood. Severe skeletal and dentoalveolar abnormalities are apparent.

standpoint) or a stable long-term occlusal result. The extraction of posterior teeth, especially of second molars, also has been suggested as a method of producing bite closure anteriorly.

Extraoral Traction

In instances in which the etiology of the open bite problem is not well defined, one typical treatment approach has been aimed at controlling the vertical growth of the patient. High-pull headgear (Fig. 8-34) has been used often in this regard, especially when posterior vertical maxillary excess is evident.[10,193-197] This type of treatment has been found to inhibit vertical maxillary development and permit forward rotation of the mandible, leading to a closure of the bite.[194,198,199] Watson[200] also has shown that if maxillary vertical growth is inhibited, but the mandibular posterior teeth are permitted to erupt further, such eruption eliminates the possibility of reducing lower facial height or changing mandibular rotation. Thus, the clinician must pay attention not only to the maxillary vertical but the mandibular vertical as well.[201-205]

One of the dilemmas faced by the orthodontist in patients with skeletal open bite is treatment timing. If treatment is initiated during the growing years, often a satisfactory occlusal result can be obtained through high-pull headgear or posterior bite block therapy combined with fixed appliance treatment. This improvement in facial and occlusal configuration has to be maintained, however, throughout the period of remaining active growth. Van der Linden[58] has noted that, following the use of a high-pull headgear in patients with a long face, suppression of vertical development unfor-

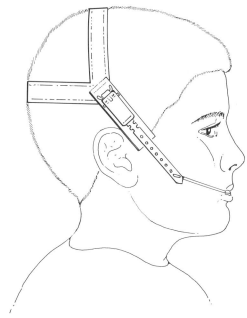

Figure 8-34. A high-pull facebow can be used to inhibit the downward and forward movement of the maxillary dentition.

tunately is followed by an excessive increase in facial height in subsequent years (Fig. 8-35).

Functional Jaw Orthopedics

In Europe, a number of investigators have treated open bite problems with various removable appliances, with the view that they were controlling "local epigenetic factors."[206,207] These appliances included the Andresen and Häupl activator,[208] the Harvold-Woodside activator,[209] the open bite Balters bionator,[210,211] and Fränkel's function regulator.[212]

As described earlier, Fränkel's approach to the treatment of skeletal open bite with the function regulator[3,4,213] (see Chapters 16 and 23), combined with rigorous lip seal training,[2] seems to have the greatest success in treating skeletal open bite patients. His data indicate that a shift in equilibrium of the soft tissues of the craniofacial complex can be obtained by orthopedic intervention based on the principles of general orthopedics. An elimination of deleterious muscle function and an exercise program of beneficial muscle training may result in a stable closure of anterior open bite in the growing individual.[2,3]

The treatment results of Erbay and co-workers[214] with the FR-IV appliance support Fränkel's approach to anterior open bite. The spontaneous downward and backward growth direction of the mandible observed in the control group changed to an upward and forward direction by FR-IV therapy. The skeletal anterior open

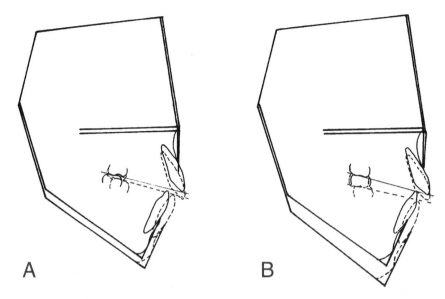

Figure 8-35. Composite cephalometric tracing of changes taking place in a patient with a Class II, division 1 malocclusion and a long face during treatment with a high-pull headgear, and of the changes in the years following. *A*, During treatment, the maxillary first permanent molars were prevented from erupting or even intruded, and lower anterior facial height increased only slightly. *B*, After treatment, the maxillary first molar erupted considerably, facial height increased markedly, and the mandibular plane became much larger. (From Van der Linden.[58])

bite was corrected successfully through upward and forward mandibular rotation.

Posterior Bite Blocks

A logical approach to the treatment of overerupted posterior teeth is dental intrusion. Experimental studies in several animal species have shown that the vertical component of skeletal and dental development can be modified with posterior bite blocks. Breitner[215,216] evaluated the effects of various block appliances in adult female rhesus monkeys and reported a favorable response in the treatment of open bite. McNamara[217] noted inhibition of molar eruption as well as a reduction in the vertical development of the maxilla in juvenile monkeys treated with posterior bite blocks that created 2 to 5 mm of bite opening. Sergl and Farmand[218] reported inhibited eruption of molars included in posterior bite blocks in growing rabbits. Woods and Nanda[219] and Hoenie and McNamara[220] described decreased posterior dental eruption and upward and forward positioning of the maxilla in growing primates treated with magnetic as well as passive posterior bite block appliances.

In clinical practice, a number of posterior bite block designs have been suggested, including both removable and fixed types. Simple removable designs (Figs. 8-36 and 8-37) are similar to the acrylic splint type of Herbst appliance, in that they consist of a wire framework and acrylic of varying thicknesses. Typically, the appliance is fabricated for the mandibular dentition, but maxillary designs similar to the acrylic splint expander made without the expansion screw also can be fabricated. This type of appliance not only can be used to help control posterior tooth eruption, but also can be incorporated into the treatment of a simple anterior crossbite (Fig. 8-38). Bonded acrylic splint expanders also have a posterior bite block effect as one of their modes of action.

With the acrylic coverage on the occlusal surfaces, the

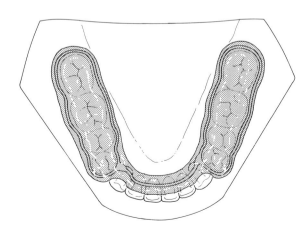

Figure 8-36. Occlusal view of the removable posterior bite block appliance.

VERTICAL DIMENSION

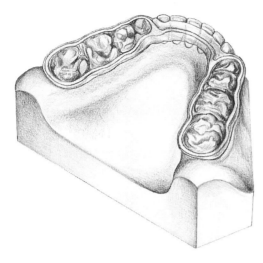

Figure 8-37. Oblique view of the removable posterior bite block appliance.

eruption of the posterior teeth is inhibited and, in some instances, slight intrusion of the posterior teeth may occur. In addition, slight extrusion of the teeth not incorporated into the expander may occur, all of which leads to a closure of the anterior open bite. In addition, after removal of the expander, slight autorotation of the mandible may occur.

If the acrylic on the occlusal surfaces is built up an additional few millimeters, the muscles are elongated and the forces against the occlusion may be increased. In addition, more than one appliance can be used at the same time to help correct the open bite problem (e.g., posterior bite block combined with a vertical-pull chin cup a belt and suspenders approach[221]). The number of clinical studies dealing with the treatment effects of posterior bite blocks (including the acrylic splint expansion appliances) has been relatively modest. Kuster and Ingervall[222] evaluated children treated with two types of bite blocks. They noted an increase in overbite during the treatment resulting from posterior dental intrusion and possibly increased mandibular growth. Sarver and Johnston[223] compared the effects of the bonded RME appliance and a Haas-type expander. They noted relative intrusion of the maxilla in the bonded group as compared to the banded expander sample. Wendling[224] evaluated the short-term cephalometric effects of the acrylic splint expander with and without concomitant Schwarz treatment in mixed dentition patients. She noted intrusion of the maxillary posterior teeth in both treatment groups.

Thus, the placement of posterior bite blocks can prevent further eruption of the posterior teeth in growing patients; however, significant tooth intrusion in adolescents or adults is difficult to verify and rarely if ever is

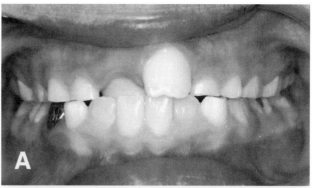
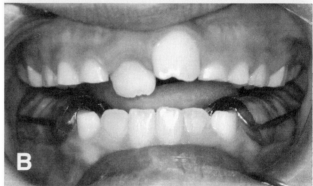

Figure 8-38. A posterior bite block appliance can be used to open the bite anteriorly to allow for the correction of an anterior crossbite. Brackets subsequently can be placed on the anterior teeth to facilitate anterior movement of the maxillary right central incisor.

achieved.[222] Furthermore, reduced vertical development by posterior bite blocks may be cancelled by excessive vertical facial growth following treatment.

Active Vertical Corrector

Another appliance that has received attention as a suggested alternative to orthognathic surgery is the Active Vertical Corrector (AVC). Dellinger[225] introduced the AVC as an appliance that incorporated repelling samarium cobalt magnets in a posterior bite block type of appliance. Dellinger's appliance (Fig. 8-39) incorporated samarium magnets into acrylic and wire posterior bite block appliances that covered the posterior dentition in both arches.

Although preliminary results appeared promising, complications were encountered.[226] Patients had difficulty in tolerating the increased vertical dimension caused by the appliance thickness, and some of the patients shifted their mandibles laterally as the repelling magnets came together. The latter finding also was noted in experimental studies of the standard design.[220, 227] In 1991, the design of the AVC was modified

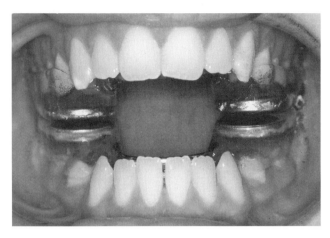

Figure 8-39. The original design of the Active Vertical Corrector™ featured samarium cobalt magnets in a repelling mode incorporated into posterior bite blocks.

so that the height of the appliance was reduced, and buccal shields were added to eliminate lateral displacement during function.

Cavanaugh and Christiansen[226] have conducted the only clinical study to date that directly compares the the original and modified designs of the Active Vertical Corrector™. They noted passive eruption of the maxillary and mandibular incisors in both appliance groups. Significant intrusion of the posterior maxillary dentition was observed with the original AVC design; significant mandibular molar intrusion did not occur in either group. Most importantly, significant skeletal changes did not occur with either AVC design. Cavanaugh and Christiansen[226] concluded, "Magnets, as used in either the original or the revised active vertical corrector, have limited value in the treatment of open-bite malocclusion." Besides, long-term follow-up studies have not been reported.

Vertical Pull Chin Cups

It is well known that the application of external forces to the dentition can lead to tooth intrusion. Perhaps the most dramatic clinical evidence that teeth can be intruded is provided by patients who wore an orthopedic collar or Milwaukee brace during treatment for scoliosis,[228,229] a procedure not used anymore today. In these patients, dramatic (and undesirable) changes in both dentoalveolar and skeletal structures occurred as sequelae of this type of orthopedic intervention (Fig. 8-40).

A more patient-friendly way of creating vertically acting forces against the craniofacial complex is the chin cup. Published cephalometric studies have indicated that open bite often is a problem of posterior vertical maxillary excess.[51,61,64,230–232] In patients who have a po-

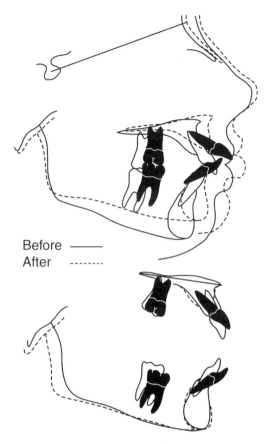

Figure 8-40. Skeletal and dentoalveolar treatment effects produced by the Milwaukee brace. Note the decrease in lower anterior facial height and closure of the mandibular plane angle, as well as the intrusion and flaring of the dentition. (Redrawn from Alexander.[212])

tential for the extrusion of posterior teeth, it is helpful to simulate another pair of masticatory muscles, thus preventing the extrusion of teeth in the buccal segments. Further, Pearson[204,205,233,234] and Speidel and co-workers[230] have stressed the importance of retarding the vertical growth vector of a backward rotating mandible by applying extraoral orthopedic forces with a vertical pull chin cup.

Vertical-pull chin cups are applicable not only in Class III patients with anterior open bite tendencies, but also can be used in patients who have an increased anterior vertical dimension. Pearson[59,205,233,234] has reported that the use of a vertical-pull chin cup can result in a decrease in the mandibular plane and gonial angles and an increase in posterior facial height, in comparison to the growth of untreated individuals.

It is very difficult to create a true vertical pull on the mandible, due to problems in anchoring the chin cup cranially. Perhaps the easiest of the orthopedic chin cups to use is that available from Unitek (Unitek Corporation, Monrovia CA), shown in Figures 8-41 and 8-42. A

VERTICAL DIMENSION

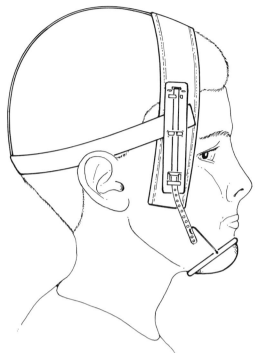

Figure 8-41. Lateral view of the vertical-pull chin cup made by Unitek.

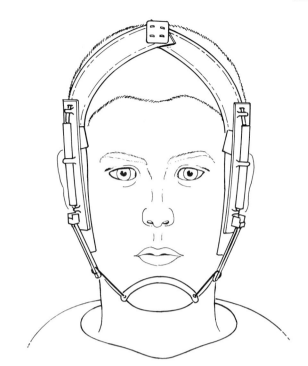

Figure 8-42. Frontal view of the Unitek vertical-pull chin cup.

padded band extends coronally and is secured to the posterior part of the head by a cloth strap. A spring mechanism is activated by pulling the tab inferiorly and attaching the tab to a hook on a hard chin cup.

Another type of chin cup that produces a vertical vector of force is available through Summit Orthodontics (Summit Orthodontics, Munroe Falls OH), shown in Figures 8-43 and 8-44. This appliance consists of a cloth headcap that curves not only around the crown of the head, but also is secured posteriorly with two horizontal straps. A throat strap also secures the appliance to the head of the patient. This particular design is useful in

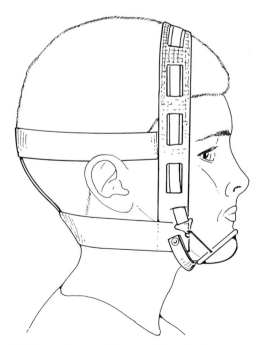

Figure 8-43. Lateral view of the vertical-pull chin cup made by Summit Orthodontics.

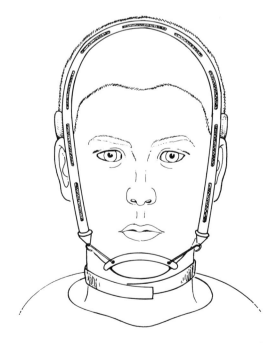

Figure 8-44. Frontal view of the Summit vertical-pull chin cup (Summit Orthodontics).

those patients in whom anchorage in the cranial region is difficult to achieve.

The wearing of a vertical-pull chin cup requires a high level of patient compliance.[234] Ideally, the vector of force should be 90° to the occlusal plane and pass through the center of resistance of the entire arch. The chin cup is fitted individually and the straps stapled as necessary to fit the patient's head. Pearson[234] recommends that patients wear the chin cup about 12 hours a day, with a force of 500 grams (18 ounces). The chin cup should be adjusted so that adequate vertical force is applied to the posterior teeth to keep them together a substantial part of the time.

Fitting the chin cup to the patient occasionally proves difficult. If a patient has an unusually shaped chin, commercially available chin cups may not be adequate, and it may be necessary to fabricate a custom-fit chin cup. By using a chin cup fitted to the morphology of the patient's chin, force levels can be increased without producing soft-tissue soreness or ulceration. In addition, the chin cup usually is lined with felt or closed-cell foam, but in some instances, it may be necessary to use other materials such as soft fabrics, facial tissue, or moleskin to prevent chin irritation.

Fitting the chin cup to the patient's head may be difficult as well. Occasionally it is necessary to trim the straps above the patient's ears for comfort. In addition, the straps of the chin cup may pull on the hair or create other discomforts. Pearson[234] recommends having several types of chin cups on hand.

Pearson[234] also recommends the use of posterior bite blocks in conjunction with a vertical-pull chin cup. Included in this category of posterior bite block appliances is the acrylic splint expander. Larger posterior bite blocks can be used as well.

Both the occipital-pull and vertical-pull chin cups presumably create pressure on the temporomandibular joint region. Although this type of therapy has been used successfully for many decades, the increased sensitivity of the orthodontic specialist toward the diagnosis and treatment of temporomandibular (TM) joint problems should lead the clinician to monitor chin cup patients on an ongoing basis for signs and symptoms of TM disorders. If any are noted, the use of the chin cup should be discontinued immediately. In general, chin cups have not been shown to produce temporomandibular dysfunction in growing patients.[235]

One of the drawbacks of chin cup wear, besides its appearance, is the potential for chin irritation. As mentioned previously, the chin cup can be lined with a variety of materials to prevent chafing and ulceration. Proffit[236] also notes that chin cup treatment may cause less irritation in cooler climates.

Orthognathic Surgery

Orthognathic surgery has become routine in patients with severe skeletal open bites, although recent problems with managed care organizations and insurance coverage in the United States has made approval of such procedures less predictable than it was a decade ago. Problems with long-term retention and stability have lead some clinicians[51,64] to conclude that in skeletal open bite cases, orthodontics without surgery should not be attempted at all, especially in all adult patients and in moderate-to-severe problems in growing children.[6,51] This approach is established more firmly as surgical procedures have become advanced and refined to the extent that they can offer the advantages of a definitive, esthetic, and stable result.[232,237]

Most of the surgical procedures for skeletal open bite involve a LeFort I osteotomy and/or a sagittal split osteotomy, although segmental osteotomies and genioplasties also often are incorporated into the overall surgical orthodontic treatment plan. Specific procedures include anterior maxillary and mandibular surgery,[238–245] surgery in the mandibular body,[238,239,246,247] mandibular ramus surgery,[248–251] posterior maxillary surgery,[240,252–254] and total maxillary surgery.[255–261] Also, various combinations of the same have been used in the treatment of skeletal open bite.

Often the treatment of skeletal open bite is postponed until growth is complete and orthognathic surgery can be performed. Evaluation of large samples of treated patients who have undergone these types of procedure reveal that the skeletal improvement generally is maintained, although a dental open bite often returns.[58] Tongue interposition between the teeth seems to persist in spite of the surgical procedure.[262]

Another surgical treatment alternative that is used for the correction of open bite is a partial glossectomy, the removal of excess lingual tissue. This procedure is performed when macroglossia, hypertonicity, or edema of the tongue is found to be a likely cause of the malocclusion and reeducation of the tongue has failed.[263] This procedure is used sparingly, usually in patients whose excessive tongue size is obviously a major etiological factor in the malocclusion.

Partial glossectomy may have a mild effect on tongue function post-surgically. Following partial glossectomy in a group of patients who presented with macroglossia as part of their craniofacial problem, Ingervall and Schmoker[264] noted a minor reduction in the ability of the patients to recognize shapes intraorally. The oral motor ability and the positions of the head, the cervical column, and the hyoid bone were unaffected. After the operation, the tongue did not fill the oral cavity as much as before, and the freeway space decreased. Patients who have undergone this procedure, however, sometimes report the inability to clean the buccal surfaces of the posterior teeth with the tongue.

TREATMENT OF DEEP BITE

The correction of deep bite is much easier when attempted in a growing child than in an adult.[265-268] A number of reasons have been suggested for the increased potential of relapse in adults, including encroachment of the therapy on the freeway space[269] against strong and mature musculature that is less adaptable to elongation.[265] Regardless of the type of malocclusion, the soft and hard tissues of the face maintain a functional homeostasis during growth.

Because opening the bite in a patient with a short vertical dimension generally is accomplished by extrusion of posterior teeth, a change in the masticatory muscle balance must occur. Four types of adaptations are possible when the functional length of a muscle is altered: within the central nervous system, within the muscle tissue itself (*e.g.*, addition of sarcomeres), at the muscle-bone interface, and within or between bony attachments.[269] It appears that adaptation within the neuromuscular system occurs more readily in a growing individual.

The suggested methods of correction of deep bite problems include intrusion of the maxillary incisors,[267,270] mandibular incisor intrusion,[267,270-275] extrusion of maxillary posterior teeth,[273, 275-277] mandibular posterior tooth extrusion,[272-275, 277] mandibular incisor proclination,[276] and increasing lower anterior facial height.[82,273,276,278-280]

Anterior Bite Plate

One of the most basic treatments proposed for overclosure associated with deep bite was suggested by Callaway[281] and Thompson,[84] who advocated stimulating the eruption of the posterior teeth as a way of "filling in" the bite (*i.e.*, opening the bite anteriorly with a bite plate, then allowing the posterior teeth to erupt into occlusion) through the reduction of excessive freeway space. A simple anterior bite plate often is used in conjunction with cervical extraoral traction to open the bite and prevent accidental incisor interference. A bite plate also is used as an adjunct to fixed appliance treatment,[282] especially in situations in which the patient otherwise would have heavy contact on brackets bonded to the mandibular teeth.[283] In recent years, either "bite turbos"[284] bonded to the lingual surfaces of the maxillary anterior teeth or build-ups of bonding material on the occlusal surfaces of the molars or premolars bilaterally have been used to clear the occlusion.

It should be remembered that increasing the vertical dimension during Class II treatment, however, will tend to mask positive anteroposterior changes in mandibular growth.[82] As a general rule, each millimeter of increase in lower anterior facial height will camouflage or mask a millimeter of increase in mandibular length by rotating the chin point downward and backward.[82]

Conventional Treatment

Conventional fixed appliance therapy often is the primary treatment of choice in patients with vertical deficiencies. If indicated, various types of intrusion arches or so-called "reverse curve" or "rocker" archwires can be used to help level an accentuated curve of Spee. This approach is similar to that used in Begg mechanics, in which bite opening bends are placed in each archwire mesial to the first molars, along with Class II elastics.[221]

In adult Class II, division 2 patients with overclosure, the extraction of two maxillary premolars to camouflage the underlying skeletal discrepancy usually should be avoided. Not only are the mechanics involved lengthy and tedious, but also the treatment often is undermined by the strength of the associated musculature.[83] In addition, the retraction of the maxillary anterior teeth often leads to bialveolar retrusion, which can result in a less than ideal esthetic result, with an increased nose and chin prominence. Thus, extraction of teeth in overclosed Class II patients often is contraindicated, particularly in the mandible.

Brankovan and co-workers[83] note that the types of patients discussed in this section often have concomitant problems in the transverse dimension. When the overclosed mandible is positioned at the proper vertical dimension, a masked transverse discrepancy may become apparent, with the maxillary arch too wide for the mandibular arch. Lowering the mandible to increase the vertical dimension will result in the mandibular dentition assuming a tendency to a lingual crossbite ("scissor-bite") relationship relative to the maxillary dentition.

In this situation, Brankovan and co-workers[83] recommend expansion of the mandibular dentition, especially in instances of a crowded dentition. This type of tooth movement can be accomplished with a number of appliances, including archwire expansion during routine fixed appliance therapy, a lower lingual or bi-helical arch, or by way of a removable lower Schwarz expansion appliance.

In short face individuals, development following treatment can be controlled more easily than in long face patients. An anterior bite plane can prevent the un-

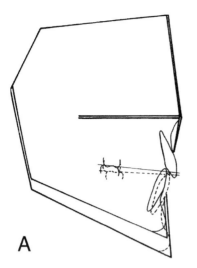 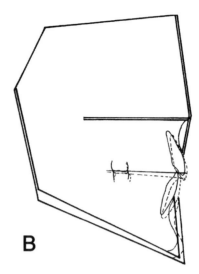

Figure 8-45. Composite cephalometric tracings of changes occurring in a patient with a Class II, division 1 malocclusion and a short face during treatment with a cervical facebow and in the years following. *A*, During treatment, the lower face height increased and the mandibular plane angle became larger. *B*, Following treatment, the mandibular plane angle became smaller and lower anterior facial height decreased. (From Van der Linden.[58])

desirable decrease in lower anterior facial height.[58, 285] Van der Linden recommends the use of a maxillary removable retainer that contacts the mandibular incisors when the appliance is worn during sleep (See Figs. 26-12 and 26-13 in Chapter 26 for the specific design recommended by Van der Linden). Such retention should be maintained until active growth has ceased, sometime until 21–22 years of age in males.[58]

Extraoral Traction

An adjunctive method of treatment in overclosed patients with maxillary skeletal protrusion is the use of a headgear, perhaps a cervical facebow combined with a bite plate, to obtain simultaneous anteroposterior and vertical correction. The clinician should monitor the width of the facebow carefully, however, so as not to produce unwanted widening of the maxillary dental arch.

Short-faced patients treated with a cervical facebow exhibit marked increase of lower anterior facial height (LAFH) during treatment, followed by little vertical growth, and a marked anterior development in the subsequent retention period. Thus, patients treated with a cervical headgear show an increase in LAFH that partially is lost in the years following treatment (Fig. 8-45).

Functional Jaw Orthopedics

If the maxillary incisors are tipped lingually, as often is the case with overclosed patients with a Class II, division 2 configuration of the maxillary incisors, the maxillary anterior teeth should be flared and aligned prior to functional appliance treatment,[286] much in the same way that a patient is prepared orthodontically for orthognathic surgery. The dental compensations should be removed before functional appliance treatment is initiated.

Several types of functional jaw orthopedic appliances can be used to increase the vertical dimension in Class II patients with a short lower anterior facial height, including the FR-2 appliance of Fränkel[4,130,213] and the twin block appliance.[287–289] For example, the treatment outcome of a 13-year-old girl is illustrated in Figure 8-46. This patient, who had a short lower anterior facial height (54 mm) and mandibular skeletal retrusion at the beginning of treatment, wore a FR-2 appliance of Fränkel for 18 months. Normally a patient of her age would have an increase in lower anterior facial height of about 1 mm per year.[82,290] During the 18 months of Frankel treatment, however, lower anterior facial height increased 6 mm.

The clinical management of the twin block appliance also facilitates opening the vertical dimension of growing patients. As will be described in detail in Chapter 15, the posterior acrylic blocks of the maxillary part of the appliance can be contoured gradually to facilitate the eruption of the mandibular permanent molars. After the molars have erupted sufficiently, acrylic can be removed from bite blocks on the mandibular part of the appliance to facilitate premolar and canine eruption. A

VERTICAL DIMENSION

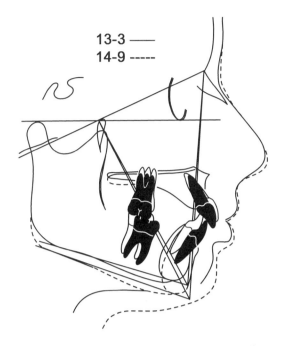

Figure 8-46. Treatment effects of the FR-2 appliance of Fränkel in a 13-year-old female patient with a short lower anterior facial height. Lower anterior facial height increased by 6 mm during the 18-month treatment period, about four times the amount of vertical increase expected without treatment.[82]

similar effect can be achieved by the clinical manipulating the eruption facets of an activator or bionator.

This type of selective leveling of the occlusal plane is indicated only in those patients who have an accentuated curve of Spee before treatment and in whom an increase in lower anterior facial height is desirable. It must be remembered once again that any increase in lower anterior facial height will camouflage concomitant increases in mandibular length,[82] which may not be advantageous in a patient with an initially short mandible.

Almost any type of functional appliance that allows for posterior tooth eruption can be used to increase lower anterior facial height. It has been our experience, however, that although the acrylic splint Herbst appliance can be used in patients with excessive vertical facial heights, this type of appliance is not indicated in overclosure patients because of the intrusive effects of the posterior acrylic. In fact, many of the increases in vertical dimension noted during Herbst therapy, regardless of the design, disappear during the post-retention period.[291]

Orthognathic Surgery

A common treatment in adult Class II short-faced individuals is orthognathic surgery. Excellent results can be obtained with a sagittal split osteotomy with reverse autorotation.[265,292] The tooth-bearing distal segment is rotated downward as it is brought forward.

In this type of patient for whom an increase in lower anterior facial height is desirable, an accentuated curve of Spee often is present in the mandible. In contrast to the usual protocol of leveling the dental arches orthodontically prior to surgery, the orthodontist should take care to maintain the accentuated curve of Spee during the presurgical phase of orthodontics. By maintaining a deep overbite, the mandible not only can be advanced, but the bite can be opened as the anterior segment is rotated downward. If a lateral open bite is created during the surgical procedure, it can be corrected during the post-surgical orthodontic phase by the extrusion of posterior teeth.

In Class II patients with extremely short lower facial dimensions, two-jaw surgery may be required. A maxillary LeFort I osteotomy can be used to move the maxilla inferiorly along with a mandibular advancement with reverse autorotation.[293–296] An interpositional genioplasty also can be performed to increase lower anterior facial height.[265,297]

Unfortunately, it appears that one of the least stable orthognathic surgical procedures is the maxillary interpositional bone graft to lengthen the vertical dimension of the face. When the maxilla is moved downward, as often is needed in the treatment of vertical maxillary deficiency, there is a strong tendency toward relapse. As demonstrated in a study conducted at the University of North Carolina by Proffit and co-workers,[298,299] if a LeFort I osteotomy alone is used to bring the maxilla downward and forward in a Class II patient with decreased lower anterior facial height, almost all of the vertical change is lost. They showed that even if this procedure was stabilized with rigid intermaxillary fixation, a strong relapse tendency still was observed.

Proffit and co-workers[299] hypothesize that the lack of stability in increasing the vertical dimension results from the forces produced against the displaced maxilla when the teeth are brought together. Three approaches toward improving the long-term stability of the inferiorly displaced maxilla have been suggested, including the use of an interpositional bone graft of synthetic hydroxyapatite to provide mechanical rigidity,[300–302] the placement of heavy fixation bars from the zygomatic arch to the posterior dentition,[300] and a simultaneous ramus osteotomy to minimize stretching of the associated elevator musculature and to decrease occlusal force until healing is more advanced.[300] It should be noted, however, that little data are available on the effectiveness of these various approaches designed to improve stability.[299]

CONCLUDING REMARKS

Of all the chapters in this volume, this chapter was by far the most difficult to write. This difficulty was not due to a lack of published material (there are literally thousands of articles in refereed journals that consider various aspects of the vertical dimension) or our inexperience in treating patients with vertical discrepancies. Rather, vertical discrepancies comprise some of the most challenging situations facing the orthodontist in everyday practice. Even the title of the 1999 Moyers Symposium,* *The Enigma of the Vertical Dimension*,[303] reflects the difficulty of dealing with these complex clinical issues.

As indicated above, many different etiological factors have been implicated in the development of hyper- and hypodivergent faces. For some of those, definitive proof has been provided, for most of them not. In addition, large variations have been reported regarding the response of the growth of the face to specific etiological factors as well as to their elimination. Most likely, all these etiological factors, each in its own way, may have only a small effect, and yet these factors can interact in ways that magnify or diminish the response.

Of prime importance in the management of vertical problems is the role of the musculature and the other soft tissues, as has been described throughout this chapter. The postural activities of the musculature that are of relatively low magnitude but are acting constantly appear to be the most important factors in determining overall facial morphology; high magnitude but short-acting phasic activities such as swallowing, chewing, and speaking have little effect.

Another important concept to keep in mind is that open bite and deep bite are the two ends of the same spectrum. For example, orthodontists recognize skeletally based open bite and deep bite as being problems difficult to treat, but these clinical conditions often are not put into the same conceptual framework. In an attempt to explain the variation in facial growth and particularly that of long and short faces, Van der Linden[58,303] has suggested the concept of interaction between what he has termed the "internal and external functional components" (Fig. 8-47). The internal components include the oral, nasal, and pharyngeal cavities, and the activities within those cavities. The external components include the masticatory and facial muscles and other soft tissues on the anterior part of the head and neck, including their behavior, particularly at rest.

The interaction between internal and external components is hypothesized to be a primary determinant of the initial facial morphology and its subsequent growth pattern. Indeed, the variations in facial patterns seen in children and adults also are found in the second half of prenatal development.[305] Furthermore, the typical hyperdivergent and hypodivergent facial patterns are

*All volumes in print from the Craniofacial Growth Monograph Series are available through Needham Press at *www.needhampress.com*.

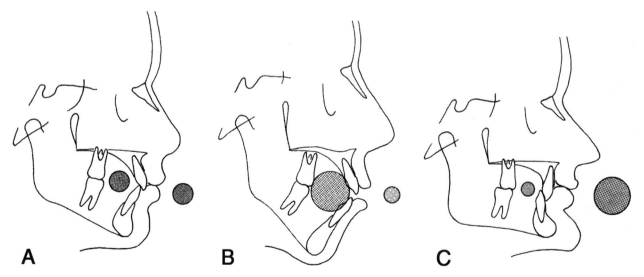

Figure 8-47. Vertical problems. *A*, In the average situation, balance exists between the internal and external functional components. Growth will conform to the average growth pattern. *B*, When internal functional components dominate over the external components, growth mainly will be in a caudal direction, leading to an increased space for the internal functional components. *C*, When external functional components dominate over the internal components and more space is available for the latter than is needed, growth will be mainly in an anterior direction, and lower anterior facial height will increase only slightly or not at all. (From Van der Linden.[58,303])

present from the beginning, but usually become more severe with continuing growth. Considering these observations, it becomes evident that the effect of the various etiological factors may have been overestimated. In addition, the limited rate of success in altering the height of the face on a permanent basis by orthodontic and facial orthopedic means supports this conclusion.

This chapter also has outlined most of the contemporary treatments of both open bite and deep bite, ranging from the management of simple dental problems in the anterior region to severe skeletal dysplasias. Generally, the more severe the skeletal imbalance, the less effective are the non-surgical approaches to correction. Often, orthognathic surgery is the only viable option in difficult open bite and deep bite situations, associated with facial disfigurations.

The duration of treatment has been cited as a critical issue in the management of vertical discrepancies, whether the appliance involved is a simple anterior bite plate in a deep bite patient or a posterior bite block or vertical-pull chin cup in an open bite patient. For example, in comparing the efficacy of vertical-pull chin cups to bite blocks, Proffit[236] states that it is important to remember what is known about the equilibrium that controls eruption. Duration of force is more important than force magnitude, so one would expect (as seems to be the case) that bite blocks would be more effective simply because they are worn more of the time. Proffit says that in order to be effective, a chin cup would have to be worn a lot more than most patients are willing to wear it each day. Given excellent patient cooperation, however, treatment with the vertical-pull chin cup or with the function regulator of Fränkel has been shown to be effective in the management of skeletal open bite in young patients.

Finally, we return to the concepts of Fränkel and his emphasis on maintaining an adequate oral seal. A regimen of lip seal training, not only in patients treated with functional appliances, but also in patients treated by other means as well as in non-patients, has been shown to produce both esthetic and functional improvements in the facial soft and hard tissue both during growth and following orthognathic surgery. Any treatment regimen that at least in part addresses problems associated with the postural activity of the facial and masticatory musculature should be more effective than those regimens that simply apply force to the craniofacial complex.

REFERENCES CITED

1. Fränkel R. A functional approach to orofacial orthopaedics. Br J Orthod 1980;7:41–51.
2. Fränkel R. Lip seal training in the treatment of skeletal open bite. Eur J Orthod 1980;2:219–228.
3. Fränkel R, Fränkel C. A functional approach to treatment of skeletal open bite. Am J Orthod 1983;84:54–68.
4. Fränkel R, Fränkel C. Orofacial orthopedics with the function regulator. Munich: S Karger, 1989.
5. Swinehart EW. A clinical study of openbite. Am J Orthod Oral Surg 1942;28:18–34.
6. Subtelny JD, Sakuda M. Open bite: diagnosis and treatment. Am J Orthod 1964;50:337–358.
7. Atkinson SR. "Open-bite" malocclusion. Am J Orthod 1966;52:877–86.
8. Bowden BD. A longitudinal study of the effects of digit- and dummy-sucking. Am J Orthod 1966;52:887–901.
9. Gershater MM. The proper perspective of open bite. Angle Orthod 1972;42:263–272.
10. Mizrahi E. A review of anterior open bite. Br J Orthod 1978;5:21–7.
11. Straub WJ. Malfunctions of the tongue. Part I. Am J Orthod 1960;46:404–424.
12. Straub WJ. Malfunctions of the tongue. Part II. Am J Orthod 1961;47:596–617.
13. Straub WJ. Malfunctions of the tongue. Part III. Am J Orthod 1962;48:486–503.
14. Straub W. Malfunctions of the tongue. Part I. The abnormal swallowing habit: its causes, effects and results in relation to orthodontic treatment and speech therapy. Am J Orthod 1979;76:565–576.
15. Lowe AA. Correlations between orofacial muscle activity and craniofacial morphology in a sample of control and anterior open-bite subjects. Am J Orthod 1980;78:89–98.
16. Linder-Aronson S. Adenoids—Their effect on mode of breathing and nasal air flow and their relationship to characteristics of the facial skeleton and dentition. Acta Otolaryngol, Suppl 265, 1970.
17. McNamara JA, Jr. Influence of respiratory pattern on craniofacial growth. Angle Orthod 1981;51:269–300.
18. Trotman CA, McNamara JA, Jr, Dibbets JMH, Van der Wheele LT. Association of lip posture and the dimensions of the tonsils and sagittal airway with facial morphology. Angle Orthod 1997;67:425–432.
19. Schudy FF. The rotation of the mandible resulting from growth: its implications in orthodontic treatment. Angle Orthod 1965;35:36–50.
20. Richardson A. Facial growth and the prognosis for anterior open-bite. Trans Europ Orthod Soc 1971;47:149–157.
21. Nanda SK. Patterns of vertical growth in the face. Am J Orthod Dentofac Orthop 1988;93:103–116.
22. Proffit WR. Equilibrium theory revisited: factors influencing position of the teeth. Angle Orthod 1978;48:175–186.
23. Swinehart EW. Relation of thumb-sucking to malocclusion. Am J Orthod 1938;24:509–521.
24. Sassouni V. A classification of skeletal facial types. Am J Orthod 1969;55:109–123.
25. Lundström A, McWilliam JS. A comparison of vertical and horizontal cephalometric variables with regard to heritability. Eur J Orthod 1987;9:104–108.
26. Strang RHW. A textbook of orthodontia. Philadelphia: Lea & Febiger, 1950.
27. Prakash P, Margolis HI. Dento-facial relations in varying degrees of overbite. Am J Orthod 1952;38:658–673.

28. Popovich F. Cephalometric evaluation of vertical overbite in young adults. J Canad Dent Assoc 1955;21:209–222.
29. Steadman SR. Predetermining the overbite and overjet. Angle Orthod 1947;19:101–105.
30. Fleming HB. An investigation of the vertical overbite during the eruption of the permanent dentition. Angle Orthod 1961;31:53–62.
31. Ludwig MK. A cephalometric analysis of the relationship between facial pattern, interincisal angulation and anterior overbite changes. Angle Orthod 1967;37:194–204.
32. Herness LE, Rule JT, Williams BH. A longitudinal cephalometric study of incisor overbite from ages five to eleven. Angle Orthod 1973;43:279–288.
33. Neff CW. Tailored occlusion with the anterior coefficient. Am J Orthod Oral Surg 1949;35:309–314.
34. Goldstein MS, Stanton FL. Various types of occlusion and amounts of overbite in normal and abnormal occlusion between two and twelve years. Int J Orthod Oral Surg 1936;22:549–569.
35. Wylie WL. The relationship between ramus height, dental height, and overbite. Am J Orthod Oral Surg 1946;32:57–67.
36. Björk A. Variability and age changes in overjet and overbite. Am J Orthod 1953;39:770–801.
37. Nanda RS, Khan I, Anand R. Age changes in the occlusal pattern of deciduous dentition. J Dent Res 1973;52:221–224.
38. Bresonis WL, Grewe JM. Treatment and posttreatment changes in orthodontic cases: overbite and overjet. Angle Orthod 1974;44:295–299.
39. Johnston LE, Jr. Personal communication, 2000.
40. Nanda S. Characteristics of the long face syndrome. In: McNamara JA, Jr, ed. The enigma of the vertical dimension. Ann Arbor: Monograph 36, Craniofacial Growth Series, Center for Human Growth and Development, The University of Michigan, 2000.
41. Sassouni V. The face in five dimensions, Morgantown: University Press, 1962.
42. Schudy FF. Vertical growth versus anteroposterior growth as related to function and treatment. Angle Orthod 1964;34:75-93.
43. Schendel SA, Eisenfeld J, Bell WH, Epker BN, Mishelevich DJ. The long face syndrome: vertical maxillary excess. Am J Orthod 1976;70:398–408.
44. Opdebeeck H, Bell WH. The short face syndrome. Am J Orthod 1978;73:499–511.
45. Isaacson JR, Isaacson RJ, Speidel TM, Worms FW. Extreme variation in vertical facial growth and associated variation in skeletal and dental relations. Angle Orthod 1971;41:219–229.
46. Karlsen AT. Craniofacial growth differences between low and high MP-SN angle males: a longitudinal study. Angle Orthod 1995;65:341–350.
47. Brunelle JA, Bhat MK, Lipton JA. Prevalence and distribution of selected occlusal characteristics in the US population. J Dent Res 1996;75:706–713.
48. Proffit WR, Fields HW, Moray LJ. Prevalence of malocclusion and orthodontic treatment need in the United States: Estimates from the N-HANES III survey. Int J Adult Orthod Orthogn Surg 1998;13:97–106.
49. Strang RHW. Textbook of orthodontia. Philadelphia: Lea & Febiger, 1933.
50. Moyers RE. Handbook of orthodontics. Chicago: Year Book Medical Publishers, 1963.
51. Nahoum HI. Anterior open-bite: a cephalometric analysis and suggested treatment procedures. Am J Orthod 1975;67:513–21.
52. Ellis E, McNamara JA, Jr. Components of adult Class III open-bite malocclusion. Am J Orthod 1984;86:277–290.
53. Van der Linden FPGM. Development of the dentition. Chicago: Quintessence, 1983.
54. Moyers RE. Handbook of orthodontics. Chicago: Yearbook Medical Publishers, 1988.
55. Daskalogiannakis J. Glossary of orthodontic terms. Chicago: Quintessence, 2000.
56. Proffit WR, Vig KW. Primary failure of eruption: a possible cause of posterior open-bite. Am J Orthod 1981;80:173–190.
57. Nielsen IL. Vertical malocclusions: etiology, development, diagnosis and some aspects of treatment. Angle Orthod 1991;61:247–260.
58. Van der Linden FPGM. The development of long and short faces, and their limitations in treatment. In: McNamara JA, Jr, ed. The enigma of the vertical dimension. Ann Arbor: Monograph 36, Craniofacial Growth Series, Center for Human Growth and Development, The University of Michigan, 2000.
59. Pearson LE. Case report KP. Treatment of a severe open-bite excessive vertical pattern with an eclectic non-surgical approach. Angle Orthod 1991;61:71–76.
60. Proffit WR, Bailey LJ, Phillips C, Turvey TA. Long-term stability of surgical open-bite correction by LeFort I osteotomy. Angle Orthod 2000;70:112–117.
61. Sassouni V, Nanda SK. Analysis of dentofacial vertical proportions. Am J Orthod 1964;50:801–823.
62. Worms FW, Meskin LH, Isaacson RJ. Open-bite. Am J Orthod 1971;59:589–595.
63. Nahoum HI. Vertical proportions: a guide for prognosis and treatment in anterior open-bite. Am J Orthod 1977;72:128–146.
64. Lopez-Gavito G, Wallen TR, Little RM, Joondeph DR. Anterior open-bite malocclusion: a longitudinal 10-year postretention evaluation of orthodontically treated patients. Am J Orthod 1985;87:175–186.
65. White E. Skeletal disharmonies associated with anterior open-bite. Angle Orthod 1957;27:212–215.
66. Hapak FM. Cephalometric appraisal of the open-bite case. Angle Orthod 1964;34:65–72.
67. Richardson A. Skeletal factors in anterior open-bite and deep overbite. Am J Orthod 1969;56:114–127.
68. Nahoum HI, Horowitz SL, Benedicto EA. Varieties of anterior open-bite. Am J Orthod 1972;61:486–92.
69. Proffit WR, Phillips C, Dann C. Who seeks surgical-orthodontic treatment? Int J Adult Orthodont Orthognath Surg 1990;5:153–160.
70. Van Spronsen PH, Weijs WA, Valk J, Prahl-Anderson B, van Ginkel FC. A comparison of jaw muscle cross-sections of long-face and normal adults. J Dent Res 1992;71:1279–1285.
71. Proffit WR, Fields HW, Nixon WL. Occlusal forces in normal and long-face children. J Dent Res 1983;62:571–574.
72. Van Spronsen PH, Weijs WA, B. P-A, Van Ginkel FC. A comparison of jaw muscle orientation and moment arms

of long-face and normal adults. J Dent Res 1996;75: 1372–1380.
73. Boyd SB, Gonyea WJ, Finn RA, Woodard CE, Bell WH. Histochemical study of the masseter muscle in patients with maxillary excess. J Oral Maxillofac Surg 1984;42: 75–83.
74. Van Spronsen PH. Kauwspieren. Deel V. Geometrie van de kauwspieren en schedelmorfologie. Ned Tijdschr Tandheelkd 1997;104:373–376.
75. Ilizarov GA, Soybelman LM. Some clinical and experimental data concerning lengthening of lower extremities. Exp Khir Arrestar 1969;14:27.
76. Ilizarov GA. The tension-stress effect on the genesis and growth of tissues. Part I. The influence of stability of fixation and soft-tissue preservation. Clin Orthop 1989;238: 249–281.
77. Ilizarov GA. The tension-stress effect on the genesis and growth of tissues. Part II. The influence of the rate and frequency of distraction. Clin Orthop 1989;239:263–285.
78. McCarthy JG, Schreider J, Karp N, Thorne CH, Grayson BH. Lengthening the human mandible by gradual distraction. Plast Reconstr Surg 1992;89:1–8.
79. Cohen SR. Distraction osteogenesis of the craniofacial skeleton—Evolving indications and techniques. In: McNamara JA, Jr, Trotman CA, eds. Distraction osteogenesis and tissue engineering. Ann Arbor: Monograph 34, Craniofacial Growth Series, Center for Human Growth and Development, The University of Michigan, 1998.
80. Molina F. Mandibular distraction in treatment of craniofacial anomalies. In: McNamara JA, Jr, ed. Distraction osteogenesis and tissue engineering. Ann Arbor: Monograph 34, Craniofacial Growth Series, Center for Human Growth and Development, The University of Michigan, 1998.
81. Molina F. Maxillary distraction: Esthetic and functional benefits in cleft and prognathic patients during the mixed dentition. In: McNamara JA, Jr, ed. Distraction osteogenesis and tissue engineering. Ann Arbor: Monograph 34, Craniofacial Growth Series, Center for Human Growth and Development, The University of Michigan, 1998.
82. McNamara JA, Jr. A method of cephalometric evaluation. Am J Orthod 1984;86:449–69.
83. Brankovan M, Woodside DG, Rossouw PE. Overclosure and its relationship to facial morphology, occlusion, orthodontic diagnosis, and treatment planning: A review. In: McNamara JA, Jr, ed. The enigma of the vertical dimension. Ann Arbor: Monograph 36, Craniofacial Growth Series, Center for Human Growth and Development, The University of Michigan, 2000.
84. Thompson JR. The rest position of the mandible and its significance to dental science. J Am Dent Assoc 1946;33: 151–180.
85. Tallgren A. Changes in adult face height due to aging, wear and loss of teeth, and prosthetic treatment. Acta Odont Scand 1957;15:Suppl 24.
86. Woodside DG. Cephalometric radiography. In: Clark JW, ed. Clinical dentistry. Hagerstown: Harper and Row, 1976.
87. Beckmann SH, Kuitert RB, Prahl-Anderson B, Segner D, The RPS, Tuinzing DB. Alveolar and skeletal dimensions associated with overbite. Am J Orthod Dentofac Orthop 1998;113:443–452.
88. Beckmann SH, Kuitert RB, Prahl-Anderson B, Segner D, The RPS, Tuinzing DB. Alveolar and skeletal dimensions associated with lower face height. Am J Orthod Dentofac Orthop 1998;113:498–506.
89. Linder-Aronson S, Woodside DG. Some craniofacial variables related to small or diminishing lower anterior face height. Swed Dent J Suppl 1982;15:131–146.
90. Muller G. Growth and development of the middle face. J Dent Res 1963;42:385–389.
91. Harvold EP, Vargervik K, Chierici G. Primate experiments on oral sensation and dental malocclusions. Am J Orthod 1973;63:494–508.
92. Ueda HM, Ishizuka Y, Miyamoto K, Morimoto N, Tanne K. Relationship between masticatory muscle activity and vertical craniofacial morphology. Angle Orthod 1998;68: 233–238.
93. Møller E. The chewing apparatus: An electromyographic study of the action of the muscles of mastication and its correlation to facial morphology. Acta Physiol Scand 1966;69:1–229.
94. Ingervall B, Thilander B. Relation between facial morphology and activity of the masticatory muscles: An electromyographic and radiographic cephalometric investigation. J Oral Rehabil 1974;1:131–147.
95. Ringquist M. Isometric bite force and its relation to dimensions of the facial skeleton. Acta Odont Scand 1973; 31:35–42.
96. Proffit WR, Fields HW, Nixon WL. Occlusal forces in normal and long-faced adults. J Dent Res 1983;62: 571–574.
97. Björk A. Facial growth in man, studied with the aid of metallic implants. Acta Odontol Scand 1955;13:9–34.
98. Björk A. Variations in the growth pattern of the human mandible: Longitudinal radiographic study by the implant method. J Dent Res 1963;42:400–411.
99. Björk A. Sutural growth of the upper face studied by the implant method. Acta Odontol Scand 1966;24:109–129.
100. Björk A, Helm S. Prediction of the age of maximum pubertal growth in body height. Angle Orthod 1967;37: 134–143.
101. Björk A. The use of metallic implants in the study of facial growth in children: Method and application. Am J Phys Anthrop 1968;29:243–254.
102. Björk A, Skieller V. Facial development and tooth eruption. An implant study at the age of puberty. Am J Orthod 1972;62:339–383.
103. Enlow DH, Hunter WS. A differential analysis of sutural and remodeling growth in the human face. Am J Orthod 1966;52:823–830.
104. Enlow DH. The human face. New York: Harper and Row, 1968.
105. Proffit WR. The development of vertical dentofacial problems: Concepts from recent human studies. In: McNamara JA, Jr, ed. The enigma of the vertical dimension. Ann Arbor: Monograph 36, Craniofacial Growth Series, Center for Human Growth and Development, The University of Michigan, 2000.
106. Lavergne J, Gasson N. A metal implant study of mandibular rotation. Angle Orthod 1976;46:144–150.
107. Angle EH. Treatment of malocclusion of the teeth. Philadelphia: SS White, 1907.
108. Rogers AP. Open-bite cases involving tongue habits. Int J Orthod 1927;13:837–844.
109. Anderson WS. The relationship of the tongue-thrust syn-

110. Massengill R, Jr, Robinson M, Quinn G. Cinefluorographic analysis of tongue-thrusting. Am J Orthod 1972;61:402–406.
111. Garliner D. Myofunctional therapy in dental practice. Abnormal swallowing habits, diagnosis, and treatment. A course of study for the dental practitioner and speech pathologist. Brooklyn: Bartel Dental Book Co, 1971.
112. Kydd WL. Quantitative analysis of forces of the tongue. J Dent Res 1956;35:171–74.
113. Parker JH. The interception of the open bite in the early growth period. Angle Orthod 1971;41:24–44.
114. Vojdani A. A simple technique for treatment of open bite due to a tongue thrust habit at an early age. Penn Dent J 1977;44:14–15.
115. Hanson ML. Oral myofunctional therapy. Am J Orthod 1978;73:59–67.
116. Frank B. A rationale for closer cooperation between the orthodontists and the speech and hearing therapist. Arch Oral Biol 1955;41:571–582.
117. Bloomer HH. Speech defects in relation to orthodontics. Am J Orthod 1963;49:920–929.
118. Proffit WR, Mason RM. Myofunctional therapy for tongue-thrusting: background and recommendations. J Am Dent Assoc 1975;90:403–411.
119. Fletcher SG, Casteel RL, Bradley DP. Tongue-thrust swallow, speech articulation, and age. J Speech Hearing Disorders 1961;26:201–208.
120. Proffit WR, Fields HW, Jr. Contemporary orthodontics, St Louis: Mosby Year Book, 1993.
121. Proffit WR, Prewitt JR, Baik HS, Lee CF. Video microscope observations of human premolar eruption. J Dent Res 1991;70:15–18.
122. Risinger RK, Proffit WR. Continuous overnight observation of human premolar eruption. Arch Oral Biol 1996;41:779–789.
123. Trentini CJ, Proffit WR. High resolution observations of human premolar eruption. Arch Oral Biol 1996;41:63–68.
124. Proffit WR, Sellers KT. The effect of intermittent forces on eruption of the rabbit incisor. J Dent Res 1986;65:118–122.
125. Haryett RD, Hansen FC, Davidson PO, Sandilands ML. Chronic thumb-sucking: the psychologic effects and the relative effectiveness of various methods of treatment. Am J Orthod 1967;53:569–585.
126. Graber TM. Thumbsucking. J Am Dent Assoc 1970;81:805.
127. Ballard CF. Variations of posture and behavior of the lips and tongue which determine the position of the labial segments: The implications in orthodontics, prosthetics and speech. Trans Europ Orthod Soc 1965;41:67–93.
128. Fränkel R. The theoretical concept underlying the treatment with functional correctors. Trans Europ Orthod Soc 1966;42:233–254.
129. Fränkel R. Funktions kieferorthopadie und der Mundvorhof als Apparative Basis. Berlin: VEB, Verlag Volk und Gesundheit, 1967.
130. Fränkel R. The treatment of Class II, Division 1 malocclusion with functional correctors. Am J Orthod 1969;55:265–275.
131. Fränkel R. The practical meaning of the functional matrix in orthodontics. Trans Eur Orthod Soc 1969;45:207–219.
132. Linder-Aronson S, Backstrom A. A comparison between mouth breathers and nose breathers with respect to occlusion and facial dimensions. Odontol Revy 1960;11:343–376.
133. Bresolin D, Shapiro PA, Shapiro GG, Chapko MK, Dassel S. Mouth breathing in allergic children: its relationship to dentofacial development. Am J Orthod 1983;83:334–40.
134. Trask GM, Shapiro GG, Shapiro PA. The effects of perennial allergic rhinitis on dental and skeletal development: a comparison of sibling pairs. Am J Orthod Dentofac Orthop 1987;92:286–93.
135. Solow B, Kreiborg S. Soft-tissue stretching: A possible control factor in craniofacial morphogenesis. Scand J Dent Res 1977;85:505–507.
136. Tomes CS. On the developmental origin of the v-shaped contracted maxilla. Monthly Rev Dent Surg 1872;1:2–5.
137. Meyer W. On adenoid vegetations in the naso-pharyngeal cavity: Their pathology, diagnosis and treatment. Medico-cherugical Trans (London) 1872;53:191–215.
138. Johnson LR. Habits and their relationship to malocclusion. J Amer Dent Assoc 1943;30:842–852.
139. Ricketts RM. Respiratory obstruction syndrome. Am J Orthod 1968;54:495–507.
140. Linder-Aronson S. Respiratory function in relation to facial morphology and the dentition. Br J Orthod 1979;6:59–71.
141. Warren DW. Dentofacial morphology and breathing: a century of controversy. In: Nelson BG, ed. Current controversies in orthodontics. Berlin: Quintessence, 1991.
142. Warren DW. Breathing behavior and posture. In: McNamara JA, Jr, ed. The enigma of the vertical dimension. Ann Arbor: Monograph 36, Craniofacial Growth Series, Center for Human Growth and Development, The University of Michigan, 2000.
143. Warren DW, Hairfield WM, Seaton D, Morr KE, Smith LR. The relationship between nasal airway size and nasal-oral breathing. Am J Orthod Dentofac Orthop 1988;93:289–93.
144. Warren DW, Hinton VA, Pillsbury HC. Analysis of simulated upper airway breathing. Arch Otolaryngol 1987;113:405–408.
145. Warren DW. Effect of airway obstruction upon facial growth. In: Koopman CF, Jr, ed. Otolaryngologic Clinics of North America. Philadelphia: WB Saunders, 1990;23:699–711.
146. Warren DW, Hinton VA, Hairfield WM. Measurement of nasal and oral respiration using inductive plethysmography. Am J Orthod 1986;89:480–484.
147. Johnston LE, Jr. The functional matrix hypothesis: Reflections in a jaundiced eye. In: McNamara JA, Jr, ed. Factors affecting the growth of the midface. Ann Arbor: Monograph 6, Craniofacial Growth Series, Center for Human Growth and Development, The University of Michigan, 1976.
148. Rubin RM. The relationship between nasal airway compromise and facial growth. In: McNamara JA, Jr, ed. The enigma of the vertical dimension. Ann Arbor: Monograph 36, Craniofacial Growth Series, Center for Human

149. Quinn GW. Personal communication, 1981.
150. Harvold EP. New treatment principles for mandibular malformations. In: Cook JT, ed. Transactions of the Third International Orthodontic Congress. St Louis: CV Mosby, 1975.
151. Miller AJ. Electromyography of craniofacial musculature during oral respiration in the rhesus monkey (*Macaca mulatta*). Arch Oral Biol 1978;23:142–152.
152. Miller AJ, Vargervik K. Neural control of oral respiration in the rhesus monkey. In: Carlson DS, McNamara JA, Jr, eds. Muscle adaptation in the craniofacial region. Ann Arbor: Monograph 8, Craniofacial Growth Series, Center for Human Growth and Development, The University of Michigan, 1978.
153. Miller AJ, Vargervik K. Neuromuscular changes during long-term adaptation of the rhesus monkey to oral respiration. In: McNamara JA, Jr, ed. Naso-respiratory function and craniofacial growth. Ann Arbor: Monograph 9, Craniofacial Growth Series, Center for Human Growth and Development, The University of Michigan, 1979.
154. Harvold EP. Neuromuscular and morphological adaptations in experimentally induced oral respiration. In: McNamara JA, Jr, ed. Naso-respiratory function and craniofacial growth. Ann Arbor: Monograph 9, Craniofacial Growth Series, Center for Human Growth and Development, The University of Michigan, 1979.
155. Harvold EP, Tomer BS, Vargervik K, Chierici G. Primate experiments on oral respiration. Am J Orthod 1981;79:359–72.
156. Miller AJ. Neuromuscular adaptation in experimentally induced oral respiration in the rhesus monkey (*Macaca mulatta*). Arch Oral Biol 1980;25:579–589.
157. Harvold EP. Experiments on mandibular morphogenesis. In: McNamara JA, Jr, ed. Determinants of mandibular form and growth. Ann Arbor: Monograph 4, Craniofacial Growth Series, Center for Human Growth and Development, The University of Michigan, 1975.
158. Miller AJ, Vargervik K, Chierici G. Sequential neuromuscular changes in rhesus monkeys during the initial adaptation to oral respiration. Am J Orthod 1982;81:99–107.
159. Balyeat RM, Bowen R. Facial and dental deformities due to perennial nasal allergy in children. Int J Orthod 1934;20:445–449.
160. McCoy JC. Applied orthodontics. Philadelphia: Lea & Febiger, 1935.
161. Todd TW, Cohen MD, Broadbent BH. The role of allergy in the etiology of orthodontic deformity. J Allergy 1939;10:246–249.
162. Marks MB. Allergy in relation to orofacial dental deformities in children. J Allergy 1965;36:293–302.
163. Quinn GW. Airway interference and its effect upon the growth and development of the face, jaws, dentition and associated parts. N Carolina Dent J 1978;60:28–31.
164. Vig PS, Sarver DM, Hall DJ, Warren DW. Quantitative evaluation of nasal airflow in relation to facial morphology. Am J Orthod 1981;79:263–272.
165. Fields HW, Warren DW, Black K, Phillips C. Relationship between vertical dentofacial morphology and respiration in adolescents. Am J Orthod Dentofac Orthop 1991;99:147–54.
166. Vig PS, Spalding PM, Lints RR. Sensitivity and specificity of diagnostic tests for impaired nasal respiration. Am J Orthod Dentofac Orthop 1991;99:354–360.
167. Kluemper GT, Vig PS, Vig KW. Nasorespiratory characteristics and craniofacial morphology. Eur J Orthod 1995;17:491–5.
168. Ketcham AH. Treatment by the orthodontist supplementing that by the rhinologist. Dent Cosmos 1912;54:1312–1321.
169. Thurow RC. The survival factor in orthodontics. In: Cook JT, ed. Transactions of the Third International Orthodontic Congress. St Louis: CV Mosby, 1975:17–25.
170. Howard CC. Inherent growth and its influence on malocclusion. J Am Dent Assoc 1932;19:642–648.
171. Leech HL. A clinical analysis of orofacial morphology and behavior of 500 patients attending an upper respiratory research clinic. Dent Pract 1958;9:57–68.
172. Huber RE, Reynolds JW. A dentofacial study of male students at the University of Michigan in the physical hardening program. Am J Orthod Oral Surg 1946;32: 1–21.
173. Quick C, Gundlach K. Adenoid facies. Laryngoscope 1978;88:327–333.
174. Stöckli PW, Ingervall B, Joho JP, Wieslander L. Myofunktionelle therapie. Fortschr Kieferorthop 1987;48:460-463.
175. Dunn GF, Green LJ, Cunat JJ. Relationships between variation of mandibular morphology and variation of nasopharyngeal airway size in monozygotic twins. Angle Orthod 1973;43:129–35.
176. Solow B, Siersbaek-Nielsen S, Greve E. Airway adequacy, head posture, and craniofacial morphology. Am J Orthod 1984;86:214–223.
177. Woodside DG, Linder-Aronson S, Lundstrom A, McWilliam J. Mandibular and maxillary growth after changed mode of breathing. Am J Orthod Dentofac Orthop 1991;100:1–18.
178. Vig PS. Respiratory mode and morphological types: some thoughts and preliminary conclusions. In: McNamara JA, Jr, ed. Naso-respiratory function and craniofacial growth. Ann Arbor: Monograph 9, Craniofacial Growth Series, Center for Human Growth and Development University of Michigan, 1979.
179. Diamond O. Tonsils and adenoids: Why the dilemma? Am J Orthod 1980;78:495–503.
180. Ung N, Koenig J, Shapiro PA, Shapiro G, Trask G. A quantitative assessment of respiratory patterns and their effects on dentofacial development. Am J Orthod Dentofac Orthop 1990;98:523–532.
181. Fricke B, Gebert HJ, Grabowski R, Hasund A, Sergl HG. Nasal airway, lip competence, and craniofacial morphology. Eur J Orthod 1993;15:297–304.
182. Gross AM, Kellum GD, Michas C, Franz D, Foster M, Walker M, Bishop FW. Open-mouth posture and maxillary arch width in young children: a three-year evaluation. Am J Orthod Dentofac Orthop 1994;106:635–640.
183. Hartgerink DV, Vig PS. Lower anterior face height and lip incompetence do not predict nasal airway obstruction. Angle Orthod 1989;59:17–23.
184. Weber ZJ, Preston CB, Wright PG. Resistance to nasal airflow related to changes in head posture. Am J Orthod 1981;80:536–545.
185. Wenzel A, Henriksen J, Melsen B. Nasal respiratory

resistance and head posture: effect of intranasal corticosteroid (Budesonide) in children with asthma and perennial rhinitis. Am J Orthod 1983;84:422–426.
186. Linder-Aronson S. Effects of adenoidectomy on the dentition and facial skeleton over a period of five years. In: Cook JT, ed. Transactions of the Third International Orthodontic Congress. St Louis: CV Mosby, 1975.
187. Fränkel R, Fränkel C. Personal communication, 1992.
188. Willmot DR. Thumb sucking habit and associated dental differences in one of monozygous twins. Br J Orthod 1984;11:195-199.
189. Justus R. Treatment of anterior openbite: A cephalometric and clinical study. ADM 1976;33:17–40.
190. Huang GJ, Justus R, Kennedy DB, Kokich VG. Stability of anterior openbite treated with crib therapy. Angle Orthod 1990;60:17–24.
191. Hellman M. Open bite. Internat J Orthod 1931;17: 421–444.
192. Weinberger BW. Practical orthodontics. St. Louis: CV Mosby, 1948.
193. Kuhn RJ. Control of anterior vertical dimension and proper selection of extraoral anchorage. Angle Orthod 1968;38:340–349.
194. Badell MC. An evaluation of extraoral combined high-pull traction and cervical traction to the maxilla. Am J Orthod 1976;69:431–446.
195. Barton JJ. High-pull headgear versus cervical traction: a cephalometric comparison. Am J Orthod 1972;62: 517–529.
196. Teuscher U. A growth-related concept for skeletal Class II treatment. Am J Orthod 1978;74:258–275.
197. Firouz M, Zernik J, Nanda R. Dental and orthopedic effects of high-pull headgear in treatment of Class II, division 1 malocclusion. Am J Orthod Dentofac Orthop 1992;102:197–205.
198. Brandt HC, Shapiro PA, Kokich VG. Experimental and postexperimental effects of posteriorly directed extraoral traction in adult *Macaca fascicularis*. Am J Orthod 1979;75:301–317.
199. Watson WG. Open-bite—a multifactorial event. Am J Orthod 1981;80:443–446.
200. Watson WG. A computerized appraisal of the high-pull face-bow. Am J Orthod 1972;62:561–579.
201. Ricketts RM. The influence of orthodontic treatment on facial growth and development. Angle Orthod 1960;30: 103–133.
202. Creekmore TD. Inhibition or stimulation of the vertical growth of the facial complex, its significance to treatment. Angle Orthod 1967;37:285–297.
203. Dougherty HL. The effect of mechanical forces upon the mandibular buccal segments during orthodontic treatment. Am J Orthod 1968;54:83–103.
204. Pearson LE. Vertical control through use of mandibular posterior intrusive forces. Angle Orthod 1973;43:194–200.
205. Pearson LE. Vertical control in fully-banded orthodontic treatment. Angle Orthod 1986;56:205–224.
206. Heckman V. Treatment of open bite with removable appliances. Trans Eur Orthod Soc 1974:173–180.
207. Fränkel R. Functional aspects of skeletal open bite. Fortschr Kieferorthop 1982;43:8–18.
208. Pancherz H. Long-term effects of activator treatment: a cephalometric roentgenographic investigation. Odont Revy 1976;27:31–42.
209. Harvold EP. The activator in interceptive orthodontics. St. Louis: CV Mosby, 1974.
210. Balthers W. Allgemeines zur Atmung und zur Atmungsstörung. Fortschr Kieferorthop 1954;15:193.
211. Balters W. Eine Einführung in die Bionatorheilmethode. Ausgewählte, Schriften und Vorträge. Heidelberg: Druckerei Hölzel, 1973.
212. Graber TM, Neumann B. Removable orthodontic appliances. Philadelphia: WB Saunders, 1984.
213. Fränkel R. Technik und Handhabung der Funktionsregler. Berlin: VEB Verlag Volk and Gesundheit, 1976.
214. Erbay E, Ugur T, Ulgen M. The effects of Frankel's function regulator (FR-4) therapy on the treatment of Angle Class I skeletal anterior open bite malocclusion. Am J Orthod Dentofac Orthop 1995;108:9–21.
215. Breitner C. Further investigations of bone changes resulting from experimental orthodontic treatment. Am J Orthod 1941;27:605–632.
216. Breitner C. Alteration of occlusal relations induced by experimental procedure. Am J Orthod 1943;29:277-289.
217. McNamara JA, Jr. An experimental study of increased vertical dimension in the growing face. Am J Orthod 1977;71:382–395.
218. Sergl HG, Farmland M. Experiments with unilateral bite planes in rabbits. Angle Orthod 1975;45:108–114.
219. Woods MG, Nanda RS. Intrusion of posterior teeth with magnets. An experiment in growing baboons. Angle Orthod 1988;58:136–150.
220. Hoenie DC, McNamara JA, Jr. The effect of interocclusal repelling magnets in a bite-opening splint on the growth of the craniofacial complex in juvenile *Macaca mulatta*. In: McNamara JA, Jr, ed. The enigma of the vertical dimension. Ann Arbor: Monograph 36, Craniofacial Growth Series, Center for Human Growth and Development, The University of Michigan, 2000.
221. Brightman BB. Personal communication, 2000.
222. Kuster R, Ingervall B. The effect of treatment of skeletal open bite with two types of bite-blocks. Eur J Orthod 1992;14:489–499.
223. Sarver DM, Johnston MW. Skeletal changes in vertical and anterior displacement of the maxilla with bonded rapid palatal expansion appliances. Am J Orthod Dentofac Orthop 1989;95:462–466.
224. Wendling LK. Short-term skeletal and dental effects of the acrylic splint rapid maxillary expansion appliance. Ann Arbor: Unpublished Masters thesis, Department of Orthodontics and Pediatric Dentistry, The University of Michigan, 1997.
225. Dellinger EL. Active vertical corrector treatment—long-term follow-up of anterior open bite treated by the intrusion of posterior teeth. Am J Orthod Dentofac Orthop 1996;110:145–154.
226. Cavanaugh CE, Christiansen RL. The effect of active vertical corrector treatment in growing anterior openbite patients. In: McNamara JA, Jr, ed. The enigma of the vertical dimension. Ann Arbor: Monograph 36, Craniofacial Growth Series, Center for Human Growth and Development, The University of Michigan, 2000.
227. Woods MG. The mechanics of lower incisor intrusion:

experiments in nongrowing baboons. Am J Orthod Dentofac Orthop 1988;93:186–95.
228. Logan WR. The effect of the Milwaukee brace on developing dentition. Pract Dent Rec 1962;12:447–454.
229. Alexander RG. The effects on tooth position and maxillofacial vertical growth during treatment of scoliosis with the Milwaukee brace. Am J Orthod 1966;52:161–89.
230. Speidel TM, Isaacson RJ, Worms FW. Tongue-thrust therapy and anterior dental open-bite. A review of new facial growth data. Am J Orthod 1972;62:287–295.
231. Schendel SA, Eisenfeld JH, Bell WH, Epker BN. Superior repositioning of the maxilla: stability and soft tissue osseous relations. Am J Orthod 1976;70:663–674.
232. Ellis E, McNamara JA, Jr, Lawrence TM. Components of adult Class II open-bite malocclusion. J Oral Maxillofac Surg 1985;43:92–105.
233. Pearson LE. Vertical control in treatment of patients having backward-rotational growth tendencies. Angle Orthod 1978;48:132–140.
234. Pearson LE. The management of vertical problems in growing patients. In: McNamara JA, Jr, ed. The enigma of the vertical dimension. Ann Arbor: Monograph 36, Craniofacial Growth Series, Center for Human Growth and Development, The University of Michigan, 2000.
235. Graber TM. Personal communication, 1997.
236. Proffit WR. Personal communication, 2000.
237. Bell WH, Proffit WR, White RP. Surgical correction of dentofacial deformities. Philadelphia: WB Saunders, 1980.
238. Köle H. Surgical operations on the alveolar ridge to correct occlusal abnormalities. Oral Surg 1959;12:277–288, 413–420.
239. Köle H. Results, experience and problems in the operative treatment of anomalies with reverse overbite (mandibular retrusion). Oral Surg Oral Med Oral Path 965;19:427-450.
240. Mohnac AM. Maxillary osteotomy in the management of occlusal deformities. J Oral Surg 1966;24:305–317.
241. Taylor RG, Mills PB, Brenner LD. Maxillary and mandibular subapical osteotomies for the correction of anterior open-bite. Oral Surg 1967;23:141–147.
242. Hinds EC, Kent JN. Diagnosis and selection of surgical procedures in management of open bite. J Oral Surg 1969;27:939–949.
243. Kent JN, Hinds EC. Management of dental facial deformities by anterior alveolar surgery. J Oral Surg 1971;29: 13–26.
244. Bell WH. Correction of skeletal type anterior open-bite. J Oral Surg 1971;29:706–714.
245. Bell WH, Dann JJ. Correction of dentofacial deformities by surgery in the anterior part of the jaws. Am J Orthod 1973;64:162–187.
246. McIntosh RB. Total mandibular alveolar osteotomy. J Maxillofac Surg 1974;22:210–218.
247. McIntosh RB, Carlotti AE. Total mandibular alveolar osteotomy in the management of skeletal (infantile) apertognathia. J Oral Surg 1975;33:921–928.
248. Kostecka F. A contribution to the surgical treatment of open-bite. Int J Orthod 1934;20:1082–1092.
249. Shira RB. Surgical correction of open-bite deformities by oblique sliding osteotomy. Oral Surg 1961;19:275–290.
250. Alfaro R, Othon LG, Levine et al. Correction of mandibular prognathism with associated apertognathia by intraoral sagittal osteotomy of rami. Opt Acta 1969; 27:285–292.
251. Kline SN, Shensa DR, Kahn M. Skeletal open-bite—surgical management: report of case. J Oral Surg 1970;28: 791–794.
252. Schuchardt K. Experiences with surgical treatment of some deformities of the jaws: prognathia, micrognathia and open bite. In: Wallace AB, ed. Transactions of the Second Congress of International Society of Plastic Surgeons. Edinburgh: Livingstone, 1961:73–78.
253. West RA, Epker BN. The posterior maxillary osteotomy: Its place in the treatment of selected dentofacial deformities. J Oral Surg 1972;30:562–575.
254. Stoker NC, Epker BN. The posterior maxillary osteotomy: A retrospective study of treatment results. Int J Oral Surg 1974;3:153–157.
255. Bell WH. Le Fort I osteotomy for correction of maxillary deformities. J Oral Surg 1975;33:412–426.
256. Wolford LM, Epker BN. The combined anterior and posterior maxillary osteotomy: A new technique. J Oral Surg 1975;33:842–851.
257. Epker BN, Schendel SA. Total maxillary surgery. Int J Oral Surg 1980;9:1–24.
258. Proffit WR, Phillips C, Turvey TA. Stability following superior repositioning of the maxilla by LeFort I osteotomy. Am J Orthod Dentofac Orthop 1987;92:151–161.
259. Denison TF, Kokich VG, Shapiro PA. Stability of maxillary surgery in openbite versus nonopenbite malocclusions. Angle Orthod 1989;59:5–10.
260. Sarver DM, Weissman SM. Long-term soft tissue response to LeFort I maxillary superior repositioning. Angle Orthod 1991;61:267–276.
261. Hack GA, de Mol van Otterloo JJ, Nanda R. Long-term stability and prediction of soft tissue changes after LeFort I surgery. Am J Orthod Dentofac Orthop 1993; 104:544–555.
262. Hoppenreijs RJM, Freihofer HPM, Stoelinga PJW, Tuinzing DB, Van't Hof MA, Van der Linden FPGM, Nottet SJAM. Skeletal and dento-alveolar stability of Le Fort intrusion osteotomies and bimaxillary osteotomies in anterior open bite deformities: a retrospective three centre study. Int J Oral Maxillofac Surg 1997;26:161–175.
263. Petit HP. Adaptation following accelerated facial mask therapy. In: McNamara JA, Jr, Ribbens KA, Howe RP, eds. Clinical alterations of the growing face. Ann Arbor: Monograph 14, Craniofacial Growth Series, Center for Human Growth and Development, The University of Michigan, 1983.
264. Ingervall B, Schmoker R. Effect of surgical reduction of the tongue on oral stereognosis, oral motor ability, and the rest position of the tongue and mandible. Am J Orthod Dentofac Orthop 1990;97:58–65.
265. Bell WH, Jacobs JD, Legan HL. Treatment of Class II deep bite by orthodontic and surgical means. Am J Orthod 1984;85:1–20.
266. Björk A. Prediction of mandibular growth rotation. Am J Orthod 1969;55:585–599.
267. Burstone CR. Deep overbite correction by intrusion. Am J Orthod 1977;72:1–22.

268. Simons ME, Joondeph DR. Change in overbite: a ten-year postretention study. Am J Orthod 1973;64:349–67.
269. McNamara JA, Jr, Carlson DS, Yellich GM, Hendrickson RP. Musculoskeletal adaptation following orthognathic surgery. In: Carlson DS, McNamara JA, Jr, eds. Muscle adaptation in the craniofacial region. Ann Arbor: Monograph 8, Craniofacial Growth Series, Center for Human Growth and Development, The University of Michigan, 1978.
270. McNamara JA, Jr. Utility arches. J Clin Orthod 1986;20:452–456.
271. Mershon JV. Possibilities and limitations in the treatment of closed-bites. Int J Orthod Oral Surg 1937;23:581–589.
272. Mitchell DL, Stewart WL. Documented leveling of the lower arch using metallic implants for reference. Am J Orthod 1973;63:526–532.
273. Otto RL, Anholm JM, Engel GA. A comparative analysis of intrusion of incisor teeth achieved in adults and children according to facial type. Am J Orthod 1980;77:437–446.
274. Greig DG. Bioprogressive therapy: overbite reduction with the lower utility arch. Br J Orthod 1983;10:214–216.
275. Dake ML, Sinclair PM. A comparison of the Ricketts and Tweed-type arch leveling techniques. Am J Orthod Dentofac Orthop 1989;95:72–78.
276. Ball JV, Hunt NP. The effect of Andresen, Harvold, and Begg treatment on overbite and molar eruption. Eur J Orthod 1991;13:53–58.
277. Schudy FF. The control of vertical overbite in clinical orthodontics. Angle Orthod 1968;38:19–39.
278. Schudy FF. Cant of the occlusal plane and axial inclinations of teeth. Angle Orthod 1963;33:69–82.
279. Nemeth RB, Isaacson RJ. Vertical anterior relapse. Am J Orthod 1974;65:565–585.
280. Engel G, Cornforth G, Damerell JM, Gordon J, Levy P, McAlpine J, Otto R, Walters R, Chaconas S. Treatment of deep-bite cases. Am J Orthod 1980;77:1–13.
281. Callaway GS. The use of bite plates. Am J Orthod Oral Surg 1940;26:120-124.
282. Menezes DM. Comparative analysis of changes resulting from bite plate therapy and Begg treatment. Angle Orthod 1975;45:259–266.
283. Cooper RB. Indirect-bonded bite plate to prevent impingement on ceramic brackets. J Clin Orthod 1992;26:253–254.
284. Mayes JH. Bite turbos... New levels of bite-opening acceleration. Clin Impressions 1997;6:15–17.
285. Björk A, Skieller V. Normal and abnormal growth of the mandible. A synthesis of longitudinal cephalometric implant studies over a period of 25 years. Eur J Orthod 1983;5:1–46.
286. McNamara JA, Jr, Huge SA. The Fränkel appliance (FR-2): model preparation and appliance construction. Am J Orthod 1981;80:478–495.
287. Clark WJ. The twin block traction technique. Eur J Orthod 1982;4:129–138.
288. Mills C, McCulloch K. Treatment effects of the twin block appliance: A cephalometric study. Am J Orthod 1998;114:15–24.
289. Toth LR, McNamara JA, Jr. Treatment effects produced by the twin block appliance and the FR-2 appliance of Frankel compared to an untreated Class II sample. Am J Orthod Dentofac Orthop 1999;116:597–609.
290. Riolo ML, Moyers RE, McNamara JA, Jr, Hunter WS. An atlas of craniofacial growth: Cephalometric standards from The University School Growth Study, The University of Michigan. Ann Arbor: Monograph 2, Craniofacial Growth Series, Center for Human Growth and Development, The University of Michigan, 1974.
291. Pancherz H. Personal communication, 1998.
292. Jager A. Longitudinal study of combined orthodontic and surgical treatment of Class II malocclusion with deep overbite. Int J Adult Orthod Orthogn Surg 1991;6:219–229.
293. Bell WH. Correction of the short face syndrome—vertical maxillary deficiency: a preliminary report. J Oral Surg 1977;35:110–120.
294. Epker BN, Fish LC, Paulus PJ. The surgical-orthodontic correction of maxillary deficiency. Oral Surg Oral Med Oral Pathol 1978;46:171–205.
295. Wessberg GA, Epker BN. Surgical inferior repositioning of the maxilla: treatment considerations and comprehensive management. Oral Surg Oral Med Oral Pathol 1981;52:349–356.
296. Wessberg GA, Fish LC, Epker BN. The short face patient: surgical-orthodontic treatment options. J Clin Orthod 1982;16:668–685.
297. Wessberg GA, Wolford LM, Epker BN. Interpositional genioplasty for the short face syndrome. J Oral Surg 1980;38:584–590.
298. Proffit WR, Phillips C, Turvey TA. Stability after surgical-orthodontic corrective of skeletal Class III malocclusion. 3. Combined maxillary and mandibular procedures. Int J Adult Orthod Orthognath Surg 1991;6:211–225.
299. Proffit WR, Turvey TA, Phillips C. Orthognathic surgery: A hierarchy of stability. Int J Adult Orthod Orthogn Surg 1996;11:191–204.
300. Wardrop RW, Wolford LM. Maxillary stability following downgraft and/or advancement procedures using rigid fixation and porous block hydroxyapatite implants. J Oral Maxillofac Surg 1989;47:326–342.
301. Moenning JE, Wolford LM. Coralline porous hydroxyapatite as a bone graft substitute to orthognathic surgery: a 24-month follow-up results. Int J Adult Orthod Orthogn Surg 1989;4:105–117.
302. Rosen HM, Ackerman JL. Porous block hydroxyapatite in orthognathic surgery. Angle Orthod 1991;61:185–191.
303. McNamara JA, Jr, ed. The enigma of the vertical dimension. Ann Arbor: Monograph 36, Craniofacial Growth Series, Center for Human Growth and Development, The University of Michigan, 2000.
304. Van der Linden FPGM. Facial growth and facial orthopedics. Chicago: Quintessence, 1986.
305. McNamara JA, Jr, Van der Linden FPGM. Unpublished data, 1970.

Chapter 9

COMPREHENSIVE FIXED APPLIANCE THERAPY

With Michael L. Swartz

"The opportunity of greatness lies in doing ordinary things extraordinarily well." This anonymous quote summarizes the purpose of this chapter, to discuss some of the "little things" dealing with the management of routine fixed appliance treatment that not only can affect the outcome of treatment, but also can make that treatment more efficient.[1]

Any individual who has been practicing clinical orthodontics for a reasonable length of time develops his or her own unique therapeutic approach. Each of us is greatly influenced, not only by our graduate and postgraduate orthodontic education, but also by our own clinical experience.

Every practitioner should have a clear understanding of the sequence of events that will lead to an excellent clinical result. An examination of transfer cases from other clinicians, however, reveals that not all share the same vision as to the sequence of events that should occur, even in relatively routine treatments. Nor do all clinicians prepare a patient for fixed appliance therapy in the same manner, as is evidenced by the wide variation observed in bracket and band placement. This variation in bracket position occurs so frequently that, when accepting a transfer patient, many orthodontists simply remove the existing appliances and replace them not only with their own specific slot size and prescription, but also place the brackets in position according to their own preference.

Radical changes in the treatment plan often occur as well. Most times, however, the details of appliance manipulation are as important as the original diagnosis and treatment plan in achieving an excellent orthodontic result. This chapter discusses many of those details.

APPLIANCE SELECTION

For the purpose of this initial discussion, a basic approach to the treatment of relatively straightforward malocclusions will be described, as used currently in our private orthodontic practice. We have found the sequence of treatment described here to be efficient and effective. Other clinicians, of course, recommend other treatment protocols. The selection of a sequence of wires should be based on a sound understanding of the characteristics of various archwire materials, but in the end, the specific details (*e.g.*, wire size and shape) of the sequence usually are based in part on the clinical experience of the practitioner.

We routinely use preadjusted appliances (Fig. 9-1), rather than standard or "neutral"[2] edgewise appliances, during comprehensive orthodontic therapy. We recommend using the "non-extraction Roth prescription" when selecting a specific prescription of a preadjusted appliance. This prescription for torque and angulation that is built into each bracket has proven satisfactory to us for nearly two decades.

It has been our choice to use brackets with a .018" slot, although a .022" slot also can be used effectively (see the discussion of the Damon 2™ self-ligating bracket system at the end of this chapter). The introduction of memory wires that have low force values over a wide range of ac-

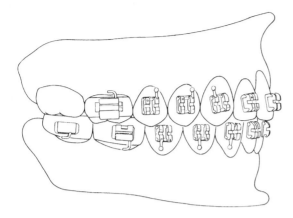

Figure 9-1. Typical bonds and bands used during fixed appliance therapy.

tivation makes the difference in slot size less important than it was two or three decades ago.

One of the primary reasons why we have selected a .018″ slot is the ability to use .016 × .022″ chrome-cobalt wires in the fabrication of utility arches.[3] We have found that size and type of wire to be much easier to manipulate clinically than the .019 × .019″ chrome-cobalt wire that is recommended for utility arch construction with a .022″ slot appliance.

When selecting molar bands, we recommend the addition of auxiliary archwire tubes on the brackets of both the upper and mandibular first molar bands or bonds (Fig. 9-1). As utility arches can be inserted at virtually any point in treatment, it is essential that these auxiliary tubes be available.

Further, the incorporation of ball hooks on the canine and premolar brackets (Fig. 9-1) is recommended. These ball hooks are available when intra- or intermaxillary elastics are incorporated into the treatment. Care must be taken, however, in the fabrication of utility arches, so that the vestibular extensions of the arch do not contact the ball hooks.

GENERAL SEQUENCE OF TREATMENT

Although no two patients are treated precisely the same way, our approach to fixed appliance therapy typically follows a prescribed sequence. In instances of significant Class II occlusal relationships, additional appliances (*e.g.*, Pendex,[4] Herbst,[5] twin block,[6] Wilson distalizing arch[7]) are used. For the purpose of the following hypothetical discussion, however, only mild sagittal occlusal problems exist.

In this consideration of routine treatment protocols, a number of specific archwires are suggested. A more general discussion of archwire properties and the rationale for their use is presented later in this chapter.

Resolution of Transverse Discrepancies

As has been described in Chapter 7 and elsewhere,[8,9] a major factor in a surprising high percentage of malocclusions is an underlying transverse discrepancy of the maxilla. If such a condition exists, rapid maxillary expansion (RME) is used to correct both posterior and anterior crossbites as well as to increase arch space in mild-to-moderate tooth-size/arch-size discrepancy patients. RME also is used to "broaden the smile" in patients with a narrow maxilla and possibly to improve nasal airflow. In any event, transverse problems always are addressed before routine fixed appliance treatment is begun.

Leveling and Aligning

The general properties that are required for the initial archwire to align all the brackets are resiliency, resiliency, and more resiliency (stored energy). The archwire need not be highly formable (assuming the treatment approach is pre-adjusted appliances with no adjustment loops). Nickel titanium wires are well suited for this application. For the majority of practitioners, nickel titanium alloy wires have become the material of choice for aligning brackets and eliminating rotations.

It has been reported that some nickel titanium wires appeared to be no more effective than a multi-stranded, inexpensive stainless steel wire[10,11] as, for example, a small diameter (.014″) superelastic nickel titanium compared to a .015″ multi-stranded stainless steel wire. The conclusions from clinical observations were that the less expensive multi-stranded wire was just as efficient as .014″ nickel titanium wire.

Round archwires usually are preferred as initial leveling wires so that unnecessary and undesirable movements of the roots of the involved teeth are avoided whenever possible. These lower load deflection rate wires can be engaged more easily in the brackets. In some situations in which the control of root torque is essential, however, the introduction of heat-sensitive copper nickel titanium (NiTi) wires has allowed the used of rectangular archwire as an initial leveling wire. We use both types of wires routinely.

In instances of severely rotated teeth, we usually place a .014″ nickel titanium wire or a .0175″ stainless steel coaxial wire (Respond™, Ormco Corp., Orange CA) for initial leveling and alignment. A .016″ NiTi

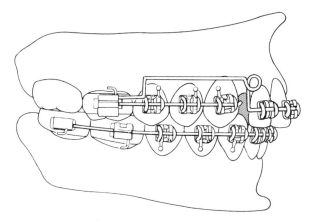

Figure 9-2. Distal rotation of the maxillary premolars and first molars typically produces small spaces distal to the maxillary lateral incisors. A retraction utility arch (shown before activation) can be used to retract the maxillary anterior teeth and close the spaces.

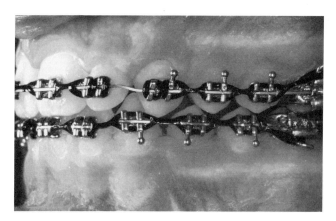

Figure 9-3. Intraoral view of a patient with elastomeric chain places in a "4-4-4" maxillary configuration (this designation refers to the number of links in each elastomeric segment). Three segments of chain with four links are placed, one from the mesial wing of the lateral incisor bracket across the central incisors to the mesial wing on the opposite lateral incisor. The other two segments extend from the distal wing of the canines to the hook on the first molar bands. Single elastomeric ties ("donuts") are places on the remaining tie wings.

wire, an archwire that may be used as the first leveling wire in less-rotated cases, usually follows the initial wire. In the later phase of initial leveling and alignment, we commonly use a .016" x .022" rectangular NiTi wire to begin adding appropriate root torque.

One of us (MLS), however, prefers a .018" NiTi archwire that is superelastic and is made from non-thermally active nickel titanium as the initial leveling wire in either a .018" or .022" slot appliance. Unpublished clinical studies[12] conducted over a ten year period have shown that a single NiTi archwire can achieve the primary objectives of this first stage of treatment, that is the elimination of all rotations and the alignment of all bracket slots to permit an easy insertion of a large diameter rectangular arch wire. This last statement assumes that the wire has superelastic properties and does not take a permanent set. A further discussion of the characteristics of NiTi archwires will appear later in this chapter.

During this early phase of fixed appliance treatment, a soldered transpalatal arch is activated sequentially to produce distal molar rotation and buccal root torque. These activations, combined with appropriate placement of brackets on the upper canines and premolars (to be discussed later) should result in spontaneous improvement in occlusal relationship. A slight opening of space anterior to the upper canines occurs frequently (Fig. 9-2). Thus, the maxillary archwire is secured to the brackets by way of "open" elastomeric chain from canine to molar bilaterally and across the four maxillary incisors.

When elastomeric chain is used segmentally, only the more proximal wing of the terminal bracket is incorporated into the chain (Fig 9-3). For example, when connecting chain from the maxillary canine to the hook on the upper first molar, the chain is attached to both pre-molar brackets, but only to the distal wing of the canine bracket; the mesial wing is secured with a single elastomeric tie. This technique of attachment prevents the unwanted rotation of the canine from occurring. Similarly, the four incisors are connected together by chaining from the mesial wing of one upper lateral incisor, around both central incisor brackets, and then around the mesial wing of the bracket on the other incisor. Single "O-rings" are placed on both distal wings, again to prevent unwanted tooth rotation. Continuous elastomeric chain is placed around the arch from first molar to first molar only after a Class I occlusion has been achieved and no further Class II correction is desired.

In the mandible, the archwire is ligated initially with single elastomeric ties and later with elastomeric chain extending from first molar to first molar (Fig. 9-3), following the insertion of a heavier rectangular archwire.

Vertical Separation (Disclusion) of the Incisors

The next goal of treatment is to provide separation of the upper and mandibular incisors, typically through maxillary and mandibular incisor intrusion. Ricketts[13] has stressed the importance of avoiding unintentional incisal contact during the subsequent correction of anteroposterior discrepancies with such auxiliary appliances as a facebow or Class II elastics.

The need to avoid incisal contact early in treatment also is illustrated by the evaluation of progress study models taken before orthognathic surgery. When preparing a patient for surgery, the incisors should be repositioned with fixed appliances so that incisal contact is reduced greatly or eliminated altogether, allowing maximal posterior contact when the presurgical study model are hand articulated to their desired postsurgical position. In this way, the surgeon is free to change the relationship of the maxilla and the mandible without encountering interferences produced by accidental anterior contact.

Correction of the Sagittal Relationship of the Posterior Teeth

The correction of any residual Class II or Class III sagittal relationships is initiated at this time. We most commonly use interarch elastics (*e.g.*, 1/4", 6 oz. elastics) to produce the necessary correction, attaching the elastic anteriorly to the ball hooks on the upper canines and posteriorly to the hooks on the mandibular first or second molars in instances of Class II correction. Class II elastics are used initially after a .016 × .022" NiTi wire is placed in both arches. Depending on anchorage requirements, a rectangular TMA™ or stainless steel wire also can be used. The use of stiffer archwires during elastic wear is required to avoid unintentional rotation of the mandibular molars, flaring of the mandibular incisors, and loss of vertical control.

When attempting to slide a tooth along an archwire during space closure, at least a .002" size difference should be maintained between the archwire and the bracket slot to facilitate sliding mechanics[14] (*e.g.*, a .016" archwire sliding through a .018" bracket). Until adequate molar correction is attained, the placement of elastomeric chain around the arch from molar to molar must be avoided, again to prevent unwanted retraction of the upper incisor and also to avert possible anchorage loss.

Retraction of Maxillary Anterior Teeth

The mechanics described thus far (even for patients treated without extraction) often will lead to the creation of small spaces distal to the upper lateral incisors (Fig. 9-2). A retraction utility arch[3,15] usually is used to intrude and retract the upper incisors (Fig. 9-4). The mandibular archwire, now a .016 × .022" TMA™ wire, typically is stepped down in the mandibular incisor region. Other types of looped closing arches, made from beta titanium, chrome cobalt, or stainless steel wire also can be inserted to retract the upper incisors. Anterior space closure typically is supported by either fulltime or nighttime wear of Class II elastics.

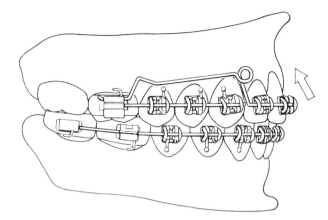

Figure 9-4. The maxillary retraction utility arch after activation. The maxillary anterior teeth have been moved superiorly and posteriorly and the space distal to the lateral incisor has closed.

Detailing the Occlusion

After the molar correction has been achieved and excess overjet and overbite have been eliminated, the finishing sequence begins. The archwires used at this time should have high formability so that precise detailing of the occlusion can be accomplished by way of first order (in-out), second order (up-down), and third order (torquing) bends. These wires also should have a high stiffness so that sufficient force is produced for final leveling and torquing movements. Archwires suitable for this purpose include rectangular wires made of beta titanium, chrome cobalt, or stainless steel. Our choice is .016 × .022" TMA™. Triangular elastics (1/4" 6 oz.) extending from the maxillary canines to the mandibular canines and mandibular first premolars, also are used to seat the occlusion before appliance removal.

As the patient nears completion of treatment, the archwires are removed and "debond evaluation" models are obtained. The models are evaluated for errors in tooth position, adjustments are made in the archwires, and then these models are sent to the laboratory for the fabrication of a tooth positioner, which is delivered at the time of appliance removal (see Chapter 26 for a discussion of finishing and retention protocols).

DETAILS OF BRACKET PLACEMENT

One of the most critical aspects of fixed appliance treatment is the position of the bracket on each tooth. Many clinicians take great pride in being known as "good wire benders." Their typical final archwires give testament to their wire-bending skills, with multiple first, second and

COMPREHENSIVE FIXED APPLIANCE THERAPY

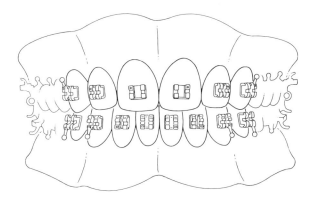

Figure 9-5. Idealized bracket placement on the maxillary and mandibular anterior teeth.

third order bends present in each wire. It is our opinion, however, that a final archwire that requires multiple artistic bends is less an indication of a clinician's prowess in archwire fabrication and more of an indication of a lack of ability in placing brackets correctly.

During the last ten years, the senior author has been involved in a group practice in which all patients are seen by multiple orthodontists. Thus, it has been very important for us to formalize our concepts of bracket position, so that usually it is impossible to tell which clinician in the practice initially placed the brackets and bands. We have tried to standardize bracket placement so that ideal bracket position can be visualized.

One of the primary goals of our comprehensive orthodontic treatment is to correct overbite before correcting overjet, as has been described above. Thus, we have emphasized mechanics that open the bite anteriorly, and this opening of the bite is incorporated into routine bracket placement. In addition, favorable rotation of the buccal segments (*e.g.*, posterior rotation of the buccal aspects of the crowns of the maxillary posterior teeth) leads to a slight, but predictable, correction in the occlusal relationship. These rotations are aided further by activating fully the soldered transpalatal arch that is placed at the beginning of treatment. Overjet is corrected only after proper vertical clearance of the incisors has been achieved and after the sagittal relationship of the posterior teeth is satisfactory. These relatively minor movements of the teeth that are crucial for the efficient treatment of the malocclusion are facilitated by proper bracket placement, the specifics of which are described in detail below.

Maxillary Incisors

The brackets are placed on the upper incisors to facilitate slight bite opening by positioning the bracket 3.5 mm to 4.0 mm above the incisal edge, as measured from the center of the bracket slot (Fig. 9-5). Each bracket is placed at the mesiodistal center of the crown of each incisor, and the wings of the bracket parallel the long axis of the crown. The incisal edge of the lateral incisors either can be maintained at the same level as the central incisor or can lie 0.5 mm gingival to the incisal edges of the central incisors and canines by placing the bracket slot 0.5 mm more incisally.

Maxillary Canines and Premolars

We recommend an alternate position of the brackets on these teeth,[16] particularly on the upper second premolars. An examination by the senior author of finished orthodontic cases both in a university orthodontic clinic and as an examiner for the Edward H. Angle Society has revealed that a common malalignment present at the end of treatment is a lack of contact of the upper second premolar with the mandibular first molar (Fig. 9-6). This lack of contact often is a result of inadequate posterior rotation of the premolar and, in great part, may be due to the initial placement of the bracket on that tooth. In addition, the retraction of anterior teeth with elastomeric chain often results in mesial rotation of the teeth in the buccal segments during treatment, especially if the upper molars are not supported by a transpalatal arch or facebow. Proper bracket position can help counteract this tendency.

When placing a bracket, particularly on the upper premolars, it is common first to determine the midline

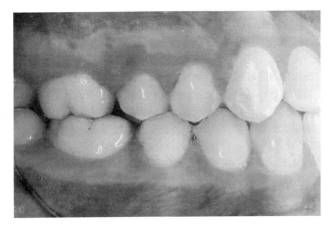

Figure 9-6. Intraoral photograph of a treated patient with incomplete correction of the sagittal malocclusion. The canines and first premolars are in a normal relationship; however, the maxillary second premolar is rotated to the mesial, due to improper bracket placement. Also, note the lack of contact of the distobuccal cusp of the maxillary first molar with the mesiobuccal cusp of the mandibular second molar, an indication that the maxillary first molar was not rotated to the posterior sufficiently around the palatal root.

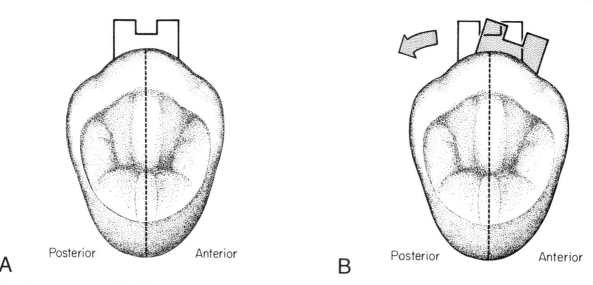

Figure 9-7. Placement of brackets on a symmetrical premolar. *A*, The long axis of the tooth (dashed line) is determined by positions of the buccal and lingual cusps. Typically, bracket placement has been based on the long axis of the tooth, by locating the center of the buccal and lingual cusps. *B*, Recommended mesial position of the bracket. Engaging the archwire into the bracket will produce a favorable posterior rotation of the crown, which is indicated during the treatment of Class I and Class II malocclusions. In Class III patients, mesial positioning of the brackets on the lower premolars is recommended.

of the tooth by examining the buccal and lingual cusps (Fig. 9-7*A*). Traditionally, the bracket is placed at the mesiodistal center of the buccal surface. We recommend routinely placing the bracket in a slightly more anterior position on the buccal surface of the upper second premolar (Fig. 9-7*B*). Such bracket positioning will result in a slight distal rotation of the upper premolar when the archwire is ligated in place.

The example shown in Figure 9-7 is of a symmetrical premolar. In clinical practice, however, it is far more common to have an upper premolar that is asymmetrical in shape, with the lingual cusp located more anteriorly (Fig. 9-8). When the midline of the tooth, as determined by the buccal and lingual cusps, is identified (Fig. 9-8*A*), and the bracket is placed according to the midline orientation, the bracket is bonded too far distally (Fig. 9-8*A*). This bracket position will cause undesirable mesial rotation of the bracket following ligation of the archwire into the bracket. This type of rotation is unfavorable except in patients having a tendency toward Class III malocclusion. If the bracket is placed more anteriorly on the upper second premolar (Figs. 9-8*B* and 9-9), automatic correction toward a Class I relationship will occur after the archwire is secured in place.

It is our opinion that more mistakes are made in the positioning of the bracket on the upper second premolar than on any other tooth. When a bracket is placed on an upper second premolar using a direct visualization technique, the clinician often will overcompensate for his or her lack of ability to see the tooth easily by placing the bracket even in a more distal position than that shown in Figure 9-8*A*. This overcompensated bracket position will result in an unfavorable mesial rotation of the premolar following archwire ligation (Fig. 9-6).

Thus, when placing a bracket on upper premolars, it is prudent to ignore the lingual cusp of these teeth altogether. Instead, first evaluate the occlusion intraorally or by way of study models, and then simply use the buccal cusp of the tooth as a guide, always remembering to place the bracket mesial to the center of the cusp of the upper second premolar and according to the needs of the occlusion when bonding the upper canine or first premolar.

The proper positions of the maxillary posterior brackets also are shown in Figure 9-10. Note the very slight mesial positioning of the premolar and canine brackets in the occlusal view.

Mandibular Incisors

The positioning of the brackets on the mandibular incisors is relatively straightforward. The brackets are placed at the mesiodistal center of the crowns (Fig. 9-11). From an incisogingival perspective, the brackets are positioned toward the incisal edge (Fig. 9-12). Only in patients with extreme deep bite are the brackets placed in a more gingival direction, an orientation that may tend to extrude these teeth, making overbite correction more difficult. In instances of excessive vertical overlap of the teeth, it is more common to place appliances on the upper arch initially and, using leveling and intrusive mechanics (*e.g.*, utility arch, anterior bite plate, "turbo-

COMPREHENSIVE FIXED APPLIANCE THERAPY

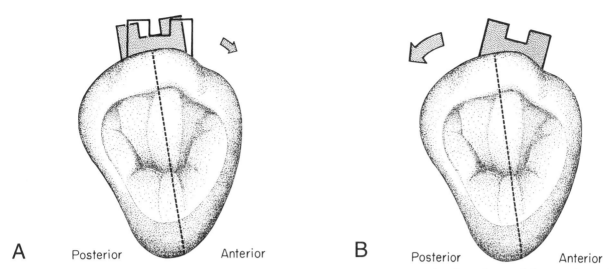

Figure 9-8. Placement of bracket on an asymmetrical premolar. *A*, The lingual cusp is oriented toward the anterior, and thus the long axis of the tooth (dashed line) is positioned more posteriorly. If the bracket is placed according to the long axis; the bracket will be located posteriorly resulting in an unfavorable anterior rotation of the premolar. *B*, In placing the bracket, the lingual cusp is ignored and only the buccal cusp is evaluated. The bracket is located anterior to the midpoint of the buccal cusp, as described in Figure 9-7*B*. Favorable posterior rotation of the premolar will occur after ligation of archwire into the bracket.

tails"), opening the bite anteriorly before mandibular bracket placement.

Mandibular Canines and Premolars

The placement of brackets on these teeth also is relatively straightforward (Fig. 9-13). Every effort should be made to place the brackets gingivally, especially in the region of the mandibular second premolar, so that the brackets are out of occlusion. Placing the brackets gingivally also aids in the leveling process.

Bracket failure is observed most frequently in this region. This failure may be due to a number of factors, including the presence of a pellicle on a recently erupted second premolar. In addition, this region is a site of frequent contamination during the bonding process. The bracket also may be dislodged due to the forces of mastication. If the mandibular premolar bond fails more than once, the placement of a band on the tooth may be indicated. Because of the frequency of loose brackets in this area, mandibular second premolars routinely are banded rather than bonded in our practice today.

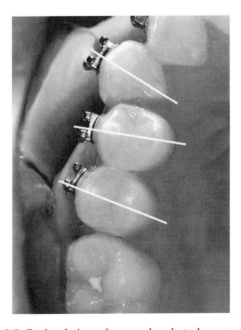

Figure 9-9. Occlusal view of proper bracket placement on the maxillary canine and premolars. The white lines indicate the long axes of the teeth. Note that the bracket on the second premolar is anterior to the midpoint of the buccal cusp. Modest adjustments have been made in the positions of the other two brackets as well.

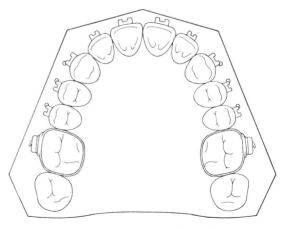

Figure 9-10. Occlusal view of idealized maxillary bracket and band position.

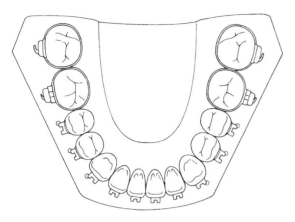

Figure 9-11. Occlusal view of idealized mandibular bracket and band position.

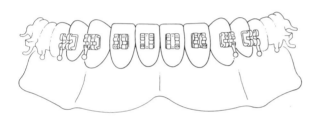

Figure 9-12. Frontal view of idealized mandibular bracket position.

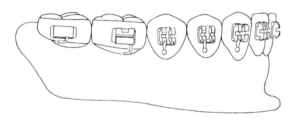

Figure 9-13. Lateral view of idealized mandibular bracket and band position.

From a mesiodistal perspective, the brackets are placed in the center of the buccal cusp in Class I and Class II patients (Fig. 9-12). In Class III patients, a more mesial placement of the bracket on the mandibular posterior teeth is indicated, as was described for Class II and Class I patients in the placement of maxillary brackets.

Overview

The placement of brackets in a patient in the early permanent dentition is shown in Figure 9-14. This clinical example illustrates the positioning of each bracket that should be placed according to the morphology of each tooth regardless of the position of that tooth within the arch.

The position of the bracket on the upper left lateral incisor in Figure 9-14A is of interest. Note that the distance of the bracket from the incisal edge is slightly greater than that of the bracket of the lateral incisor on the opposite side. In this instance, the bracket on the left lateral intentionally was placed slightly more gingivally because of the morphology of the incisal edge of that tooth. The incisal edge of the left lateral was modified later to eliminate the small bump (mamelon). Judicious enamoplasty before bracket placement is recommended in instances of abnormal tooth morphology or wear.

BAND SELECTION

The placement of bands is considered "common knowledge" among orthodontists and thus will not be described in detail here. Only a few remarks concerning the placement of separators and the selection and cementation of bands are in order.

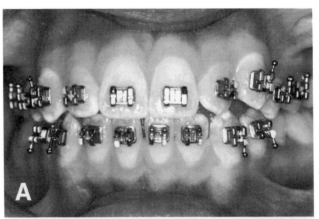

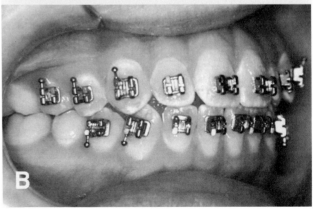

Figure 9-14. Intraoral views of a patient following bracket placement. Appliances shown are the midsize "Tru-Straight-wire™" brackets from Ormco Corp., Orange CA (.018″ slot, non-extraction Roth prescription). See text for specific comments about bracket position. A, Frontal view. B, Right lateral view.

COMPREHENSIVE FIXED APPLIANCE THERAPY

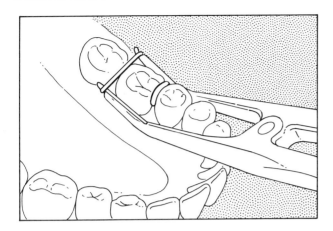

Figure 9-15. Placement of elastomeric separators using separating pliers. The separator is stretched and then one side of the separator is passed through the contact.

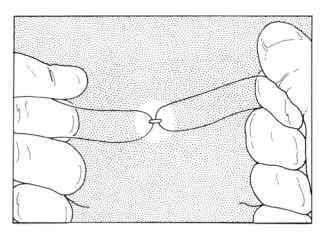

Figure 9-16. Placement of elastomeric separators using dental floss. Two pieces of floss are placed through the hole in the center of the separator and are held one in each hand.

Separators

Although there are a wide variety of materials that have been used for the separation of teeth, including brass wire, we normally use two types of separators: elastomeric separators and spring-type separators made from stainless steel wire.

Elastomeric Separators

For most patients, particularly patients who began treatment in the mixed dentition, the clinician will experience little difficulty in placing separators. Routinely, separating pliers can be used to stretch the separator and place it interproximally (Fig. 9-15).

An alternative method (that also is easily performed by a patient or parent) is the placement of the elastomeric separator using dental floss. Two pieces of dental floss are threaded through the center of the separator (Fig. 9-16). A hemostat and a piece of floss also can be used. The separator is stretched and placed through the contact point (Fig. 9-17). The dental floss then is removed. If an elastomeric separator continues to break on tight contacts, a piece of floss can be snapped through the contact and the separator is pulled under the contact, stretched, and snapped through the contact superiorly.

As the loss of elastomeric separators is a common occurrence, the patient can be instructed on the proper method of replacement using dental floss if a separator is lost before the banding appointment.

Spring-type Separators

Only in patients in whom there are extremely tight or gingivally positioned contacts (common in adult patients) is

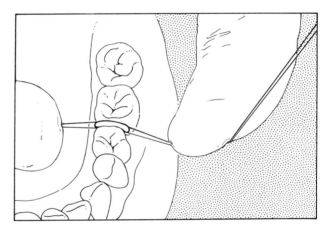

Figure 9-17. The placement of the elastomeric separator through a contact point with dental floss.

the spring-type separator (TP Laboratories, LaPorte IN) used. A Weingart plier is used to grasp the short arm of the separator (Fig. 9-18). The long, hooked arm of the separator is placed under the contact point and the short arm pried open with the plier. The separator is rotated into position with the short arm lying under the contact point and the long arm lying over the contact point.

The removal of the spring-type separator is accomplished most easily using two hooked scalers. The tip of one scaler is placed through the center of the spring while the tip of another scaler is placed in the hooked portion of the long arm. The spring-type separator then is pulled laterally, dislodging it from the contact point.

Band Placement

In our practice, bands usually are placed on both mandibular permanent molars and on the mandibular second premolars. As mentioned before, the latter teeth

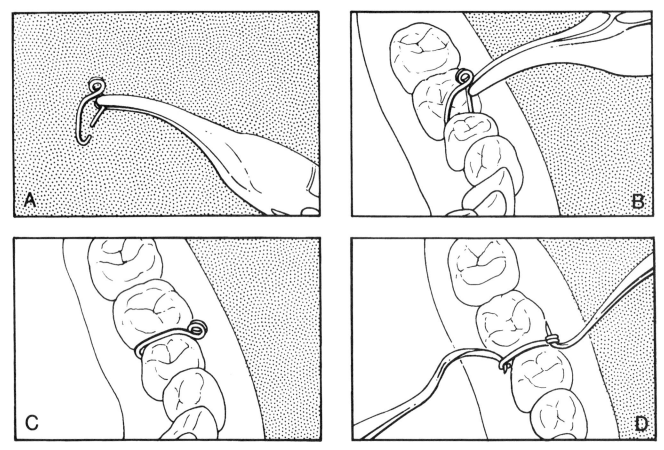

Figure 9-18. Placement of spring-type separators. *A*, The short arm of the separator is held in Weingart pliers. *B*, The long, hooked arm is placed under the contact point and the short arm is pulled laterally by the pliers. *C*, The separator is rotated into position with the long, hooked arm of the separator over the contact point and the short arm under the contact point. *D*, Removal of separators using two hooked scalers.

are banded rather than bonded because of the forces of mastication tend to dislodge the brackets on the mandibular posterior teeth. Bands also are placed on the upper first permanent molars, usually connected by a transpalatal arch. The upper second molars are banded only in instances in which there are obvious abnormalities in tooth position (*e.g.*, rotation, flaring, crossbite).

The bands are placed symmetrically on the teeth, particularly with respect to the contours of the marginal ridges. In addition, the bands should be large enough to fit teeth adequately. A band that is too small may appear to fit the tooth snugly but will result in a bracket or tube position that is too occlusal. On the other hand, a band that does not fit tightly will have more cement between the band and the tooth, a situation that leads to the increased probability of washed-out cement and subsequent decalcification of the tooth. In addition, loose-fitting bands obviously have to be recemented more frequently.

Bands usually are cemented using a resin band cement that is filled with glass beads (BandLok™, Reliance Orthodontics, Itasca IL). We prefer cement that is not tooth colored (as, for example, blue BandLok™), because we have found that it is much easier for the clinician to differentiate cement from tooth material during cement cleanup and following band removal.

In instances in which bands are to be recemented intentionally within a few weeks or months (*e.g.*, following further activation of the soldered transpalatal arch), the use of resin band cement with high cohesive strength is not recommended. Rather, a polycarboxylate cement such as Durelon™ (Premier Dental, Frankfurt, Germany) is used to minimize patient discomfort during band removal, due to the lower cohesive strength of the cement.

ARCHWIRE SELECTION

During the last thirty years, a number of new materials have become available to the orthodontist, with several titanium alloys supplementing stainless steel wire and chrome-cobalt wire. A brief discussion of the major

COMPREHENSIVE FIXED APPLIANCE THERAPY

types of arch wires previously and currently used in orthodontic treatment is provided below.

Gold-Nickel Archwires

In the early 1900s, the archwires used for tooth movement generated extremely high orthodontic forces over very short distances (*i.e.*, very high load deflection rates). By today's standards, the materials and techniques used were extraordinarily inefficient, as the orthodontic appliances were not resilient, having a low level of springback and little stored energy. As a result, patients had to be seen often, sometimes daily.

With the non-extraction doctrine that was in fashion at that time, a primary function of the archwire was to form a rigid base against which teeth could be expanded facially. For example, the so-called E-Arch of Angle[17] served this purpose; it was formed from gold-nickel alloy, .030–.036″ in diameter. The E-Arch evolved to the ribbon arch, also intended to be a rigid wire with which teeth could be moved facially.

The first edgewise archwires (.022″ × .030″) simply were ribbon arches placed on edge (hence, the term "edgewise"). Angle[17] intended these gold-nickel wires, at least initially, to facilitate his non-extraction dogma, with the archwires rigid enough to allow for the expansion of the dental arches. Teeth first were tipped facially toward the archwire and subsequently engaged into the rectangular, edgewise appliance.

With the shift away from non-extraction and expansion protocols in later years, the function of the archwire changed as well. The archwire no longer was intended to serve as a rigid, non-yielding base, but rather the archwire was deflected into the bracket slots. In order to do so, the load deflection rate had to be reduced, and this demand for archwire flexibility resulted in the use of *wire progressions*. Smaller diameter wires and wires with adjustment loops (Fig. 9-19) could be engaged into the bracket without permanent deformation. Sstainless steel, which is 20% stiffer than gold-nickel, has a higher load deflection rate than the latter type of wire. Due to wire progressions, the overall treatment could be performed by means of stainless steel with lower load deflection rates. The use of wire progressions led to increased treatment efficiency, with patients routinely seen for appointments less frequently.

Stainless Steel Archwires

Beginning in 1929 and continuing into the mid 1930s, stainless steel began to replace gold-nickel arch wires. Because stainless steel was about 20% stiffer than comparably sized gold-nickel wires, the wire size would have to be reduced by about 20% in order to stay in the same force range as was being used previously. A 20% reduction in .022″ yields .018″. Thus, the introduction of the .018″ slot bracket occurred.

The stress-strain curve of stainless steel (Figure 9-20) shows a steep slope. It has a modulus of elasticity of 25×10^6 psi and a relatively short elastic range, thus taking a permanent set (deformation) easily. With a small elastic range and a high modulus, it is a relatively non-resilient material with relatively low springback of 15%. It has an extended plastic range with good formability.

Stainless steel wire often is used in a multistranded configuration and is available commercially as Respond™ wire (Ormco Corporation, Orange CA) or Wildcat™ wire (GAC International, Central Islip NY). These wires, which have a low level of stiffness and being composed of stainless steel and being mulitstrand, they are highly formable. They are not resilient. These types of wires often are used as initial leveling and alignment

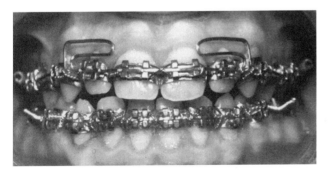

Figure 9-19. Intraoral view of a patient with adjustment loops in the archwire. The loops increase the length of the wire between brackets, increasing the resiliency of the wire.

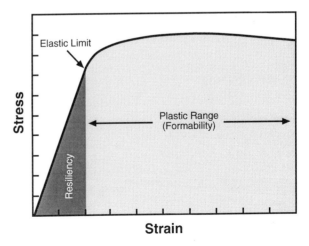

Figure 9-20. Load deflection of stainless steel wire. Deformation in the resilient range is reversible, whereas deformation in the non-linear portion of the curve is permanent.

wires, especially in dental arches that have a significant number of rotations present. These wires have a very low stiffness and are not suitable for any significant tooth movement such as space closure, as they cannot resist the side effects of tipping and arch collapse.

Chrome-Cobalt Alloy Archwires

The primary use of chrome-cobalt alloy (Elgiloy™, Rocky Mountain Orthodontics, Denver CO; Azurloy™, Ormco Corp.) is in the fabrication of utility arches and anterior sectional arches. The chrome-cobalt alloy, in its supplied un-annealed state, is easier to deform than is stainless steel. The force levels produced by unheat-treated .016 × .022″ wire are ideal for the fabrication of utility arches. The level of force generated is predictable, and intraoral activation of the utility arches can be performed routinely. Although chrome-cobalt wires can be heat-treated to increase stiffness, it has been our experience that heat-treating these wires usually is not necessary.

Titanium Alloy Archwires

In the 1980s, titanium alloy archwires began to replace stainless steel in many orthodontic applications. With the use of titanium alloys, load/deflection rates were reduced greatly (Fig. 9-21), and their highly resilient nature provided the opportunity for greater efficiency and for further extending appointment intervals. With titanium alloy wires, it was possible to treat comprehensive full appliance patients in half the number of office visits and in the same or shorter total treatment time, with improved treatment results.

Until the development of new alloys, there were only two possible ways of altering the load/deflection rate of an archwire: changing the wire diameter or cross sectional area and changing the wire length by incorporating adjustment loops (Fig. 9-19). In 1977, two variations from solid stainless steel became available to the profession, a rectangular braided stainless steel wire (D-Rect™, Ormco Corp.) and Nitinol™ (Unitek Corp., Monrovia CA). In 1980, an alloy of titanium and molybdenum (TMA™, Ormco Corp.) was introduced. Since then, there has been a great proliferation of titanium alloys.

Nickel-titanium archwires now exist that are super-elastic and also may be activated by temperature changes. It also is possible to have archwires with such a low load deflection rate as to be apparently ineffective. As a result, we now have, for the first time in orthodontics, forces that clinically appear to be below the thresh-

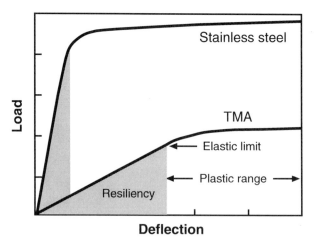

Figure 9-21. Load deflection of stainless steel and TMA wire.

old of efficient tooth movement, which tells us a great deal about optimal force ranges for tooth movement.

Wire Stiffness

As the varieties of new archwire alloys were introduced, the confusion concerning archwire selection increased. To aid orthodontists in relating the newer wires to a known entity, stainless steel, Burstone[18] developed wire stiffness values. The wire stiffness, Ws, relates other wire alloys and compositions to solid stainless steel. First, the modulus of elasticity is related to that of stainless steel. The modulus of elasticity provides the material stiffness value, Ms. Next, to relate one size wire to another, the wire's cross-sectional stiffness, Cs, must be considered. The cross-sectional stiffness value will vary for the first and second order dimensions of the wire. The bar graphs in Figure 9-22 show the relative wire stiffness (Ws) of several wires.

In comparing the relative wire stiffness of the titanium alloy wires with stainless steel, it is of value to note the relatively low stiffness (forces) of all sizes of the nickel titanium wires. A wire progression in stainless steel accounts for a significant increase in forces (Fig. 9-23). Conversely, a size progression in a nickel titanium wire has significantly less change in force levels and at forces that are but a fraction of those that are delivered in stainless steel.

Stress-Strain Curves

The wire stiffness comparisons can provide relative values of force levels that a wire might exert. They do not convey, however, other important material properties. Other descriptions of the material properties of archwires can be illustrated with stress-strain curves.

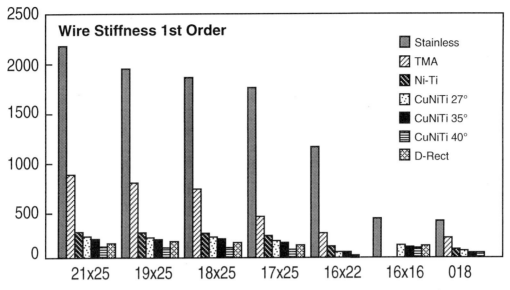

Figure 9-22. Wire stiffness of first order bends for various types of archwires.

As the level of force is increased on a wire (as represented in Figure 9-20), the wire initially springs back to its original position until the *elastic limit* is reached. If a wire is deflected past the elastic (proportional) limit, permanent deformation of the archwire occurs, as would be necessary when placing first, second, and third order bends. The wire then remains in a plastic state until the point of *ultimate strength* is reached, at which the wire fractures (*e.g.*, bending a wire paperclip or coat hanger until it breaks).

Beta Titanium. In 1980, a variation from stainless steel and nickel-titanium was introduced. Developed for orthodontic use by Burstone and Goldberg,[18-20] ß-titanium is an alloy composed of titanium and molybdenum (11% molybdenum, 6% zirconium, and 4% tin. Note: There is no nickel in TMA™). It has a material stiffness of 0.42 (42% the stiffness of stainless steel).

Quoting Burstone and Goldberg:[19]

"It has been our aim to develop an orthodontic alloy which offers an over-all balance in superiority of properties over those that are currently in use. Although the properties required in an orthodontic wire will vary, depending upon its application, generally three characteristics are important for a superior wire. First, it should be possible for the wire to be deflected over long distances without permanent deformation; hence, a large springback. This ensures that the clinician can activate his appliances without permanent deformation, which assures better control over tooth movement and minimizes intervals for adjustment. Second, the wire should have a stiffness that is lower than that of stainless steel, which would allow wires to fill the bracket for control and at the same time produce lighter forces. Third, the wire should be highly formable, that is, capable of being easily shaped, bent, and formed into complicated configurations, such as loops, without fracture."[19]

A comparison of stress-strain plot for stainless steel and TMA (Fig. 9-21) demonstrates the unique properties of TMA, which has more than twice the resiliency of stainless steel. It has a good plastic range and like stainless steel, it is formable. As TMA is a softer alloy, however, it must be bent with greater care. TMA has a recovery on deformation (springback) of about 35% or approximately 90–110% greater than stainless steel. Titanium alloys cannot be soldered, but TMA may be welded to itself, with some extra care. Welding TMA requires special electrodes and technique.

Nickel Titanium Alloys. Nitinol, an acronym for *Ni-*

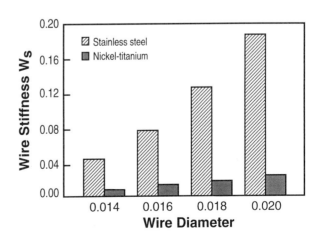

Figure 9-23. Relative wire stiffness of round stainless steel and NiTi wire.

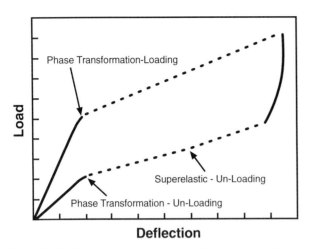

Figure 9-24. Diagrammatic representation of stress induced phase transformation of NiTi wire. A shift from one crystal structure to another (between martensitic and austenitic phases) occurs when there is a stress induced phase transformation.

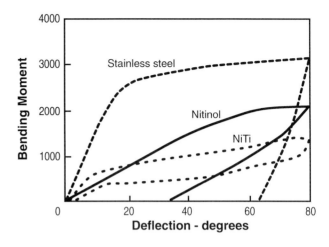

Figure 9-25. Bending moment, deflection characteristics of stainless steel, Nitinol and NiTi wires. Both loading (activation) and unloading (deactivation) curves are shown. NiTi wire produces lower moments and forces than Nitinol wire (after Burstone et al.,[22] and Proffit[14]).

nickel, *ti*-titanium, *n*-Navy, *o*-ordnance, *l*-laboratory, was the first nickel titanium alloy for orthodontics. The research for this class of material originally was performed by the US Navy, NASA, and the University of Iowa in 1971. Its original purpose was for use in Navy communication satellites.

The satellites were powered by large solar panels, with the nickel titanium wire forming the frame for these panels. At ambient earth temperatures, the wire was designed to be dead soft (below its designed temperature transition range or *TTR*). When exposed to the radiant heat of the sun in outer space, the wire heated up, passed through its TTR and became a resilient wire with a shape that was predetermined on earth. The wire expanded, opening up the solar panels. This property of temperature induced phase transformation is referred to as *shape memory*. Andreasen[21] was the first to recognize the potential for this wire in orthodontics. Since its introduction in 1977, the technology and manufacture of nickel-titanium alloys for use as an orthodontic arch wire has evolved considerably.

The metallurgical properties of shape memory (Fig. 9-24) are the result of a phase shift from one crystal structure to another (the austenitic, body-centered cubic form and the martensitic hexagonal form). This phase transformation (shifting between martensitic and austenitic phases) occurs when a material, in this instance a nickel-titanium alloy, either passes through its TTR, a temperature induced phase transformation, or when there is a stress induced phase transformation.

Whereas the first nickel-titanium wire to be introduced in orthodontics was Nitinol™, this material does not have the same physical properties of many of the more recent nickel-titanium wires. The purpose for raising this issue is that often the name "Nitinol" is used generically to refer to other nickel-titanium wires. The orthodontic literature frequently contains references to other nickel-titanium wires that have been referred to as a Nitinol. While most nickel-titanium wires are composed of about 55% nickel and 45% titanium, each manufacturer's brand of nickel-titanium will have different properties. Many of these differences can be significant, with important clinical implications. The original Nitinol wires (1977–1990) were work hardened and did not have the special property of superelasticity.

To clarify this increasingly complex subject, it is appropriate to look at the unusual stress-strain plots for nickel-titanium alloys. A major difference in the stress-strain curve (Fig. 9-25) of nickel-titanium to other alloys is that it is not linear within its elastic range. This non-elastic type of behavior is called *psuedoelastic*. The reason for this disproportionality is that the wire is shifting between phases because of the stress applied (*i.e.*, stress induced phase transformation). A material that is proportional in its elastic state (*i.e.*, a single phase alloy) essentially will have a single plot for stress-strain under load as when the load is released during unloading. Due to the stress induced phase transformation of nickel-titanium, the unloading curve is different from and at a lower force than the loading curve (Fig. 9-25). Because the force that the wire exerts on the bracket and tooth is the primary factor, the unloading curve takes on added significance.

Superelasticity

Nickel-titanium wire can, with additional manufacturing care, include the physical property of *superelasticity*. Super elasticity is the property of having force relatively independent of deflection; that is, a constant force generated over a large range of deflections. On the stress-strain curve, this property is represented by a relatively flat portion of the unloading curve. To achieve superelasticity, the wire must be primarily in its austenitic phase at its normal operating temperature.

The manufacture of orthodontic wires requires the drawing of a larger size bar or wire. The wire is drawn a number of times to achieve the desired size and shape of the end product. Each drawing can work-harden the alloy. To achieve the desired finished properties, which include a final heat treatment, the starting alloy ingot must factor in all the manufacturing steps along the way as well as the work hardening. The first nickel-titanium, Nitinol, was work hardened, martensitic (TTR 48°) and thus did not have the desirable property of superelasticity (Nitinol SE is superelastic).

An article by Burstone and co-workers[22] helped to define the significance of superelasticity. This publication first pointed out the differences between work-hardened martensitic Nitinol and the superelastic Chinese NiTi.*

Why is superelasticity of importance? In the same 1985 publication, Burstone and co-workers[22] tested and demonstrated significant differences between identical compositions of nickel and titanium, one with superelastic behavior (Chinese NiTi) and the other, work hardened and non-superelastic (Nitinol) (Figure 9-25). The non-superelastic nickel titanium took a permanent set and did not exhibit unloading phase transformation.

As shown in Figure 9-26, the Chinese NiTi (marketed by Ormco Corp. as Ni-Ti™) was deflected (cantilever bending) 20°, 40°, 60°, and 80° and the unloading measured at each deflection. Two important properties are displayed. At higher deflections (60° and 80°) the greater the energy that is released on unloading, and as the wire approaches its original austenitic shape, the stiffer the NiTi wire becomes. At large deflections, the wire exerts less force than at smaller deflections. At large deflections, NiTi is 7% as stiff as stainless steel,

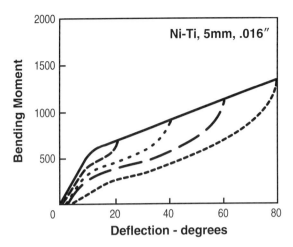

Figure 9-26. Bending moments of NiTi wire (after Burstone et al.[22]).

whereas at smaller deflections it is 28% as stiff as stainless steel.

The other property demonstrated by this test is that if a wire is superelastic, it will become more efficient the closer it gets to its original shape. This observation indicates that the wire could be left in until it is passive, if it does not undergo time dependent stress relaxation, and if the force delivered is adequate for the desired tooth movement.

Temperature Sensitivity

All materials will undergo phase transformations at several temperature transition ranges (TTR). The transition from ice to water to steam causes H_2O to change phases at the TTR at 0°C and 100°C. When the material passes through a TTR that is above ambient temperatures, the material is said to be thermally active. The wires on the satellite solar panels were thermally active above 200°C. A thermally active orthodontic wire must pass through a TTR above room temperature (~22°C) and ideally have its TTR near mouth temperature, 35–37°C. The temperature transition range represents the lower temperature at which the alloy begins its phase transformation and the higher temperature at which it completes its transformation.

Below its TTR, nickel-titanium alloy is primarily in its martensitic phase. After passing through its TTR, it enters into its austenitic phase. It is in the austenitic phase that it recovers the shape (in this case the arch form) that was built-in at the time of heat treatment (above 450°C). This recovery is the property of shape memory.

In 1991, an article comparing various nickel-titanium wires[26] identified the different properties that can exist between brands of nearly identical compositions of

---

*The literature refers to Chinese nickel titanium and Japanese nickel titanium. While these categories have little significance now, they initially referred to alloys developed primarily by Burstone[22] working with Chinese metallurgists and to those of Miura[23-25] working with Japanese metallurgists. The Chinese NiTi was not designed to be thermally active (TTR at or below ambient temperatures), whereas the Japanese nickel titanium wires were designed to be thermally active.

nickel and titanium. This same study pointed out the significance of superelasticity relative to springback (recovery from deformation). Superelastic wires had springback values of 65 to 70% versus non-superelastic wires with springback ranging from 40 to 60%.

Overview

Just as our world in general has become more technologically oriented, so to have orthodontic biomaterials. The introduction of titanium to archwire materials has expanded greatly the possibilities of routine orthodontic mechanics. The resiliency (stored energy) of nickel titanium, when used as an initial leveling wire, has allowed for greater appointment intervals and increased patient comfort. Titanium molybdenum alloys can be used during the final stages of treatment to align and detail the occlusion. In addition, the recent introduction of lower load/deflection wires, composed of copper, nickel, and titanium, has made it possible to engage a large diameter rectangular wire as the initial leveling and alignment wire. This option is advantageous when facial-lingual moment (torque) is critical. By understanding and maximizing the capabilities of the varieties of titanium alloy wire, there is a significant labor savings. This savings in time and energy more than compensates for any additional cost of these more complex and exotic alloys.

NEW TECHNOLOGY: SELF-LIGATING BRACKETS

We have chosen to include a short synopsis of a new technology that has the potential of positively influencing the treatment efficiency of routine orthodontic practice while maintaining or enhancing treatment quality. The use of active and passive self-ligation in an orthodontic bracket requires a shift in paradigm away from elastomeric chain and stainless steel ligation, as described earlier in this chapter.

The general concept of self-ligating brackets is not new, but rather has been part of the orthodontic literature for many years. The Edgelock™ bracket system was developed by Ormco Corporation in 1968, and Hanson[27] introduced the first self-ligating bracket in 1980. He described the primary components of the SPEED™ appliance and provided an explanation of the manner in which it functions. Hanson stated that the bracket body, the mounted spring clip, and the bonding pad assemblies permitted the application of corrective forces to teeth and their supporting structures without the need for archwire-ligating materials. The spring and arch slot geometry has been designed to reduce sliding friction and to enhance the three-dimensional control of tooth movement. He also stated that despite their small size, SPEED brackets have provision for a wide variety of auxiliaries. It was possible to secure uprighting springs and several types of elastic hooks to individual brackets.

The SPEED™ (Strite Industries Ltd, Cambridge, Ontario) and Sigma™ (American Orthodontics, Sheboygan WI) brackets (Fig. 9-27A) are examples of an *active* self-ligation system, in that a mounted spring clip is used to secure the archwire in the bracket slot. The primary objective of active ligation is to seat the archwire against the back of the slot for torque and rotation control. Damon[28, 29] has raised concerns about this type of spring clip activation by stating that the slot size of active ligation brackets actually is reduced in a passive state. As a result, the smaller the lumen size, the greater that level of friction. He contends that the seating action of the active clip nearly replicates the action of conventional ligature ties, as is shown in Figure 9-27A.

Damon[28-30] advocates *passive* self-ligation and has developed a bracket that has a low level of friction. He recommends using small diameter nickel titanium archwires as initial wires in this bracket system to decrease treatment time and chair time with longer appointment intervals. He also states that this type of approach improves treatment quality and control, while increasing patient comfort significantly.

The Damon 2™ bracket (Ormco Corp., Orange CA) is shown in Figure 9-28. It is a fully programmed Straight-Wire™ appliance with a twin bracket configuration. The slide on the bracket, which opens and closes with an audible click, opens away from the clinician in both arches, so that the clinician can determine easily if

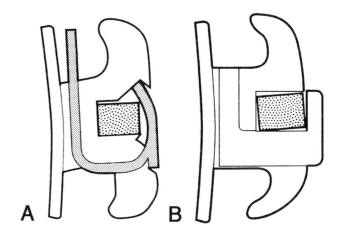

Figure 9-27. A comparison of an active (Sigma™) and a passive (original Damon SL™) bracket. Active self-ligation forces the wire into the slot, whereas the passive system does not "seat" the wire, thus reducing the friction on the archwire (from Damon[28]).

COMPREHENSIVE FIXED APPLIANCE THERAPY

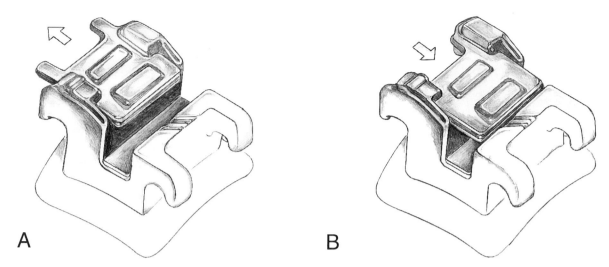

Figure 9-28. Schematic drawings of the Damon 2 bracket. The reduced thickness of the bracket facilitates placement of the brackets on malposed teeth. *A.* Bracket slide in open position. *B.* Bracket slide in closed position. (Modified from a drawing from Ormco Corp.)

the archwire is engaged in the slot. The closed slide (Fig. 9-28*B*) forms a complete tube that facilitates rotational control. When the slide is closed, the lumen of the bracket remains at full size. The combination of such bracket design and superelastic archwires allows filling of the slot buccolingually.[28]

The bracket is opened by way of specially designed pliers (#801-2100, Ormco Corp.) that is angled at 45" to the face of the bracket (Fig. 9-29). The slide is pushed down with the beaks of the pliers. When closing the slide (Fig. 9-30), the pliers are angled in the opposite direction, and the beaks of the pliers are used to push the slide over the archwire.

The Damon 2 bracket can be opened and closed with special instruments developed specifically for that purpose. The bracket can be opened with special tweezers (#801-2100, Ormco Corp.) that have been modified so that one of the ends is bent 90" to contact the bracket base (Fig. 9-31*A*). The other end is used to move the slide away from the archwire (Fig. 9-31*B*).

Another tweezer-like tool has been developed for closing the slide after the archwire has been pushed into the bracket slot (Fig. 9-32). One end of the tool has been modified to hold the archwire in the slot, as the other end is used to push the slide over the archwire, closing the bracket. Another instrument that has been devel-

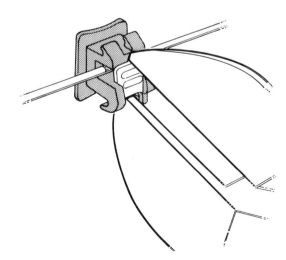

Figure 9-29. Opening the slide of the Damon 2 bracket with a specially designed plier. (Modified from a drawing from Ormco Corp.)

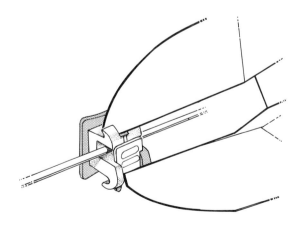

Figure 9-30. Closing the slide of the Damon 2 bracket with the Damon plier. (Modified from a drawing from Ormco Corp.)

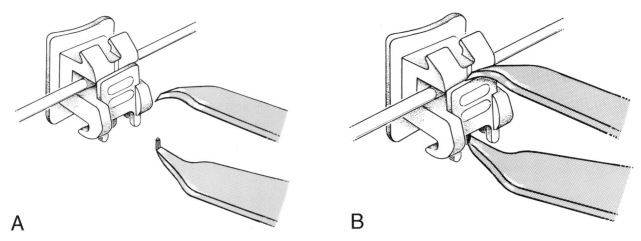

Figure 9-31. Opening the Damon 2™ bracket with tweezers (Ormco Corp.) *A*. The vertical tip of the lower arm of the tweezers is placed under the bracket. *B*. The upper arm of the Tweezers is used to open the slide (Modified from drawings from Ormco Corp.)

oped is the Cool Tool™ (#866-4003, Ormco) that, as the name implies, can be chilled or frozen to assist in the placement of NiTi wires (Fig. 9-33).

Damon[30] states that the most obvious advantage of self-ligation is the time saved during archwire changes. Using this type of bracket also allows placement of such low force high technology wires as nickel titanium. Reduced friction allows lower force wires to operate at their peak expression, thereby stimulating more biologically compatible tooth movement.

A number of studies have shown a reduction in friction when self-ligating brackets are compared to conventional bracket systems.[31-35] Voudouris[34] measured friction produced by three types of brackets: conventional twin brackets with O-rings and stainless steel ligatures, active self-ligation brackets, and passive self-ligation brackets, including the original Damon SL™ design. The conventional brackets tied with O-rings produced 500 times the friction of either passive self-ligating bracket tested, and brackets with stainless steel ligature produced 300 times greater friction. Further, the active self-ligating bracket produced 216 times greater friction.

Kapur and co-workers,[35] compared the original Damon SL™ bracket to conventional mini-twin brackets. They reported that the frictional forces produced when a NiTi wire was pulled through a conventional bracket tied with elastomeric power modules was

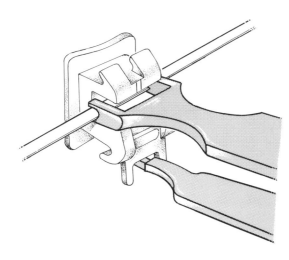

Figure 9-32. The upper arm of the modified tweezers is used to insert the wire into the bracket slot. The lower arm is used to close the bracket slide over the archwire. Modified from a drawing from Ormco Corp.)

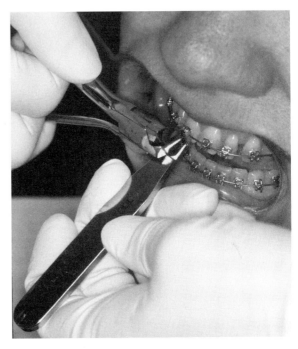

Figure 9-33. The Cool Tool™ can be chilled or frozen to facilitate the placement of NiTi wires.

nearly three times greater than that produced when the passive self-ligating bracket was used. When a stainless steel wire was tested, the conventional bracket produced over 15 times as much friction. They concluded that this type of self-ligation bracket not only makes archwire placement more convenient and secure, but also produces a lower friction level that is a substantial advantage to orthodontists using sliding mechanics.

Damon[30] recommends the .022" slot passive self-ligating appliance. He uses a progression of three wires, beginning with a .014" Align™ SE nickel titanium (Ormco), a wire selected for its surface characteristics and its observed clinical performance. Damon[30] maintains "starting with a small wire in a large lumen diminishes the divergence of the angles of the archwire slots in malaligned teeth, diminishing friction forces greatly." Proffit and co-workers[36] have shown that in conventionally tied .018" and .022" brackets, the same archwires aligned mandibular anteriors in the .022" slots in less time.

Damon[30] recommends appointment intervals of 10 weeks to allow the archwires to work fully without interrupting the biological processes involved in tooth movement. According to Proffit and Fields,[37] "Activating an appliance too frequently, short circuiting the repair process, can produce damage to the teeth or bone that a longer appointment cycle would have prevented or at least minimized."

The second archwire in the sequence is a .016 × .025" Align™ SE (Ormco) nickel titanium archwire.[30] This archwire enable the clinician to gain rotational control of the dentition. Both Proffit and Fields[37] and Damon[30] recommend maintaining at least .002" clearance between the slot of the bracket and the archwire. In this instance, the .025" depth of the archwire fits into the .027" deep slot with ample clearance to reduce friction as rotations are corrected. Damon stresses that it is imperative that rotated teeth be corrected fully before the final archwire in the sequence is inserted. If problems in bracket positioning become evident during treatment, brackets should be repositioned as soon as possible.

The third and final archwire, a "pre-posted" .019 × .025" stainless steel wire (Ormco), provides the opportunity for fine detailing the occlusion, completing torquing and leveling, and also helping control the vertical dimension. Space closure typically is achieved by way of intraarch or interarch elastics connected anteriorly to the soldered or crimped posts that are located distal to the lateral incisors.

From a clinical research perspective, passive self-ligation is in its infancy. From a common sense point of view, this system seems reasonable, and our initial exposure to the Damon 2 protocol has been positive. As with all new procedures, however, and considering the learning curve that is involved with mastering any new clinical approach, data is required to determine the types of patients in which the Damon protocol is indicated.

CONCLUDING REMARKS

The intent of this chapter is not to provide a comprehensive discussion of all possibilities using fixed appliances. We have presented a few representative treatment protocols that have proven successful in patients undergoing comprehensive orthodontic treatment, either as a single-phase patient or as a patient undergoing Phase II treatment.

We have emphasized the importance of proper bracket position as well as the use of the transpalatal arch and the utility arch as routine parts of orthodontic mechanics. We also have tried to present several logical progressions of archwires, primarily using "memory wires." We have found these wires to have a long period of activation, while providing minimal discomfort to the patient.

It is assumed that the reader is well versed in the various orthodontic treatment mechanics available today and that he or she will make use of whatever techniques or protocols are appropriate for a given patient.

REFERENCES CITED

1. McNamara JA, Jr. Ordinary orthodontics: Starting with the end in mind. World J Orthod 2000;1:45-54.
2. Vaden JL, Dale JG, Klontz HA. The Tweed-Merrifield edgewise appliance: Philosophy, diagnosis, and treatment. In: Graber TM, Vanarsdall RL, Jr, eds. Orthodontics: Current principles and practices. St Louis: CV Mosby, 2000.
3. McNamara JA, Jr. Utility arches. J Clin Orthod 1986;20: 452–456.
4. Hilgers JJ. The pendulum appliance for Class II non-compliance therapy. J Clin Orthod 1992;26:706–714.
5. Pancherz H. The mechanism of Class II correction in Herbst appliance treatment. A cephalometric investigation. Am J Orthod 1982;82:104–113.
6. Clark WJ. The twin block traction technique. Eur J Orthod 1982;4:129–138.
7. Wilson RC, Wilson WL. Enhanced orthodontics. Denver: Rocky Mountain Orthodontics, 1988.
8. McNamara JA, Jr. The role of the transverse dimension in orthodontic diagnosis and treatment. Ann Arbor: Monograph 36, Craniofacial Growth Series, Center for Human Growth and Development, The University of Michigan, 1999.
9. McNamara JA, Jr. Maxillary transverse deficiency. Am J Orthod Dentofac Orthop 2000;117:567–570.
10. Jones ML, Staniford H, Chan C. Comparison of super-

elastic NiTi and multistranded stainless steel wires in initial alignment. J Clin Orthod 1990;24:611–613.
11. Kusy RP, Stevens LE. Triple-stranded stainless steel wires—evaluation of mechanical properties and comparison with titanium alloy alternatives. Angle Orthod 1987; 57:18–32.
12. Swartz ML. Unpublished data, 1998.
13. Ricketts RM. Personal communication, 1974.
14. Proffit WR. Contemporary orthodontics. St Louis: CV Mosby Co, 1986.
15. McNamara JA, Jr., Brudon WL. Orthodontic and orthopedic treatment in the mixed dentition. Ann Arbor: Needham Press, 1993.
16. Jensen JL. Personal communication, 1976.
17. Angle EH. Treatment of malocclusion of the teeth. Philadelphia: SS White, 1907.
18. Burstone CJ. Variable-modulus orthodontics. Am J Orthod 1981;80:1–16.
19. Burstone CJ, Goldberg AJ. Beta titanium: a new orthodontic alloy. Am J Orthod 1980;77:121–132.
20. Burstone CJ, Goldberg AJ. Maximum forces and deflections from orthodontic appliances. Am J Orthod 1983;84:95–103.
21. Andreasen GF, Brady PR. A use hypothesis for 55 Nitinol wire for orthodontics. Angle Orthod 1972;42:172–177.
22. Burstone CJ, Qin B, Morton JY. Chinese NiTi wire—a new orthodontic alloy. Am J Orthod 1985;87:445–452.
23. Miura F, Mogi M, Ohura Y, Hamanaka H. The super-elastic property of the Japanese NiTi alloy wire for use in orthodontics. Am J Orthod Dentofac Orthop 1986;90:1–10.
24. Miura F, Mogi M, Ohura Y, Karibe M. The super-elastic Japanese NiTi alloy wire for use in orthodontics. Part III. Studies on the Japanese NiTi alloy coil springs. Am J Orthod Dentofac Orthop 1988;94:89–96.
25. Miura F, Mogi M, Okamoto Y. New application of superelastic NiTi rectangular wire. J Clin Orthod 1990;24:544–548.
26. Khier SE, Brantley WA, Fournelle RA. Bending properties of superelastic and nonsuperelastic nickel-titanium orthodontic wires. Am J Orthod Dentofac Orthop 1991; 99:310–8.
27. Hanson GH. The SPEED system: a report on the development of a new edgewise appliance. Am J Orthod 1980; 78:243–265.
28. Damon DL. The rationale, evolution and clinical application of the self-ligating bracket. Clin Orthod Res 1998;1: 52–61.
29. Damon DH. The Damon low-friction bracket: A biologically compatible straight-wire system. J Clin Orthod 1998; 22:670–679.
30. Damon DH. Introducing the Damon System II. Clin Impressions 1999;8:2–9, 31.
31. Berger JL. The influence of the SPEED bracket's self-ligating design on force levels in tooth movement: a comparative in vitro study. Am J Orthod Dentofac Orthop 1990;97:219–28.
32. Kemp DW. A comparative analysis of frictional forces between self-ligating and conventional edgewise orthodontic brackets. Toronto: Unpublished Master's thesis, Department of Orthdontics, The University of Toronto, 1992.
33. Shivapuja PK, Berger J. A comparative study of conventional ligation and self-ligation bracket systems. Am J Orthod Dentofac Orthop 1994;106:472–480.
34. Voudouris JC. Interactive edgewise mechanisms: Form and function comparisons with conventional edgewise brackets. Am J Orthod Dentofac Orthop 1997;111:119–139.
35. Kapur R, Sinha PK, Nanda RS. Functional resistance of the Damon SL bracket. J Clin Orthod 1998;32:485–489.
36. Cobb N, Kula KS, Phillips C, Proffit WR. Efficiency of multi-stranded steel, super elastic NiTi and ion-implanted NiTi archwires for initial alignment. Clin Orthod Res 1998;1:12–19.
37. Proffit WR, Fields HW, Jr. Contemporary orthodontics. St Louis: Mosby Year Book, 1993.

Chapter 10
ORTHODONTIC BONDING

With Paul A. Gange

During the last 30 years, there has been an increased use of bonding during routine orthodontic and orthopedic protocols. Orthodontists place brackets to atypical enamel (*e.g.*, hypocalcified, fluorosed, aprismatic) on a broader spectrum of surfaces (*e.g.*, porcelain crowns, composite restorations, amalgam restorations, gold crowns, dentin) under a wider range of conditions (*e.g.*, dry and wet fields). Yet there are few areas in orthodontics that are more technique sensitive than orthodontic bonding—a mistake in a single step of a multistep protocol can result in bond failure.

This chapter will outline the principles of bracket bonding and band cementation as applied to everyday orthodontic therapy. In addition, specialized situations in which advancements in bonding technology allow the placement of orthodontic attachments on surfaces other than enamel and in conditions in which a dry field cannot be maintained are discussed. The bonding of lingual retainers also is described; the bonding of large acrylic appliances (*e.g.*, acrylic splint rapid maxillary expanders) is presented in Chapter 13.

One of us (PAG) has had nearly three decades of experience with orthodontic adhesives, and many of the products mentioned in this chapter are from the company (Reliance Orthodontic Products, Itasca IL) that he heads. There are a variety of good orthodontic adhesives available today. We will mention those products in each category that are well known to orthodontic clinicians in the text, but we will describe in detail those materials with which we are most familiar* and whose properties we know best.

*All products without a company designation are from Reliance Orthodontic Products, Itasca IL.

ROUTINE ORTHODONTIC BONDING

Two of the more perplexing problems encountered in everyday clinical practice are loose brackets and bands. Overall, a 5% or less failure rate is considered satisfactory, whereas a failure rate of greater than 8% is cause for concern. This section will discuss the basic steps in bonding brackets to tooth enamel. Each phase is critical, and each step in the sequence must be followed carefully.

Preparation of the Enamel

Prophylaxis

The first step in any successful bonding procedure is a thorough coronal polish; teeth must be clean if the acid is to act properly. The media used (typically medium grit pumice) should not contain oil, often present in flavored pumice, that will leave a film on the enamel surface that the acid cannot penetrate. Thoroughness in the polishing process is critical in this initial step. Whatever time is spent polishing in the anterior aspect of the mouth should be doubled posteriorly.

Even though either a rubber cup or a bristle brush may be used (Fig. 10-1), generally the bristle brush is more effective, especially when removing the pellicle that may be present on posterior teeth. The operator should take special care to make sure that the bristle brush does not contact the gingiva; trauma and laceration of gingival tissue may occur.

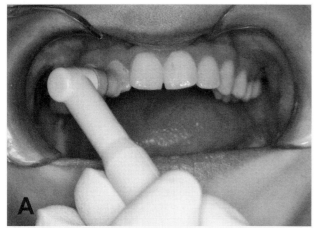

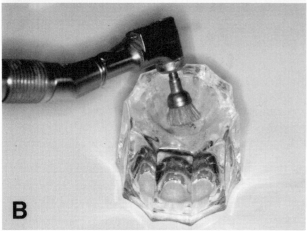

Figure 10-1. Prophylaxis can be accomplished with A, a rubber cup or B, a bristle brush in a low speed handpiece. Typically, medium grit pumice that does not contain oil is used.

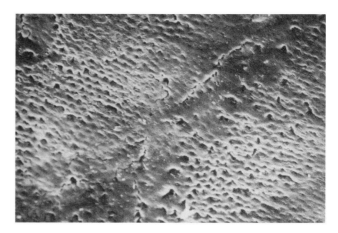

Figure 10-2. Scanning electron micrograph of enamel before etching.

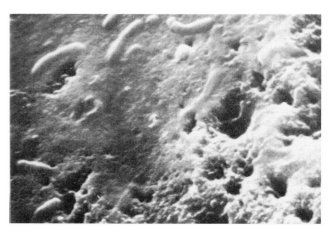

Figure 10-3. Etched enamel with inadequate prophy. Calculus remains on some of the enamel rods, potentially reducing bond strength.

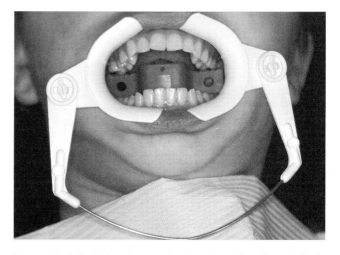

Figure 10-4. Isolation for routine bonding. Petroleum jelly is rubbed on the tissue at the corners of the mouth to improve patient comfort. Adequate isolation for the bonding procedure is obtained by positioning a cheek retractor after Dri-Angles™ have been placed over the openings of the parotid ducts. A Tongue-Away™ bite block is seen posteriorly.

After the teeth have been cleaned, the pumice and debris should be removed thoroughly from the enamel surface with a water/air spray. Insufficient rinsing after coronal polishing can reduce bond strength. Figure 10-2 shows the enamel rods after the prophy has been completed and before etching. Figure 10-3 shows a tooth that was not thoroughly prophied but then was acid etched. The enamel rods still are covered by calculus, potentially reducing the bond strength. Thus, to ensure a good etch on the majority of teeth, a clean surface is necessary, and that can be accomplished with a thorough prophylaxis.

Isolation

The teeth must be isolated properly prior to the etching procedure (Fig. 10-4). Petroleum jelly (*e.g.,* Vaseline™) can be placed in the corners of the mouth before positioning the lip/cheek retractor. Dri-angles™ or cotton rolls should be placed over the openings of the parotid ducts before the placement of the cheek retractor (*e.g.,*

ORTHODONTIC BONDING

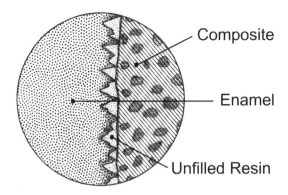

Figure 10-5. Diagrammatic representation of acid-etched surface. An unfilled resin sealant is used to prepare the enamel surface for the composite resin bonding agent.

Access™, Reliance; Dry Field™ System, Nola, Hilton Head SC; Cottonmouth™ System, Orthoarch Co, Schaumburg IL). In most instances, this type of isolation is sufficient to allow for preparation of both dental arches for the placement of bonded brackets.

In instances of excessive saliva flow, an antisialogue such as atropine sulfate (0.4 mg per patient's 100 pounds) can be given to the patient one hour before the bonding procedure. In addition, tilting the patient's head to one side allows the operator to bond the maxillary and mandibular right quadrants, while the saliva drains to the left side of the mouth.

Acid Etch

The process of acid etching (Fig. 10-5) removes the fluoride-rich surface layer that leaves the etched enamel prone to bacterial buildup and makes the enamel amenable to bonding. To reduce decalcification, only the area of each tooth surface on which the bracket will be placed should be etched. Safety glasses must be worn by the patient and orthodontic staff.

Most orthodontic adhesives are sold with a 37% concentration of phosphoric acid with the minimum etching time on normal permanent enamel given as 15 seconds.[1] Research conducted at the University of Michigan shows that etching with a 37% concentration of phosphoric acid provides the most consistent surface on a majority of teeth.[2-4] A more realistic etching period for permanent teeth is 30 seconds and deciduous teeth 60–90 seconds. It is unlikely that the clinician could dab acid effectively on each tooth in a quadrant and then return to the first tooth to rinse within a 15-second interval. There is no evidence that indicates any significant increase in bond strength between 15 and 90 seconds of permanent tooth etching.[3] It is possible, however, to "over-etch" enamel. If the crown of the tooth is etched

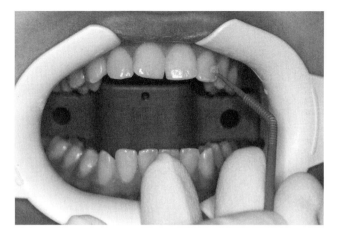

Figure 10-6. Etching of the enamel with a solution of 37% phosphoric acid. The etchant is dabbed on the tooth surface by way of a flexible Kerr Applicator™. A small sponge or cotton pellet held in cotton forceps also can be used.

for more than 90 seconds, an insoluble calcium phosphate salt crystal forms on the enamel that is impervious to rinsing, resulting in reduced bond strength.

In general, either a liquid etch or a gel etch may be used. A gel etch is indicated when the etching is in an isolated area or where control of the etching material is imperative.

Liquid Etch

The liquid etching material should be *dabbed* on the enamel surface with a small sponge or cotton pellet (Fig. 10-6). The acid etch never should be *rubbed* on the enamel (Fig. 10-7), because the moment the phosphoric acid contacts the enamel, the rods are exposed. The enamel rods are the delicate "fingers" to which the adhesive will bond mechanically. Rubbing the acid on the

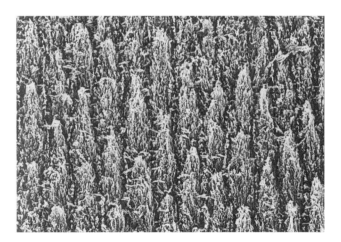

Figure 10-7. Scanning electron micrograph of enamel rods at the completion of the etching process following dabbing of the acid on the teeth.

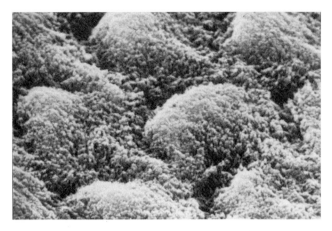

Figure 10-8. Scanning electron micrograph of enamel rods at the completion of the etching process after the etchant was rubbed on the teeth. Note the morphological changes in the structure of the enamel rods.

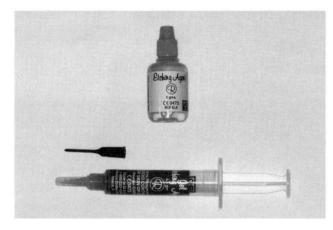

Figure 10-9. The dispensing of gel etch in a syringe. Due to its consistency, this type of etch is ideal for use in areas where there is concern about the etch flowing onto the associated soft tissue.

crown surface can cause the enamel rods to fracture and weakening the surface area where the bonding will occur (Fig. 10-8).

Gel Etch

Gel etch is used when the clinician wants to etch a concentrated area of the tooth or prevent the acid from contacting the gingiva. Glycerin is added to the liquid etch as a thickening agent. The gel etch typically is packaged in a syringe that dispenses the gel directly onto the enamel surface (Fig. 10-9). The dispensing needle of the syringe should not be used to move the acid around the tooth, because that movement also can fracture the fragile enamel rods. A small sponge held in locking cotton forceps should be used to dab the acid into each tooth to achieve proper penetration. The action of the sponge pellet is important because the gel etch is very heavy and does not wet the enamel surface as well as a liquid etch.

Rinsing and Drying

The two most neglected steps in the tooth preparation technique are rinsing and drying. There is a common misconception that rinsing (Fig. 10-10) is performed simply to remove the acid from the teeth. In fact, acid removal is a secondary reason for rinsing. The primary reason for the rinse is to remove the calcium phosphate salt crystals, byproducts of the phosphoric acid on the enamel, as well as the demineralized particles that were loosened from around the enamel rods. Thus, a thorough rinse is imperative. We recommend using a water spray for 10–15 seconds per tooth with a liquid etch, and

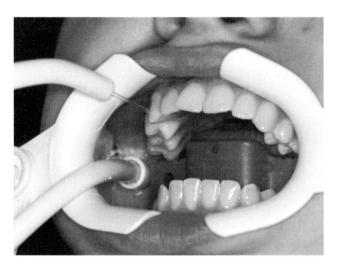

Figure 10-10. Rinsing of the etched surfaces with water from an air/water syringe.

20 seconds per tooth with a gel etch. The operator never should take a wet cotton roll and attempt to wipe the acid off the tooth. This procedure will fracture the enamel rods and weaken bond strength.

A concentrated drying of each tooth with oil-free air should follow the thorough rinsing. Before blowing air on the teeth, the purity of the air should be checked. The chairside assistant should blow air on the patient's napkin or a mouth mirror (Fig. 10-11), exposing condensation or oil. Contamination in the airline usually can be corrected by installing a chairside filter. An alternative means of drying is with a warm air source (Fig. 10-12) sold by Nola (Hilton Head SC). This dryer ensures that no contaminants are in the system. In the posterior region, it is recommended that the air be directed

ORTHODONTIC BONDING

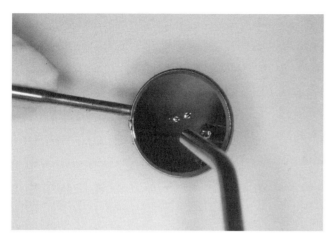

Figure 10-11. Spraying compressed air on a mouth mirror can reveal the presence of condensation or oil in the system. The patient's napkin can be used in the same manner to detect contaminants in the air line.

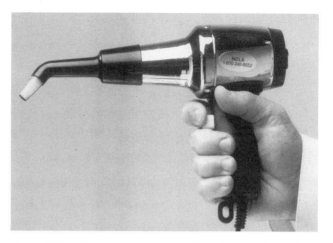

Figure 10-12. A warm air source, such as the one shown here (Nola, Hilton Head SC) can be used to dry the teeth with no risk of moisture contamination of the etched and rinsed enamel surface.

toward the gingiva to prevent subgingival saliva from contacting the enamel.

At this point, the enamel should be checked to make sure that it is dull and frosty white, not yellowish in appearance (Fig. 10-13). A yellowish cast indicates the presence of calculus that must be removed by scaling, requiring that the enamel be re-etched. If the enamel appears dull in some areas and shiny in others, a pellicle probably is present, again requiring scaling and re-etching.

From this point forward, care should be taken that saliva not touch the enamel, because saliva contains proteins that will remineralize the enamel during the bonding process. If saliva contamination is suspected after etching, the contaminated enamel must be re-etched for 20 seconds, rinsed, and dried thoroughly. If this procedure is not performed, bond failure will result.

Preparing a tooth for bonding involves getting the tooth surface chemically clean. A chemically clean surface, however, cannot be seen with the naked eye. Simply because an etched tooth appears dull and frosty white does not necessarily make it an ideal surface for bonding. Only the operator knows if all steps in the preparation process were performed correctly and thoroughly.

Adhesion Booster

Hypocalcified, fluorosed, excessively chalky, and deciduous enamel do not present ideal surfaces for bonding. Enhance™ adhesion booster was created to increase adhesion on these types of teeth or on any enamel surface where bond failure has occurred previously. An adhesion booster, as the name implies, increases bond strength. Some offices, including ours, apply adhesion booster to all patients.

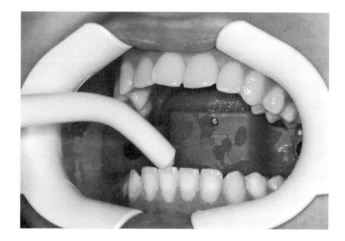

Figure 10-13. The appearance of the enamel after the etching, rinsing, and drying steps have been completed. The enamel should appear dull and chalky white.

When using an adhesion booster, the clinical crown of the tooth initially should be polished, etched, rinsed, and dried according to routine protocol. Next, the two equal parts (Part A and Part B) of Enhance™ should be combined in a mixing well (Fig. 10-14) and four generous coats should be applied to the enamel. After waiting ten seconds, the material then should be dried lightly with compressed air. This system can be used with any chemical, light, or dual cure adhesive.

All the aforementioned boosters* also will maintain optimal bond strength on a saliva-contaminated tooth without re-etching. All but Assure™ are used in con-

---

*For those practitioners using light-cure systems, Enhance LC™ and Assure™ are single step systems that do not require mixing, but they must be used under light-cure adhesives.

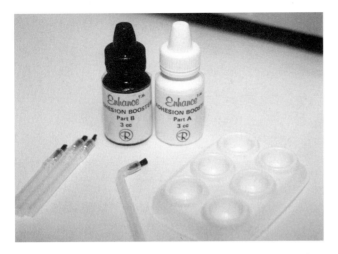

Figure 10-14. The use of Enhance™ adhesion booster to improve bond strength. Equal amounts of parts A and B are blended together in a mixing well.

junction with a sealant; it is an extra step after etching and before the bonding resin is applied.

Bonding Adhesives

The four types of adhesives currently available for direct bonding appliances can be divided into three categories: chemical cure, light cure, and dual cure. The first two systems to be discussed (mixed and no-mix systems) fall into the chemical cure category, in which two components of the adhesive interact with each other. A light cure system is polymerized via exposure to a high intensity visible light. Working time is unlimited and an active archwire can be placed immediately. A dual cure system will cure with or without exposure from a visible curing light. A short exposure from a visible light source will protect the adhesive from saliva and start the polymerization that the chemical cure will finish.

The choice of bonding system depends on the personal preference of the orthodontist and staff. All four systems described below offer adequate strength when used properly. Keep in mind, however, that orthodontic adhesives are low-film thickness materials, meaning that they have a higher strength in a thin layer than in a thick layer.[5]

Chemical-Cure Adhesives

A chemical cure system has two components that react with each other when they come into contact. When the two components are mixed (Fig. 10-15), the working time begins. During this time, brackets can be placed or moved without weakening the bond. When the start of the gel period begins, the working time is over. Brackets

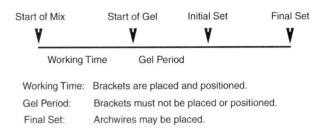

Figure 10-15. Stages of mixed adhesive curing from the start of the mix to the final set.

cannot be moved during this period, or the bond will be weakened significantly. The manufacturer's guidelines for working time should be followed closely. At the start of the initial set, the adhesive is hard to the touch, and the brackets can become wet with saliva without difficulty. Five minutes thereafter, an active archwire can be inserted.

Mixed Adhesives

Mixed adhesives are composed of equal parts of A and B pastes that are blended together and then applied to the bracket base (Fig. 10-16), after the two parts of the bonding resin have been combined and applied to the tooth. Two of the most commonly used mixed adhesives are Phase II™ (Reliance) and Concise™ (3M Company). In our private practice, a two-paste mix system (Phase II™) is used routinely for orthodontic bonding.

The first step in this procedure is to mix a drop of ac-

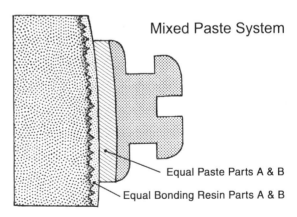

Figure 10-16. Diagrammatic representation of a mixed adhesive system. Parts A and B of the sealant are painted on the enamel surface. Parts A and B of the adhesive are mixed together, placed on the mesh of the bracket, and the bracket is pressed to place. Excess material is removed immediately.

ORTHODONTIC BONDING

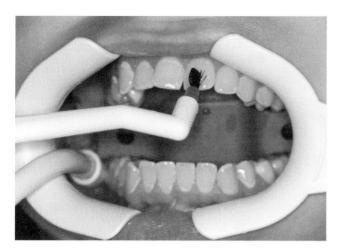

Figure 10-17. Application of sealant to the prepared enamel surface. The clinician can blow air on the sealant to ensure that the sealant is applied in a thin coat.

celerator and base bonding resin (*i.e.,* Part A and Part B) in a mixing well, and a thin layer is applied to each tooth with a brush (Fig. 10-17). The operator should be careful to avoid saliva contamination by beginning the application of the bonding resin from the gingival edge of the clinical crown and moving the brush incisally. At this point, there are two options: the teeth can be bonded immediately, or if the teeth can be kept saliva free, several minutes can elapse without risk of compromising bond strength.

The next step in the procedure is to mix equal parts of the A and B pastes together on a mixing pad. The two pastes should be spatulated together for 10 seconds. A one-to-one mixing ratio produces a two-minute working time. The bonding paste is applied firmly to the mesh side of the bracket (Fig. 10-18), When the bracket is pressed to place on the tooth (Fig. 10-19), minimal adhesive is extruded from under the bracket. The bracket is pressed into position by means of a gold foil knife (#850-05, Zulauf Co, Lubbock TX) or other bracket-seating instrument.

After the bracket is positioned properly, the excess adhesive should be removed carefully with a gold foil knife or a straight explorer. The chemical-cure nature of this type of product makes immediate cleanup mandatory. If cleanup is not initiated at the time each bracket is placed, the excess material will set, making removal of excess material difficult and sometimes impossible.

After two minutes, the bracket cannot be moved because the adhesive has entered the gel period (Fig. 10-15). Any movement of the bracket after the two-minute working-time period will weaken the bond strength significantly. An active archwire can be placed five minutes after the last bracket has been positioned.

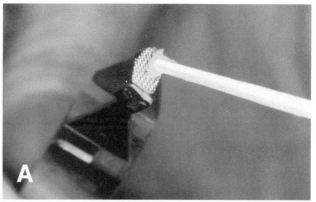
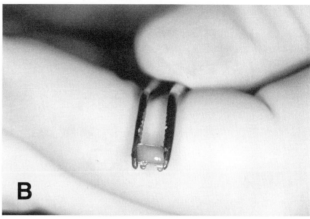

Figure 10-18. Placement of adhesive on bracket. *A,* the adhesive is worked into the mesh with a toothpick and or small spatula. *B,* Proper amount of adhesive has been applied to the bracket.

In our practice, individual mixes of adhesive are made for each pair of brackets placed. Small dabs of A and B paste are placed on the mixing pad (Fig. 10-20), and one dab of each type of paste are mixed together

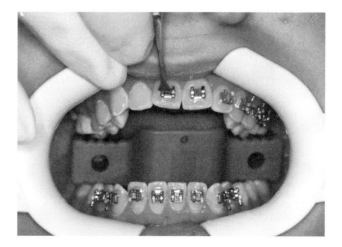

Figure 10-19. Positioning a bracket. After the bracket has been placed on the tooth, a gold foil knife (trimmer) can be used for bracket positioning and for adhesive flash removal.

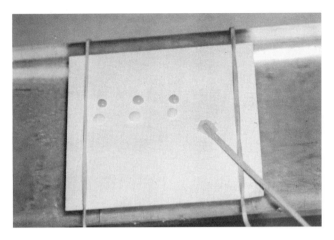

Figure 10-20. Preparation of mixed adhesive on a mixing pad. Small dabs of A and B paste are mixed together for each bracket placed. If extending the working time of the paste is desired, a single waxed sheet of paper from the mixing pad can be fastened to a frozen glass slab with rubber bands. The curing time of the adhesive is doubled.

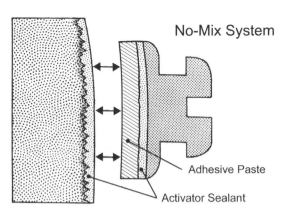

Figure 10-21. Diagrammatic representation of a no-mix adhesive system. The catalyst is painted on the mesh surface of the bracket pad and on the enamel of the tooth. The paste is worked into the mesh and the bracket is pushed to place. Excess material may be removed after the last bracket is bonded. It is essential that the bracket be contoured to the enamel surface; bond strength is weakened if the adhesive layer is too thick.

for each bracket placed. Some clinicians, however, prefer to bond multiple brackets with each mix. To double the working time of the adhesive, a sheet of waxed paper from the mixing pad can be affixed to a frozen glass slab (Fig. 10-20). The A and B paste can be placed on this paper, and a minute should elapse to allow the paste to chill. By doing so, the working time of the adhesive is doubled (four minutes) without compromising the chemistry of the paste. If an individual mix of adhesive is made for each bracket, the extended working time is not necessary. It should be noted, however, that the most common operator errors seen with the two-part mix system are applying an excessive layer of sealant on the tooth and placing brackets after the adhesive gel period has begun. Therefore, we recommend that a separate mix be made for each bracket.

No-Mix Adhesives

A no-mix adhesive system (Fig. 10-21) relies on the catalyst or primer to initiate the polymerization process. The bond strength of a no-mix adhesive system is dependent on the thickness of the adhesive layer between the bracket base and the tooth enamel, with a thin layer preferable. Therefore, when using a no-mix adhesive (*e.g.*, Rely-a Bond™, Reliance; System 1™, Ormco; Right-On™, TP Orthodontics), we strongly recommend that each bracket be placed against the appropriate tooth on a study model to make sure that the curvature of the bracket corresponds to the crown anatomy of the tooth to be bonded. If there are any large gaps present, bird-beak or three-pronged pliers can be used to contour the bracket base appropriately to ensure a flush fit.

After the tooth has been etched, rinsed and dried, a thin coat of no-mix primer should be placed on each bracket base and each tooth (Fig. 10-21). With a toothpick or syringe, a small quantity of adhesive paste should be applied to the mesh side of the bracket (Fig. 8-18). The working time for most no-mix adhesives is 30 seconds (the time begins when paste is placed on the bracket base). The bracket then should be placed on the tooth and pressed into position (Fig. 10-19). The primer will be forced into the paste, increasing bond strength and insuring the paste is in a uniform layer. In contrast to brackets placed with a mixed adhesive system, excess bracket adhesive can be removed easily from the periphery of the bracket bases after all brackets have been placed. An archwire can be inserted and ligated in place five minutes after the last bracket has been positioned.

The most common operator errors noted with the no-mix system are applying an excessive layer of primer on the tooth or bracket and placing an excessive amount of paste on the bracket.

Light-Cure Adhesives

The third system that has become popular is a light cure adhesive (Fig. 10-22). This material utilizes a visible light source to polymerize the material. Popular light-cure bonding agent include Light-Bond™ (Reliance), Transbond XT™ (Unitek), and Enlight™ (Ormco).

The curing light (Fig. 10-23) used in this protocol

ORTHODONTIC BONDING

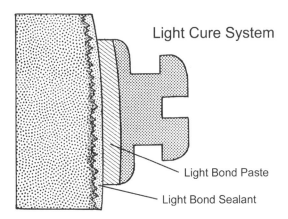

Figure 10-22. Diagrammatic representation of a light-cure adhesive system. Light-cure sealant is applied to the enamel surface and cured for 10 seconds. Light-cure paste is worked into the mesh and the bracket is pressed to place. Excess bonding material is removed before the curing light is applied.

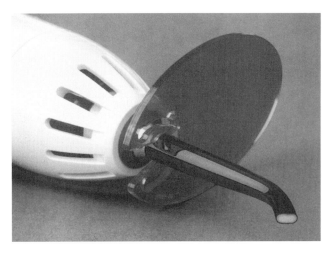

Figure 10-23. Curing light with Power Slot™ light director.

should be capable of providing a minimum of 400 milliwatts of continuous output to cure material properly during the manufacturer's recommended time interval for each product. The curing light should be checked monthly with a radiometer to verify the light intensity. Clear plastic sleeves placed on the curing light tip that are used for infection control may affect the intensity of the light negatively.

Curing Lights

Due to a demand to cure light-cure adhesives quickly, several new fast cure light devices have been intriduced, including the laser, Plasma Arc™, turbo tip, and Power Slot™.

Laser. The laser cures light-cure adhesive in five seconds because the photons that activate the adhesive catalyst are released in a collimated beam that concentrates a larger number of photons in one area.

Plasma Arc™. Camphoquinone, the most popular catalyst used in light-cure orthodontic adhesives, optimally cures at a wavelength of 468 nanometers. The wavelength emitted by standard curing lights is between 400–500 nanometers. The plasma arc light filters the wavelength to between 440–480 nanometers and utilizes a higher watt bulb to cure standard composite in 10 seconds.

Turbo Tip. The Turbo tip light director simply reduces the size of the director from 11 mm to 8 mm. As a result, more energy (photons) attacking the composite beneath the bracket base, resulting in a 10 second cure time.

Power Slot™. The Power Slot™ is a light director that fits the Demetron, Unitek, Vivadent, and Caulk curing lights (Fig. 10-23). Its unique patented shape con-

centrates the energy where it is most effective—beneath the bracket base—resulting in a cure of 10 seconds for standard light-cure adhesives.

Bonding Protocol

The first step in the protocol is to paint a very thin coat of light-cure sealant on the tooth. A drop or two of sealant resin is dispensed on the mixing pad, and a brush can be used to apply a thin uniform layer of sealant on the etched enamel. At this point, the operator either can cure the sealant (Fig. 10-24) or leave it uncured. The preferred practice is to cure the sealant because if the sealant is cured for 10 seconds (20 seconds for a filled sealant), the enamel rods are sealed off, protecting the enamel from saliva contamination. The con-

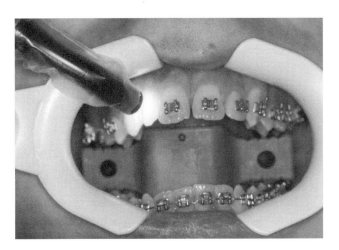

Figure 10-24. Light cure sealant. After the sealant has been applied with a brush, the sealant is cured for 10 seconds with a curing light.

taminated tooth can be cleaned by dabbing the surface lightly with 100% alcohol.

Curing the sealant before bracket placement also is recommended to reduce the risk of bracket flotation. The sealant makes the bracket more likely to move following placement because of its fluid nature in the uncured state.

Next, the paste is applied to the back of the bracket. It is important to work the paste into the mesh of the metal bracket with the flat head of a toothpick or a plastic mixing spatula to insure a strong mechanical bond between paste and mesh. The bracket should be placed on the tooth, pressed into final position, and the flash of bonding material removed before the curing of the adhesive with a curing light (Fig. 10-25).

We recommend curing a metal bracket with a standard curing light for a total of 30 seconds; 20 seconds from the incisal, and 10 from the gingival or mesial edge. It is imperative that the light director be placed as close to the bracket base as possible when curing. A ceramic or paste bracket can be cured through the archwire slot from the facial surface for 30 seconds. Archwire placement is immediate.

A light-cure system can be used very efficiently in routine orthodontic bonding. One of the drawbacks of direct bonding of brackets is the concentrated chair time (4–8 minutes per arch) needed by an experienced orthodontist to place brackets after the patient has been prepared for bonding. With the advent of more powerful curing lights, the brackets in one arch initially can be positioned by the chairside assistant.[6] Having the orthodontic assistant push the brackets to place after curing the sealant minimizes bracket floatation, and the staff member then can remove the obvious flash before the orthodontist positions the brackets in their final position. By having the brackets on the teeth and the excess removed before the orthodontist sees the patient, the time the orthodontist spends positioning brackets is reduced considerably. The assistant then cures the adhesive with a fast-curing light, usually 10 seconds per tooth.

The most common errors encountered in clinical practice associated with this type of bonding agent include not properly working the paste into the metal mesh base and second, holding the light director position too far from the bracket base when curing.

Dual-Cure System

Another form of direct bonding is a dual cure system (*e.g.*, Phase II™ Dual Cure, Reliance) in which curing occurs with or without exposure to a visible curing light. The enamel is conditioned, sealed with a light cure sealant, and light cured as usual. Equal portions of A and B

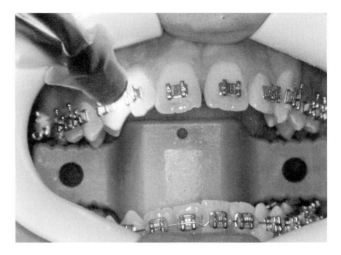

Figure 10-25. Curing two brackets that have been bonded with light cure adhesive.

dual cure paste are placed on the mixing pad, using opposite ends of the spatula to avoid cross contamination if the paste is dispensed in jars. The two pastes are mixed together for 10 seconds and applied to the bracket base. A one-to-one catalyst to base ratio produces a three minute working time, allowing several brackets to be placed from one mix of paste. The mixed paste should be shielded from intense direct light.

When a bracket is in the final position, a five-second exposure incisally from a curing light initially will tack set the adhesive, making it impervious to saliva. This curing starts the final polymerization, which will occur chemically. Excess bonding material must be wiped clean from the placement instrument before it polymerizes. An archwire can be placed five minutes later.

If only one bracket is to be bonded and immediate ligation of an archwire is desired, Paste A alone can be used to bond the bracket. The bracket can be placed on the sealed tooth and light cured for 20 seconds from the incisal edge and 10 seconds from the mesial or distal edge.

The most common operator error occurring with this system is failure to wait five minutes to ligate the archwire in place after light curing the paste for five seconds.

BAND CEMENTATION

Successful band cementation is dependent on several factors, the most important of which is fit. The better the fit of the band, the less chance for failure. Most bands today are mechanically roughened or microetched on the inside to increase adhesion between the cement and the band material (Fig. 10-26), thus reducing the incidence of cement washout. If the orthodontist has band

ORTHODONTIC BONDING

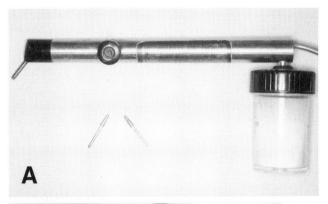

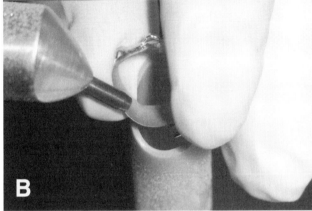

Figure 10-26. A microetcher (*A*) can be used to etch the inner surface of a molar band (*B*). Microetching improves adhesive strength.

inventory that has not been prepared mechanically, we suggest that the insides of these bands be prepared with a microetcher (Danville Engineering, Danville CA) or a green stone.

The first products used for band cementation were polycarboxylate and zinc phosphate cements. Recently, glass ionomer cements (*e.g.*, Fuji Ortho LC™, GC America, Ketac™, ESPE, Germany; Protech™, Ormco; Precedent™, Reliance) became popular because they can be used in a wet environment, release fluoride, and have high compressive strength. None of these cements, however, bond chemically to metal, which means that cement cleanup often is tedious and time consuming, because the aPdhesive stays bonded to the tooth rather than remaining in the band as the band is removed.

The state of the art for band cement today is compomer cement that has chemical adhesion to the band material, exhibits high compressive strength, and releases fluoride. BandLPPok™, a two paste dual cure adhesive and Ultra BandLok™, a single paste light cure adhesive, were the first cements of this type. These products show higher compressive strength and better chemical adhesion to the band material than zinc phosphate or glass ionomer cements, resulting in fewer loose bands. The recommended technique for successful band cementation is described below.

When BandLok™ is used, the inside of the bands should be roughened lightly with a fine diamond bur or microetcher. Ideally, the tooth to be banded should be prophied, flossed, rinsed, dried, and isolated. Then equal parts of BandLok™ Pastes A and B should be placed on a mixing pad (Fig. 10-27). We have found that a one inch strip of each part will provide enough cement for four bands and a ¼″ strip of each will cement one band. The operator should make sure that if the paste is not going to be mixed immediately, the paste should be shielded from light. The two portions of the adhesive are mixed together for ten seconds, and then the internal side of each band is covered with cement. The band is seated, and excess adhesive is removed before the material is light cured (Fig. 10-28).

One of the advantages of this type of cement is that the material can be mixed and the bands filled without it being necessary for immediate band placement. We have found it very convenient to have the chairside assistant place one or more bands under an alginate mixing bowl or an orange covered plastic box[11] to protect the material from ambient light. Several minutes can elapse between the mix and loading procedures and the actual band cementation by the orthodontist, a significant advantage in a busy practice.

We suggest the use of a non-tooth colored band cement, such as Blue BandLok™. We have found that the use of a colored adhesive facilitates the cleanup process after the bands are removed. We also suggest that to prevent BandLok™ from sticking to metal instruments, the instruments should be wiped in wax before touching the cement, because Bandlok™ adheres chemically to

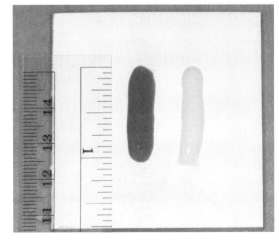

Figure 10-27. One inch strips of BandLok™ A and B pastes provides sufficient adhesive to cement four bands.

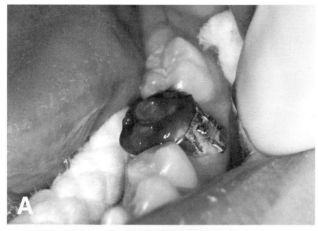

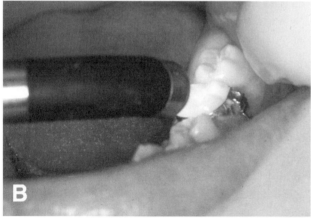

Figure 10-28. Cementing bands with a compomer cement. Blue colored BandLok™ is used to cement the band. *A*, After cementation and removal of excess cement. *B*, Curing the BandLok™ with a curing light.

metal. Alternatively, Pam™ cooking spray (International Home Foods, Parsippany NJ) can be applied to the instruments for the same reason.

BONDING IN A WET FIELD

There are occasions during which it is impossible to maintain a perfectly dry field. These instances require the use of a hydrophilic bonding agent or cement.

Moderate Contamination

There are two degrees of wetness encountered: moderate and excessive. A moderate amount of moisture is comparable to a smear layer of water or saliva. This situation can be bonded to successfully with a hydrophilic product such as Assure™. The steps are outlined below.

The teeth are prophied, flossed, etched, rinsed, and dried in the usual manner. With a brush or sponge pellet, a generous coat of Assure™ sealant is applied to each prepared tooth. After ten seconds, the sealant should be lightly dried for five seconds with contaminant free air. Then light cure each tooth for ten seconds. It should be noted that in difficult atypical enamel situations, it is recommended to use two coats of sealant.

Using the Assure™ syringe tip or a spatula, the paste is worked into the bracket base. The bracket is placed on the tooth and pressed to the desired position. With a metal bracket, the curing light should be positioned to shine from the incisal edge and illuminate the bracket for 20 seconds and then for 10 additional seconds from the gingival, mesial, or distal bracket edge. A ceramic bracket should be cured directly through the bracket from the labial for 20 seconds. The light director must be placed as close to the bracket base as possible during the curing. Once the paste has been cured properly, an active archwire can be placed immediately.

Excessive Contamination

Excessive contamination involves an uncontrollable, copious amount of saliva or water, generally found in the mandibular second molar region. For this procedure, a powder and liquid glass ionomer cement such as Fuji Ortho LC™ (GC America) or Precedent™ (Reliance) should be used as directed, except that the teeth first should be cleaned with pumice, acid etched for 30 seconds with a phosphoric acid, then rinsed and excess moisture blown away (Fig. 10-29). The enamel should be moist when the appliance is applied with the glass ionomer cement. Even though etching intuitively seems counterproductive because the enamel will become recontaminated, etching is mandatory to produce an adequate level of bond strength.

Bonding in any type of wet conditions, no matter how slight will *not* produce the same level of bond strength as in a dry field. There are two categories of glass ionomer cements: chemical cure and dual cure. The dual cure Fuji Ortho LC™ glass ionomer cement contains a light cure photo-initiator that cures the material quicker than chemical cure cements and reaches a higher strength quicker. Being able to reach an adequate strength level quickly is vital when bonding individual orthodontic brackets and buttons.

SPECIAL BONDING SITUATIONS

There are a number of special situations in orthodontics that require specific bonding protocols. For example, the increased incidence of adult orthodontic treatment in the last decade, particularly those patients undergoing complex interdisciplinary treatment, has led to an

ORTHODONTIC BONDING

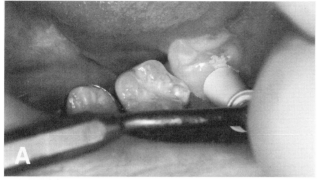
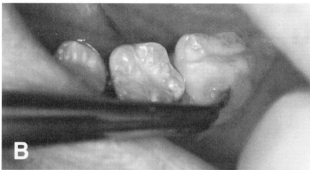
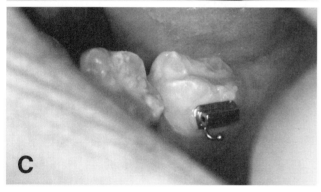

Figure 10-29. Use of a hydrophilic bonding agent. Fuji LC™ cement is used to bond a bracket on a mandibular molar. *A*, Prophy with pumice. *B*, Acid etch for 30 seconds. *C*, placement of bracket on the tooth. The cement is light-cured for 40 seconds. Some clinicians add cement to the mesial and distal incisal portions of the bracket for an additional mechanical lock.[11]

increased necessity of bonding to restored teeth. In addition, as children have become more exposed to fluoride through the intake of vitamins, drinking water, toothpaste and preventive treatments, hypocalcified, fluorosed, and aprismatic enamel is encountered more frequently than in the past. These and other special situations are discussed below.

Acrylic Jacket or Composite Restoration

For this procedure, the material required is a plastic conditioner (Reliance Plastic Conditioner™) or an adhesion booster (Enhance™). The composite should be

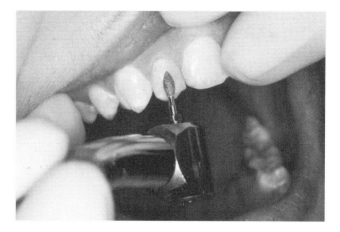

Figure 10-30. A fine diamond is used to lightly roughen the surface of an acrylic or composite restoration at the beginning of the bonding sequence.

roughened lightly with a fine diamond bur (Fig. 10-30). A carbide bur should not be used to roughen the surface, as it will leave a smear layer on the composite that will weaken the bond. The enamel surface should be etched for 30 seconds, rinsed, and dried thoroughly. At that point, a drop of Part A and a drop of Part B of Enhance™ adhesion booster are placed in a mixing well and combined for five seconds. Three or four thin coats are applied per tooth. After the last coat, the surfaces then should be lightly air dried with compressed air. Bonding then proceeds as usual.

If a no-mix adhesive is used, a thin coat of no-mix primer should be applied to the tooth. If a light cure system is used, a thin coat of light cure sealant should be applied. With a mixed system, a thin coat of mixed sealant should be painted on the tooth surface.

Porcelain Crown

Adequate bonding to a porcelain crown can be achieved if the suggested protocol is followed. First, the glaze of the porcelain should be removed with a green stone or fine diamond bur by lightly roughening the porcelain surface (Fig. 10-31*A*). A microetcher also can be used. The exposed gingiva adjacent to the tooth should be coated with a barrier gel (Fig. 10-31*B*), because of the highly caustic nature of the acid to be used during the etching process. Alternatively, a rubber dam can be placed.

A thin coat of hydrofluoric acid (Porc-Etch™) is applied carefully to the crown (Fig. 10-31*C*). The hydrofluoric acid is left in place for three minutes, and then the etch is rinsed thoroughly (Fig. 10-31*D*) and removed through suction. The tooth is dried, and a generous coat of porcelain conditioning material is applied to the

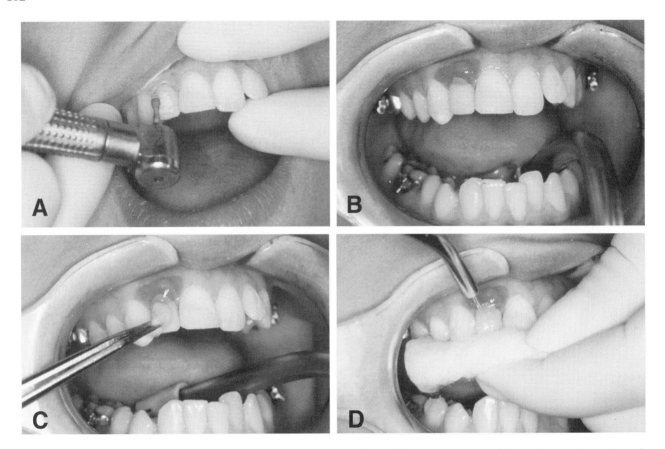

Figure 10-31. Bonding a bracket to a porcelain restoration. *A*, A fine diamond bur (or green stone) is used to roughen the surface of the restoration. *B*, Barrier gel is placed. *C*, The tooth surface is etched with hydrofluoric acid. *D*, The tooth is rinsed thoroughly and carefully, making sure that the residue does not contact the soft tissue during the rinsing process.

crown with a brush or small sponge. After 60 seconds, the same bonding technique as described above for bonding to composite is followed. After debonding, the luster of the porcelain can be restored by means of a diamond polishing paste.

Metal Surface (Gold, Amalgam or Stainless Steel)

The process of bonding to a metal surface requires a metal primer and a mixed sealant. The metal surface should be prepared by micro-etching the tooth surface (Fig. 10-32*A*), after which the microetching particles are blown clean (Fig. 10-32*BC*). If a microetcher is not available, the surface should be roughened with a medium diamond stone.

Microetching will double the strength value of the bond over roughening.[7] A uniform coat of metal primer then is painted on the sandblasted surface. After 30 seconds, the two-part sealant is mixed and applied in a thin coat to the conditioned surface. At that point, the bracket is placed with the adhesive paste of choice.

If enamel is present, the surface should be etched for 30 seconds with phosphoric acid, rinsed, and dried. Several coats of adhesion booster should be painted on the roughened metal surface. After waiting for ten seconds, the metal is air dried for five seconds. If Enhance LC™ is used, three coats are applied to the roughened metal surface. After ten seconds, the area is lightly air dried for five seconds. Then a thin coat of light-cure sealant is painted on the conditioned surface and the sealant is cured for 10 seconds (20 seconds for filled sealant). Light-cured adhesive can be used to bond the bracket (Fig. 10-32*D*).

Rebonding a Metal Bracket

Today many orthodontists charge for the repair of broken brackets, some of which actually may be due to improper technique. If composite remains only on the bracket, then an error in bonding technique occurred. If composite remains on the tooth, then the patient usually caused the failure.

One of the obvious consequences of bond failure is the need to rebond the bracket. If a micro-etcher is available, simply sandblast the composite off the bracket base

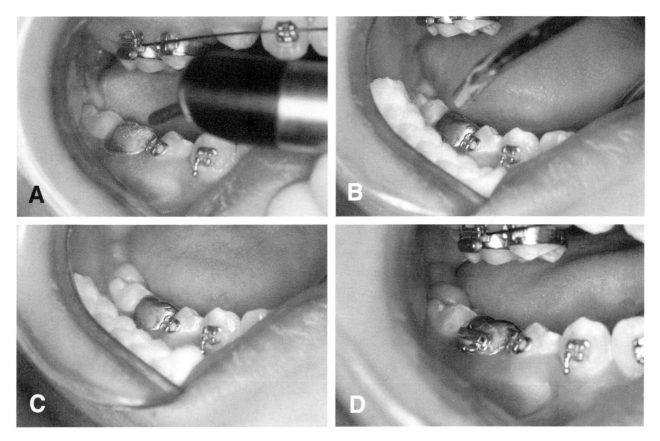

Figure 10-32. Bonding a bracket to a stainless steel crown. *A*, Sandblasting the buccal surface. *B*, removing the residue. *C*, Surface after sandblasting and cleanup. *D*, Bonding of the bracket with light cure adhesive. Adequate isolation should be maintained through the procedure.

if it is not distorted (Fig. 10-33) and bond the bracket as if it were a new bracket.

If a sandblaster is not available, the composite on the bracket base should be roughened lightly with a fine diamond, taking care not to expose the mesh. A generous coat of plastic conditioner or Enhance™ Adhesion Booster is painted on the bracket base. After 10 seconds, the bracket base can be lightly air-dried. The enamel then should be polished, etched, rinsed, and dried as previously described, making sure that the old adhesive is removed. Several coats of Enhance™ adhesion booster are applied to the prepared enamel. After 10 seconds, the surface is dried lightly with air (the use of Enhance™ will ensure a successful rebond to the enamel).

When a no-mix adhesive is used, the bracket and tooth should be primed as usual, the paste is applied to the bracket, and the bracket is positioned on the tooth. With a mixed or light cure system, a thin coat of sealant is applied to the tooth and the bracket base. The paste is worked into the bracket mesh, and the bracket is seated on the tooth. If a light cure system is used, the sealant and paste are cured in the usual manner.

Plastic Brackets

Brackets made of plastic once again are becoming popular. The plastic used in the formulation of the latest generation of brackets is more durable and consequently more difficult to bond. To ensure a successful bond with any plastic bracket, a generous coat of plastic conditioner is painted on the bracket base and allowed to dry thoroughly (generally 30 seconds).

With a no-mix adhesive, the bracket and tooth are primed as usual. The paste is applied to the bracket and the bracket is positioned on the tooth. With a mixed or light cure system, a thin coat of sealant is applied to the tooth and the bracket base. Paste is worked into the bracket mesh, and the bracket is seated on the tooth. When a light cure system is used, the sealant and paste are cured as usual.

BONDING LINGUAL RETAINERS

Lingual retainers are used commonly in orthodontics as a permanent form of retention.[8-10] The bonding of these retainers is described below.

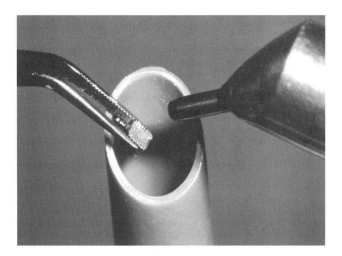

Figure 10-33. Sandblasting a loose bracket.

Prophylaxis

Using a slow-speed handpiece and a rubber cup or bristle brush, the enamel or dentin surfaces to be bonded should be polished with plain pumice. With a green stone or preferably a microetcher, the lingual surfaces of the mandibular anterior teeth then should be roughened lightly. A prophy paste that contains oil should not be used because of the potential for leaving a film on the tooth that will inhibit the etch.

Special attention should be paid to the buildup of calculus that may occur on the lingual surfaces of the teeth. If calculus is present, it should be removed through scaling. The teeth then should be polished, rinsed, and dried with moisture-free compressed air.

Etch, Rinse, and Dry

The etching agent, which can be either liquid or gel, is dispensed onto the mixing pad. After adequate isolation has been achieved, the etching agent should be applied to the entire area to be bonded. The operator should be careful not to flow the etchant onto the adjacent soft tissue. A thirty second etching period should be adequate in most situations.

The area to be bonded should be rinsed thoroughly to cleanse the enamel surface. Copious amounts of water are used, with each tooth rinsed for 10–15 seconds to stop the etching process and remove the demineralized particles. The bonding area is dried thoroughly with moisture-free air, and the area is reisolated. The patient should not be allowed to rinse or otherwise contaminate the etched surface. The etched teeth should appear frosty white; if specific areas appear shiny, those surfaces should be re-etched for 20 seconds. Adhesion booster is applied to the conditioned enamel as per instructions, and the Enhance™ is dried to increase bond strength further.

Bonding Procedure

Retainer with Bonding Pads

The retainer should fit the anatomy of the teeth as closely as possible. The lingual retainer should be placed back on the construction model to make sure that there are not any obvious gaps between the lingual pads and the teeth. Any irregularities should be corrected, if possible. The pads then should be microetched to increase bond strength.

Two types of adhesive can be used to secure the lingual retainer: light-cure adhesive and chemical-cure adhesive. Typically, light-cure adhesive is preferred because the pads can be cured from the labial, due to the relative thinness of the enamel in the incisor regions. A thin coat of light-cure sealant is painted on the lingual surface of each tooth. Using a syringe tip or a spatula, the paste is worked into the mesh of each bonding pad. The appliance is seated and pressed into place. The light cure director is used to cure the adhesive for forty seconds from the incisal edge or directly through the labial enamel.

If a mixed adhesive is used (*e.g.,* Excel™, Phase II™), equal portions are mixed together, and a small but adequate portion is placed on each pad, insuring proper penetration into the mesh base. The appliance is seated and stabilized in place until the initial set of the material has occurred (five minutes). The appliance then is inspected for adhesive flash, and dental floss is used to determine the patency of the interproximal contacts. All excess bonding material is removed.

Retainer without Bonding Pads

The first step in bonding a lingual wire is to make sure that the wire fits the lingual contour of the teeth. If a work model is available, the wire should be burnished to insure a flush fit. The wire also should be microetched in the areas to be covered by the adhesive (Fig. 10-34A).

If a light-cured adhesive is used, light-cure sealant is applied to each etched tooth. The wire then is placed into the desired position and secured with dental floss or elastic rings. The wire is covered by light-cure paste and shaped and smoothed as desired (Fig. 10-34B). We recommend that at least four teeth, and preferably all the teeth, be incorporated into the anchorage system. The adhesive on the lingual of each tooth then is cured for 30 seconds.

ORTHODONTIC BONDING

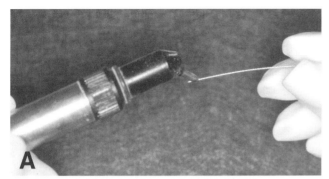

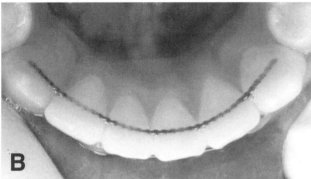

Figure 10-34. Bonded lingual retainer. *A*, The ends of the wire are microetched to increase adhesive retention to the wire. *B*, Bonding adhesive is added over the wire to each tooth.

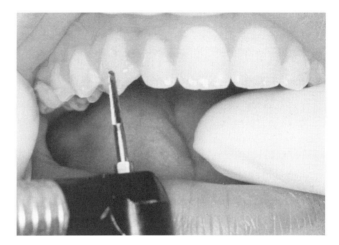

Figure 10-35. A finishing bur in a high-speed handpiece can be used to remove excess acrylic following debonding. Rinsing with warm water during this procedure has been advocated by some clinicians.[12]

When bonding a lingual wire with a mixed system, the sealant is placed on each etched tooth. Equal portions of the A and B of the mixed adhesive are mixed and placed over the lingual wire. The mounds of adhesive should be shaped and smoothed as desired within the working time of the selected adhesive. After the adhesive has hardened, the patient should be checked for adhesive excess and obstructed interdental contacts.

DEBONDING BRACKETS AND ADHESIVE REMOVAL

Debonding brackets is a routine part of orthodontic treatment. The following are a few comments about efficient and effective debonding and cleanup procedures.

When removing metal brackets, we have found it easiest to physically remove the metal bracket by applying a pinch or torque to the bracket base. This procedure can be accomplished using bracket removing pliers, a ligature cutter, or Weingart pliers. For easy bracket removal, the tie wings of the bracket can be pinched together, breaking the adhesive bond.

Any bulk residue adhesive can be removed from the tooth surface with a finishing bur (*e.g.*, #118S bur, Reliance; #12 fluted steel bur, Brassler) in a high-speed handpiece (Fig. 10-35). For tight areas and to polish the tooth surface, the use of another finishing bur (#383) in a low speed handpiece is recommended. The cleaned enamel surface then should be smoothed with pumice to complete the removal sequence. A polishing paste such as Restore™ can be used to regain the smooth, shiny finish after debonding a bracket from a porcelain jacket, composite restoration, or metal crown.

The removal of ceramic or liquid sapphire brackets can pose particular problems for the clinician, although many advances have been made in this technology, including less dependence on silane as a chemical bond to enamel.* When removing these types of brackets, the operator should follow the recommendations of the manufacturer regarding the proper method and debonding instrument. Any flash around the bracket base should be removed with a finishing bur (#118S) before attempting bracket removal. Eliminating flash facilitates the placement of the debonding instrument so that it firmly grips the bracket base and prevents the plier from riding up the bracket base and shearing off the tie wings when pressure is applied. Once the bracket is removed, the conventional cleanup protocol is followed.

CONCLUDING REMARKS

As is obvious from the multiple protocols described in this chapter, the bonding of orthodontic appliances is no

---

*The original liquid sapphire brackets were attached to the enamel by way of a silane bond that was stronger than the enamel, occasionally resulting in enamel fracture during the debonding procedure. Removing the brackets in a conventional fashion often proved difficult, resulting in the need literally to grind off the bracket from the enamel with a diamond stone.

simple matter. Attention to detail is the order of the day, and failure to do so results in increased chair time, prolonged treatment, increased overhead, and patient discomfort and dissatisfaction.

This chapter has not presented a detailed description of the biomaterial theory and research that underlie the bonding protocols described above. Rather, we have chosen to focus on a somewhat pragmatic approach to this most precise subject. Most of the protocols described in this chapter have been used clinically for many years in offices both in the United States and elsewhere and have produced satisfactory results in a variety of bonding situations.

REFERENCES CITED

1. Silverstone LM. The acid etch technique: In vitro studies with special reference to the enamel surface. Proceedings of an International symposium on acid etch technique. St Paul: North Central Publishing Co, 1975.
2. Gange PA. Unpublished data, 1995.
3. Barkmeier WW, Gwinnett AJ, Shaffer SE. Effects of reduced acid concentration and etching time on bond strength. J Clin Orthod 1987;21:395–398.
4. Brännström M, Nordenvall KJ, Malmgren O. The effect of various pretreatment methods of the enamel in bonding procedures. Am J Orthod 1978;74:522-30.
5. Jost-Brinkmann PG, Schiffer A, Miethke RR. The effect of adhesive-layer thickness on bond strength. J Clin Orthod 1992;26:718–720.
6. Nolan PJ, Starr GM. Personal communication, 2000.
7. Jost-Brinkmann PG, Miethke RR. Personal communication, 1995.
8. Zachrisson BU. Clinical experience with direct-bonded orthodontic retainers. Am J Orthod 1977;71:440–448.
9. Zachrisson BU. Third-generation mandibular bonded lingual 3-3 retainer. J Clin Orthod 1995;29:39–48.
10. Krause FW. Bonded maxillary custom lingual retainer. J Clin Orthod 1984;18:734–737.
11. Brightman BB. Personal communication, 2000
12. Burkhardt DR. Personal communication, 2000.

Chapter 11
UTILITY ARCHES

One of the most versatile auxiliary archwires that can be used in either mixed or permanent dentition treatment is the utility arch. The utility arch is a continuous wire that extends across both buccal segments, but engages only the first permanent molars and the four incisors. This archwire originally was developed to provide a method of leveling the curve of Spee in the mandible, but, through the incorporation of loops, has been adapted to perform additional functions in addition to incisor intrusion in both arches.

This auxiliary archwire has been developed according to the biomechanical principles described by Burstone[1,2] and has been popularized as an integral part of Bioprogressive therapy.[3-5] Most commonly, these archwires are made of rectangular chrome-cobalt alloy (*e.g.*, Elgiloy™, Azurloy™), although other archwire materials also can be used.

BASIC COMPONENTS

Regardless of the presence or absence of loops, all utility arches have a common design (Fig. 11-1). First, the *molar segment* extends into a tube on the first molar (Fig. 11-1*A*). This segment may be cut flush with the end of the tube or may be bent gingivally, if the utility arch is to be tied back. When utility arches are used in combination with full arch appliances, it is necessary to have auxiliary tubes located in a gingival position on the first molar bands. If the premolars and canines are not banded, the main archwire tube on the first molar can be used to anchor the utility arch posteriorly.

The *posterior vertical segment* (Fig. 11-1*B*) is formed by making a 90° bend with 142 arch-forming pliers (Fig. 11-2*A*). This posterior step typically is 3–4 mm in length in the mandible and 4–5 mm in the maxilla. It often is necessary to place a third order (torquing) bend at the junction of the molar segment and the posterior vertical segment to avoid impingement of the utility arch on the adjacent gingiva.

The *vestibular segment* is formed by placing a right-angle bend at the inferior portion of the posterior vertical segment (Fig. 11-1*C*). The wire then passes anteroinferiorly along the gingival margin. If the patient has fixed appliances that contain ball hooks, the utility arch should not interfere with these gingivally directed extensions of the bracket.

The *anterior vertical segment* should be about 4–5 mm in length when the utility arch is used in the mandible and about 5–8 mm in length when the arch is used in the maxilla (Fig. 11-1*D*). The depths of the maxillary and mandibular vestibules of the individual patient, along with the design of the fixed appliances used during treatment, determine the specific lengths of both vertical segments.

A final 90° bend creates the *incisal segment* that should lie passively in the brackets of the anterior teeth (Fig. 11-1*E*). Any irregularities in the position of the maxillary and/or mandibular anterior teeth usually are corrected before the placement of the utility arch, by means of sectional leveling arches (*e.g.*, .0175″ co-axial wire followed by a .016″ × .022″ blue Elgiloy™ sectional wire).

Figure 11-3 can be used as the basis of wire bending exercises in the fabrication of the various types of utility arches, as will be described later.

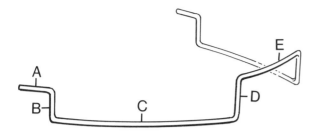

Figure 11-1. Generic design of the utility arch. *A*, Molar segment. *B*, Posterior vertical segment. *C*, Vestibular segment. *D*, Anterior vertical segment. *E*, Incisal segment. Loops also may be incorporated into this design.

WIRE SELECTION

As is advocated by Ricketts and co-workers,[4] it is our strong preference to fabricate utility arches from chrome-cobalt wire (*e.g.*, blue Elgiloy™ wire, Rocky Mountain Orthodontics, Denver CO; blue Azurloy™ wire, Ormco Corp., Orange CA). In contrast to stainless steel wire, chrome-cobalt wire is manipulated easily, and loops can be formed in the wire with little difficulty. *Heat-treating the wire is not recommended,* because the force generated by the wire is increased greatly following heat-treatment. Because a low amount of force (*e.g.*, 60 gm) has been advocated by Bench[5] among others for intrusion of incisors, unheat-treated chrome-cobalt wire provides an optimal level of force, based on empirical evidence. The clinician can activate the utility arch easily by way of an intraoral adjustment without removing the arch wire from the brackets, in a procedure to be described in detail below.

With regard to the selection of the appropriate size of wire for a .018″ slot appliance, the recommended wire for the mandibular utility arch is either .016″ × .022″ or .016″ × .016″ wire. For most maxillary arches, .016″ × .022″ wire is recommended. With a .022″ slot appliance, .019″ × .019″ wire can be used in either arch. Generally, a rectangular wire is preferable to a round wire to control torque and to prevent unwanted tipping of incisors. Other types of arch wires (*e.g.*, TMA™) also can be used in utility arch fabrication, sometimes eliminating the need for loops.

TYPES OF UTILITY ARCHES

Although many configurations for utility arches have been described,[4] four types of utility arches can be defined, based on their use.[6]

Passive Utility Arch

The passive utility arch (Fig. 11-4) is ideal for stabilization or space maintenance in either the mixed or permanent dentition. A passive utility arch can be used in the mixed dentition to maintain arch length during the transition to the permanent dentition. In many respects, the

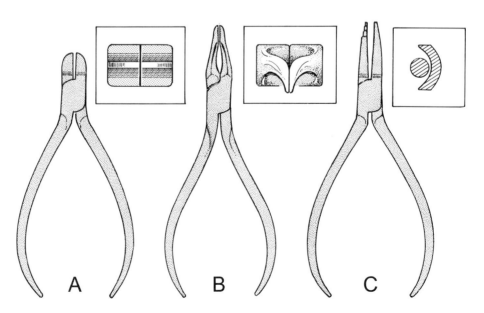

Figure 11-2. Instruments used in utility arch fabrication. *A*, 142 arch-bending pliers. *B*, Weingart pliers with narrow tip. *C*, Loop-bending pliers (#881, Masel Orthodontics, Bristol PA). Note that the surface opposite the turret is concave, allowing for intraoral activation of the utility arch.

UTILITY ARCHES

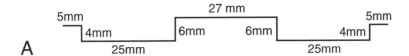

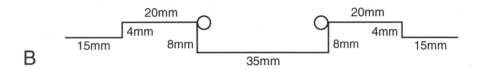

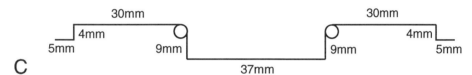

Figure 11-3. Typical dimensions of utility arches. *A*, Passive mandibular utility arch. *B*, Retrusive maxillary utility arch. *C*, Protrusive maxillary utility arch. These illustrations can be used in wire bending exercises of utility arch fabrication. The dimensions given are arbitrary; exact dimensions must be determined for each patient.

utility arch acts in the same manner as a lingual arch, because the passive utility arch prevents the mesial migration of the molars, particularly in the mandibular arch. The utility arch also may influence the eruption of the posterior teeth by holding the cheek musculature away from erupting teeth, allowing for spontaneous arch widening.

The passive utility arch also is used in the permanent dentition, primarily for the maintenance of anchorage. In non-extraction patients, the passive utility arch is useful particularly after molar distilization has been completed (Fig. 11-5). With many techniques (*e.g.,* Pendulum appliance, Wilson distalizing arch, NiTi coils), a large space is opened posterior to the maxillary second premolars as the first permanent molar is distalized (Fig. 11-5*A*). One of the challenges to the clinician is to maintain molar anchorage while the maxillary premolars and canines are being retracted. In combination with a transpalatal arch, extraoral traction, or a Nance holding arch, a passive utility arch can be used to incorporate the anterior teeth as anchor units (Fig. 11-5*A*). "Driftodontics" (*i.e.,* tooth movement produced without active orthodontic forces being applied) is used to allow the premolars to migrate posteriorly without active orthodontic treatment (Fig. 11-5*B*). This movement occurs due to the pull of the transseptal fibers that have been stretched as the molars move distally.

Passive utility arches also are used as anchorage appliances in patients whose treatment includes the extraction of permanent teeth (Fig. 11-6). Before canine retraction is initiated, a passive utility arch that extends from the first molars to the incisors is placed. Canine retraction then is begun, using the incisors as additional anchor units.

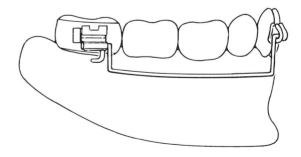

Figure 11-4. Passive utility arch. Note that the posterior vertical segment fits snugly against the auxiliary tube of the mandibular molar band.

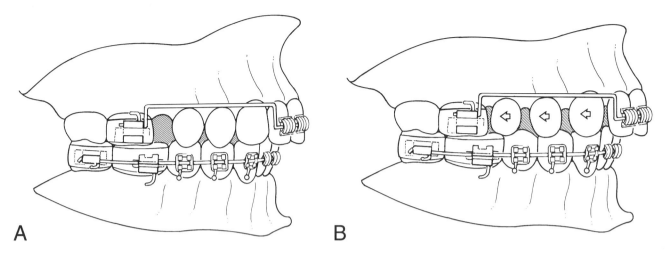

Figure 11-5. *A*, Passive utility arch used after molar distalization. A transpalatal arch or Nance holding arch often is used to provide additional molar stabilization. *B*, Note the spontaneous distal movement of the premolar and canine teeth after 3–4 months of passive maintenance of molar position. Fixed appliances then can be placed to further retract the premolars and canines. Class II elastics also may be used in the retraction of the canines and premolars.

Fabrication

The basic design of the passive utility arch is demonstrated in Figs. 11-3*A* and 11-4. The molar segment of the arch extends into the auxiliary tube. There is no need for a tieback when this arch is placed, because the arch is formed to fit passively to the existing contours of the dental arch. The posterior vertical segments, the vestibular segments, and the anterior vertical segments then are bent according to the needs of the individual patient.

Activation

No activation of the passive utility arch is required.

Intrusion Utility Arch

The intrusion utility arch (Fig. 11-7) is similar in design to the passive utility arch, except that the posterior vertical segment does not lie against the auxiliary tube on the first molar bracket. This arch is activated to intrude the anterior teeth.[7] After activation, the vestibular segments and anterior and posterior vertical segments, which serve as long lever arms from the molars to the incisors, deliver a light continuous force.

The utility arch should produce 60–100 gms of force on the mandibular incisors, a force level considered ideal for mandibular incisor intrusion.[3] The overall effect is intrusion and possible torquing of the mandibular incisors (Fig. 11-8) as well as a tipping back of the mandibular molars (Fig. 11-9). Widening or narrowing the archwire can achieve expansion or contraction of intermolar width. Molar rotation is produced through the activation of the molar segments of the arch as appropriate.

Fabrication

As with the passive arch, the intrusion arch is stepped gingivally at the molars (Fig. 11-7*A*), passes through the buccal vestibule, and then is stepped occlusally at the incisors to avoid distortion from occlusal forces. In contrast to the passive utility arch that fits flush against the auxiliary tube of the molar, there is at least a 5 mm

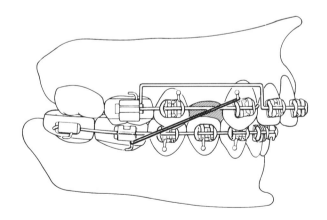

Figure 11-6. Passive utility arch used for maximum anchorage in extraction cases. In this Class II division 1 patient in whom maxillary first premolars have been extracted, canine retraction is initiated with either Class II elastics and/or elastomeric chain. The passive utility arch incorporates the maxillary incisors into the anchor unit. A transpalatal arch or a Nance holding arch also may be used for maximum anchorage, in addition to extraoral traction.

UTILITY ARCHES

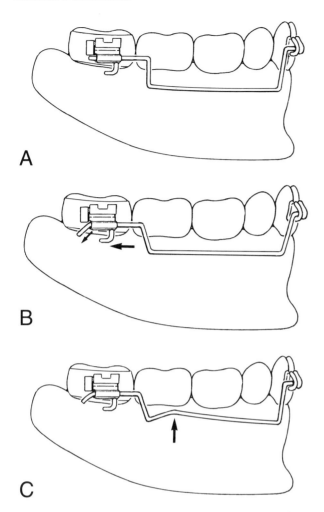

Figure 11-7. Intrusion utility arch. *A*, The intrusion utility arch first is bent passively to the existing occlusion. Note that the posterior vertical segment lies at least 5 mm ahead of the auxiliary tube on the mandibular first molar band. *B*, Retraction of the mandibular incisors is produced by grasping the distal end of the molar segment with a pair of small Weingart pliers, pulling the segment posteriorly, and then turning the segment gingivally. *C*, Intrusive forces are produced by using loop-forming pliers to place an occlusally directed gable bend in the posterior aspect of the vestibular segment.

space between the anterior border of the auxiliary tube and the posterior vertical segment of the utility arch (Fig. 11-7*A*). This configuration allows tying back the utility arch, as is described below.

Activation

Two types of forces can be produced using this design: retraction and intrusion. With a simple utility arch, a modest amount of incisor retraction can be achieved by grasping the end of the molar segment with small Weingart pliers (Fig. 11-2*B*) distal to the molar tube and bending this segment gingivally after pulling the wire

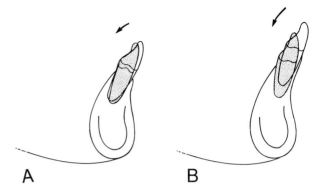

Figure 11-8. Intrusion of the mandibular incisor produced by the intrusive utility arch. *A*, Mild intrusion and retraction. *B*, Additional intrusion and retraction.

posteriorly through the tube (Fig. 11-7*B*). Care must be taken that the protruding end of the wire does not encroach on the soft tissue of both the cheek and gingiva. This type of activation prevents proclination of the mandibular incisors during intrusion.

Intrusion of the anterior teeth can be produced in one of two ways. First, the utility arch can be bent passively to fit the existing occlusion, as has been described previously. After ligating the utility arch into the anterior brackets, an intrusive force can be produced by placing an occlusally directed gable bend (similar to the angle formed between two slopes of a pitched roof) in the posterior portion of the vestibular segment of the archwire (Fig. 11-7*C*). A specific type of loop-forming plier (Fig. 11-2*C*), such as #881 loop-forming pliers (Masel Orthodontics, Bristol PA), is used for this type of intraoral activation. These loop-bending pliers must have a concave surface next to the loop-forming portion

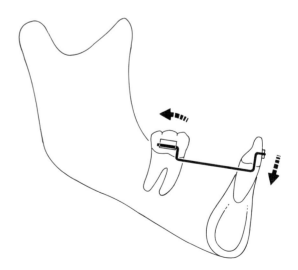

Figure 11-9. Forces produced by utility arch activation. The lower incisors are intruded, and the lower first molars are uprighted as they tip distally.

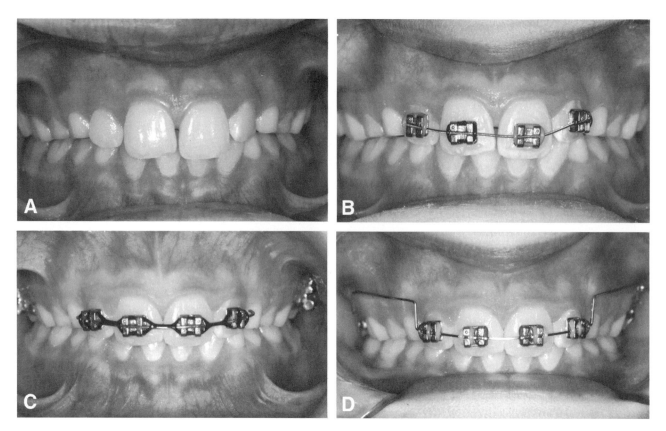

Figure 11-10. Intrusion utility arch in a mixed dentition patient. *A*, Initial malocclusion before treatment. *B*, Placement of brackets and .0175" coaxial wire to achieve initial incisal alignment. *C*, A .016" × .022" chrome cobalt wire used for further alignment. *D*, Placement of the intrusion utility arch.

of the plier; therefore, not all loop-bending pliers, such as omega loop-forming pliers, can be used for intraoral activation of the utility arch.

Bench[5] has advocated an alternative method of activation of the utility arch to produce intrusion. This type of activation involves placing a tip-back bend in the molar segment. The tip-back bend causes the incisal segment of the archwire to lie in the vestibular sulcus. The intrusion force is created by placing the incisal segment of the utility arch into the brackets of the incisors. This activation creates a moment that allows for the long action of the lever arm of the utility arch to intrude the mandibular incisors. It has been our experience, however, that placing distal crown torque in the molar segment occasionally leads to an unintentional posterior tipping of the first molars. Thus, activating the utility arch by placing a gable bend the posterior aspect of the vestibular segment (Fig. 11-7*C*) seems to avoid unwanted molar tipping. With the maxillary utility arch, tipping of the molars also is reduced through the concurrent use of a transpalatal arch.

Bench[3,5] also recommends the placement of buccal root torque in the mandibular molar region to anchor the roots of the molars in cortical bone. This type of force produces lingual crown torque that is counterbalanced by placing 10 mm of expansion in the molar region of the utility arch during appliance fabrication.

The intrusion utility arch can be used in both the mixed and permanent dentition. Figure 11-10 illustrates the typical sequence in a mixed dentition patient who presents with a moderately deep overbite (Fig. 11-10*A*). First, brackets are placed on the maxillary anterior teeth and a .0175" coaxial wire is inserted to achieve initial alignment (Fig 11-10*B*). Next, a contoured .016" × .022" chrome cobalt wire is used to align the maxillary incisors further (Fig. 11-10*C*). An intrusion utility arch is inserted (Fig. 11-10*D*) and then activated sequentially (Fig. 11-11) to produce the desired incisor intrusion.

The intrusion utility arch also can be used to improve a Class II molar relationship in patients with a deep overbite (Fig. 11-12). In such situations, the intrusive force that is generated by the anterior portion of the maxillary utility arch produces a distalizing force posteriorly in the region of the maxillary first molar. As the bite is opened anteriorly, molar correction is achieved posteriorly by a distal tipping of the maxillary first molar. Thus, a patient with a Class II malocclusion and an impinging overbite is an excellent candidate for this

UTILITY ARCHES

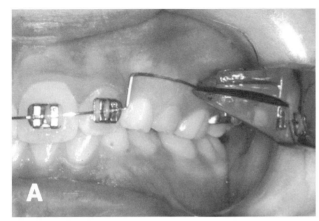

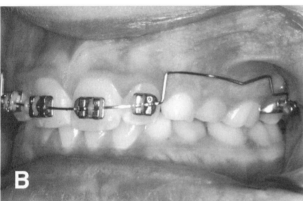

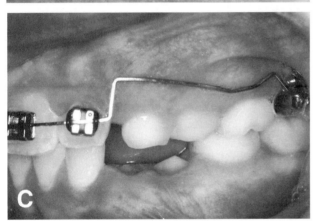

Figure 11-11. Intraoral activation of the intrusion utility arch. *A*, A loop bending plier is used to activate the arch by creating an occlusally-directed gable bend about two-thirds or three-quarters of the distance posteriorly. *B*, After the first activation. *C*, After the second activation.

protocol, a type of treatment requiring minimal patient compliance.

Retraction Utility Arch

The most common type of utility arch used in our practice is the retraction utility arch (Fig. 11-13*A*). This type of utility arch can be used in both the mixed and the permanent dentitions to achieve retraction and intru-

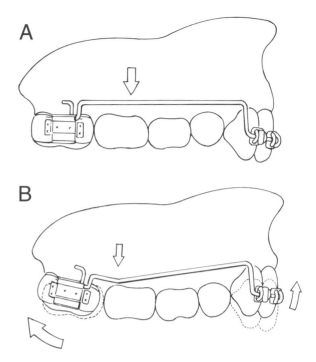

Figure 11-12. Spontaneous improvement of Class II molar relationship during incisor intrusion. *A*, Intrusion utility arch placed in deep bite patient (before activation). *B*, Activation of the utility arch not only results in incisor intrusion but also some posterior relocation of the maxillary first molars.

sion of the incisors. Loops are incorporated in the archwire anterior to the anterior vestibular segment. The loops add additional wire to the utility arch, facilitating retraction (Fig. 11-13*B*) and intrusion (Fig. 11-13*C*) of the anterior teeth. These movements can be produced by activating the retraction arch in a manner described previously for the intrusion utility arch.

Perhaps the most common use of the retraction utility arch is during the final stages of comprehensive edgewise treatment. In extraction patients, in whom the canines have been retracted, space opens distal to the maxillary lateral incisors. In non-extraction patients, a similar but smaller space often is present distal to the lateral incisors due to molar and premolar rotation (see Chapter 9) as well as a result of Class II mechanics (Fig. 11-14*A*). A retraction utility arch can be used to close this space by retracting the maxillary incisors (Fig. 11-14*B*). This arch also provides the necessary intrusion that often must precede the retraction of anterior teeth.

In some instances, the maxillary canines may become flared during the retraction of the maxillary incisors with a utility arch. After adequate retraction of the maxillary incisors has been achieved, the sectional wires are removed and an overlay ("piggyback") wire is placed over the utility arch anteriorly and into the bracket slots posteriorly (Fig. 11-15). Typically, in a .018" slot appli-

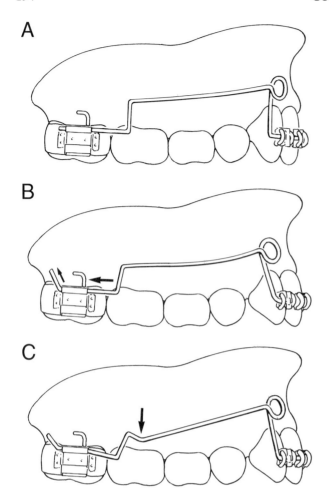

Figure 11-13. Sagittal view of maxillary retraction utility arch. *A*, Before activation. *B*, Retraction of the molar segment of the archwire. *C*, An occlusally directed gable bend has been placed in the vestibular segment of the archwire to produce incisor intrusion.

Figure 11-14. The use of a retracting utility arch during comprehensive orthodontic treatment. *A*, A retraction utility arch is bent passively to the existing occlusion. Note space distal to the maxillary lateral incisor. Intraoral activation then is performed. *B*, Retraction and intrusion of the maxillary incisors after utility arch treatment.

ance, the wire of choice is either a .016″ stainless steel or NiTi wire.

The retraction utility arch is used less commonly in the mandible. It may be placed, however, in patients with dentoalveolar anterior crossbite in whom there is some proclination and spacing of the mandibular incisors. In these situations, the anterior crossbite can be corrected using a retraction utility arch, whereas the spacing between the incisors is eliminated with elastomeric chain.

Utility arches also can be combined with bonded orthopedic appliances. For example, buccal tubes can be incorporated into a variety of acrylic splint appliances. Following expansion with a bonded RME, for example, a utility arch can be fabricated so that it is anchored posteriorly in the buccal tubes of the bonded appliance and then can be used to move the anterior teeth in all three planes of space.

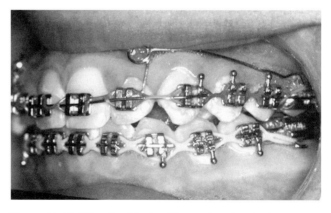

Figure 11-15. "Piggyback" wire. The sectional archwires are removed and a light (*e.g.*, .016″) round NiTi or stainless steel wire is placed on top of the utility arch and in the bracket slots posteriorly. This type of archwire is used to consolidate the arch and tuck in the maxillary canines that often become flared during incisor retraction.

UTILITY ARCHES

Fabrication

Used most often in the maxilla, the retraction utility arch originates in the auxiliary tube on the molar band, and 5–8 mm of wire should protrude anteriorly before a posterior vertical step of 3–4 mm is placed (Fig. 11-3B, Fig. 11-13A). The vestibular segment extends anteriorly to the interproximal region between the maxillary lateral incisor and the canine.

At this point, a 90° bend is placed with 142 arch-forming pliers. Loop-bending pliers (Fig. 11-2C) are used to form a loop in the archwire, with the end of the anterior leg crossing lingual to the posterior leg (Figs. 11-3B and 11-13A). After a 5–8 mm vertical segment is formed, another right angle bend carries the wire across the anterior teeth. A gentle anterior contour is placed in the wire to simulate arch form, and an offset is placed in the canine region.

On the other side of the arch, the anterior vertical step is created in the interproximal area between the lateral incisor and canine. The retraction loop is formed with loop-bending pliers, and then loop-bending pliers (rather than arch-forming pliers) are used to create the 90° bend in the horizontal vestibular segment (Fig. 11-2C). The wire extends to the posterior vertical segment at the middle of the second premolar. In most instances, the length of the horizontal vestibular segment can be estimated, based on the length of the horizontal segment on the opposite side. Care must be taken to make sure that the utility arch does not encroach on any fixed appliances present, including ball hooks or Kobayashi hooks (Fig. 11-14).

Activation

As with the intrusion utility arch, there are two possible types of activation. First, Weingart pliers are used to grasp the extension of the utility arch posterior to the auxiliary tube. The wire is pulled 3–5 mm posteriorly and then bent upward at an angle (Fig. 11-13B). Care must be taken that this protruding end of the utility arch does not impinge on the cheek or gingiva. Second, an occlusally directed gable bend in the vestibular segment is used to produce intrusion, as has been shown previously in Figure 11-13C.

Protraction Utility Arch

The protraction utility arch (Fig. 11-16) can be used to procline and intrude maxillary and mandibular incisors. In the permanent dentition, this type of archwire commonly is used for proclining and intruding maxillary incisors in Class II, division 2 patients, especially in those with an impinging overbite (Fig. 11-17). This archwire is used to provide clearance between the maxillary and mandibular incisors to allow for placement of brackets on the mandibular dental arch. The protraction utility arch also is used during the presurgical orthodontic phase of treatment to decompensate the position of the maxillary incisors in patients undergoing a mandibular advancement.

In addition, this type of utility arch can be inserted during the mixed-dentition period before functional jaw orthopedic appliance therapy. In Class II patients who have retruded maxillary incisors, brackets can be placed on the maxillary anterior teeth and bands on the maxillary first molars (perhaps supported by a transpalatal arch). A utility arch can be used to procline and intrude the incisors as necessary. Often a simple intrusion arch without loops is all that is required in the mandibular arch.

Fabrication

In contrast to the retraction utility arch and similar to the passive utility arch, the posterior vertical step of the protraction arch must be made flush with the auxiliary tube. The posterior vertical segment should be about 4 mm in length (Fig. 11-3C). The vestibular segment traverses anteriorly to the interproximal region between the canine and the lateral incisor. Loop-bending pliers (Fig. 11-2C) then are used to place a loop distal to the anterior vertical segment and occlusal to the vestibular segment. The anterior leg of the loop should be positioned medially, thus providing some canine offset.

The anterior vertical step typically is 5–8 mm in length, depending on patient tolerance. The incisal segment courses through the incisor brackets, and the utility arch is completed in a similar manner on the other side.

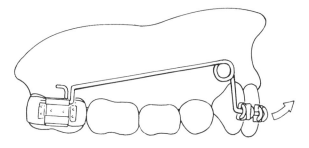

Figure 11-16. Protraction utility arch. Note that the posterior vertical segment is flush against the auxiliary molar tube. When passive, the anterior portion of the utility arch should lie approximately 2–3 mm ahead of the incisor brackets.

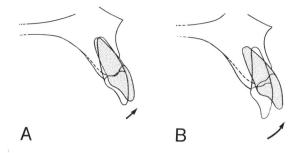

Figure 11-17. Movement of maxillary incisors using a protraction utility arch. *A*, Simple flaring. *B*, Protrusion and intrusion.

Activation

When the protrusive utility arch is passive, the anterior segment lies about 2–3 mm anterior to its ultimate position in the incisor brackets. Tying the anterior segment of the utility arch into the anterior brackets produces the protrusive force. An occlusally directed gable bend in the posterior aspect of the vestibular segment produces intrusion.

The protrusion arch is reactivated by removing the anterior segment from the brackets, bending the posterior vertical step forward from 90° to 45°, and replacing the arch wire in the brackets. Other adjustments can be made in both the anterior and posterior vertical steps to produce further activation.

CLINICAL PROBLEMS

By far, the major complications associated with the use of utility arches involve the soft tissue. One of the difficulties in fabricating the utility arch, whether it is for the maxilla or the mandible, is in placing the horizontal vestibular segment between the gingival and buccal tissues. If the posterior step is too long, or if the horizontal segment encroaches on the gingival tissue, the wire can become embedded easily. If the horizontal vestibular segment is placed too far laterally, tissue irritation and a buildup of fibrous tissue along the inside of the cheek can occur (Fig. 11-18). In instances in which tissue irritation occurs in the areas adjacent to the vestibular portion of the utility arch, clear or gray sleeving ("bumper sleeve") may be used to shield the tissue from the edges of the wire (Fig. 11-19).

Another major area of concern is the formation of the loops of the retraction utility arch. If these loops extend too far into the vestibular area or protrude anteriorly, severe irritation can result and patient discomfort can occur. The patient should be given wax at the delivery appointment to aid in the break-in period after the utility arch has been inserted. The patient and parent, if the patient is a child, should be advised that problems can arise during the firsr few days after the utility arch is delivered. They should notify the office immediately to prevent significant soft tissue impingement.

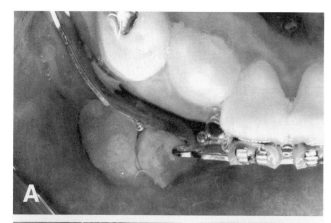
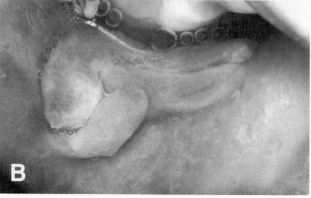

Figure 11-18. Soft tissue impingement by the utility arch can lead to tissue hyperplasia that may be asymptomatic to the patient. *A*, Epulis adjacent to utility arch. *B*, Another example of tissue hypertrophy caused by a utility arch.

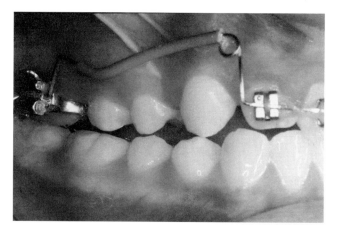

Figure 11-19. "Bumper sleeve" can be used in some patients to prevent the utility arch from impinging on the soft tissue, especially in the maxillary posterior regions.

OTHER CONSIDERATIONS

The above descriptions represent our recommendations concerning the clinical management of utility arches. Other clinicians have mentioned various modifications of these arch wires.

If one is concerned about unwanted posterior tipping of the molar, this tipping can be reduced significantly by placing buccal root torque in the molar segments bilaterally so the roots of the molars are moved buccally into the buccal cortical plate.[3–5] This so-called "cortical anchorage" is reported to be effective, particularly in the mandible. As mentioned earlier, expansion of the utility arch is recommended to offset lingual crown torque that can occur.

Utility arches can be designed differently for use in extraction and non-extraction patients.[3,4] In patients treated with extraction, the forces generated on the molars often are directed mesially and occlusally. A distolingual bend in the molar segment of the utility arch prevents this mesial rotation of the first molars. Such a bend may not be necessary in non-extraction patients or in patients in whom a transpalatal arch or a Nance holding arch is used.

Bench[5] also notes that rotation of molars can play an important role in determining anchorage requirements. When using retracting mechanics in which maximum anchorage is required, Bench recommends that molar rotation should be built either into the auxiliary tube or, if not present, into the archwire. The molar segment of the utility arch should have a 15° lingual offset bent into it. If no anchorage is to be maintained, the offset is not used.

Bench[5] also recommends tying back the utility arch when mandibular anterior intrusion is being produced. This protocol prevents the trapping of the mandibular incisors against the lingual cortical bone of the symphysis. Bench also suggests that 5–15° of buccal root torque is placed in the incisal segment of the utility arch during intrusion. The incisors cannot be torqued if the utility arch is formed from round wire.

CONCLUDING REMARKS

Utility arches are an integral part of our orthodontic protocols used in mixed-dentition and permanent-dentition patients. They are efficient in intruding maxillary and mandibular incisors and are effective especially in retracting and protruding anterior teeth.

One of the major difficulties in correcting anteroposterior discrepancies (particularly in Class II malocclusion) is an impairment of the anteroposterior tooth movement by unintentional anterior vertical interferences. Utility arches can be used, both in orthopedic and orthognathic surgery therapy, to move maxillary and mandibular incisors gingivally so that tooth positions can be corrected properly.

REFERENCES CITED

1. Burstone CJ. The mechanics of the segmented arch techniques. Angle Orthod 1966;36:99–120.
2. Burstone CR. Deep overbite correction by intrusion. Am J Orthod 1977;72:1–22.
3. Bench RW, Gugino CF, Hilgers JJ. Bioprogressive therapy. Part 12. J Clin Orthod 1978;12:569–586.
4. Ricketts RM, Bench RW, Gugino CF, Hilgers JJ, Schulhof RJ. Bioprogressive therapy. Denver: Rocky Mountain Orthodontics, 1979.
5. Bench RW, McNamara JA Jr. Fabrication of utility arches (videotape). Ann Arbor, Department of Orthodontics and Pediatric Dentistry, University of Michigan, 1988.
6. McNamara JA Jr. Utility arches. J Clin Orthod 1986;20:452–456.
7. Otto RL, Anholm JM, Engel GA. A comparative analysis of intrusion of incisor teeth achieved in adults and children according to facial type. Am J Orthod 1980;77:437–446.

Chapter 12
TRANSPALATAL ARCH

The transpalatal arch (TPA) has become an integral part of our approach to fixed appliance therapy. This type of arch, which spans the palate between the maxillary first molars, has been shown to be effective as an active orthodontic appliance as well as an anchorage maintenance device.

Since the introduction of the TPA (Fig. 12-1) by Robert A. Goshgarian[1] of Waukegan, Illinois in 1972, there have been surprisingly few articles in the orthodontic literature that have dealt directly with the clinical management of this particular appliance. Burstone and Koenig[2] and Baldin[3–5] have considered many of the biomechanical aspects of activating the transpalatal arch. Cetlin and Ten Hoeve[6] discussed the use of this appliance as part of non-extraction orthodontic treatment. The effect of the TPA on tongue function also was considered in two unpublished Master's theses by Lazzara[7] and Weisenberg.[8] All of the above investigations evaluated the removable transpalatal arch; the clinical management of the soldered transpalatal arch has not been described previously, not even by Goshgarian.

USES OF THE TRANSPALATAL ARCH

Several functions have been ascribed to the transpalatal arch, including the correction of molar rotation and the production of buccal root torque. Other functions such as molar stabilization and anchorage, maintenance of leeway space, and molar distalization and intrusion also have been suggested.[6,9]

Correction of Molar Rotation

In the evaluation of an orthodontic patient before treatment, attention should be paid to the position of the maxillary first molars. In particular, this is true in patients with Class II malocclusion. Lemons and Holmes[10] have indicated that, in the majority of Class II patients, the maxillary first molars are rotated mesially around the palatal root. A gain of 1–2 mm of arch length per side may be achieved following correction of these rotations (Fig. 12-2). Partial Class II correction also may be noted. If a correction of molar rotation is desired, this movement can be achieved through sequential activation of the transpalatal arch, as is described in detail below.

Clinicians have advocated various methods of determining the correct or ideal position of the molars. Andrews[11,12] has published his "six keys to optimal occlusion" (described in Chapter 26), a general scheme against which an occlusion can be compared. Andrews stated that the maxillary first molar should have a three-point contact with opposing teeth. The distal surface of the distobuccal cusp of the maxillary first molar should contact the mesial surface of the mesiobuccal cusp of the mandibular second molar (Fig. 12-3). In addition, the mesiobuccal cusp of the maxillary first molar should fall within the groove between the mesiobuccal and distobuccal cusps of the mandibular first molar.

When evaluating molar position, another evaluation technique can be used to determine whether or not molar rotation is desirable. Cetlin[13,14] has stated that, in

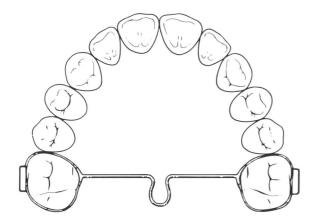

Figure 12-1. The soldered transpalatal arch used in the permanent dentition.

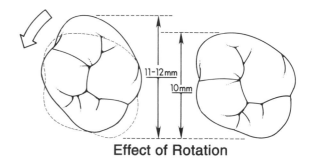

Effect of Rotation

Figure 12-2. Occlusal view of correction of molar rotation. This movement usually is achieved by rotating the maxillary right first molar in a distolingual direction around the palatal root. A gain of 1–2 mm of arch length can be achieved bilaterally when molar rotation is corrected.

an ideal occlusion, the buccal surfaces of the maxillary first molars usually are parallel to one another (Fig. 12-4). The orientation of the buccal surfaces of the first molars relative to one another can be determined visually through intraoral inspection.

Figure 12-5A demonstrates a common clinical condition, that is a patient who presents with first molars that are rotated mesially around the lingual root. Figure 12-5B shows the pretreatment maxillary study model of the same patient. Based on the imprints of the upper second deciduous molars that still were visible, the molars appear to have been rotated mesially before the recently lost maxillary deciduous second molars were exfoliated. The fitting of a facebow in this patient, for example, would be difficult because of the converging buccal tubes.

A transpalatal arch can be used effectively in correcting this type of unwanted molar rotation. The TPA is activated unilaterally to produce rotation of the maxillary first molar around the palatal root by grasping the solder joint with the beaks of small Weingart pliers (Fig. 12-6) and pushing the palatal wire posteriorly with finger pressure. By convention, the right side is activated initially, and the left side is activated in the same manner 6–8 weeks later.

Application of Buccal Root Torque

Another common observation when evaluating a patient's occlusion is lateral flaring of the maxillary buccal segments (Fig. 12-7). As discussed in Chapter 7, this flaring often is dentoalveolar compensation for a maxilla that is constricted (*i.e.*, reduced transpalatal width). One of the goals of fixed appliance treatment usually is flattening the curve of Wilson, often by applying buccal root torque to the maxillary first molars.

This type of torquing movement is accomplished

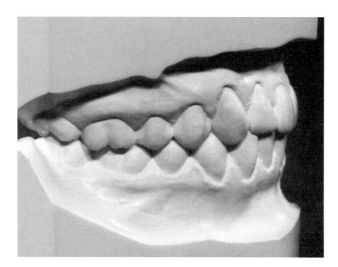

Figure 12-3. Normal occlusion. The distobuccal cusp of the maxillary first molar should contact the mesiobuccal cusp of the mandibular first molar.

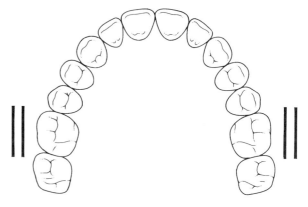

Figure 12-4. Evaluation of molar position. The buccal surfaces of the maxillary first molar should be parallel to each other in an ideal occlusion (after Cetlin[13]).

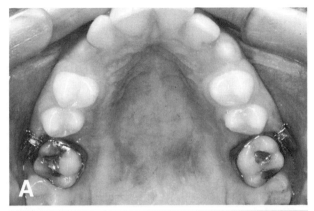

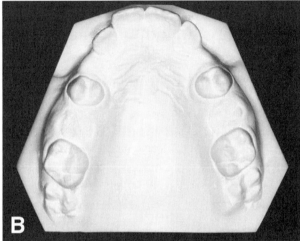

Figure 12-5. *A*, Intraoral view of patient with preadjusted bands and facebow tubes on maxillary first molars that are rotated mesially. *B*, Pretreatment maxillary study model of the same patient. The mesial rotation of the molars makes the fitting of a facebow or an archwire difficult.

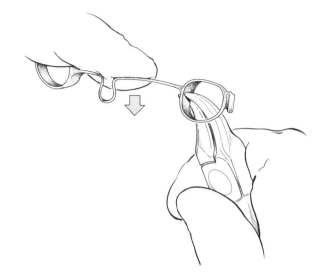

Figure 12-6. Routine rotational/anteroposterior activation of the transpalatal arch. Weingart pliers are used to hold the molar band at the solder joint. Rotational movements are produced by applying finger pressure against the TPA.

that buccal root torque is produced on the activated maxillary first molar after the TPA is cemented.

The activation sequence of the transpalatal arch is shown in Figures 12-9 and 12-10. First, the three-dimensional bends are placed in the transpalatal wire immediately adjacent to the right solder joint, as described above. Then Durelon™ (Premier Dental, Frankfurt, Germany) is used to cement the TPA temporarily. Durelon™ is used for all but the final activation because this type of cement allows for easy removal of the

easily through the three-dimensional activation of the transpalatal arch (Fig. 12-8), by adding an additional bending movement at the solder joint. In this movement, the transpalatal wire is bent toward the tongue, so

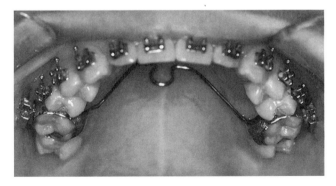

Figure 12-7. An example of a malocclusion characterized by a narrow transpalatal width and flared maxillary posterior teeth. The lingual cusps of the premolars and molars are inferior to the buccal cusps. Before activation, the transpalatal arch fits passively to the existing malocclusion.

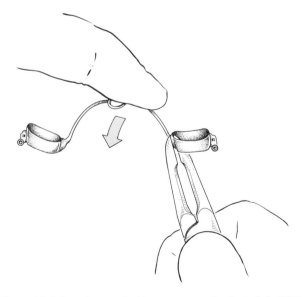

Figure 12-8. Routine vertical/transverse activation of the TPA. Weingart pliers are used to hold the molar band at the solder joint. Finger pressure is directed inferiorly, producing buccal root torque.

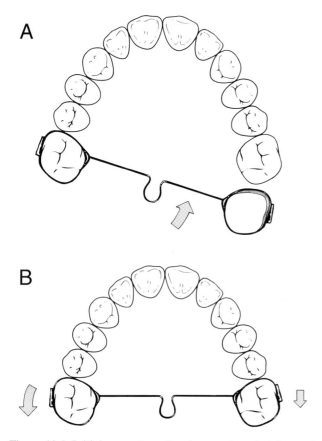

Figure 12-9. Initial correction of molar rotation. *A,* After activating the TPA on the right side, the band is seated on the right first molar. The molar band on the opposite side now lies in the second molar region below the occlusal plane. *B,* After the left molar band has been moved anteriorly and pushed into position, a rotational movement of the right molar is produced and a slight distal force is applied to the left molar.

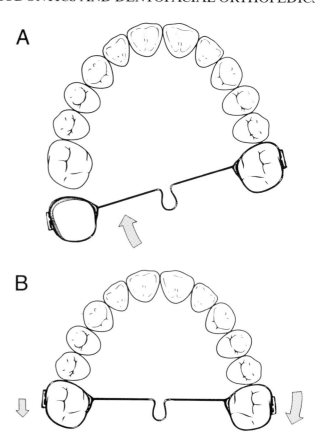

Figure 12-10. Subsequent activation. *A,* At the next appointment, the transpalatal arch is removed from the mouth and the left side of the appliance is activated. The left molar band is seated first, and the right molar band now lies in the region of the maxillary right second molar. *B,* After seating the molar band on the right side, a rotational movement of the left molar is produced and a slight distal force is applied to the right molar.

bands for reactivation. Cement is placed in both maxillary molar bands, and the right band is pushed into position (Fig. 12-9*A*). The left molar band now lies in the second molar position, below the maxillary occlusal plane toward the tongue. The left molar band is moved forward and upward and then is seated on the maxillary first molar (Fig. 12-9*B*). This movement produces distal rotation and buccal root torque on the activated right molar. Cetlin[9] also states that this type of unilateral activation produces a distalizing force on the opposite first molar, pushing the tooth distally. The slight extrusive force produced on the left molar is counterbalanced by the forces of occlusion.

Six to eight weeks later, the TPA is removed and the left side is activated. The same seating sequence is used, except in reverse. A three-dimensional activation bend is placed in the transpalatal wire adjacent to the solder joint on the maxillary left first molar band. Cement is placed in both bands (if this is the final activation, compomer cement such as Bandlok™, Reliance Orthodontic Products, Itasca IL, is used), and the left band is seated on the maxillary left first molar (Fig. 12-10*A*). The right molar band usually lies inferiorly in the right second molar position. The right band is pushed anteriorly and seated on the maxillary first molar (Fig. 12-10*B*), again producing distal rotation and buccal root torque movements in the right molar.

Why not activate both sides as the same time? This question is answered easily. If both sides are activated, the initial molar band seats without difficulty, but the second molar band to be cemented will be very difficult if not impossible to push into position because of the bend made at the adjacent solder joint. Routine unilateral activation of the TPA is recommended strongly.

Stabilization and Anchorage

Once the position of the molars has been corrected, the transpalatal arch serves as a stabilizing appliance by connecting the two first molars together with the palatal wire. An anchorage unit is formed that resists the mesial rotation of the molars. This type of anchorage is helpful when elastomeric chain is applied to a continuous arch wire. The transpalatal arch resists the tendency of the molars to rotate in a mesial direction around the palatal root.

A transpalatal arch also can be used as an anchorage appliance in those extraction patients with minimal to moderate anchorage requirements. Maximum anchorage cases that utilize the TPA should be supported by extraoral traction. The transpalatal arch also may be used as a bilateral space maintainer following the premature loss of a maxillary deciduous second molar.

Intrusive Movements

Cetlin[13] maintains that the transpalatal arch can prevent molar extrusion and perhaps can encourage molar intrusion (Fig. 12-11). By enlarging the midline omega loop and directing the loop mesially, the force of the tongue may produce an intrusive force on the teeth to which the transpalatal arch is anchored.

The effect of the transpalatal arch on tongue function has been evaluated in two clinical studies. Lazzara[7] evaluated vertical tongue pressure in 11 adolescent subjects who exhibited steep mandibular plane angles. He noted a greatly increased force of the tongue against the transpalatal arch following insertion. Although there was a drop in forces produced against the transpalatal arch at the end of one week, the force levels remained above normal values previously reported by Kydd[15,16] and others. Weisenberg[8] studied 12 subjects with steep mandibular plane angles and concluded that the anteroposterior positioning of the tongue was not affected significantly by the Goshgarian transpalatal arch. Definitive studies of the relationship between lingual function and the forces produced against the transpalatal arch have not been reported. Thus, we do not anticipate molar intrusion as a routine treatment effect of the TPA.

INDICATIONS AND CONTRAINDICATIONS

The transpalatal arch has become a routine part of our treatment protocol in both the permanent and late mixed dentitions, with a frequency of use well above 90%. This usage not only includes both extraction and non-extraction orthodontic patients, but the TPA usually is indicated in orthognathic surgery patients, especially in patients in whom severe malocclusions are going to be corrected. Once again, if an ideal occlusion is the goal, the achievement of this goal is enhanced by

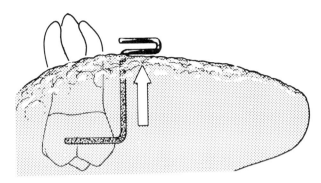

Figure 12-11. Proposed intrusive effect of the TPA. According to Cetlin,[13] molar extrusion can be prevented by placing the omega loop so that it is directed mesially. Tongue pressure then can be used to place an intrusive force on the transpalatal arch and subsequently to the molars.

molar rotation and the application of appropriate buccal root torque.

The routine use of the transpalatal arch also is recommended during the transition from the mixed dentition to the permanent dentition. This type of appliance can be used at the end of the mixed dentition period not only to rotate molars but to stabilize molar position, allowing for the retention of the leeway space that usually is available during the transition from the second deciduous molar to the second premolar (Fig. 12-12).

The transpalatal arch is contraindicated in two types of malocclusions, certain Class II malocclusions in which maxillary first premolars are removed and most Class III non-surgical patients. In instances of Class II malocclusion, the decision whether to use a TPA depends on the severity of the Class II molar relationship. If the molars are in a solid Class II position and no molar anchorage loss is desired, a TPA without activation can be used to maintain anchorage, as described previously. End-to-end molars, however, contraindicate the use of a TPA in

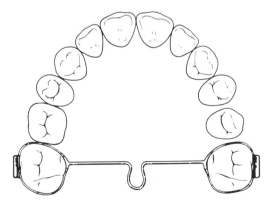

Figure 12-12. The transpalatal arch can maintain the leeway space that is available when the maxillary deciduous second-molar is lost and the maxillary second premolar erupts.

maxillary premolar extraction patients, in that a mesial rotation and migration of the molars into a solid Class II molar relationship is desirable. If a fully activated TPA is used in these instances, the complete closure of the extraction spaces may be impossible to achieve.

The use of the transpalatal arch as a molar rotating appliance also is contraindicated in Class III patients in whom orthognathic surgery is not undertaken and in whom permanent teeth are not extracted. A more mesial position of the buccal segments, including the molars, is desired to help camouflage any underlying anteroposterior jaw discrepancy. Thus, the transpalatal arch should not be used routinely in these types of patients.

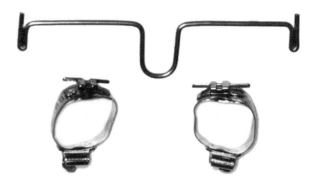

Figure 12-13. Components of the removable transpalatal arch. Lingual sheaths are welded to the lingual surfaces of the maxillary first molar bands.

FABRICATION OF TRANSPALATAL ARCHES

Transpalatal arches either can be fixed or removable, depending on the preference of the clinician. Both types of arches are described below.

Removable Transpalatal Arch

The original type of transpalatal arch was developed by Goshgarian[1] and refined by Cetlin[6] (Fig. 12-13). If this type of arch is to be used, a sheath must be attached to the lingual aspect of each molar band at the same occluso-gingival height and the same mesiodistal position as the buccal tube on the opposite side of the band. These sheaths receive the doubled-over .036″ terminals of the transpalatal arch. In doubling-over the ends of the arch, a rectangular insert of .036″ × .072″ is formed to control molar position in all dimensions.

Theoretically, there should be little difference in the adjustment of the removable and soldered transpalatal arches. At first glance, the removable TPA is easier to adjust because it can be removed from the sheaths and adjusted outside of the mouth. It has been our experience, however, that the routine adjustment of the removable TPA is less accurate than is that of the soldered TPA because the orientation of the bands is used as the primary reference for TPA adjustment. Thus, we strongly recommend the soldered version of the TPA as the appliance type of choice.

Fixed (Soldered) Transpalatal Arch

This type of transpalatal arch is made from .036″ stainless steel wire and features the soldering of the palatal wire to the lingual surfaces of the molar bands (Fig. 12-14). The specific sequence of three dimensional activation of the soldered TPA is shown in detail in Figures 12-15 and 12-16, including the application of molar rotation and buccal root torque forces.

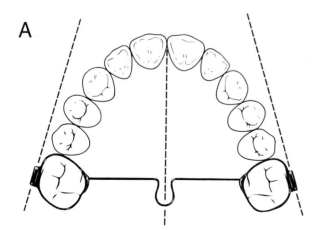
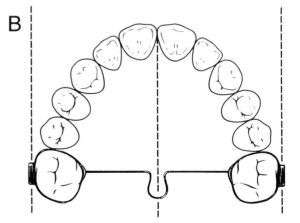

Figure 12-14. Evaluation of transpalatal arch activation. A, Before activation. Note the convergent orientation of the tubes on the maxillary first molars. B, After final activation. Clinically, the facebow tubes on the molar bands should be parallel to each other.

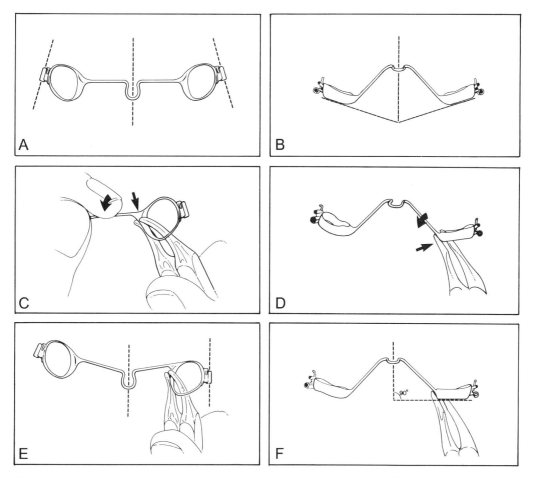

Figure 12-15. Initial activation of the transpalatal arch. By convention, the right side of the appliance is activated first. *A*, Occlusal view before activation. *B*, Posterior view before activation. *C*, Molar rotation and *D*, buccal root torque are produced by a bend at the solder joint. After the first activation, *E*, the right buccal tube is parallel to the midline, and *F*, the occlusal surface of the right molar band is parallel to the lower lingual edge of the left molar band.

Fabrication

When fabricating the appliance, bands are fitted on the maxillary molars. An alginate impression is made; the bands are removed from the teeth, placed in the impression, and secured with sticky wax. After the work model is poured and rough-trimmed, the lingual attachments of the bands (if present) are removed. A crosscut fissure bur then is used to remove 1–2 mm of stone lateral to the lingual surfaces of the bands, unless wax previously has been placed in those areas. Removing stone from the lingual surfaces of the molar bands facilitates the soldering process. The transpalatal arch then can be formed out of .036″ stainless steel wire, maintaining a 1.0–1.5 mm clearance in the palatal area. Right angle bends are placed in the arch so that the wire follows the lingual contour of the molar bands. The wire initially should contact the molar band at the mesiolingual line angles to facilitate the production of rotational movements.

After the transpalatal arch has been formed, it is secured in the palatal area using mortite or modeling clay, attaching the wire to the work model in the palatal area. Low-fusing solder is used to attach the constructed transpalatal arch to the bands. The bands are removed from the work model, and the entire appliance is smoothed, polished, and disinfected.

DELIVERY AND ACTIVATION

In most instances in which a transpalatal arch is used, the maxillary first molars are rotated mesially around the palatal root. The degree of molar rotation can be determined clinically by comparing the direction of the facebow tube on the molar bands with the midline of the palate (Fig. 12-14*A*). The ultimate goal of adjusting the transpalatal arch is to have the facebow tubes on the molar bands oriented parallel to the midpalatal suture (Fig. 12-14*B*). If the facebow tubes have a prescribed ro-

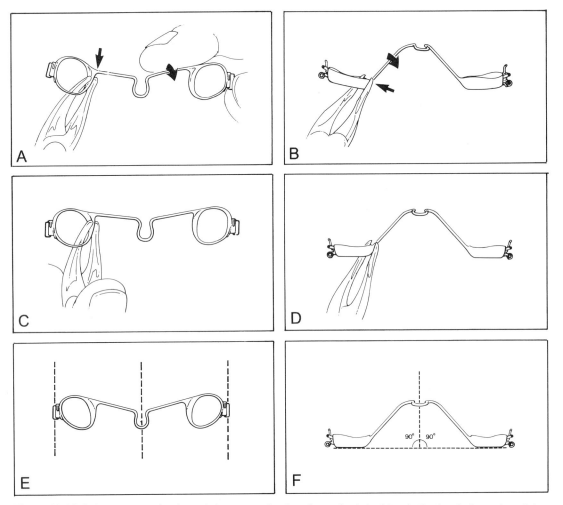

Figure 12-16. Subsequent activation of the transpalatal arch on the left side. *A*, Occlusal view of applying molar rotation to the left molar band *B*, Posterior view of application of buccal root torque to the left molar band. *C* and *D*, Fully activated TPA. After the final activation, *E*, both buccal tube are parallel to the midline and to each other, and *F*, the occlusal surface of both molar bands are parallel to each other.

tation incorporated into the band/tube assembly, as for example the 15° molar offset built into many preadjusted appliances, this angulation also must be taken into consideration. In most instances, however, making sure that the facebow tubes are parallel to each other and to the midline at the end of the final activation seems to be satisfactory, even the molars may be slightly over-rotated after full molar movement has been achieved. Routine orthodontic mechanics, especially those involving elastomeric chain, will tend to rotate the molars mesially during treatment.

SEQUENCE OF ACTIVATION

Because of the three-dimensional nature of the activation of the transpalatal arch, an attempt will be made to integrate the activation of the appliance as shown in Figures 12-15 and 12-16, which illustrate the initial and subsequent activation sequences.

Initial Activation

As mentioned previously, the first step in delivering the appliance is to place the TPA passively in the mouth. After the proper fit of the bands and the transpalatal wire has been verified, the arch should be removed from the mouth and evaluated. Normally, mesial rotation of the maxillary molars will be evident, as indicated by the orientation of the molar tubes relative to the mid-sagittal plane (Fig. 12-15*A*). In addition, the need for buccal root torque also is evident (Fig. 12-15*B*).

The initial activation of the TPA is made simply by grasping the solder joint with the ends of Weingart pliers. The anteroposterior activation is accomplished using finger pressure (Fig. 12-15*C*), whereas buccal root

TRANSPALATAL ARCH

torque can be produced by bending the transpalatal arch occlusally (Fig. 12-15*D*). At the end of the activation, the right buccal tube is oriented parallel to the midsagittal plane (Fig. 12-15*E*), and the occlusal surface of the right molar band is perpendicular to the midsagittal plane (Fig. 12-15*F*).

Subsequent Activation

About six to eight weeks is required for the molar rotation to take place on the activated side. Removing the appliance before that time may cause some discomfort to the patient, because tooth movement still may be occurring. As mentioned earlier, the clinician is cautioned against using a highly adhesive cement (*e.g.*, glass ionomer or compomer cement) except during final cementation after full activation, because of the difficulty (*e.g.*, pain to the patient) of removing the appliance.

After the appliance has been removed from the mouth, the bands and teeth are cleaned of all remaining cement. Then the previously passive side of the appliance is activated at the solder joint, again using Weingart pliers. Molar rotation is produced by bending the transpalatal arch posteriorly (Fig. 12-16*A*), and buccal root torque is incorporated into the appliance by pushing the wire occlusally (Fig. 12-16*B*).

Before cementing the TPA, the clinician should make sure that the buccal tubes are parallel to each other and to the midsagittal plane (Fig. 12-16*C*) and that the occlusal surfaces of the molar bands are parallel (Fig. 12-16*D*). If the appliance cannot be activated fully because of excessive tooth rotation or tooth tipping, additional activations may be necessary.

The transpalatal arch is activated fully and needs no

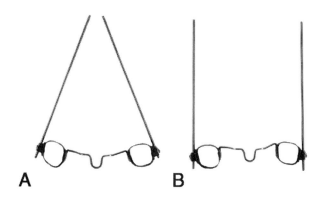

Figure 12-17. Indicator wires, made from .045″ stainless steel wires can be used to check the parallelism of the buccal tubes. *A*, Before activation. *B*, After full activation.

further adjustment when the buccal tubes approximate the midsagittal plane (Fig. 12-16*E*) and when the occlusal surfaces of the bands are perpendicular to the midsagittal plane and parallel to each other (Fig. 12-16*F*). The TPA can be left in place for the duration of fixed appliance treatment as both an intra-arch stabilization appliance and as an appliance serving as anchorage for other orthodontic movements.

EVALUATION OF ACTIVATION

The easiest way to determine if the transpalatal arch requires activation is to place two 4–5″ sections of .045″ round stainless steel wires in the facebow tubes, either before or after the TPA is cemented (Figs. 12-17 and 12-18). When the clinician is learning the technique of sequentially activating the TPA, these wires can be used to

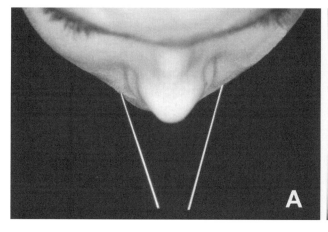
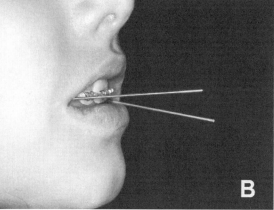

Figure 12-18. Indicator wires used intraorally. *A*, Evaluation of patient from above; tip of nose is seen. Note the convergence of the wires, indicating that the molars need to be rotated distolingually. *B*, Frontal view. Variation in molar angulation is noted. The two indicator wires should be at the same level when the TPA is activated properly.

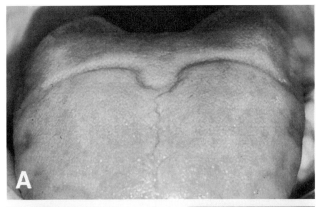
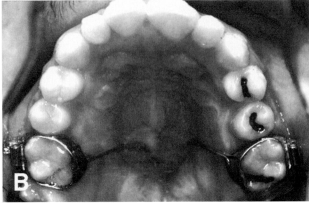

Figure 12-19. Soft tissue impingement. *A*, Indentation on tongue. *B*, Tissue of palate overgrowing the TPA at the midline.

indicate the orientation of the buccal tubes in three dimensions. Before activation, the wires are placed in the facebow tubes (Fig. 12-17*A*), usually converging anteriorly. After full activation, the wires are parallel to each other (Fig. 12-17*B*) and to the midline omega loop.

This technique also can be used during treatment by placing the indicator wires in the facebow tubes. Looking from above the patient (Fig. 12-18*A*), a TPA that is not fully activated will result in the indicator wires converging anteriorly. Problems in molar angulation will be identified as well (Figs. 12-18*B*). After full activation, the wires should remain parallel to each other in the same plane. Intraorally, the occlusal surfaces of the bands on the maxillary first molars should be parallel to each other.

CLINICAL PROBLEMS

The most common clinical problem is soft tissue irritation. Because of the variable tolerance of patients to this type of appliance, the transpalatal wire should not encroach either on the tongue or on the tissue of the hard palate. Whereas slight grooving of the tongue is common and is asymptomatic to the patient, it is possible to produce ulcerations of or a deep groove on the tongue within a few days of cementation (Fig. 12-19*A*). On the other hand, if the transpalatal arch passes too closely to the tissue of the palate, the TPA may become embedded in the palatal tissue (Fig. 12-19*B*) and must be removed to allow for healing.

With proper fabrication of the soldered transpalatal arch, it is uncommon to see breakage of this appliance. It is slightly more common to see problems with appliance loosening using a removable transpalatal arch, especially if the TPA is not ligated in place. Also removing the latter type of TPA may irritate or impinge on the palatal mucosa.

CONCLUDING REMARKS

The transpalatal arch has become an integral part of both mixed-dentition and permanent-dentition treatment. We strongly prefer the soldered transpalatal arch rather than the removable transpalatal arch. Part of the reason for this choice is based on the belief that a more precise activation of the appliance can be achieved if the TPA is removed from the mouth for reactivation. Although the "removable TPA" obviously can be taken from the mouth, it is only the arch that is removable, not the bands. The bands are the landmarks that determine proper activation.

We have found that the routine use of the soldered transpalatal arch to be an important adjunct to our fixed appliance treatment. If used after existing transverse problem has been corrected, the sequential activation of the TPA allows for the proper positioning of the maxillary first molars within a few appointments, so that the rest of the patient's fixed appliance treatment can proceed smoothly and efficiently.

REFERENCES CITED

1. Goshgarian RA. Orthodontic palatal arch wires. United States Government Patent Office, 1972.
2. Burstone CJ, Koenig HA. Precision adjustment of the transpalatal lingual arch: computer arch form predetermination. Am J Orthod 1981;79:115–133.
3. Baldini G. Wechselwirkung zwischen bukkalem Wurzeltorque und Expansion beim Palatinalbogen nach Goshgarian. Informat Orthodont Kieferorthopäd 1981;3:181–6.
4. Baldini G. Apparative Messung der durch die Torquebiegungen am Palatinalbogen entstehenden Drehmomente und der durch die Torqueapplikation entstehenden expansiven Kraft. Informat Orthod Kieferorthopäd 1981;3:187–198.

5. Baldini G, Luder HU. Influence of arch shape on the transverse effects of transpalatal arches of the Goshgarian type during application of buccal root torque. Am J Orthod 1982;81:202–208.
6. Cetlin NM, Ten Hoeve A. Nonextraction treatment. J Clin Orthod 1983;17:396–413.
7. Lazzara DJ. Lingual force on the Goshgarian palatal bar. Chicago: Unpublished Master's thesis, Department of Orthodontics, Loyola University, 1976.
8. Weisenberg MJ. The influence of the Goshgarian palatal bar on the anterior-posterior positioning of the tongue. Chicago: Unpublished Master's Thesis, Department of Orthodontics, Loyola University, 1976.
9. Cetlin NM. Syllabus of Cetlin-Ten Hoeve treatment mechanics, 1992.
10. Lemons FF, Holmes CW. The problem of the rotated maxillary first permanent molar. Am. J. Orthod. 1961;47:246–272.
11. Andrews LF. The six keys to normal occlusion. Am J Orthod 1972;62:296–309.
12. Andrews LW. Straightwire: The Concept and Appliance. San Diego, CA: L.A. Wells Company, 1989.
13. Cetlin NM. Personal communication, 1984.
14. Cetlin NM. Personal communication, 1990.
15. Kydd WL. Quantitative analysis of forces of the tongue. J Dent Res 1956;35:171–74.
16. Kydd WL. Maximum forces exerted on the dentition by perioral and lingual musculature. J. Am Dent. Assoc. 1957;55:646–651.

Chapter 13
RAPID MAXILLARY EXPANSION

In recent years, there has been increased interest among many members of both the professional and lay populations in treatments that do not involve the extraction of permanent teeth. This interest is based on many concerns, both real and perceived (*e.g.*, avoidance of unfavorable facial changes, fear of litigation). Non-extraction protocols also have become increasingly popular, in part, because of changes in orthodontic technology and procedures, such as bonded brackets and judicious interproximal reduction.

Another protocol that has been incorporated into non-extraction treatment is rapid maxillary expansion (RME). Although used traditionally as a method of crossbite correction, this procedure now is intended to increase arch perimeter in the maxilla, level the Curve of Wilson, "broaden the smile," and perhaps increase airway patency (see Chapter 7 for a discussion of these issues). According to the *1996 Study of Orthodontic Diagnosis and Treatment Procedures* published by the *Journal of Clinical Orthodontics*,[1] over half of the orthodontic practitioners surveyed use RME appliances routinely; relatively few report never using this type of appliance at all.

This chapter will consider several types of rapid expansion appliances, both banded and bonded. Of all the areas of the craniofacial complex, perhaps the most readily adaptable is the transverse dimension of the maxilla. Generally, RME appliances are fixed and generate 3–10 pounds of force.[2] Once activated, RME produces a net increase in the transverse width of the maxillary basal bone, thereby leading to the correction of preexisting crossbites as well as increasing available arch length. Adkins and co-workers[3] have determined that every millimeter of posterior expansion produces about 0.7 mm of additional arch perimeter.

MECHANISM OF ACTION

The mechanism of action of RME initially became clarified in the 1950s through studies of cats[4] and pigs.[5] Both of these investigations demonstrated that the midpalatal suture was opened using this technique. The monkey studies of Starnbach and colleagues[6] demonstrated that the effect of this technique was not only on the midpalatal suture but also on the circummaxillary sutural system.

These findings were supported by the later investigations of Biederman,[7] Brossman and co-workers,[8] Chaconas and Caputo,[9] and Tanne and associates.[10] Gardner and Kronman[11] reported opening of the spheno-occipital synchondrosis. In general, these investigators reported an increase in the cellular activity of the sutural system as well as a widening of the bony nasal airway, a treatment effect that served as a popular rationale for RME during the first part of this century.

Melsen described midpalatal sutural morphology and postnatal palatal development based on human autopsy material[12,13] and on biopsies performed on children.[14] Her work is critical to our understanding of age-related responses to RME. Because of the increasing complexity of the sutural system, fewer skeletal and more dentoalveolar adaptations are observed in older patients, particularly in adults. Similar findings have been reported by Murray and Cleall[15] and Ten Cate and associates.[16] Thus, the literature argues that the age and maturational level of the individual patient is an important factor when considering the effect of RME on craniofacial structures.

BANDED EXPANDERS

Generally, there are two types of banded expanders that are used routinely in both mixed dentition and early permanent dentition patients to produce orthopedic expansion of the maxilla. In adults, these appliances also are used to produce major skeletal changes, but only if the expansion is surgically assisted.

Types of Banded Expanders

Two types of fixed banded expanders are recognized, the Haas-type and the Hyrax-type. Both of these designs can be used to widen the maxillary sutural system, but they differ as to the amount of transverse expansion produced relative to lateral tooth tipping.

Haas-type Expander

The first type of expansion appliance was popularized by Haas.[17-20] This appliance consists of bands placed on the maxillary first premolars and maxillary first molars (Fig. 13-1). A midline jackscrew is incorporated into the two acrylic pads that closely contact the palatal mucosa. Support wires also extend anteriorly from the molars along the buccal and lingual surfaces of the posterior teeth to add rigidity to the appliance.

Haas[17] states that more bodily movement and less dental tipping is produced when acrylic palatal coverage is added to support the appliance, thus permitting forces to be generated not only against the teeth but also against the underlying soft and hard palatal tissues. Inflammation of the palatal tissue, however, has been reported as an occasional complication.

A review of the literature concerning RME appliances has been presented in Chapter 7. A more detailed description of one Haas-type studies is presented here. Herberger[21] evaluated 55 RME subjects who had been treated with a Haas-type expander as part of their fixed appliance therapy. The average patient was 11.0 years of age at the time that the initial records were obtained. Records were taken immediately post-treatment at 14.4 years and about six years later at 21.0 years. The long-term effects of treatment were determined by analyzing serial dental casts and posteroanterior cephalograms.

Herberger[21] noted an increase in transpalatal width

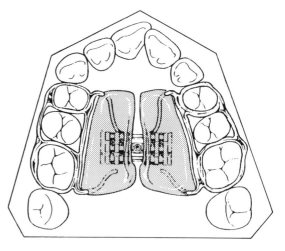

Figure 13-1. The Haas-type expander with an expansion screw incorporated in the palatal acrylic.

of 4.5 to 6.8 mm following the removal of the appliances, depending on the region measured (Fig. 13-2). After analyzing the long-term records, Herberger noted that 85 to 94% of the increases in arch width present at the end of treatment still were evident six years after appliance removal. He also noted an increase in maxillary bony base width, as viewed in the P-A cephalogram, of about 3.9 mm, a value that increased slightly during the post-treatment period (Fig. 13-3). Herberger concluded that the use of a tooth- and tissue-borne RME appliance combined with fixed appliances was reasonably stable during the post-treatment period studied.

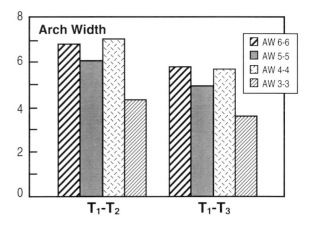

Figure 13-2. Changes in the transverse dimension following RME treatment using an expander of the Haas-type design. T_1-T_2, changes between the initial and post-treatment records. T_1-T_3, changes between initial and long-term records. AW 6-6, arch width changes between the upper molars; AW 5-5, between the upper second premolars; AW 4-4, between the upper first premolars, AW 3-3, between upper canines (Adapted from Herberger [21]).

RAPID MAXILLARY EXPANSION APPLIANCES

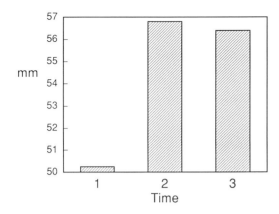

Figure 13-3. Transverse skeletal dimensional changes between Point Mx bilaterally on the lateral outline of the maxilla as viewed in the posteroanterior cephalogram T_1, before treatment; T_2, after treatment; T_3, six years following appliance removal (adapted from Herberger [21]).

A recent study by Cameron[22] investigated the short-term and long-term effects of rapid maxillary expansion with the Haas appliance by way of posteroanterior headfilms. The treated sample consisted of 42 patients (9–15 yeas old) who underwent rapid maxillary expansion followed by standard edgewise therapy. The RME sample was compared to a group of 20 subjects from the *University of Michigan Elementary and Secondary School Growth Study* who did not undergo any orthodontic treatment. The groups were analyzed at three intervals: T_1, pretreatment (11 years 10 month of age for both groups), T_2, immediately post-expansion, and T_3, long-term follow-up (20 years, 6 months for the treated group and 17 years, 8 months for the control group).

Cameron[22] reported that the maxilla split in triangular fashion. This morphologic change confirmed the assumption that the skeletal response was greater near the screw and decreased toward the cranial base. The increases from pre-treatment were 9.1 mm, 3.5 mm, and 3.0 mm for maxillary first molar width, maxillary width, and nasal width respectively. In the long-term, a nasal width that exceeded the expected growth increment of the control sample by 2.7 mm was observed. Not only were the changes in dental dimensions greater in the treated group, but a larger nasal width was observed in the treated group as well.

Other studies dealing with the long-term treatment effects produced by rapid maxillary expansion include Stockfisch,[23] Wertz and Dreskin,[24] Linder-Aronson,[25] Herold,[26] and Fenderson.[27] The results of these investigations reinforce the importance of appliance design as well as patient age and maturation in the determination of the treatment effects produced by rapid maxillary expansion.

Hyrax-type Expander

The more commonly used type of banded RME appliance is the Hyrax-type expander (Fig. 13-4), the design of which has been credited to Biederman.[7,28] This type of expander is made entirely of stainless steel. This design does not include palatal acrylic and thus has been considered more hygienic by many practitioners. Bands are placed on the maxillary first molars and first premolars. The expansion screw is located in the palate in close proximity to the palatal contour. Buccal and lingual support wires also may be added for rigidity (Fig. 13-4).

One of the concerns about the Hyrax design is that the appliance may be more flexible than the Haas design, thus producing more dental tipping and less sutural separation. Ralph,[29] using a theoretical model (*i.e.*, finite element analysis), tested whether there was an appreciable difference between the Hyrax and Haas RME appliances in affecting the midpalatal suture, teeth, and attached structures. Ralph reported that the average tipping effects are 2.5 to 3 times greater in the Hyrax model compared to the Haas model and that the Haas appliance displaces teeth an average of 26% more than the Hyrax appliance in the transverse dimension. Larger sutural displacement occurred in the Haas model compared to the Hyrax. The Hyrax expander also deformed to a greater extent than the Haas-type, resulting in appreciably less energy available in affecting sutural tissues immediately after activation. The effective result was sutural strain energy density (stored energy) being seven times greater in the Haas model suture.

The concern about the flexibility of banded expanders without rigid support is illustrated by the investigations of Timms,[30] who examined RME subjects out of retention for twelve months or more and noted an average relapse in transpalatal width of 41% with a range of 31–82%. Unfortunately, this study was flawed in several

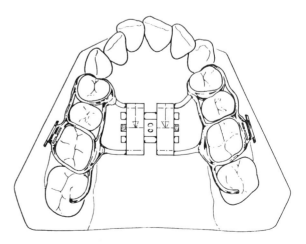

Figure 13-4. Hyrax-type expander.

respects. First, Timms used a non-rigid expansion appliance and found that the molar teeth tipped buccally during the treatment period but returned approximately to pretreatment values during retention, a finding that indicated that a substantial amount of tooth movement (*i.e.*, tipping) was produced by this appliance. Second, Timms reported that some of the patients in his study had histories of poor cooperation during the early retention period. He concluded that it was probable that "a few of the relapse cases are artificially high . . ." and attributed the high amount of relapse, in part, to "a few bad cases." A later study by Timms[31] also showed a significant amount of relapse. The differences between the Timms studies and the Herberger[21] and Cameron[22] studies of the Haas expander may be due to variations in appliance design, another factor that must be considered in the evaluation of the long-term treatment effects of RME.

When making the decision about which of the two designs to select when choosing a banded RME appliance, the age and anchorage requirement of the patient must be taken into consideration. In patients with mild-to-moderate transverse constriction in the late mixed or early permanent dentition, a time during which the sutures presumably are reasonably patent, the Hyrax design can be used successfully with little difficulty. In patients with severe maxillary constriction in the early permanent dentition or who have moderate maxillary constriction in late adolescence, however, the Haas expander is the design of choice. When considering surgically assisted expansion, a procedure that frees the sutural system in late adolescence or adulthood, both designs can be used effectively.

Clinical Management of Banded Expanders

A rapid palatal expansion appliance normally is the first appliance used when palatal expansion is planned for a patient in the permanent dentition. To ensure maximum orthopedic effect, the abutment teeth incorporated into the expander should not have undergone prior orthodontic movement. If teeth have been aligned before the placement of the expander, the periodontal membrane usually is widened and the likelihood of tooth movement rather than orthopedic movement of the maxilla is increased.

Impression

The maxillary first premolars and first molars are separated at the previous appointment so that there is adequate space interproximally for the placement of bands. The bands selected for this appliance ideally are made from heavy band material, adding rigidity to the appliance. The bands selected should be slightly oversized to allow for the path of insertion of the appliance.

After band fitting is completed, an alginate impression is made with a standard aluminum tray. It is essential to have an adequate reproduction not only of the teeth, but also the entire palatal region, regardless of appliance design. The bands are removed from the mouth of the patient and placed in their appropriate positions in the impression. The bands are secured to the alginate with sticky wax to ensure that they are not displaced during the pouring of the work model. Band movement during pouring can result in the fabrication of an appliance that does not fit.

Fabrication

It has been our experience that Haas-type expander is best made by a commercial laboratory. The Hyrax expander, because of its less complex design, can be constructed in-office or by a laboratory. The following describes the fabrication of the latter type of expander.

After the work model has been poured and trimmed, the position of the bands on the work model are checked. If there is any obvious malalignment of the bands due to movement during pouring, fabrication of the appliance should not proceed. Usually, another impression of the patient must be made at a subsequent appointment. In rare instances, the proper position of the band is obvious, and adjustments in band position can be made on the work model.

The first step in the fabrication of the expander is to cut to proper size the four legs (struts) of the expansion screw assembly. We recommend the use of Leone expansion screws (Leone Co, Florence, Italy). This type of screw can be activated about 50 times without disassembling, resulting in about 10 mm of expansion. Sections of .036″ stainless steel wire are used for the fabrication of the lingual support wire that extends between the maxillary first molar and the first premolar on both sides (Fig. 13-4). The support wires are attached to the work model using MDS Adhesive™ (Great Lakes Orthodontic Products, Tonawanda NY) prior to soldering. A small mound of stone or plaster also can be placed in the palate to provide a reference matrix for the expansion screw.

Every attempt should be made to place the palatal screw within 2–4 mm of the palatal mucosa so that tongue function is interrupted minimally. Lingual support wires are added as well. After the expander is soldered, the appliance is removed from the work model by grinding away the plaster holding the bands. The appliance is finished and polished in an appropriate manner and, after disinfection, the appliance is ready for delivery.

Delivery of the Appliance

Separators are left in place between the fabrication appointment and the delivery appointment. The separators are removed and a preliminary try-in of the appliance is attempted. Occasionally, the clinician will experience difficulty during the initial placement of the appliance. Because of the diverging paths of withdrawal of the four anchoring bands, it is necessary to allow the expander to remain in place for a few minutes, with the patient applying gentle pressure against the expander, sometimes biting against a tongue depressor or cotton rolls placed over the appliance. As long as the bands have not been distorted during the pouring of the work model, the appliance usually will seat into place gradually.

The cementation of the banded expander is accomplished using a glass ionomer or compomer cement (*e.g.*, blue BandLok™, Reliance Orthodontic Products, Itasca IL). Because very heavy forces are generated, adequate adhesion of the cement to both the expander and the teeth is essential. The use of glass ionomer or compomer for cementing bands presents one important advantage when compared to the traditional use of zinc phosphate cement. The release of fluoride decreases the risk of decalcification due to microleakage at the interface between the band and the enamel surface.[32,33]

Delivery Instructions

The patient is instructed to expand the appliance once per day until the appropriate amount of expansion is produced. We prefer a once per day protocol because occasionally some nasal distortion occurs. The appearance of a "saddle-nose deformity" is very rare, but this sinking of the nasal septum between the two halves of the maxilla typically has been associated with a two-expansions-per-day protocol. If this situation occurs, simply removing the appliance usually resolves the problem.

We attempt to maintain contact between the lingual cusps of the maxillary teeth and the buccal cusps of the mandibular teeth in most instances (Fig. 13-5). On the other hand, Haas[34] recommends expanding the patient 10.5–11.0 mm, an amount of expansion that usually results in the occurrence of a buccal crossbite posteriorly.

After an adequate amount of expansion has been achieved, the appliance is left in place for an additional three to five months to allow for adequate reossification of the involved sutural systems.[17] In patients whose treatment is delayed due to the transition of the dentition (*e.g.*, late eruption of a premolar), the expander can be left in place longer.

In instances in which there is some suspicion that the screw is "backing off" or becoming unwound, a piece of

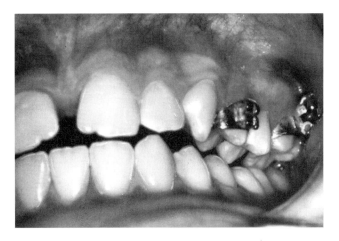

Figure 13-5. Adequate expansion is achieved when the lingual cusps of the upper posterior teeth approximate the buccal cusps of the lower posterior teeth.

ligature wire can be passed through one of the small holes in the palatal screw. Usually, this is not possible until the expander has been widened for 30–35 activations. Alternatively, cold-cure acrylic can be applied to the screw to stabilize the appliance.

Expander Removal

An ordinary pair of posterior band removing pliers can be used to remove the expander. The associated teeth should be cleaned and any residual cement removed. In most instances, it is essential that fixed appliances be placed on the involved teeth within a very short period. Depending on the severity of the original maxillary skeletal constriction, either brackets can be placed on the maxillary first and second premolars at the removal appointment or a transpalatal arch can be fabricated for delivery within a few days. Usually, most arches that have been expanded using a banded-type expander will be stabilized during treatment with a transpalatal arch (See Chapter 12). If fixed appliances are not to be used immediately, an acrylic stabilization plate is fabricated and is worn by the patient full-time.

BONDED ACRYLIC SPLINT EXPANDER

The foundation of early orthopedic treatment in patients with tooth-size/arch-size discrepancy problems is the bonded rapid maxillary expansion appliance. A number of articles have appeared in the literature that have described various types of bonded acrylic splint appliances that are used either alone as expanders[35–39] or in combination with other appliances.[40–45]

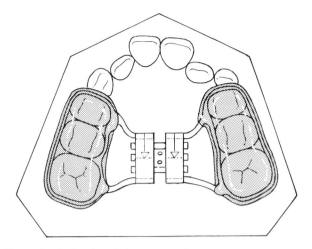

Figure 13-6. The bonded acrylic splint rapid maxillary appliance made with a wire framework and 3.0 mm thick splint Biocryl™.

The acrylic splint expander (Fig. 13-6) widens the maxilla (Fig. 13-7) by separating the midpalatal suture and activating the circummaxillary sutural systems. In young patients, the effect of the appliance primarily is orthopedic in nature. Brust[46] has shown that little tooth tipping is observed during expansion, presumably due to the rigid framework of the appliance and the bonding of the appliance to the posterior dentition.

The bonded expander not only widens the transverse dimension, but it produces changes in the vertical and anteroposterior dimensions as well. The posterior occlusal coverage of the acrylic (the acrylic parts of the appliance are made from 3 mm splint Biocryl™ or cold-cure acrylic) acts as a posterior bite block, inhibiting the eruption of the posterior teeth during treatment and making possible the use of this appliance in patients with long lower anterior facial heights. The acrylic occlusal coverage also opens the bite posteriorly, facilitating the correction of anterior crossbites.

The expansion of the maxilla during the early mixed dentition also may lead to a spontaneous correction of malocclusions that tend toward Class II or Class III. As has been described in detail in Chapter 4, the widening of the maxilla of a Class II patient into an overexpanded position may lead to the forward repositioning of the lower jaw, ultimately resulting in a solid Class I occlusion. This type of occlusal change occurs during the *retention* period. In contrast, spontaneous correction of Class III tendency relationships may occur during the *active* phase of treatment, presumably due to the slight forward displacement of the maxilla during orthopedic expansion.[17,18,47]

As was discussed in Chapter 7, rapid maxillary expansion is used to correct a unilateral or bilateral posterior crossbite. The patient whose maxillary dental casts are seen in Figure 13-8A presented with a narrow maxilla (transpalatal width 30.4 mm) and a posterior crossbite on the left side. Six months of rapid maxillary expansion not only corrected the crossbite but also overexpanded the maxilla slightly (38.5 mm; Fig. 13-8B) relative to the mandibular dental arch. As no arch length discrepancies existed in the maxilla after expansion, the use of transpalatal arch to maintain arch length was not needed during the further transition of the dentition (Figs. 13-8C and 13-8D).

Figure 13-9 represents the corresponding series of mandibular dental casts from the patient described in Figure 13-8. A mild arch length discrepancy was present initially, as evidenced by the lingual eruption of the lower left lateral incisor (Fig. 13-9A). Spontaneous unraveling of the dental arches occurred in the mandible during the transition to the permanent dentition (Fig. 13-9BCD). A slight increase in transmandibular width also was noted. A lower lingual arch was not needed for this patient.

A patient with an obvious tooth-size/arch-size dis-

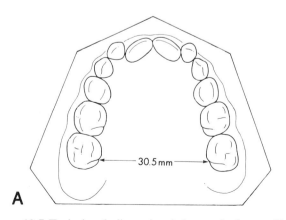

A

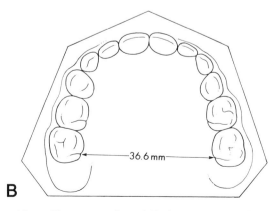

B

Figure 13-7. Typical arch dimensional changes in the maxilla following rapid maxillary expansion. *A*, Before treatment. *B*, Immediately following the removal of the acrylic splint expander.

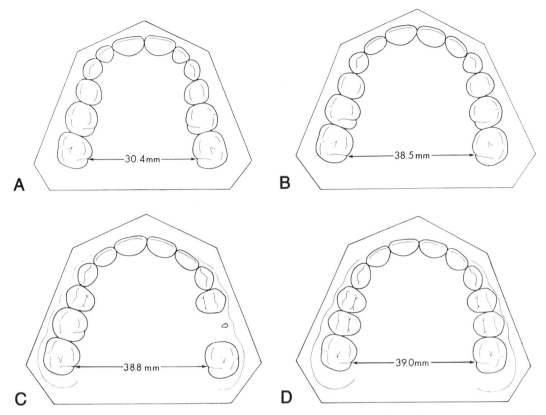

Figure 13-8. Typical arch dimensional changes in a patient with a crossbite on the left side. *A*, Before treatment. *B*, One year later. *C*, After the eruption of the first premolars. *D*, After the eruption of the second premolars. The use of a transpalatal arch to maintain arch length was not necessary in this patient.

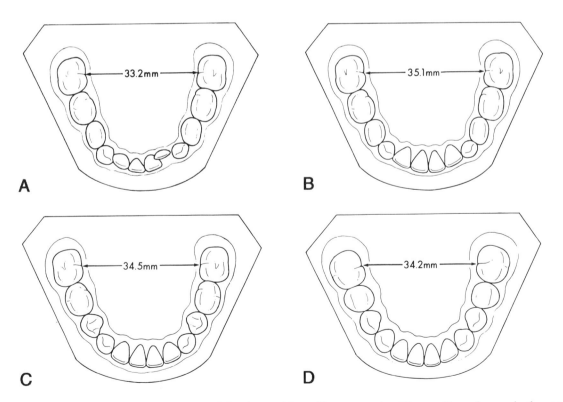

Figure 13-9. Mandibular arch dimensional changes following rapid maxillary expansion. The maxillary changes in the same patient are shown in Figure 13-8. *A*, Immediately before treatment. *B*, One year post-expansion. *C*, After the eruption of the lower first premolars. *D*, After the eruption of the lower second premolars.

crepancy is shown in Figure 13-10. The palate is narrow (transpalatal width 30.5 mm) and there is crowding of the upper anterior teeth. This patient was treated by way of a bonded rapid maxillary expansion appliance, as well as the placement of brackets on the upper incisors to achieve alignment (Fig. 13-10*B*). A transpalatal arch was placed before the eruption of the upper second premolar so that arch space was maintained posteriorly during transition to the permanent dentition (Figs. 13-10*CDE*) Adequate arch length still was available following the final phase of comprehensive orthodontic therapy (Fig. 13-10*F*).

Clinical Management of the Acrylic Splint Expander

The clinical success of bonded expanders is dependent on the technique used in bonding the appliance. This section will cover the specifics of appliance management in detail.

Impressions

Standard aluminum trays normally are used for impression taking. A medium mix of alginate impression ma-

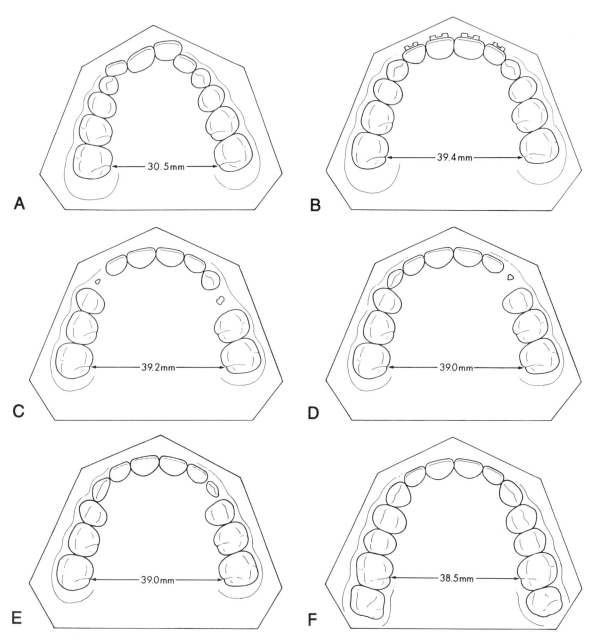

Figure 13-10. Maxillary arch dimensional changes in a patient with anterior crowding. *A*, Pre-expansion. *B*, After one year. Brackets were placed on the upper anterior teeth initially to align the incisors. *C*, At the time of eruption of the first premolars. *D*, After the eruption of the second premolars. *E*, After the eruption of the canines. *F*, Following Phase II treatment.

terial is placed into the tray, and the impression is taken in the usual manner.

No bite registration is needed. In fact, the acrylic splint almost always is delivered without any occlusal adjustment. When used in juveniles, no difficulty is encountered even if the bite is prompted open posteriorly at the time of delivery. The bite settles within a few weeks, a desired treatment effect.

Fabrication

The acrylic splint expander also incorporates a Hyrax-type screw (Leone Orthodontics, Florence, Italy) into a wire framework made from .040″ stainless steel. The framework extends around the buccal and lingual surfaces of the dentition, with the wire crossing the occlusion between the upper deciduous canines and the deciduous first molars (Fig. 13-6). The wire also curves around the distal aspect of the upper first molars. Adequate solder should be applied to the junctions of the wires to prevent breakage of the solder joint during the expansion procedure.

A small mix of stone or plaster is placed in the palate of the work model to provide a reference matrix for the expansion screw. The screw is positioned in the palate with the midline of the screw aligned with the palatal midline and about 2 mm away from the surface of the palate. After the mix has hardened, the screw is removed from the plaster, and a reference position for the screw is established. The wire extensions (struts) of the screw are adjusted to contact the lingual surfaces of the first deciduous molars and the distolingual cusps of the permanent first molar. The four struts are soldered to the framework after they have been tack-welded or bonded temporarily with MD™ adhesive (Great Lakes Orthodontic Products, Tonawanda, NY). If the soldering is performed on the work model, another model may be required for acrylic fabrication, as the work model can be damaged during the soldering procedure.

We recommend the use of a thermal pressure machine (e.g., Biostar™, Great Lakes Orthodontic Products, Tonawanda NY) for the fabrication of this type of appliance. Three millimeter splint Biocryl™ is heated in a Biostar™ and then, through the application of five atmospheres of pressure, the softened acrylic is pushed into place on the wire framework. While the acrylic is softening, a small mix of clear cold-cure acrylic is applied to the wire framework to assure the adherence of the acrylic to the framework.

The acrylic also can be added using a "salt and pepper" application of methyl methacrylate monomer and polymer. It has been our experience, however, that the acrylic produced using this method is more difficult to manipulate clinically. First, the occlusal surfaces of the acrylic tend to be flat, making chewing more of a problem for the patient. We also have found that the removal of appliances made from cold-cure acrylic tend to be more difficult. The acrylic is more rigid and thus does not spring free from the dentition, as usually occurs with Biocryl™.

We recommend the fabrication of all bonded expanders from clear acrylic. Although we use colored acrylic routinely in the fabrication of Schwarz appliances and maintenance plates, it is best to fabricate acrylic splint expanders with clear Biocryl™. By doing so, possible leakage under the expander can be detected clinically. Colored acrylic usually obscures subtle changes in the occlusal surfaces of the teeth incorporated in the acrylic splint.

Appliance Delivery

Generally, a tray set-up that has all the instruments and other material needed for the bonding procedure is used. If a patient has heavy, copious saliva, an anti-sialogogue can be used to reduce saliva flow. For example, atropine sulfate given at a dosage of 0.4 mg per 100 lbs. has been shown to be effective. The drug usually is taken by the patient one hour before the appointment. Of course, an anti-sialogogue should not be used in patients who have glaucoma or heart problems or who wear contact lenses.

Preparation of the Expander

The first step in the delivery of the expander is to check the integrity of the screw. If there is any doubt concerning adequate friction being present in the screw mechanism to prevent "backturning" (i.e., the screw becomes loose in the screw housing, and the expansion is not maintained), a heavy pair of wire cutters can be used to gently indent the casing against the threads of the screw (Fig. 13-11). This procedure also can be performed during treatment if back turning is detected. The expander is removed, the casing squeezed, and the expander then can be rebonded. Alternatively, the expander then can be worn as a removable appliance.

The second step involves preparing the expander for placement of the bonding agent. The acrylic of the expander must be softened to enhance the cohesion of the bonding agent to the plastic. We recommend the use of methyl methacrylate liquid (commonly known as "plastic bracket primer"). This material is painted on the inside of the appliance at the start of the procedure

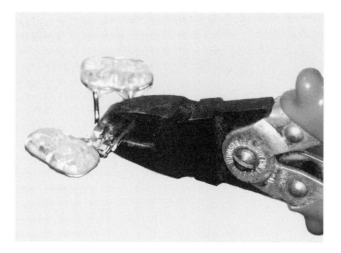

Figure 13-11. Crimping the screw casing. A heavy pair of wire cutters can be used to compress the screw casing against the screw in instances when there is insufficient friction to prevent "back-turning" of the screw during treatment.

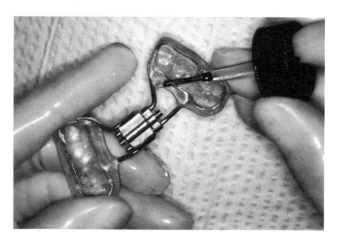

Figure 13-12. The preparation of the appliance using "plastic bracket conditioner." The conditioner should be applied twice, at the start of the procedure and immediately before bonding the appliance.

(Fig. 13-12). An additional coat of conditioner is applied just prior to the placement of the bonding agent in the appliance.

Preliminary Try-in

The next step in the bonding procedure is to ensure that the appliance fits the patient properly. Because this procedure normally is performed by a chairside assistant, any problems with appliance fit (*e.g.*, undercuts, loose-fitting appliance) should be called to the attention of the orthodontist.

In addition, a thorough check for caries is made at this time. Occasionally, a carious lesion will be overlooked during the record-taking process and is discovered at the time of bonding. In this instance, the patient should be dismissed and sent to the family or pediatric dentist for proper care.

Pumice

The teeth are cleaned with an oil-free abrasive material, usually flour of pumice. Routinely, the pumice is applied to the teeth using a rubber cup in a contra-angle handpiece. If any pellicle still is present on recently erupted teeth, the use of a rotating bristle brush may be necessary.

After the teeth have been properly cleaned, the teeth are rinsed thoroughly using water with either a high-speed or low-speed evacuation system (Fig. 13-13). The teeth should be thoroughly cleaned and rinsed before bonding.

Placement of Cheek Retractors

Adequate isolation is essential for a successful bonding procedure. Thus, a cheek retractor should be selected that will isolate the oral field adequately.

The patient should be told to moisten his or her lips. In instances of dry lips, a liberal application of petroleum jelly (*e.g.*, Vaseline™) is recommended. Dri-Angles™, which are absorbent and triangular, are placed in the maxillary vestibule adjacent to the parotid duct (Fig. 13-14). The use of the Dri-Angles™ will absorb saliva in these regions. A cheek retractor (*e.g.*, Clear and Dry™ lip and cheek retractor, L.C. Caulk

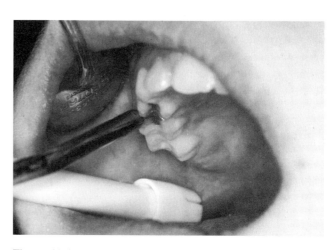

Figure 13-13. All involved teeth must be rinsed thoroughly with water to remove pumice before placing the cheek retractors.

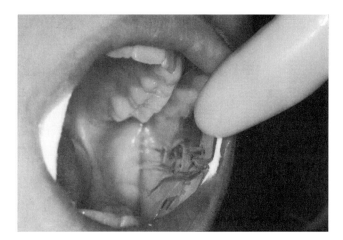

Figure 13-14. Placement of Dri-Angles™ in each vestibule to block the saliva flow from the parotid gland.

Company, Milford DE) is placed into position according to the manufacturer's instructions (Fig. 13-15).

In most orthodontic offices, the initial phase of patient preparation is performed as a two-handed procedure. We have found it helpful to have the patient serve as a "third hand" during the etching and sealing procedures. Two absorbent triangles can be stapled to a tongue blade using a heavy-duty stapler so that the absorbent side of the triangles face away from the tongue blade (Fig. 13-16). The patient can then hold the Dri-Angles™ against the tongue, helping to keep the tongue out of the field of operation.

Etching

A 37% solution of phosphoric acid is used during orthodontic bonding procedures, including the bonding of large acrylic appliances. The etching agent, either in liquid or gel form, is applied liberally with a dabbing motion to the involved teeth (Fig. 13-17). The acid should not be rubbed on the enamel surfaces.

All buccal and lingual surfaces of the posterior teeth are etched, as well as the mesial surface of the most anterior tooth (usually the first deciduous molar) and the distal surface of the last molar tooth (usually the upper first permanent molar). It is extremely important to note that *the occlusal surfaces of the posterior teeth are not etched*. This recommendation is made to facilitate removal of the appliance at the end of treatment. We have found that the deep grooves on the occlusal surfaces of many posterior teeth make appliance removal more difficult if the occlusal surfaces are etched.

We recommend etching permanent teeth for up to 60 seconds and deciduous teeth for up to 120 seconds. The specific etching time is dependent, in part, upon the nature of the enamel of the patient. Increased etching time may be necessary in instances of high fluoride concentration in the drinking water.

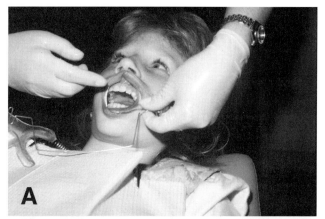
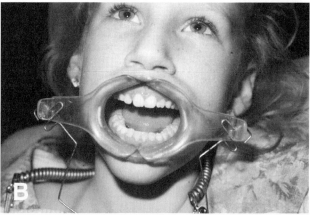

Figure 13-15. Placement of cheek retractors. *A*, Application of Vaseline to the patient's lips. *B*, Dri-Angle™ and cheek retractors in place.

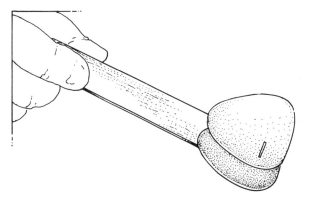

Figure 13-16. Two Dri-Angles are stapled to a tongue depressor. This device can be held by the patient or the chairside assistant to assist in keeping the tongue out of the field of operation.

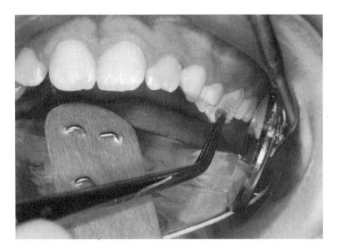

Figure 13-17. The application of 37% phosphoric acid to the involved teeth.

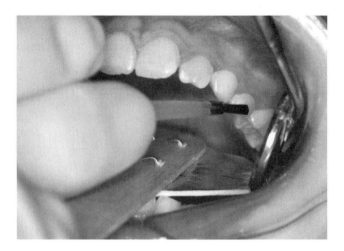

Figure 13-18. The application of sealant to the etched teeth. The tongue is held down by the tongue depressor.

Rinsing and Drying the Etched Teeth

After the etching procedure has been completed, the involved teeth are rinsed thoroughly with water. One major source of contamination is residual etching solution on the teeth. Rinsing with water for 10–20 seconds per tooth is recommended.

The teeth then are air-dried. In instances in which air/water syringes are used, the air first should be tested for water contamination by blowing air onto the patient's napkin or a piece of tissue. No indication of moisture or other contamination should be evident. After the involved teeth are dried thoroughly, the enamel surfaces are checked for a chalky white appearance. In instances in which it appears that the etching procedure was not totally successful, the procedure is repeated by applying additional etchant to the teeth for approximately 20 seconds. In instances of contamination following etching, a 20-second etching period also is recommended.

Application of Sealant

In most instances, the teeth are sealed immediately after the etching procedure has been completed. Sealing of the involved teeth usually involves the placement of a non-filled resin on all of the etched tooth surfaces (Fig. 13-18). The placement of a sealant is optional, but it is believed that such a sealant may help protect the teeth and may, in fact, enhance the bonding procedure.

Usually, the sealant is comprised of two types of liquid that are mixed together (*i.e.*, cemical cure) at the time of application. A bristle brush is used to apply the sealant directly to the teeth, usually beginning at the gingival margin and brushing occlusally (Fig. 13-18). In this way, contamination of the tooth surface with saliva is avoided.

Preparing the Appliance for Bonding

As mentioned earlier, the acrylic on the expander must be softened in order to maximize the bonding adhesion. If the plastic is not conditioned, the bonding agent will remain on the teeth rather than in the appliance at the time of RME removal. At this time, a second coat of conditioner should be applied to the inside of the appliance (see Fig. 13-12).

Bonding Procedure

Two types of bonding agents can be used for securing the acrylic RME to the maxillary dentition: a chemical-cured adhesive and a light-cured adhesive. Each of these two substances have advantages and disadvantages that are discussed below.

Chemical-Cure Adhesive

We have had more experience dealing with chemical-cure rather than light-cure adhesives in bonding large acrylic appliances. In many respects, the chemical-cured adhesive is similar to a two-part adhesive used for the bonding of orthodontic brackets. There are two major differences, however: the adhesive used in bonding brackets should have a high viscosity and a fast setting time in order to prevent brackets from drifting. These two features are not desirable in a bonding agent that is used for attaching a large acrylic appliance to the teeth. A long working time is necessary for proper clean-up, and low viscosity is desirable when the appliance is

RAPID MAXILLARY EXPANSION APPLIANCES

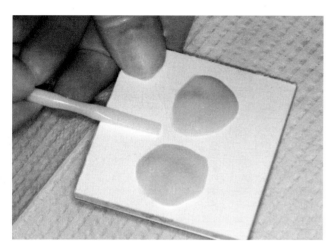

Figure 13-19. Preparation of the chemical-cure adhesive on a mixing pad prior to mixing.

being seated into place to ensure thorough wetting of the internal surface.

The use of a product that has been formulated specifically for the bonding of large acrylic appliances is recommended (*i.e.*, Excel™, Reliance Orthodontic Products, Itasca IL). This type of adhesive is composed of two parts that are mixed together to initiate the chemical reaction (Fig. 13-19). Approximately three minutes of working time are available before the material begins to set.

Figure 13-20 presents two rheograms, graphic representations of the setting time of two bonding agents, one (Ortho Concise™ at two parts base to one part catalyst) used for bonding brackets and one (Excel™) specifically formulated for the bonding of large acrylic appliances. Figure 13-20*A* indicates that the gel phase of Concise™ begins about one minute after the start of mixing. A final set occurs at about four minutes. In contrast, Excel™ has been designed to provide a much longer working time (Fig. 13-20*B*). The gel phase begins at about three minutes, giving the clinician ample time to cleanup the excess material. The gel phase lasts another minute, during which the Excel™ becomes doughy and easy to remove from the borders of the acrylic splint. The final set occurs at about four minutes.

The following outlines the specific steps involved in the bonding of the acrylic splint expander. After the two parts of the chemical-cured adhesive are mixed together for ten to twenty seconds, the adhesive then is placed into the appliance, filling the occlusal area completely (Fig. 13-21). The chairside assistant passes the appliance to the clinician, who seats the appliance on the maxillary posterior dentition with firm finger pressure (Fig. 13-22). This pressure extrudes the excess bonding material from under the appliance.

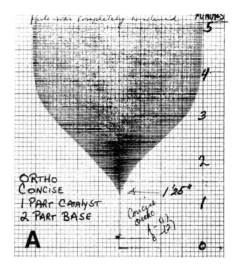

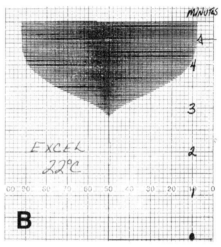

Figure 13-20. Rheograms of two types of adhesive. *A*, A chemical-cure adhesive (Orthodontic Concise™) that is formulated for the bonding of brackets. *B*, A chemical-cure adhesive (Excel™) that has been formulated for the bonding of large acrylic appliances.

The clinician then uses five or six cotton-tipped applicators (*e.g.*, Q-Tips™) to clean up the excessive adhesive (Fig. 13-23). Particular care should be taken to remove adhesive excess from the margins of the appliance, especially under the arms of the expansion screw. After the gross excess is removed, a small cotton pellet or a small sponge held in angled cotton forceps can be used to remove remaining bonding material from the lingual surfaces of the appliance, particularly under the screw arms (Fig. 13-24).

As the material begins to become doughy during the gel phase, a universal scaler is used to clean the appliance further (Fig. 13-25), with attention being paid to the distal aspect of the first molar (Fig. 13-25*B*). Because the bonding material is clear, excesses sometimes are not apparent until after the cleanup has been completed and the material has hardened. If excesses are

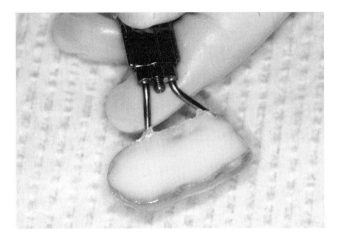

Figure 13-21. The appliance is filled with adhesive. Excess adhesive will lead to problems during cleanup, but insufficient adhesive may result in appliance leakage during treatment.

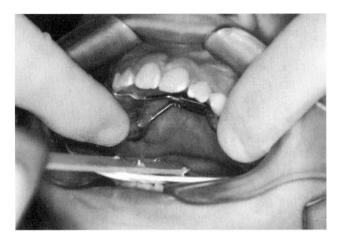

Figure 13-22. The appliance is seated by applying firm pressure to the occlusal surfaces of the appliance. Excess bondinng material is expelled.

detected after the adhesive has set, it is difficult, if not impossible, to flick the excess material from the appliance as with typical orthodontic cements. Usually a bur and a handpiece are necessary to reduce acrylic excess. Sometimes it is advisable to let the excess remain, if it is not bothering the patient.

If facial mask hooks are attached to the anterior portion of the bonded RME (see Chapter 22 for a discussion of the facial mask), the clinician should check these hooks thoroughly with a piece of dental floss to make sure that no acrylic has become incorporated into the inside of the hooks. If excess bonding material is present, it may be very difficult to attach the elastics of the facial mask to the hooks later. Once again, if the bonding agent has set within the hooks, removing the excess is difficult, but necessary.

After the material has set, the appliance is checked thoroughly for any excesses or voids. If voids along the margins of the appliance are identified, an additional mix of bonding agent can be made and the voids eliminated. The appearance of the bonded expander after cleanup is shown in Figure 13-26.

Light-cured Adhesive

Light-cured adhesive also can be used successfully in bonding the acrylic RME appliance. For this purpose, several such adhesives are available (*e.g.*, Light-Bond™, Reliance Orthodontic Products, Itasca IL). After sealing the etched teeth with a light-cured bonding agent, the light-cured adhesive is injected into the occlusal portion of the acrylic expander. The expander then is placed over the maxillary dentition and pressed firmly to place.

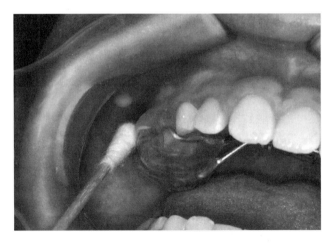

Figure 13-23. Initial cleanup of the excess bonding agent with cotton applicators. Both the buccal and lingual surfaces are wiped.

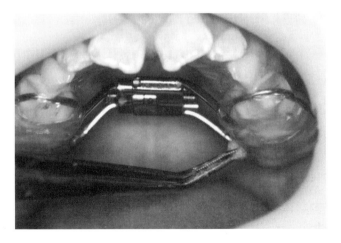

Figure 13-24. Small cotton pellets held in locking forceps are used to clean excess adhesive from around the struts on the lingual surface of the appliance.

RAPID MAXILLARY EXPANSION APPLIANCES

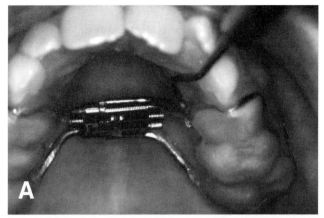

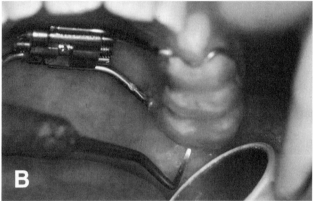

Figure 13-25. Cleanup of the bonding agent as it begins to harden, using a universal scaler. *A*, Under the arms of the expander. *B*, Along the posterior aspect of the appliance.

Excess bonding material once again is expelled from the expander. Cotton applicators and small cotton balls in angle forceps are used to remove the excess bonding material. In contrast to the chemical-cured bonding agent that becomes firmer with time, the excess light-cured adhesive stays relatively pliable until it is cured with visible light. The soft nature of this material sometimes poses problems during cleanup, because not all of the material can be wiped from the margins of the appliance.

After the appliance has been checked thoroughly for excess bonding agent, a visible light source is used to cure the adhesive (Fig. 13-27). Generally, light is applied to each side of the appliance for 60–120 seconds. As the acrylic of the bonded expander is clear, the light source can be applied directly to the occlusal surfaces of the RME appliance.

In general, we prefer using a chemical-cured bonding agent when securing a large acrylic appliance. In part, this may be due to our extensive experience working with this type of material. One advantage of using a chemical-cured adhesive is that the working time is reasonably well defined (*i.e.*, three to four minutes). Although the clinician controls the setting time when using a light-cure system, the actual curing time usually is longer using light-cure adhesive. Inexperienced operators may desire a longer clean up period or may prefer to verify that the appliance has been properly cleaned before initiating the curing of the adhesive.

Home Care Instructions

After the appliance has been bonded and checked thoroughly for voids, the cheek retractors are removed and the patient rinses his or her mouth thoroughly. The parent then is brought into the operatory so that both the patient and the parent can be instructed concerning the proper method of activating and maintaining the appliance.

The patient is told to activate the appliance one turn per day for a prescribed period. Our routine protocol is

Figure 13-26. Occlusal view of the bonded acrylic splint expander after cleanup.

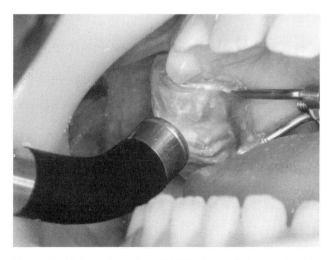

Figure 13-27. Bonding of the RME using a light-cured adhesive system.

to have the appliance activated once per day for four weeks (*i.e.*, twenty-eight turns), after which time the patient is evaluated for the need for further expansion. We do not say, "Expand your appliance once per day until your next appointment" because of the danger in having the patient expand the appliance excessively if an appointment is missed or postponed.

The key used by the parent for expansion is shown in Figure 13-28. This key has a short piece of wire that is inserted into the screw hole and is connected to a long plastic handle. We prefer this key holder to the traditional expansion key that is composed only of a formed segment of wire. If only the traditional key is available, it should be ligated with a long piece of dental floss to prevent aspiration by the patient (Fig. 13-28).

The diet of the patient also is discussed. The patient is given a list of foods to avoid that includes those foods generally avoided during orthodontic treatment (*i.e.*, hard and sticky foods). The patient also is asked to use a fluoride mouthwash (*e.g.*, Listermint™, Fluorigard™, Act™) as part of the home-care regimen. The parent is told that if the patient complains of a bad taste in the mouth or develops an offensive breath, a call to the office should be made immediately. In addition, the office should be notified if the patient feels that his or her appliance has become loosened.

The clinician also should make a careful notation as to the appearance of the appliance following bonding. As there always is the risk of decalcification under the appliance, the RME routinely is removed within a few weeks if there is a suspicion of leakage. Leakage often is determined by discoloration occurring under the appliance, particularly along the occlusal surface of the posterior teeth. As these areas are not etched, it is possible that saliva or other oral fluids can leak into the space between the teeth and the appliance, usually resulting in discoloration (Fig 13-29). If this type of discoloration is noted, the appliance should be monitored and probably removed within a short period. The patient can wear the appliance on a removable basis, making sure that the teeth and the appliance are properly cleaned several times a day.

If there is any discoloration present under the appliance at the time of bonding (*e.g.*, enamel stain, amalgam restoration) these observations should be noted in the patient's chart as being the normal appearance of that patient's expander. If these findings are noted later, the previous description of the appliance in the chart should be checked to avoid unnecessary removal of an otherwise satisfactory appliance.

Appointment Intervals

After the bonding procedure has been completed, the patient is appointed four weeks later, at which time the amount of further expansion is determined. The average amount of expansion with this type of appliance is 6–9 mm, which translates into approximately 28–45 activations or about four to six weeks of active expansion treatment. The patient then is seen every 6–8 weeks for an additional five months to allow for the reossification and reorganization of the midpalatal suture to occur.

Usually, a diastema opens between the upper central incisors (Fig. 13-5). This space may become pronounced

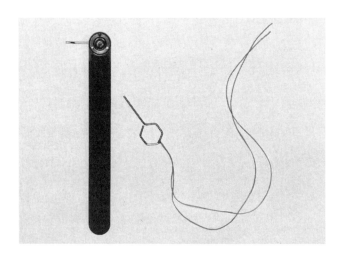

Figure 13-28. Types of keys used to activate the RME screw. Left, extended safety key with acrylic handle. Right, traditional wire key. A piece of dental floss should be attached to this latter type of key to prevent the patient from inadvertently swallowing the key.

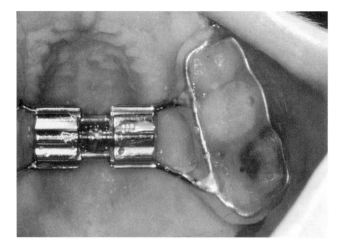

Figure 13-29. Occlusal view of a leaking expander. The dark discoloration can be seen on the occlusal surface of the upper left first molar. If any discoloration is present at the time of appliance placement (*e. g.*, amalgam restoration), it should be noted in the chart.

RAPID MAXILLARY EXPANSION APPLIANCES

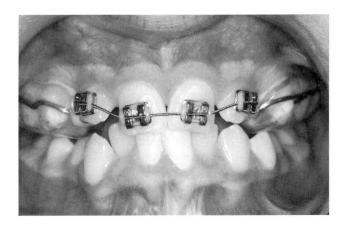

Figure 13-30. Placement of brackets on the upper anterior teeth, usually two appointments following the termination of expansion. A coaxial segment of archwire has been ligated into the brackets with O-rings.

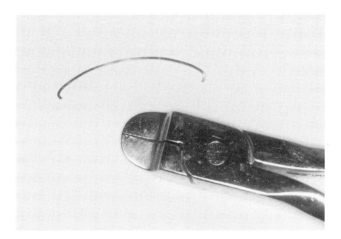

Figure 13-31. After initial incisor alignment, a contoured section of rectangular chrome cobalt wire is placed in the upper incisor brackets. The wire is bent with a pair of 142 arch forming pliers.

by the end of the active phase of expansion. During the period when the appliance is not activated further, however, a gradual closure of the diastema usually occurs that is characterized by a mesial tipping of the upper incisor teeth. Parents often interpret this normal change in tooth position, produced by pull of the transseptal fibers, as "relapse." Parents and patients should be cautioned beforehand about this phenomenon.

During the latter part of the time that the expander is in place, the clinician may elect to place brackets to align and upright the incisor teeth (Fig. 13-30). Usually a flexible .0175" coaxial archwire is placed to attain initial incisal alignment, followed by a segment of .016 × .022" chrome cobalt (*e.g.*, Elgiloy™, Azurloy™) archwire that has been contoured to the desires arch form (Fig 13-31). The placement of brackets also is indicated in patients who lack space for unerupted canines.

Appliance Removal

The bonded rapid maxillary expansion appliance is removed easily in most early mixed dentition patients (6–9 years of age). These patients normally do not have loose deciduous posterior teeth, and thus removal of the appliance is accomplished swiftly and easily.

The first step in the debonding procedure is the placement of a topical anesthetic (Fig. 13-32) along the margin of the appliance in the region of the deciduous molars. Although not essential, we have found that this relatively straightforward procedure reduces patient discomfort.

The instrument of choice in removing any bonded large acrylic appliance is anterior bracket-removing pliers (Fig. 13-33), such as ETM 349 pliers (Ormco

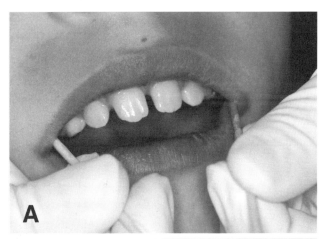

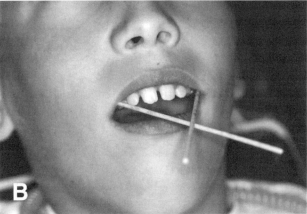

Figure 13-32. Topical anesthetic is applied to the gingival margins of the appliance in the region of the upper deciduous molars a few minutes before appliance removal.

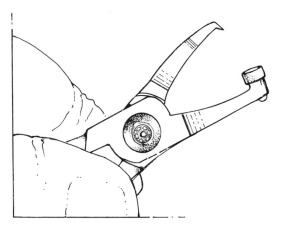

Figure 13-33. An anterior bracket removing plier (ETM 349, Ormco Corp., Orange CA) is recommended for routine expander removal.

Corp, Orange CA). These pliers have a sharp-angled tip on one side that can be hooked at the gingival margin of the appliance between the first and second deciduous molar (Fig. 13-34). The other arm of the pliers has a Teflon-coated pad that can rest against the occlusal surface of the expander. The expander is removed easily by simply torquing the appliance laterally and inferiorly on one side, usually the side opposite to the handedness of the operator (e.g., left side first if the clinician is right-handed).

Usually both sides can be loosened with one pull on the appliance; if only one side is loosened, the operator should put down the pliers and place his or her hands on the loosened edge of the appliance. Usually a firm downward pull will result in the dislodging of the remaining bonded side. If there still is difficulty in removing the appliance, ETM 349 pliers are used in the manner described previously to loosen the remaining side.

In the late mixed dentition, it is common to find resorbed deciduous teeth in the expander upon removal (Fig. 13-35). In all instances of patients with potentially loose deciduous teeth (e.g., patients 10–13 years of age) and in all patients with permanent dentitions, the use of local anesthesia is recommended strongly. Of course, the parent should be informed of the possible need for local anesthetic before its administration. The use of anesthesia with a simple local injection in the area of the roots of the first and second premolars usually is sufficient. One half of a carpule of local anesthetic can be administered bilaterally using a short needle. The area of injection should have been prepared previously by topical anesthesia.

In instances in which the clinician is experiencing difficulty in removing the bonded appliance, one additional step is taken, that is the cutting of the base wire of the appliance using a high-speed handpiece and a cross-cut fissure bur. If the base wire is sectioned on the labial side, usually between the upper first and second premolars or deciduous molars, appliance removal becomes easier. It is unusual for difficulty to be encountered in mixed dentition patients; however, removing a bonded expander in permanent detition patients can pose a challenge because of the naturally occurring undercuts in the posterior regions.

It should be noted that it is common for significant

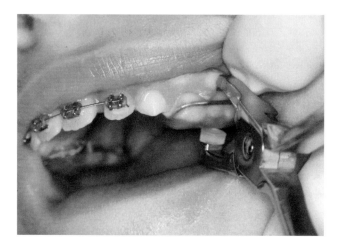

Figure 13-34. Removal of the bonded expander. The Teflon pad of the plier is placed on the occlusal surface, and the hooked edge of the plier is placed at the gingival margin between the upper first and second premolars. A quick forceful movement in an occlusal direction is used to break the seal of the adhesive. Usually both sides of the appliance can be loosened in one pull.

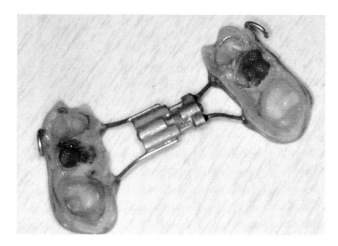

Figure 13-35. The extraction of two second deciduous molars during appliance removal. (This appliance has facial mask hooks attached to the framework.) In patients in the late-mixed dentition and in patients in the permanent dentition, the administration of local anesthetic is recommended prior to the removal of a bonded acrylic splint expander. Anesthetic is injected above the premolar roots.

RAPID MAXILLARY EXPANSION APPLIANCES

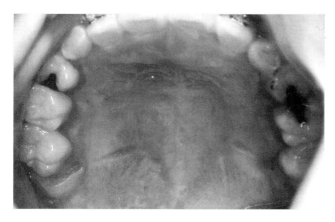

Figure 13-36. Typical gingival irritation following expander removal, including irritated gingival around posterior teeth. Usually, all evidence of gingival hypertrophy and irritation disappears within a few days of expander removal.

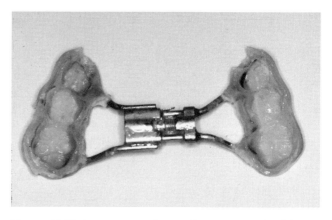

Figure 13-37. Appearance of expander at removal. All bonding material should line the acrylic of the expander. If the prescribed protocol is followed, no bonding adhesive is left on the teeth.

gingival irritation and redness to occur at the time of appliance removal (Fig. 13-36). The degree of irritation is, of course, dependent upon the level of hygiene of the patient during treatment as well as the susceptibility of the patient to localized gingivitis. Usually, all evidence of inflammation will disappear from the patient's gingiva within 72 hours after the appliance has been removed. Long-term gingival problems have not been observed.

Retention Appliances

The appearance of the debonded appliance is shown in Figure 13-37. In spite of the best cleanup efforts at the time of delivery, there always will be excess bonding material evident when the appliance is removed. The appliance is cleaned as much as possible, and any excess material is removed from the expander by way of an acrylic bur (Fig. 13-38). The appliance is returned to the patient with instructions to wear the appliance fulltime until the maintenance plate is delivered, typically one week later. The removable expander is worn fulltime except during oral hygiene.

At the time of appliance removal, an alginate impression is taken for the maintenance plate. The appliance most typically used is a simple palatal plate that has ball clasps between the upper first and second deciduous molars and the upper first permanent molar.

The patient is instructed to wear the removable palatal plate on a full-time basis (except mealtimes). It is advisable to maintain the achieved expansion for at least one year if not longer, in order to facilitate changes that might be occurring in the mandibular dentition or in the maxillomandibular relationship (*e.g.*, spontaneous correction of Class II).

In instances in which several deciduous teeth have been lost during the removal of the expander, a transpalatal arch can be used as a retention appliance. Usually, the transpalatal arch is not activated at the time of appliance delivery but may be activated at subsequent visits, depending upon the needs of the given patient.

CONCLUDING REMARKS

Some comment should be made regarding the use of the two types of banded appliances during the mixed dentition period. We have found that the banded-type of expander, although used routinely in adolescent patients, is much more prone than the bonded-type to becoming dislodged when used in the mixed dentition. In addition, it appears that a greater amount of tooth tipping occurs with a banded-type appliance than with the

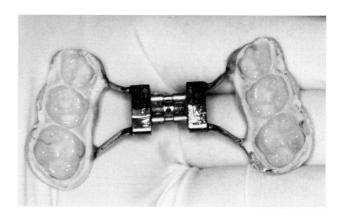

Figure 13-38. The expander is cleaned and any excess bonding material is removed before returning the expander to the patient. The expander is worn as a removable appliance until the maintenance plate is delivered, usually within one week.

bonded-type of appliance. In general, we use the banded-type appliance primarily in the permanent dentition and rely on the bonded-type expander for mixed dentition treatment.

In conclusion, we have found that the incorporation of RME into many of our fixed appliance protocols to be very beneficial, not only with regard to treatment outcome, but also to treatment efficiency. The use of the bonded appliance in the mixed dentition, particularly in instances of crossbite or arch length discrepancies has led to a relatively straightforward management of these problems. Similarly, the incorporation of the hyrax-type expander in the management of routine transverse skeletal problems and the use of the Haas-type in those adolescent patients in whom maximum skeletal expansion is desired have proven to increase treatment efficiency while reducing overall treatment time as well.

REFERENCES CITED

1. Gottlieb EL, Nelson AH, Vogels DS. 1996 JCO study of orthodontic diagnosis and treatment procedures. Part I. Results and trends. J Clin Orthod 1996;30:615–629.
2. Zimring JF, Isaacson RJ. Forces produced by rapid maxillary expansion. Angle Orthod 1965;35: 178–186.
3. Adkins MD, Nanda RS, Currier GF. Arch perimeter changes on rapid palatal expansion. Am J Orthod Dentofac Orthop 1990;97:194–199.
4. Debbane EF. A cephalometric and histologic study of the effect of orthodontic expansion of the midpalatal suture of the cat. Am J Orthod 1958;44:187–219.
5. Haas AJ. Gross reactions to the widening of the maxillary dental arch of the pig by splitting of the midpalatal suture. Am J Orthod 1959;45:868–869.
6. Starnbach H, Bayne D, Cleall J, Subtelny JD. Facioskeletal and dental changes resulting from rapid maxillary expansion. Angle Orthod 1966;36:152–164.
7. Biederman W. Rapid correction of Class III malocclusion by midpalatal expansion. Am J Orthod 1972;63:47–55.
8. Brossman RE, Bennett CG, Merow WW. Facioskeletal remodeling resulting from rapid palatal expansion in the monkey (*Macaca cynmologus*). Arch Oral Biol 1973;18: 987–994.
9. Chaconas SJ, Caputo AA. Observation of orthopedic force distribution produced by maxillary orthodontic appliances. Am J Orthod 1982;82:492–501.
10. Tanne K, Sachdeva R, Miyasaka J, Yamagata Y, Sakuda M. A study of strain and stress levels in the circummaxillary sutural systems during rapid maxillary expansion: An approach using both the strain gauge technique and the theoretical stress analysis. J Osaka Univ Dent Sch 1986;26: 151–165.
11. Gardner GE, Kronman JH. Cranioskeletal displacements caused by rapid palatal expansion in the rhesus monkey. Am J Orthod 1971;59:146–155.
12. Melsen B. Palatal growth studied on human autopsy material. A histologic microradiographic study. Am J Orthod 1975;68:42–54.
13. Melsen B, Melsen F. The postnatal development of the palatomaxillary region studied on human autopsy material. Am J Orthod 1982;82:329–342.
14. Melsen B. A histological study of the influence of sutural morphology and skeletal maturation of rapid palatal expansion in children. Trans Europ Orthod Soc 1972;48: 499–507.
15. Murray J, Cleall JF. Early tissue response to rapid maxillary expansion in the midpalatal suture of the rhesus monkey. J Dent Res 1971;50:1654–1660.
16. Ten Cate AR, Freeman E, Dickinson JB. Sutural development: structure and its response to rapid expansion. Am J Orthod 1977;71:622–636.
17. Haas AJ. Rapid expansion of the maxillary dental arch and nasal cavity by opening the mid-palatal suture. Angle Orthod 1961;31:73–90.
18. Haas AJ. The treatment of maxillary deficiency by opening the mid-palatal suture. Angle Orthod 1965;35:200–217.
19. Haas AJ. Palatal expansion: just the beginning of dentofacial orthopedics. Am J Orthod 1970;57:219–255.
20. Haas AJ. Long-term posttreatment evaluation of rapid palatal expansion. Angle Orthod 1980;50:189–217.
21. Herberger TA. Rapid palatal expansion: long term stability and periodontal implications. Philadelphia: Unpublished Master's thesis, Department of Orthodontics, University of Pennsylvania, 1987.
22. Cameron CG. Short-term and long-term effects of rapid maxillary expansion: A posteroanterior cephalometric and morphometric study. Ann Arbor: Unpublished Master's thesis, Department of Orthodontics and Pediatric Dentistry, The University of Michigan, 2000.
23. Stockfish H. Rapid expansion of the maxilla-success and relapse. Trans Europ Orthod Soc 1969;45:469–481.
24. Wertz R, Dreskin M. Midpalatal suture opening: a normative study. Am J Orthod 1977;71:367–381.
25. Linder-Aronson S, Lindgren J. The skeletal and dental effects of rapid maxillary expansion. Br J Orthod 1979;6: 25–29.
26. Herold JS. Maxillary expansion: a retrospective study of three methods of expansion and their long-term sequelae. Br J Orthod 1989;16:195–200.
27. Fenderson FA. Long-term post-retention comparison of two methods of maxillary expansion. Ann Arbor: Unpublished Masters thesis, Department of Orthodontics and Pediatric Dentistry, The University of Michigan, Ann Arbor, 1998.
28. Biederman W. Rapid correction of Class 3 malocclusion by midpalatal expansion. Am J Orthod 1973;63:47–55.
29. Ralph SW. A comparison of two rapid maxillary expansion appliances using three-dimensional finite element analysis. Ann Arbor: Unpublished Master's thesis. Department of Orthodontics and Pediatric Dentistry, The University of Michigan, 1998.
30. Timms DJ. An occlusal analysis of lateral maxillary expansion with mid-palatal suture opening. Dent Pract 1968; 18:435–440.
31. Timms DJ. Long-term follow-up of cases treated by rapid maxillary expansion. Trans Europ Orthod Soc 1976;52: 211–215.
32. Hallgren A, Oliveby A, Twetman S. Caries associated mir-

croflora in plaque from orthodontic appliances retained with glass ionomer cement. Scand J Dent Res 1992;100: 140–143.
33. Serra MC, Cury JA. The *in vitro* effect of glass-ionomer cement restoration on enamel subjected to a demineralization model. Quintessence Internat 1992;23:143–147.
34. Haas AJ. Personal communication, 1992.
35. Howe RP. Palatal expansion using a bonded appliance. Report of a case. Am J Orthod 1982;82:464–468.
36. Spolyar JL. The design, fabrication, and use of a full-coverage bonded rapid maxillary expansion appliance. Am J Orthod 1984;86:136–145.
37. Sarver DM, Johnston MW. Skeletal changes in vertical and anterior displacement of the maxilla with bonded rapid palatal expansion appliances. Am J Orthod Dentofac Orthop 1989;95:462–466.
38. Spillane LM, McNamara JA, Jr. Maxillary adaptations following expansion in the mixed dentition. Sem Orthod 1995;1:176–187.
39. Brust EW, McNamara JA, Jr. Arch dimensional changes concurrent with expansion in mixed dentition patients. In: Trotman CA, McNamara JA, Jr, eds. Orthodontic treatment: Outcome and effectiveness. Ann Arbor: Monograph 30, Craniofacial Growth Series, Center for Human Growth and Development, The University of Michigan, 1995.
40. Howe RP. The bonded Herbst appliance. J Clin Orthod 1982;16:663–667.
41. Howe RP, McNamara JA, Jr. Clinical management of the bonded Herbst appliance. J Clin Orthod 1983;17:456–463.
42. McNamara JA, Jr. An orthopedic approach to the treatment of Class III malocclusion in young patients. J Clin Orthod 1987;21:598–608.
43. McNamara JA, Jr. Fabrication of the acrylic splint Herbst appliance. Am J Orthod Dentofac Orthop 1988; 94:10–18.
44. McNamara JA, Jr, Howe RP. Clinical management of the acrylic splint Herbst appliance. Am J Orthod Dentofac Orthop 1988;94:142–149.
45. Wendling LK. Short-term skeletal and dental effects of the acrylic splint rapid maxillary expansion appliance. Ann Arbor: Unpublished Masters thesis, Department of Orthodontics and Pediatric Dentistry, The University of Michigan, 1997.
46. Brust EW. Arch dimensional changes concurrent with expansion in the mixed dentition. Ann Arbor: Unpublished Masters thesis, Department of Orthodontics and Pediatric Dentistry, The University of Michigan, 1992.
47. Dellinger EL. A preliminary study of anterior maxillary displacement. Am J Orthod 1973;63:509–516.

Chapter 14
THE SCHWARZ APPLIANCE

This chapter concerns the use of a specific type of active plate, the Schwarz appliance. This removable expansion plate can be used in the early stages of the mixed dentition to produce orthodontic tooth movement in the mandible or maxilla. Generally, we use this appliance in the mandible to upright posterior teeth and to create additional arch length anteriorly.

The terms "Schwarz plate" and "Schwarz appliance," in fact, may be inappropriately attributed to Professor A.M. Schwarz, because this appliance was mentioned over 100 years ago in an article by Kingsley.[1] In that article, Kingsley describes the use of a jackscrew in a lower removable plate that was made from vulcanite, a hard rubber often used for bite splints. Instead of a midline split, the appliance was divided bilaterally in the region of the mandibular canines. Other removable expansion appliances for the mandibular dental arch have been described by Badcock,[2] Crozat,[3] Nord,[4] and Hotz.[5]

The term "Schwarz appliance" often is considered synonymous with any removable expansion appliance that incorporates one or more expansion screws. Perhaps the underlying reason is that in 1938 Schwarz published a text that became the so-called "orthodontic bible" of Europe.[6] Schwarz had taken the myriad of appliances that currently were in use in Europe, organized them into an orderly system, and stressed treatment objectives.

The specific appliance to be discussed in this chapter (Fig. 14-1) has been described in a number of orthodontic publications, including those of Schwarz and Gratzinger,[7] Adams,[8] Hotz,[5] and Houston and Isaacson.[9] These authors consider this type of appliance an active plate appliance, one that uses forces generated within the appliance by devices such as screws, labial wires, springs, or elastics to produce orthodontic tooth movement. Active plate appliances are contrasted with the various functional appliances[10–14] in which intrinsic muscle forces are used to promote changes in the skeletal, dentoalveolar, and soft tissue environment.

PARTS OF THE APPLIANCE

The appliance (Fig. 14-1) is made from wire, acrylic, and a midline screw. Simple ball clasps can be placed in the embrasures between the first and second deciduous molars and between the deciduous second molars and the permanent first molars. In general, we have found that the ball clasps serve as "handles" when the patient removes the appliance. These ball clasps frequently become distorted during mastication. No attempt usually is made to adjust the ball clasps unless they become severely distorted and prevent appliance wear. If additional retention is needed (which usually is not the case), an Adams clasp[8] can be used on the mandibular first molars.

The expansion screw[15] is located in the midline and is embedded almost entirely in acrylic (Fig. 14-1). It usually is activated once per week until 4–5 mm of anterior expansion has been gained (Fig. 14-2). The acrylic is applied to the work model on the lingual surfaces of the teeth and the associated alveolar area (Fig. 14-3). Additional acrylic also can be placed on the occlusal surfaces of the posterior teeth in instances in which a posterior bite block effect is desired.

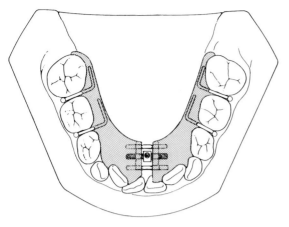

Figure 14-1. Mandibular occlusal view of the lower Schwarz appliance that is used to upright the posterior dentition and create a modest amount of arch length anteriorly.

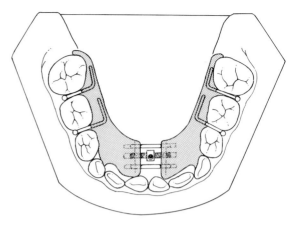

Figure 14-2. Mandibular occlusal view of the lower Schwarz appliance after activation for 4–5 months. Some spontaneous "decrowding" of the lower anterior teeth may occur.

USE OF THE SCHWARZ APPLIANCE

As has been described in Chapter 4, we use the appliance in patients who have arch length deficiencies and/or posterior teeth that have an abnormal lingual inclination (Fig. 14-4A). The gradual expansion of the Schwarz appliance, produced by the activation of the midline expansion screw, simply tips the posterior teeth in a lateral direction (Fig. 14-4B). This type of movement is followed by rapid maxillary expansion (Fig. 14-4C), the results of which tend to stabilize mandibular dentoalveolar position during the retention period (Fig. 14-4D).

It is rare that we would use the lower Schwarz appliance as the sole appliance to produce orthodontic tooth movement. An exception is the treatment of a patient with a posterior buccal crossbite (scissor bite, "Brodie bite"), in whom the mandibular teeth lie lingual to the maxillary dentition.[16] In this type of patient, the mandibular teeth are uprighted by the Schwarz appliance relative to a normally positioned maxillary dentition.

A question often arises regarding the sequencing of Schwarz and RME treatments: Why not initiate both treatments simultaneously? The answer to this question is related to the frequency of appliance activation. The Schwarz appliance is activated once per week, whereas the RME appliance is expanded once per day. The simultaneous use of both appliances would result in the completion of maxillary expansion within four to six weeks, with the mandibular dental arch being expanded only 1.0 to 1.5 mm during that time. We recommend the completion, or near completion, of Schwarz activation prior to the onset of RME, so that the mandibular teeth are positioned properly by the time expansion therapy is begun. We have found that by eliminating mandibular dentoalveolar compensations before rapid maxillary expansion (RME) is begun, a greater transverse expansion of the maxillary dental arch can be attained. Eliminating the compensations lessens the need for an additional phase of RME later in severely constricted individuals.

A patient with moderate mandibular incisor crowding is shown in Figure 14-5. In this clinical example, a mandibular expansion appliance was worn to upright the posterior teeth and create additional arch length anteriorly. It should be noted, however, that no attempt was made to align the incisors completely. Later in treatment, a lower lingual arch was used to maintain arch length posteriorly during the transition from the

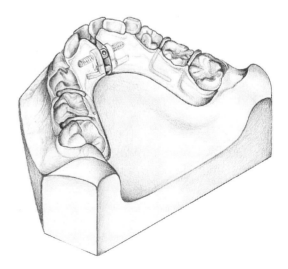

Figure 14-3. Oblique view of the mandibular Schwarz appliance. Note the contact of the acrylic with the lingual surfaces of the teeth and adjacent alveolus.

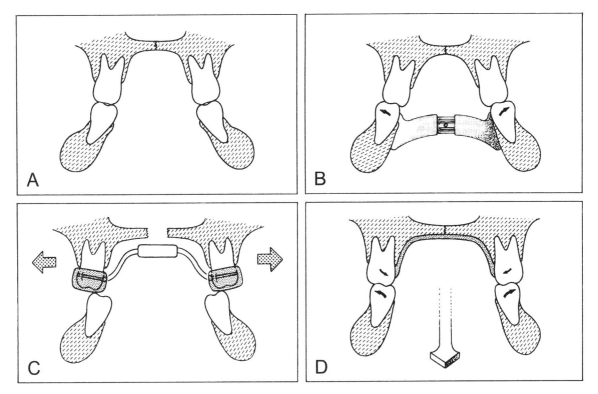

Figure 14-4. Cross-sectional view of a patient with narrow maxillary and mandibular dental arches. *A*, Before treatment. *B*. The lower Schwarz appliance simply tips the posterior teeth laterally, sometimes producing a tendency toward a posterior crossbite. *C*, A bonded rapid maxillary expansion appliance is used to widen the maxilla, aiding in the stability of the dental change in the mandible. *D*. A removable maintenance plate (shown in cross-section) is used to stabilize the achieved result in the maxilla. In some instances a spontaneous improvement in the sagittal jaw relationship may occur (see arrow).

second deciduous molars to the second premolars. During the fixed appliance phase, mild interproximal reduction was used to create additional arch space in the premolar region.

The use of this appliance is not recommended in patients with severe mandibular incisor crowding or in patients who have proclined lower incisors. In these instances, a protocol of serial extraction may be appropriate, as the objective of such treatment is to align the mandibular incisors over basal bone. (See Chapter 4 for a discussion of serial extraction.)

STUDIES OF MANDIBULAR DENTAL EXPANSION

One of the major concerns that exists regarding the use of any removable expansion appliance is the long-term stability of the achieved expansion. Research on this topic, particularly regarding the protocols advocated within this text, is limited. The research that does exist, particularly the German literature, generally indicates that expansion of the dental arches using *removable* appliances is not very stable. For example, Schwarze[17,18] reported on about 500 patients treated with removable expansion appliances. He stated that the average amount of expansion was 3.7 mm during the treatment period. The average amount of transverse relapse was 2 mm. These type of observations have been made by a number of individuals including Tulley and Campbell,[19] Graf and Ehmer,[20] and Ülgen and associates.[21]

For an orthodontist who received a traditional orthodontic education, one of the "cardinal rules" of orthodontics is that expansion of the distance between the mandibular canines is relatively unstable, as has been illustrated in the recall studies published at the University of Washington.[22] Given the rather negative outcome concerning expansion, why is the treatment with the Schwarz appliance advocated at all?

As was mentioned earlier, we began using the bonded rapid palatal expansion appliance in the mixed dentition in the early 1980s. After analyzing the results of our first five years of treatment, it became obvious that some spontaneous widening in the mandibular dental arch was occurring. The nature of this widening was variable, however, with some individuals experiencing expansion, whereas others did not. Given our background using the Fränkel appliance[13,14] and hav-

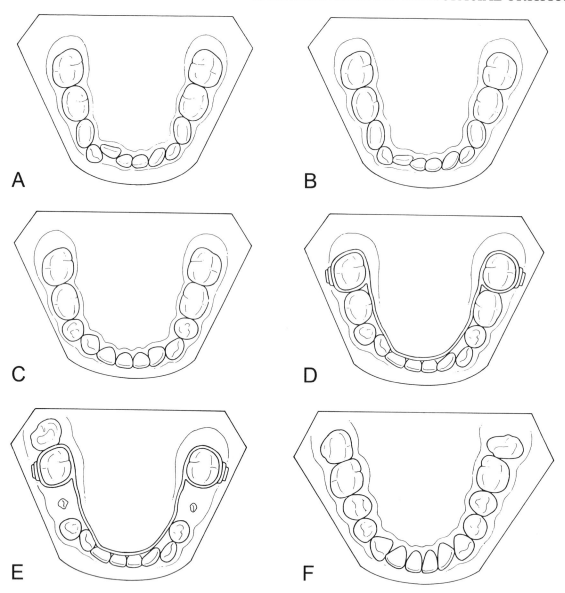

Figure 14-5. The use of a Schwarz appliance in a patient with moderate mandibular incisor crowding. *A,* Pretreatment. *B,* After six months of appliance wear. *C,* After the eruption of the mandibular first premolars. *D* and *E,* A lower lingual arch is used to maintain the "leeway space." *F,* Following the eruption of the mandibular second premolars, but prior to Phase II treatment. A mild amount of interproximal stripping was necessary to align the teeth during the later final phase of fixed appliance therapy.

ing observed our own patients who underwent spontaneous arch expansion using the FR-2 appliance,[23] it seemed logical to consider active mandibular expansion and the uprighting of the posterior dentition as an initial means of treatment prior to rapid maxillary expansion.

There are very few studies, particularly in the English literature, that have considered the effects of mandibular expansion. Lutz and Poulton[24] evaluated 13 patients (ages 4–7 years) who had a minimum of 3 mm of mandibular intercanine arch length deficiency and who were expanded with removable appliances. Annual recordings taken over a six-year period indicated a stable increase in arch width of 5.6 mm between the primary second molars, whereas a transient increase occurred between the primary canines.

Bruno[25] investigated mandibular arch expansion using Crozat, Jackson, and Schwarz appliances in a sample of 38 patients who began treatment in the primary or early mixed dentition (average age was 7 years at the beginning of treatment). All patients were significantly narrower in arch width and shorter in arch length and depth than was the control group. Three years after appliance removal, no significant differences existed in mandibular arch width between the treated and control group except between the mandibular first premolars. Increases in mandibular arch width were greater in the treated group than in the control group.

An investigation of Schwarz appliance therapy as advocated in this text was carried out by Brust[26,27] who studied a sample of patients on whom treated records were gathered prolectively. Thirty-six of these mixed dentition patients underwent Schwarz appliance therapy prior to rapid maxillary expansion. Brust found an average increase of 2.3 mm in arch perimeter at the end of RME therapy in the RME/Schwarz group. At the time of Phase II records, there was an average increase in arch perimeter of 1.7 mm in comparison to initial values. In contrast, the untreated control group experienced a naturally occurring *net decrease* in mandibular arch perimeter of 1.6 mm. This relatively modest difference in arch dimension (3.3 mm) indicates that the Schwarz appliance may be useful in patients with mild-to-moderate mandibular incisor crowding, but will not satisfy the arch length requirements of a patient with severely crowded mandibular incisors.

One of the concerns that is expressed about Schwarz appliance therapy is that this type of treatment might produce an undesirable proclination of the mandibular incisors during treatment. Wendling[28] conducted a prospective clinical study that evaluated the short-term treatment effects of acrylic splint rapid maxillary expansion used alone or in conjunction with lower Schwarz appliance therapy. Pretreatment and post-treatment lateral cephalograms were available for 25 RME-only patients and 19 Schwarz-RME patients. The average time between films was 8.7 months for the RME group and 12.1 months for the Schwarz-RME group. Among other findings, it was interesting to note that the group of patients treated with the Schwarz appliance in conjunction with RME showed no significant differences from the control sample for any of the mandibular dental measures, including mandibular incisor proclination, at least as observed cephalometrically.

A related investigation was the retrospective clinical analysis of Wright[29] who compared the treatment effects of the Schwarz appliance and the lower lingual holding arch. One hundred patients were divided into four groups: patients treated with a Schwarz appliance followed by RME, RME patients treated with a lower lingual holding arch, patients treated with a combination of both appliances, and patients who received no treatment. Mandibular study casts were analyzed at two time periods: in the mixed dentition, prior to placement of any appliances (T_1) and in the early permanent dentition, prior to Phase II orthodontics (T_2). Arch parameters including arch perimeter, arch width, arch depth, incisor irregularity, and molar angulation were examined.

A comparison of the two appliances showed that both maintained arch perimeter during the transition to the permanent dentition, though the method of preservation differed between the two treatment modalities. Those patients treated with a Schwarz appliance gained significant arch width, but lost arch depth. In addition, the incisor irregularity was reduced significantly. In contrast, the patients who were treated with a lower lingual holding arch showed a less pronounced increase in arch width, and less decrease in arch depth. There was little change in the alignment of the incisors when using a lower lingual holding arch.

Wright[29] concluded that both the Schwarz appliance and the lower lingual holding arch were effective methods of preserving arch perimeter during the transition of the dentition. Arch width increased in both the Schwarz group and the lower lingual holding arch group, with a greater effect seen in the Schwarz group. Arch depth was maintained in the lower lingual holding arch group, whereas the Schwarz appliance had no effect on arch depth. Finally, the Schwarz appliance resulted in a reduction of incisor irregularity, whereas the lower lingual holding arch had little effect on incisor alignment.

CLINICAL MANAGEMENT

Impression Taking

A standard aluminum tray and alginate can be used to make an impression for the work model. The impression should be extended into the lingual region to ensure that an adequate reproduction of the soft tissue including the lingual frenum is obtained.

No bite registration is necessary because there is no articulation with a maxillary model during appliance fabrication.

Appliance Fabrication

After the impression has been poured in stone, a work model is made. The Schwarz appliance is fabricated directly on the work model. First, the model should be checked for bubbles and other surface defects; and they should be repaired, if present. Areas of significant undercuts are filled with wax and then separating medium is placed on the model.

A midline expansion screw (#600-151-3, Dentaurum, Newtown PA) is secured into position on the work model by warming the wax on the back of the screw and pressing the screw into position on the work model as close to the midline as possible. A bead of wax can be placed on the work model before screw placement to aid in the retention of the screw. Additional wax is added to the model, extending from the wax on the top of the screw to the lingual portion of the anterior teeth and to the bottom of the screw to avoid any undercuts. When the wax is applied properly, wax from the screw should extend from the incisal edges of the incisors to the lingual area as one continuous piece of wax.

The work models are modified in interdental areas where clasps are to be placed. These interdental areas are relieved on the work model so that clasps can be adapted well into the embrasures. Four ball clasps, made from .028″ or .032″ stainless steel, are placed between the mandibular first and second deciduous molars and between the mandibular second deciduous molars and the mandibular first permanent molars. The clasps are held in place with sticky wax.

The work model is placed in water and is soaked until the model becomes completely moist. The acrylic can be applied using the traditional "salt and pepper" method of applying polymer and monomer. The acrylic must incorporate the clasps thoroughly and encompass the screw. As the acrylic begins to set, the work model and appliance are placed in a pressure pot for at least 10–15 minutes. The work model and appliance are removed from the pressure pot, and the Schwarz appliance is removed carefully from the work model. The wax covering the screw is discarded, and the appliance is smoothed and polished. The appliance then is disinfected, using appropriate immersion or spray techniques.

In recent years, various types of neon and "glow-in-the-dark" acrylics have become available and are popular with young patients. Similar types of bright-colored acrylics also can be used for maintenance plates.

Home Care Instruction

The Schwarz appliance is easily managed clinically, except in instances of severe undercuts due to pronounced lingual tipping of the mandibular posterior teeth. Usually, the appliance is delivered without adjustment. In instances of hard or soft tissue impingement, an acrylic bur can be used to remove excess acrylic.

The patient is instructed to wear the appliance on a full-time basis except during tooth brushing. Most patients are instructed to leave the appliance in place during most meals because of a concern about misplacing or damaging the appliance when it is not in the mouth.

TYPICAL TREATMENT PROTOCOL

Figures 14-6 to 14-10 demonstrate a typical treatment sequence involving Schwarz-RME therapy in a patient with a moderately severe tooth-size/arch-length discrepancy. The patient presented with a chief concern of mandibular incisor crowding (Fig. 14-6). Her maxilla

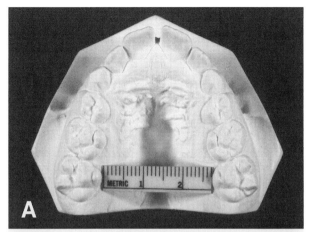
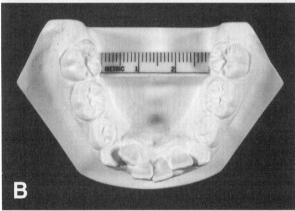

Figure 14-6. Occlusal views of the study models of a patient with moderately severe mandibular incisor crowding. Transpalatal width between the lingual surfaces of the maxillary first molars was 27 mm at the start of treatment, an indication of signifi-cant maxillary transverse constriction. A, Maxilla. B, Mandible.

also was narrow, with a transpalatal width of 27 mm as measured from the closest points between the maxillary first molars.

The patient and parent were instructed to expand the Schwarz appliance once per week. As about 1 mm of expansion was produced with every five turns, slightly less than one millimeter of expansion occurred during each month of wear. The appliance was worn as an active appliance for 5–6 months, at the end of which a tendency toward a lingual crossbite was observed intraorally (Fig. 14-7).

Because of the severity of mandibular incisor crowding in this patient, no attempt was made to resolve all of the arch length discrepancy by means of lower arch expansion, and some minor residual crowding remained when the active turning of the appliance was terminated (Fig. 14-8). An acrylic splint maxillary expander was bonded and activated one turn per day for 40 days (Fig. 14-9A). The RME appliance then was left in place passively for an additional five months, as was the Schwarz

SCHWARZ APPLIANCE

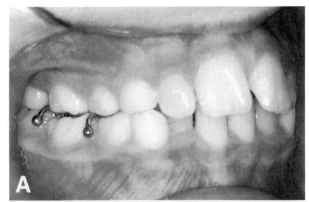

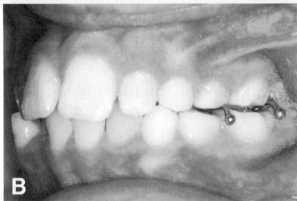

Figure 14-7. After 4–5 months of fulltime wear of the Schwarz appliance, a tendency toward a lingual crossbite is evident bilaterally. *A*, Right sagittal view. *B*, Left sagittal view. Even though the clasps obviously are distorted, no attempt to adjust the clasps is made, except in instances of patient discomfort. Adjusting the clasps often results in breakage. The clasps are used primarily as handles when dislodging the appliance, not for retention.

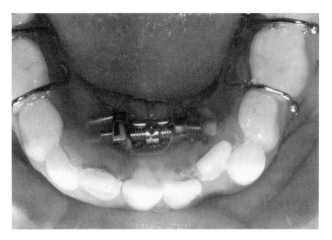

Figure 14-8. Occlusal view of the Schwarz appliance in place at the end of the active period of expansion. Note that some residual crowding remains. This remaining tooth-size/arch length discrepancy will be eliminated through the maintenance of the leeway space bilaterally.

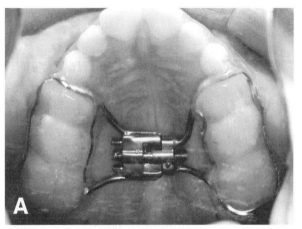

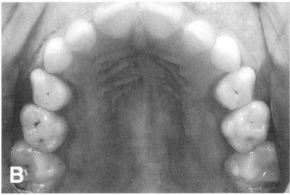

Figure 14-9. *A*, Maxillary view of the bonded acrylic splint rapid maxillary expander prior to activation. *B*, Maxillary view after RME has been removed.

appliance. Schwarz wear ended at the time of maxillary expander removal (Fig. 14-9*B*).

The interim phase of treatment involved the initial placement of a simple maxillary maintenance plate (Fig. 14-10*ACE*). The patient preferred to wear the maintenance plate on a fulltime basis throughout the transition to the permanent dentition. Typically, a soldered transpalatal arch is delivered before the loss of the maxillary second deciduous molars occurs.

Because of the severity of the original crowding in the mandibular anterior region, brackets were placed temporarily on the mandibular incisors for esthetic reasons after the exfoliation of the mandibular deciduous canines (Fig. 14-10*B*). Later a lower lingual arch maintained the leeway space that was gained in the transition of the mandibular second deciduous molars to the mandibular second premolars (2.5 mm per side,[30] on average; Fig. 14-10*D*). At the end of the interim period, sufficient space was available to allow for the alignment of the mandibular dentition without extraction or interproximal reduction (Fig. 14-10*F*). This case example illustrates how the Schwarz appliance can be used in conjunction with the lower lingual arch in managing significant crowding problems that are recognized in the early mixed dentition.

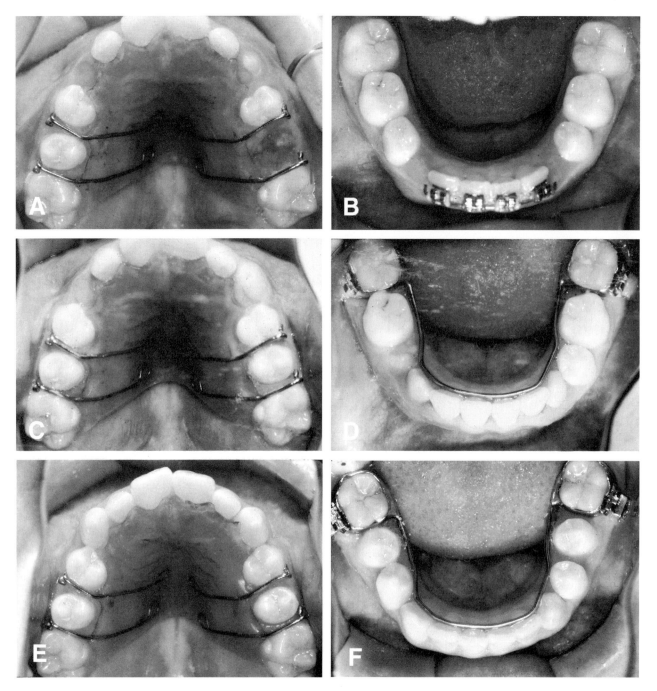

Figure 14-10. Transition of the dentition during the interim period. *A*, A simple maxillary maintenance plate was worn full time. The position of the maxillary molars was maintained by the posterior clasps. *B*, Brackets were placed on the mandibular incisors after exfoliation of the mandibular deciduous canines. *C* and *E*, Emergence of the maxillary premolars is complete. Typically, a transpalatal arch would have been placed before the loss of the maxillary second deciduous molars. *D*, A lower lingual arch was cemented before the exfoliation of the mandibular second deciduous molars. *F*, Adequate space now is available for the alignment of the mandibular teeth over basal bone without extraction.

CONCLUDING REMARKS

As has been stated many times throughout this text, the use of the lower Schwarz appliance as a mandibular "dental decompensation" appliance should be viewed as just that, an appliance that produces orthodontic (not orthopedic) movement of the mandibular dentition. In order for this therapy to be successful over the long term, orthopedic expansion of the maxilla and widening of the maxillary bony base is essential for this therapy to have long-term stability.

Our clinical studies of this appliance have indicated

that on average about 3–4 mm of additional arch length can be gained on a routine basis. Thus, the use of this appliance is not recommended in the treatment of gross tooth size/arch length discrepancy problems; rather, a serial extraction procedure may be indicated. Used with caution, however, this relatively simple and straightforward technique has proven to be a valuable adjunct in mixed dentition therapy.

REFERENCES CITED

1. Kingsley NW. Regulating teeth. Johnston Dental Miscellany 1877.
2. Badcock JH. The screw expansion plate. Trans Brit Soc Orthod 1911:3–8.
3. Crozat GB. Possibilities and use of removable labiolingual spring appliances. Am J Orthod 1920;6:1–6.
4. Nord CFL. Loose appliances in orthodontia. Dental Cosmos 1928;70:681–687.
5. Hotz R. Orthodontics in daily practice: Possibilities and limitations in the area of children's dentistry. Bern: Hans Huber Publishers, 1974.
6. Graber TM, Neumann B. Removable orthodontic appliances. Philadelphia: WB Saunders, 1977.
7. Schwarz AM, Gratzinger M. Removable orthodontic appliances. Philadelphia: WB Saunders, 1966.
8. Adams CP. The design and construction of removable orthodontic appliances. Bristol: J Wright and Sons, 1977.
9. Houston WJB, Isaacson KG. Orthodontic treatment with removable appliances. Bristol: J Wright and Sons, 1977.
10. Andresen V. The Norwegian system of gnatho-orthopedics. Acta Gnathol 1936;1:4–36.
11. Andresen V, Häupl K. Funktions-Kieferorthopädie: die Grundlagen Des Norwegischen Systems. Leipzig: JA Barth, Verlag, 1945.
12. Andresen V, Häupl K, Petric L. Funktions-Kieferorthopädie. Munich: JA Barth, 1957.
13. Fränkel R. Technik und Handhabung der Funktionsregler. Berlin: VEB Verlag Volk and Gesundheit, 1976.
14. Fränkel R, Fränkel C. Orofacial orthopedics with the function regulator. Munich: S Karger, 1989.
15. Haynes S, Jackson D. A comparison of the mechanism and efficiency of 21 orthodontic expansion screws. Dent Prac 1962;13:125–133.
16. Ogihara K, Nakahara R, Koyanagi S, Suda M. Treatment of a Brodie bite by lower lateral expansion: a case report and fourth year follow-up. J Clin Ped Dent 1998;23:17–21.
17. Schwarze CW. Dokumentation und Analyse von Langzeitstudien. Über das transversale und sagittale Positionsverhalten der Zähne im kieferorthopädisch behandelten Gebiss. Cologne: Habilitations-Schrift, 1969.
18. Schwarze CW. Expansion and relapse in long term follow-up studies. Trans Eur Orthod Soc 1972;48:275–284.
19. Tulley WJ, Campbell AC. A manual of practical orthodontics. Bristol: J Wright and Sons, 1960.
20. Graf H, Ehmer U. Das Rezidiv der transversalen Erweiterung bei Kompressionen mit frontalem Engstand. Fortschr Kieferorthop 1970;31:175–186.
21. Ülgen M, Schmuth GPF, Schuhmacher HA. Dehnung und Rezidiv. Fortschr Kieferorthop 1988;49:324–330.
22. Little RM. Stability and relapse of dental arch alignment. Br J Orthod 1990;17:235–241.
23. McDougall PD, McNamara JA, Jr, Dierkes JM. Arch width development in Class II patients treated with the Fränkel appliance. Am J Orthod 1982;82:10–22.
24. Lutz HD, Poulton DR. Stability of dental arch expansion in the deciduous dentition. Angle Orthod 1985;55: 299–315.
25. Bruno EC. Evaluation of post-retention mandibular arch dimensions following expansion in the deciduous or early mixed dentition. Unpublished Master's thesis, Department of Orthodontics, University of the Pacific, San Francisco, 1990.
26. Brust EW. Arch dimensional changes concurrent with expansion in the mixed dentition. Ann Arbor: Unpublished Master's thesis, Department of Orthodontics and Pediatric Dentistry, The University of Michigan, 1992.
27. Wendling LK. Short-term skeletal and dental effects of the acrylic splint rapid maxillary expansion appliance. Ann Arbor: Unpublished Master's thesis, Department of Orthodontics and Pediatric Dentistry, The University of Michigan, 1997.
28. Wright NS. A comparison of the treatment effects of the Schwarz appliance and the lower lingual holding arch. Ann Arbor: Unpublished Master's Thesis, Department of Orthodontics and Pediatric Dentistry, The University of Michigan, 2000.
29. Moyers RE, Van der Linden FPGM, Riolo ML, McNamara JA, Jr. Standards of human occlusal development. Ann Arbor: Monograph 5, Craniofacial Growth Series, Center for Human Growth and Development, The University of Michigan, 1976.

Chapter 15

THE TWIN BLOCK APPLIANCE

A functional appliance system that has grown in popularity during the last decade is the twin block appliance. This appliance was developed by William J. Clark of Fife, Scotland, for the correction of Class II malocclusions characterized in part by mandibular skeletal retrusion. Clark introduced his appliance in 1982 in an article in the *British Journal of Orthodontics*,[1] with a later article appearing in the *American Journal of Orthodontics and Dentofacial Orthopedics*[2] in 1988. Subsequent publications by Clark primarily have been case reports,[3,4] although recently Clark has published a textbook[5] and a book chapter[6] describing his treatment technique.

This chapter is based in part on two previous publications on the twin block appliance,[7,8] and it is the first in a series of chapters that consider the family of functional jaw orthopedic (FJO) appliances. Thus, before describing the design and clinical management of the twin block appliance in detail, a brief overview of the historical background and the biological basis underlying the twin block and other such functional appliances is in order.

HISTORICAL PERSPECTIVE

The concept of advancing the mandible by way of inclined planes is not new, with the notion of "jumping the bite" (*i.e.*, posturing the mandible forward) being traced back to the 1880 writings of Kingsley.[9] Kingsley was a dentist who developed a maxillary vulcanite plate that guided the mandible into a forward position during mandibular closure. Initial clinical investigations demonstrated the difficulty in maintaining a forward position of the lower jaw;[10] therefore, this technique fell into disuse.

One of the few direct descendants of this approach was the "Vorbissplatte" of Schwarz.[11] Hotz[12] also used a modified Kingsley plate in the treatment of Class II patients with deep bites, especially in instances of lingual inclination of the mandibular incisors due to hyperactivity of the mentalis muscle.

The Oliver "guide plane"[13,14] also was used to jump the bite in association with the labiolingual technique. Instead of a removable plate, however, this guide plane consisted of a maxillary lingual arch to which had been soldered auxiliary wires in the canine regions. The height of the bite plane was determined by the amount of bite-opening that was desired. In recent years, DeVincenzo and co-workers[15–17] have used an appliance similar to that developed by Clark, except that the bite blocks were angled 90° to the occlusal plane, as opposed to the 70° orientation ultimately recommended by Clark.[5]

BIOLOGICAL BASIS

All functional jaw orthopedic (FJO) appliances, including the activator, bionator, function regulator, Herbst and twin block, have as a common element, the forward positioning of the lower jaw produced by the appliance. Of all the major functional appliances, however, it can be argued that the twin block appliance appears to be the most direct clinical extension of the experimental

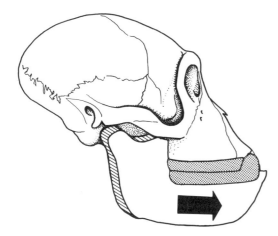

Figure 15-1. Diagrammatic representation of the functional protrusion experiments in non-human primates. After the placement of the intraoral appliances, the mandible is prompted forward and downward.

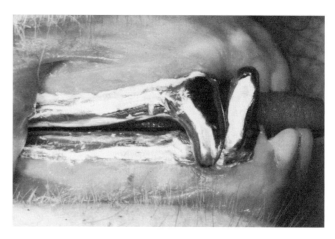

Figure 15-2. Intraoral view of the cast protrusive appliances at the time of placement. The maxillary and mandibular splints were bonded in place after grooves were made on the buccal and lingual surfaces of the posterior teeth.

studies of functional protrusion conducted in many laboratories since the early 1930s. These investigations, primarily in rat and non-human primate models, have considered the effect of mandibular protrusion (Figs. 15-1 and 15-2) on the growth of the mandible at various maturational levels, with specific emphasis on the growth and adaptation of the temporomandibular joint in juveniles and adolescents.

In contrast to the correction of a Class II malocclusion to Class I, as occurs with FJO therapy, the experiments typically altered the normal occlusion of the experimental animal to a protrusive Class III relationship (Fig. 15-3). Although the findings from these experimental studies are applicable in a general way to all FJO appliances, we have chosen to review and summarize these research efforts within this chapter.

Breitner[18-20] was the first to conduct investigations on non-human primates with this experimental model of functional protrusion. These studies were followed by those of Häupl and Psansky,[21] Hoffer and Colico,[22] Derichsweiler and Baume,[23,24] Hiniker and Ramfjord,[25] Joho,[26] and Stöckli and Willert.[27] These studies, conducted primarily in non-human primates, were characterized by occlusal alterations from a normal occlusion to a Class III relationship, similar in concept but different in specifics from the correction of a Class II occlusal relationship to a normal occlusion.

A number of these early investigators[18-22,24,27] demonstrated that the condylar cartilage is capable of exhibiting compensatory tissue responses following experimental alteration of the mandibular functional position. Breitner[18-20] also noted significant adaptive changes in the temporal bone following functional protrusion, concluding that "a mesial migration of the glenoid fossa" had occurred. Similar findings were reported by Häupl and Psansky,[21] but other investigators[22,24,28] observed that significant forward migration of the glenoid fossa did not occur.

A later study by Woodside and co-workers[29] investigated the treatment effects of the Herbst appliance in a non-human primate model. The issue of temporal bone adaptations once again was raised, as bony and soft-tissue adaptations were noted within the glenoid fossa. Although an incremental ("step-by-step") bite advancement was performed on these animals, ultimately the bite was brought forward 7–10 mm in a few months, an amount greater than that usually observed in other non-human primate studies.

One of the most comprehensive series of investigations dealing with the issue of altering mandibular growth has been conducted by Petrovic, Stutzmann and

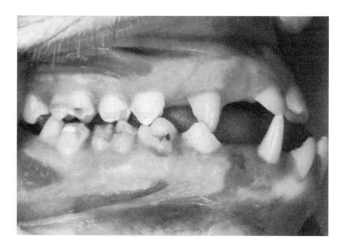

Figure 15-3. Class III malocclusion evident after appliance removal.

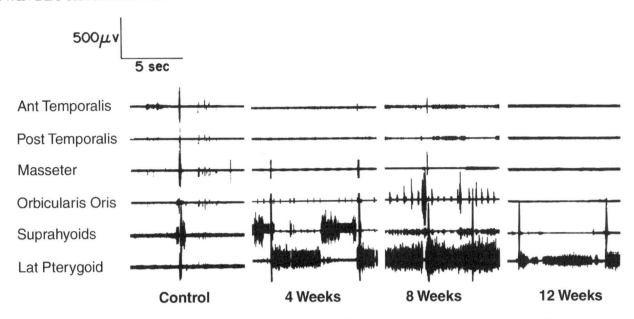

Figure 15-4. Electromyographic recordings of experimental monkey before and after appliance placement. Note the increase in the activity of the superior head of the lateral pterygoid muscle, especially at the four and eight week intervals.

colleagues at the University of Strasbourg. Their initial studies[30–32] demonstrated that anterior displacement of the mandibular condyle in rats resulted in increased growth of the condylar cartilage. Charlier and Petrovic[30] reported that the condylar cartilage did not appear to have an independent growth potential when isolated from its environmental structures. After the mandible was displaced anteriorly, however, increased condylar growth occurred through stimulation of the prechondroblastic or proliferative layers of cells.[30,31] A later study by Petrovic[33] indicated that mandibular growth augmentation can be achieved in rats when appliances simulating those used in clinical treatment of humans (e.g., bionator, Fränkel appliance) are used.

Our group at the University of Michigan also has conducted a series of studies that have considered craniofacial adaptations to protrusive function. To study functional adaptations to changes in mandibular postural position in the rhesus monkey, we have employed many experimental designs, the one most frequently used being the model of functional protrusion[34-38] (Figs. 15-1 to 15-5). One unique aspect of these investigations is that both structural and functional adaptations were studied simultaneously. For example, an increase in lateral pterygoid activity was associated with the forward positioning of the lower jaw. This new functional pattern was noted, first with such phasic activities as swallowing and subsequently with such tonic functions as maintenance of the mandibular postural position (Fig. 15-4). As the experimental period progressed, however, there was a gradual return toward the pre-appliance levels of muscle activity. This change was correlated in time with the skeletal and dental adaptations observed in the same animals.

In another study of functional protrusion,[36] the sequence of adaptation within the condylar cartilage was examined on a cross-sectional basis. Proliferation of the condylar cartilage was observed as early as two weeks after appliance placement (Fig. 15-5). Maximum cartilage proliferation was observed at six weeks after appliance placement, after which time there was a gradual return to a condylar morphology similar to that observed in the temporomandibular regions of control animals (Fig. 15-5). A later cephalometric investigation by McNamara and Bryan[38] indicated that the condylar cartilage proliferation was followed by increased bone deposition (i.e., bone eventually replaced most of the proliferated cartilage), leading to a lengthened mandible.

A summary of the overall temporal sequence of adaptation is shown in Figures 15-6 and 15-7. The placement of the protrusive appliance causes an immediate disruption of normal neuromuscular activity, but within a few days or weeks the animal adapts to the permanent change in the occlusion produced by the cementation of the appliance (Fig. 15-6). The exteroceptive and proprioceptive inputs of the teeth, gingiva, tongue, palate, and temporomandibular joints transmit the altered sensation to the central nervous system. The animal responds by altering the way its muscles function, typically posturing the mandible forward.

Structural adaptations typically take weeks or months to occur. Such induced changes include increased condy-

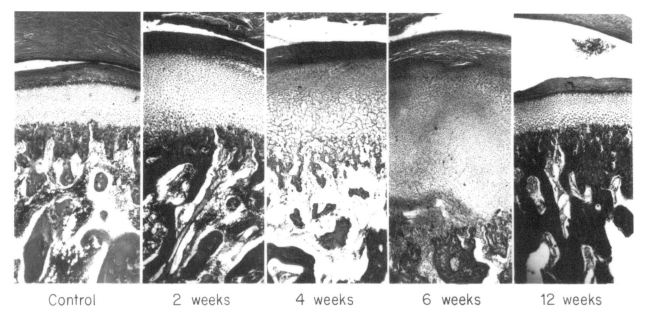

Figure 15-5. Response of the condylar cartilage to protrusive function. A proliferation of the condylar cartilage was evident at two weeks, with the peak response at six weeks. By twelve weeks, the thickness of the condylar cartilage was diminished as the calcified cartilage matrix was replaced by new bone.

lar cartilage proliferation and subsequent bony adaptations in the temporomandibular joints of growing animals,[36] as well as forward movement of the mandibular dentition (Fig. 15-7). Other more subtle changes occur throughout craniofacial region as well. As structural adaptations occur in the animal, the level of neuromuscular function tends to return to pretreatment levels (Fig. 15-4), even though the appliances remain in place.

The results of these studies seem to indicate that the growth of the temporomandibular joint in young animals is somewhat adaptive in nature and that the condylar cartilage is responsive to changes in function. The question of whether or not these mandibular adaptations are transient or permanent, however, still is open to question. Only two research groups have addressed this issue directly. Petrovic and co-workers,[39] using their version of a protrusive appliance, which they termed the postural hyperpropulsor, on young male rats, evaluated the growth rate of the condylar cartilage by counting the total number of cells that incorporated tritiated thymidine. In rats that wore the postural hyperpropulsor until the end of their growth period, the overall length of the mandible was greater than that of the controls. In addition, when the appliance was removed, no relapse occurred.

In a later study in rats by the same group,[33] long-term wear of the postural hyperpropulsor produced a 5–8% increase in mandibular length, whereas long-term wear of a modified bionator produced a 4–8% increase in mandibular length. Long-term wear of a simulated Fränkel appliance as well as of Class II elastics produced the greatest response: a 14% increase. The results of these studies led Petrovic and his associates to state that the final length of the mammalian mandible can be increased over its "genetically-determined length".

The Michigan group also has examined this question experimentally. McNamara and Bryan[38] monitored increments of mandibular growth in 11 experimental and 12 control male monkeys from the early mixed dentition until young adulthood. A series of protrusive appliances were placed in these animals throughout their growth period. After 48 weeks, significant increases in mandibular condylar growth and in overall mandibular length were noted in the treated animals. At the end of the three year experimental period (equivalent to 9–10 years in human terms), the mandibles of the treated animals were nearly 7 mm longer than those of the controls.

The results of this study, combined with the findings of Petrovic and co-workers,[33] indicate that significant adaptations can occur in the temporomandibular joint region of a growing animal. These adaptations are more observable when the animal is in the mixed dentition stage and tend to become less dramatic as the animal matures. It should be stressed, however, that these studies were conducted in a controlled experimental environment characterized by maximum "patient cooperation," in that the appliances were cemented in place in the experimental animal. The relevance of this research to the clinical situation of correcting Class II malocclu-

TWIN BLOCK APPLIANCE

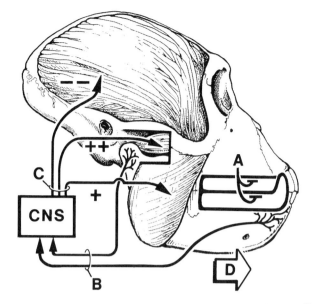

Figure 15-6. Short-term adaptations to the protrusive appliance. *A*, Placement of the cast appliance; *B*, Input from the periodontium and temporomandibular joint (TMJ) region is transmitted to the central nervous system (CNS); *C*, CNS regulates activity of the muscles of mastication, including increasing lateral pterygoid and masseter function and decreasing the activity of the posterior temporalis muscle; *D*, The postural position of the mandible is altered anteriorly. These short-term changes in muscle activity occur within days or weeks of appliance placement.

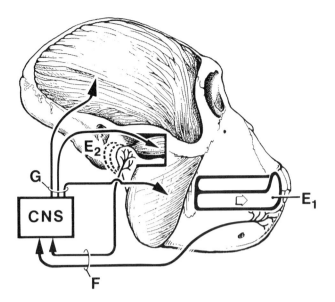

Figure 15-7. Long-term adaptations to the protrusive appliance. E_1, Anterior movement of the mandibular incisors, especially in more mature animals; E_2, Adaptations within the temporomandibular joint, especially in growing animals; *F*, The resulting change in sensory input is transmitted to the CNS, resulting in *G*, a gradual return of muscle activity to pretreatment levels. These long-term structural adaptations usually occur after several months of appliance placement.

sion in humans is indirect at best; the extrapolation directly to the orthodontic patient should be avoided.

PARTS OF THE TWIN BLOCK APPLIANCE

Perhaps of all the functional appliances routinely in use today, the twin block appliance may be most similar in design to the functional protrusion appliances evaluated in the previously mentioned experimental investigations. The twin block appliance (Fig. 15-8) is composed of maxillary and mandibular retainers that fit tightly against the teeth, alveolus and adjacent supporting structures. In his book, Clark[5] describes a variety of designs of the twin block appliance. In this chapter, both the original design of Clark (Figs. 15-9) and our modified design that incorporates a lower labial wire covered with acrylic (Figs. 15-8 and 15-10) will be described in detail.

Maxillary Appliance

The maxillary part of the twin block typically consists of a split plate design (Figs. 15-11), with one or two midline screws (6 mm expansion screw, Leone Co., Florence,

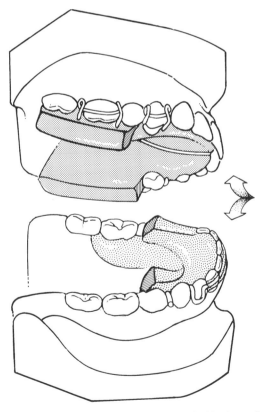

Figure 15-8. Book view of the modified twin block appliance. Bilateral bite blocks are located posteriorly in the maxillary appliance and anteriorly in the mandibular appliance.

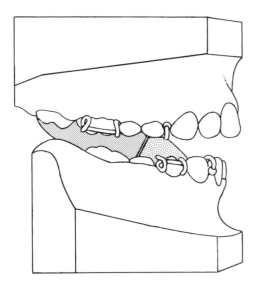 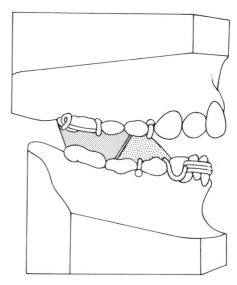

Figure 15-9. Traditional design of the appliance according to Clark.[1,2,5] Note that ball clasps are used to provide anterior retention in both arches. The inclined planes of the posterior bite blocks are oriented at 70 degrees to the occlusal plane. Ball ended clasps and delta clasps are used for retention.

Figure 15-10. Preferred modified twin block design. The anterior ball clasps are replaced by a labial bow to which clear acrylic has been added, increasing anterior retention of the lower appliance, especially during the period of the transitional dentition.

Italy). The plate also can be made without a midline screw if there is no need for maxillary expansion during treatment (*e.g.*, the patient underwent Phase I rapid maxillary expansion). The use of the two-screw design is encouraged in order to avoid unwanted flexibility of the maxillary appliance during treatment as the appliance is expanded. Our experience has shown that in those patients in whom significant expansion is desired during twin block treatment, the appliance becomes unstable and too flexible if only one midline screw is used. Each screw is activated once per week (~0.2 mm) until adequate expansion is attained.

Clark[5] also suggests the incorporation of sagittal screws in instances of retroclination of the maxillary incisors. Our approach to this problem, however, is to treat the patient with "temporary" fixed appliances (4–8 months) before twin block therapy, eliminating the need for the sagittal screws.

The maxillary plate is anchored to the dentition by way of delta clasps[5] (Figs. 15-8 and 15-9) or alternatively Adams clasps,[40] made from .030″ stainless steel wire, on the maxillary first molars. Ball clasps made from .030″ stainless steel typically contact the interproximal area between the maxillary premolars (Fig. 15-11A), although delta clasps also can be used to anchor the upper appliance against the first premolars (Fig. 15-

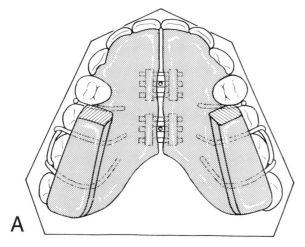 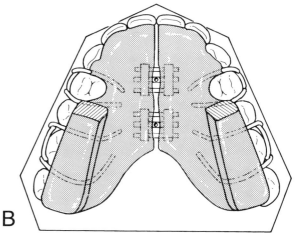

Figure 15-11. Maxillary occlusal view of the twin block appliannce. Two expansion screws are placed in the midline. Delta clasps are used to secure the appliance to the molars posteriorly, whereas A, ball clasps or B, delta clasps are used to anchor the plate in the premolar/deciduous molar region.

TWIN BLOCK APPLIANCE

11B). The precise clasp configuration depends on the type (deciduous or permanent) and number of teeth present at the time of appliance construction.

The maxillary appliance contains two bite blocks that cover the medial aspects of the posterior teeth (Fig. 15-11). The lateral aspects of the posterior teeth are not covered, so that the clasps can be adjusted during treatment. It is very important to make sure that the upper and lower parts of the appliance fit tightly against the dentition, so that the parts do not "float" during normal oral activities such as speech and mastication.

The anterior part of the maxillary bite block terminates in an inclined plane, against which the lower bite block functions (Figs. 15-12). The bite blocks are trimmed so that the inclined planes are at a 70° angle with the occlusal plane. The integrity of the incline planes is maintained throughout treatment, in spite of acrylic recontouring and possible reactivation that occur during the treatment of deepbite patients (to be discussed in detail later).

Mandibular Appliance

A number of different designs have been proposed for the mandibular part of the appliance. All designs feature bilateral anterior bite blocks that terminate in posteriorly directed inclined planes above the mandibular second premolars.

Original Design of Clark

The original design of Clark[5] is a horseshoe of acrylic that extends posteriorly to the mandibular second premolars bilaterally (Figs. 15-13 and 15-14). The lingual surfaces of the mandibular molars are not contacted by the appliance to allow for the unimpeded eruption of these teeth during treatment. The lower appliance is anchored to the dentition by means of delta clasps that contact the mandibular first premolars bilaterally. In addition, a series of ball clasps lie in the interproximal areas between the canines and mandibular incisors (Figs. 15-9 and 15-13). Additional ball clasps can be placed between the incisors if appliance retention is thought to be a problem.

Modified Design

We have modified the original design of Clark by placing a labial bow anterior to the mandibular incisors that has labial acrylic similar to that of a lower spring retainer[41] (Fig. 15-15). In contrast to the spring retainer, however, the positions of the mandibular incisors are not altered in the work model prior to appliance construction. This .030″ wire extends laterally from the acrylic distal to the canines and then after curving inferiorly in the canine region (as in a Hawley loop). The wire crosses the clinical crowns of the mandibular incisors just below their midpoints (Fig. 15-16). The acrylic used usually is clear and fills the interproximal areas below the contact points of the mandibular incisors.

The overall shape of the modified lower appliance is very similar to the Schwarz appliance described in Chapter 14; the appliance extends posteriorly to the mandibular first molars and mandibular second molars, if present (Fig. 15-17). Posteriorly, the acrylic should be trimmed so as not to impede the eruption of the mandibular permanent molars, as the maxillary bite blocks are contoured (see below). Our routine use of

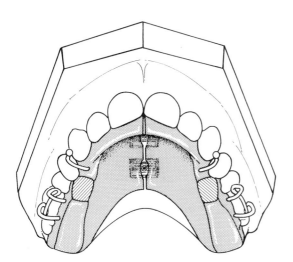

Figure 15-12. Oblique view of the maxillary part of the twin block appliance. Note the inclined planes on the anterior aspect of the posterior bite blocks.

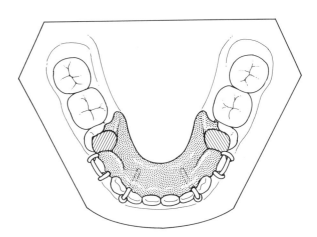

Figure 15-13. Mandibular view of the original twin block appliance of Clark[5] that incorporates acrylic on the lingual surfaces of the teeth anterior to the first permanent molars.

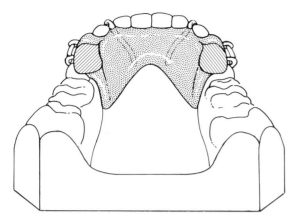

Figure 15-14. Posterior oblique view of the mandibular part of the original twin block appliance of Clark.[5] Note the inclined planes along the posterior aspect of the bite blocks. With this design, no acrylic touches any aspect of the mandibular permanent first molars.

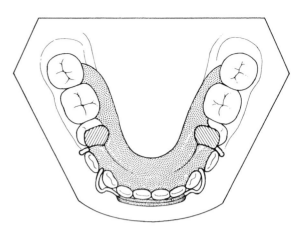

Figure 15-15. Preferred modified design of the lower appliance in which the lower lingual acrylic extends posteriorly into the permanent molar region. The lower labial bow with clear acrylic covering extends anteriorly to cover the labial surfaces of the mandibular anterior teeth.

this design has shown that the lower labial bow provides increased retention if the appliance is used in mixed dentition patients during the transition to the permanent dentition.

Other Mandibular Designs

If a modest increase in mandibular arch perimeter is desired, the lower appliance can be fabricated with a Schwarz-type design (Fig. 15-18). In this instance, a labial wire is not present because of the desired expansion in the mandibular incisor region. The need for this design can be eliminated, however, during prior Phase I treatment by way of combined Schwarz and acrylic splint expander therapy (see Chapter 4).

Another design that has evolved is based on the acrylic splint Herbst appliance[42-44] (Figs. 15-19 and 15-20). An acrylic cap is used to anchor the mandibular appliance anteriorly. Ball clasps lie in the interproximal area between the mandibular first and second premolars.

Regardless of the specific design chosen, special care should be taken in the fabrication of the posterior bite blocks, particularly in the mandible. As mentioned earlier, the mandibular blocks originate in the mandibular canine region. The blocks gradually increase in height posteriorly and extend to the middle of the mandibular second premolar or mandibular second deciduous molar, at which point the blocks terminate. Two to three millimeters of tooth surface anterior to the embrasure with the mandibular first permanent molar should be visible (Fig. 15-18A), so that contact can be maintained

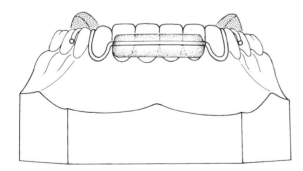

Figure 15-16. Anterior view of the modified appliances that illustrates the labial bow that contacts the labial surfaces of the mandibular anterior teeth. In contrast to the typical spring retainer of Barrer,[41] the positions of the mandibular incisors on the work model are not adjusted in wax prior to appliance construction. Typically, clear acrylic is used in the fabrication of the lower labial bow.

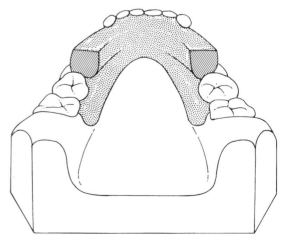

Figure 15-17. Oblique view of the modified mandibular appliance. The acrylic extends posteriorly to the permanent molars.

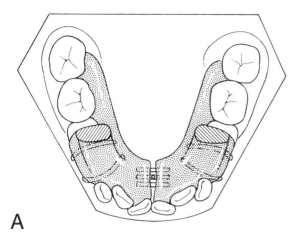 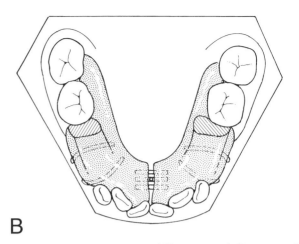

Figure 15-18. Alternative (Schwarz-type) design of the mandibular appliance that incorporates a midline screw. *A*, Proper appliance design in which the posterior bite block terminates 2–3 mm anterior to the mandibular first molars; *B*, Improper appliance design in which the acrylic extends to the mandibular first molar.

between the mandibular second premolar/deciduous molar and the maxillary bite block during the acrylic contouring process. If the mandibular bite block extends too far posteriorly (Fig. 15-18*B*), it is impossible to allow for the eruption of the mandibular first molar while still maintaining contact with the inclined planes of the maxillary part of the appliance as acrylic contouring occurs (to be discussed in detail below).

CLINICAL MANAGEMENT

Preparation of the Dental Arches

Our usual protocol involves the decompensation of the dental arches with fixed appliances prior to twin block treatment if there are significant dental irregularities, such as retroclined or rotated maxillary incisors or protruded or extruded mandibular incisors. In addition, rapid maxillary expansion often is initiated prior to twin block therapy if transpalatal width is narrow. Thus, in many respects, the twin block patient is treated conceptually the same as a surgical orthodontic patient, in that all major dentoalveolar obstructions to mandibular advancement are eliminated prior to the initiation of twin block treatment.

The first aspect to be considered when evaluating a twin block patient for prior Phase I intervention is the transverse dimension of the maxilla. Although some expansion is possible with this appliance (the midpalatal screws opens 6 mm), patients who are diagnosed as having a significant transverse maxillary discrepancy initially should receive a rapid maxillary expansion appliance prior to the fabrication of the twin block. This is especially true with patients in the mixed dentition, as RME with the acrylic splint expander has been shown to be effective in eliminating transverse problems.[45,46] In mixed dentition patients (typically those with a transpalatal width of less than thirty mil-

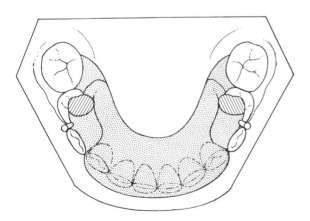

Figure 15-19. Occlusal view of an alternative (Herbst-type) design for the mandibular appliance based on the acrylic splint Herbst.[65]

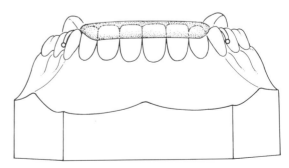

Figure 15-20. Frontal view of the mandibular appliance shown in Figure 15-19. The acrylic incisal cap covers the superior aspect of the incisors and canines. Ball clasps are included posteriorly to aid retention.

limeters, as measured from the closest points between the maxillary first permanent molars) may be considered for this type of early orthopedic intervention. Additionally, in instances of moderate crowding of the mandibular incisors, a removable lower Schwarz appliance can be used to upright the mandibular posterior teeth and to gain a modest amount of arch length anteriorly. By necessity, the use of any of these preparatory procedures will increase treatment time. Thus, the cost (*e.g.*, time, expense) of these preliminary procedures must be judged against the potential benefits to the patient.

Dental decompensation, especially of the maxillary incisors often is necessary prior to functional appliance therapy. The results of a cross-sectional study of Class II mixed dentition patients prior to treatment[47] indicated that about 30% of the patients had retroclined maxillary incisors relative to ideal values. Many methods can be used to correct the horizontal and vertical position of these teeth, including utility arches[48] and other "2×4" intrusion arches.[49–51] The correction of extruded mandibular incisors concomitant with an accentuated curve of Spee in a patient with a normal or long lower anterior facial height prior to the onset of treatment also is beneficial in avoiding unwanted increases in the vertical dimension. Ideally, the maxillary and mandibular dental arches should fit together in a satisfactory manner with the occlusion in a Class I or slightly overcorrected relationship prior to the fabrication of the twin block appliance.

Impression Technique

Impression-taking and work model preparation for the twin block appliance is relatively straight-forward, in comparison to that required for the FR-2 appliance of Fränkel[52] described in the next chapter. If decompensation of the dental arches has been undertaken, all fixed appliances are removed prior to obtaining the impressions. The only exception is the placement of brackets on the maxillary four anterior teeth, appliances that may be left in place during appliance fabrication. Removal of the incisor brackets typically is recommended at the time of appliance delivery, however, so as to facilitate patient comfort during twin block treatment.

After the teeth are cleaned, accurate bubble-free alginate impressions are obtained of both arches and the associated soft tissue. Particular attention should be paid to the lingual extensions of the mandible, as the mandibular acrylic extends inferiorly in this region.

If major changes in the occlusion have been achieved during a preparatory phase of fixed appliance treatment, it is prudent to take an additional set of impressions and fabricate a pair of transitional retainers (*i.e.*, invisible retainers made from 1 mm thick splint Biocryl™; see Chapter 27) to prevent unwanted tooth movement during the time of appliance fabrication. If the patient has undergone rapid maxillary expansion just prior to twin block treatment, the expander can be worn as a removable appliance during the time of appliance construction.

Bite Registration

There is no universal agreement as to the amount of bite advancement that should be used with the construction of the twin block appliance (or for any other function appliance for that matter). Clark[5] recommends that in a growing child with an overjet of up to 10 mm, the patient should be postured forward to an edge-to edge incisal relationship if the patient maintains a forward mandibular position comfortably. He recommends that larger discrepancies require a sequential activation of the appliance. In contrast, Fränkel[53] recommends a "step-by-step" activation of his functional appliances, with increments as little as 2.0–2.5 mm. Using a third protocol, the amount of forward bite advancement is based on the range of forward mandibular movement, with the maximum one-step bite advancement being no more that 70% of the protrusive path.

Our current recommendation regarding the amount of bite advancement varies according to the severity of the original problem, although some practitioners[5,54] with long-term experience with the twin block advocate an edge-to-edge bite advancement, except in extreme cases. We recommend that in patients with an overjet of 7 mm or less, the bite registration is taken in an incisal end-to-end position. In those patients with overbites greater than 7 mm, the bite should be taken half way between centric relation and an incisal end-to-end position, with a subsequent advancement of the mandible to an edge-to-edge relationship 2–4 months later.

The importance of another aspect of the bite registration, that is the amount of vertical bite opening, cannot be overestimated. Our clinical experience has shown that in order for twin block therapy to be effective, the bite blocks must be at least 5–7 mm thick vertically (Fig. 15-21*A*). The blocks must encroach on the resting lengths of the elevator musculature to insure that the mandible continues to be postured forward, even though the anterior teeth are not touching. Depending on the amount of vertical opening, the patient must open the mouth 10–14 mm before the posterior bite blocks become disengaged (Fig. 15-21*B*).

TWIN BLOCK APPLIANCE

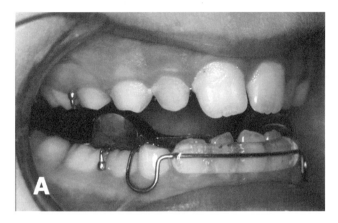 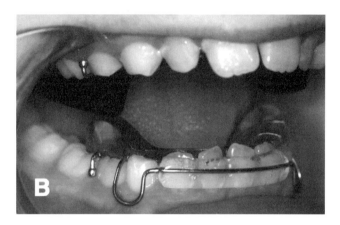

Figure 15-21. Intraoral view of the modified version of the twin block appliance. *A*, In occlusion. Note the 7 mm of bite block height in the premolar region. *B*, Patient opening vertically. The patient must open about 14 mm before disengaging the maxillary and mandibular bite blocks.

If the vertical opening is not sufficient, the inclined planes of the posterior bite blocks are too short (Fig. 15-22), and the patient can posture the mandible posteriorly by disengaging the maxillary and mandibular inclined planes. In contrast to intuitive logic, patient wearing an appliances that is constructed with blocks that are too short vertically (<5 mm) are prone to more cooperation problems than those with taller bite blocks. Surprisingly, increasing the heights of the blocks typically improves the level of patient cooperation.

To assure an adequate bite registration, the technique advocated by Clark is recommended.[5,6] The Projet™ Bite Gauge (Great Lakes Orthodontic Products, Tonawanda NY) is ideal for construction of a bite registration. This bite fork (Fig. 15-23) is available in two colors: blue (2 mm bite opening) and white (formerly yellow; 4 mm bite opening). Typically the latter bite fork is recommended, as there must be 5–7 mm of height to the bite blocks posteriorly. The blue bite gauge can be used in patients with a deep bite and an accentuated curve of Spee.

The anterior segment of the bite gauge has a single large groove on one side and three serrations on the other (Fig. 15-23). We prefer to use the bite gauge with the serrated side up. The clinician should determine the amount of bite advancement for the specific patient and then have the patient practice posturing his or her jaw forward the specified amount by looking in a hand-held mirror with the bite gauge in place. The serrated edge should be held against the maxillary incisors, with the incisal edges of the maxillary central incisors placed in one of three possible positions (Fig. 15-24), as determined by the clinician. With the bite gauge held in the proper position against the maxillary teeth, the patient is instructed to close into the large groove on the underside of the gauge with the skeletal midlines symmetrical.

After the patient has become accustomed to biting into the bite fork, medium hard pink wax is softened

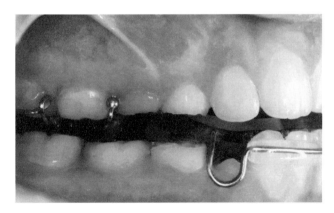

Figure 15-22. Intraoral view of a twin block made with inadequate vertical opening. The posterior bite blocks should be about 7 mm in height in the premolar region.

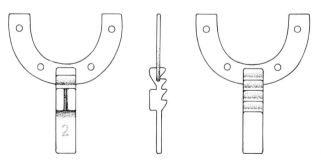

Figure 15-23. The Projet™ bite registration fork. This bite fork is available in two sizes, 2 mm thick (blue) and 4 mm thick (yellow or white). In most instances the latter size is recommended for use in order to assure adequate bite opening in the posterior bite block regions. (Great Lakes Orthodontic Product, Inc., Tonawanda NY.)

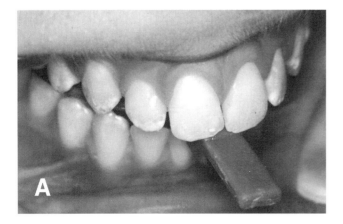

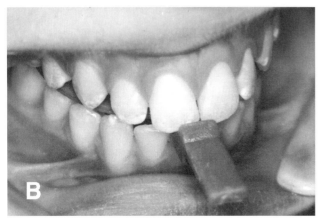

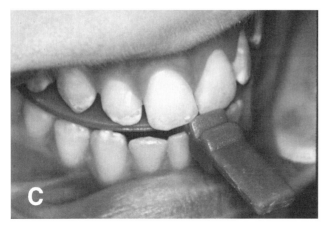

Figure 15-24. Preliminary bite registration with the bite fork in place. The three photographs from top to bottom show increasing amounts of bite advancement. The bite can be advanced in increments by placing the maxillary incisors between or in front of the serrations on the upper surface of the bite fork. *A*, modest advancement; *B*, intermediate advancement; *C*, incisal edge-to-edge advancement.

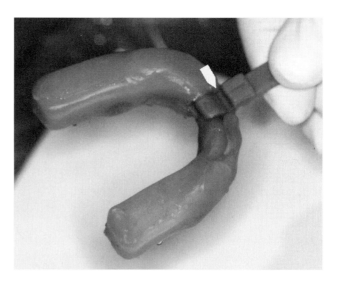

Figure 15-25. Medium hard pink wax is placed around the bite fork after softening. The single large "V" on the inferior surface of the bite fork (see white arrow) is used to register the position of the mandibular incisors once the bite fork is positioned against the maxillary dentition.

and placed around the arms of the bite fork (Fig. 15-25). The clinician places the bite fork and wax into the patient's mouth, securely against the maxillary teeth with the midline of the fork coincident with the midline of the maxilla. The patient is instructed to bite into the wax, with the mandibular teeth guided into the position determined by the large groove on the underside of the bite fork. The midline alignment is checked, and then the lateral aspects of the softened wax are pushed medially against the teeth, so that a true three-dimensional bite registration is obtained (Fig. 15-26). The wax bite is removed from the mouth and chilled, so that the dimensional stability of the bite registration is attained.

In patients who do not have a deep bite at the beginning of treatment, the bite registration procedure is essentially the same, except that a greater incisal opening is necessary in order to achieve an adequate height of the bite blocks. Once again, opening the vertical dimension beyond the freeway space is essential.

Laboratory Prescription

In ordering a twin block appliance, almost always the modified design is prescribed. The key features are the double midline screw in the maxilla portion of the appliance and the lower labial bow in the mandible. The appliance can be ordered in a variety of colors and patterns, so the patient can customize the appliance to his or her desires (*e.g.*, school or team colors, glow-in-the-dark, speckled, multicolor). Participation in this treatment decision by the patient has been shown to increase the level of patient enthusiasm and cooperation. It is recommended, however, that the acrylic on the lower labial bow be clear in most instances for cosmetic purposes.

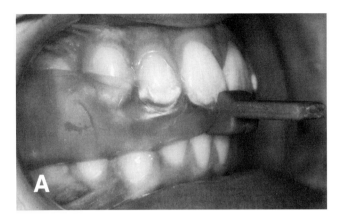 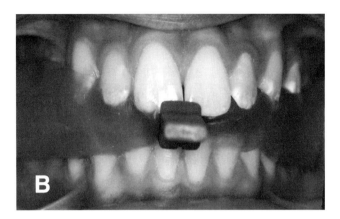

Figure 15-26. A three-dimensional registration is obtained with the bite fork in position by pressing the softened wax laterally against the teeth after the wax registration is obtained. *A*, Lateral view. *B*, Frontal view. The midlines should be aligned.

Appliance Delivery

After the twin block appliance has been returned by the laboratory, the appliance should be examined thoroughly to make sure that it has been fabricated correctly. Usually the work models are damaged during the fabrication process, but these models should be stored for future reference in case of appliance breakage.

The patient is shown how to place the appliance in the mouth properly (Fig. 15-21*A*). The upper and lower halves of the appliance are tried in the mouth separately to check the fit of the appliance to each dental arch. The delta clasps and ball clasps should be adjusted so that each portion of the appliance fits securely against the adjacent teeth. In addition, the lower labial bow and the adjacent anterior acrylic should be pinched together so as to increase resistance to dislodging.

Both parts of the appliance should be anchored in place and should not float loosely in the mouth. If retention of the lower appliance remains a problem in spite of clasp and bow adjustments, composite resin also can be added to the buccal surfaces of the premolars or deciduous molars to create undercuts for increased retention.[5]

Clark[5] stresses that patient compliance is a major key to treatment success, and patient education and motivation must be continued at the delivery appointment. The patient is shown his or her appliance out of the mouth, illustrating the importance of having the patient posture the jaw anteriorly when wearing the appliance. If the appliance is constructed properly with adequate vertical opening, the patient will do so automatically. The bite is brought forward as the patient closes into the appliance, a concept easily grasped even by young mixed dentition patients.

Patient education often is the primary responsibility of the chairside auxiliary. The auxiliary should show the patient and parents how to properly wear the appliance, with the patient looking in a hand-held mirror. Typically an improvement in facial appearance can be seen. If lip strain or other soft tissue distortions are evident, the patient is told that the function of the orofacial muscles will improve with time, within a few months given excellent patient compliance. Lip seal exercises [55] (see also Chapter 8) may be prescribed at this time if needed. Although the twin block appliance does not have the direct muscle retraining effect of the FR-2 appliance, the principles of Fränkel in retraining the orofacial musculature should be remembered and used whenever possible.

The twin block appliance is designed to be worn full-time. Thus, the patient is instructed to wear the appliance at all times, especially during eating. Normal speech patterns will be interrupted for the first few days after appliance delivery. Similarly, the patient may experience difficulties in swallowing during the same period. One clever suggestion is that of Leishman,[54] who recommends that, with parental approval, the patient be permitted to eat as much ice cream as desired during the first few days after appliance placement. Allowing such soft cold food *ad libitum* not only facilitates the recovery of normal orofacial reflexes; it also improves patient enthusiasm for the twin block dramatically. As with any intraoral appliance, speech can be improved by having the patient read out loud for a week or so after delivery, once again restoring oral reflexes.[52]

Clark[5] has suggested that one method of improving patient compliance is to cement or bond the appliance in place for 7–10 days. Glass ionomer can be used for cementation. In addition the clasps can be bonded to the adjacent teeth by adding composite to the buccal surfaces of the premolars or deciduous molars. Later the appliances are made removable, but by this time patient compliance with full-time wear has been achieved.

Our experience with cementing or bonding the appliance at the time of delivery has been limited to date, and we have met with mixed results. It seems that the best way to assure proper compliance is to deliver a well-fitting appliance that fits snugly to the adjacent dental arches. If the patient has been given an appliance that does not float in the mouth, reasonable masticatory patterns can be established when wearing the twin block.

Appointment Scheduling

The following appointment schedule is recommended for the typical patient:

Interval	Week No.	Procedure
0	0	Delivery of appliance
2	2	Begin contouring
6	8	Reactivate (if needed); contour
6	14	Contour
6	20	Reactivate (if needed); contour
6	26	Maintenance
6	32	Maintenance
6	38	Impression for stabilization plate
4	42	Deliver stabilization plate
8	50	Check stabilization plate

Contouring the Bite Blocks

A typical sequence of contouring and advancement in a Class II patient in the mixed dentition (Fig. 15-27A) will be illustrated here. The delivery appointment should be used to make sure that the appliance fits properly and that the patient feels comfortable with the appliance in place (Fig. 15-27B). Beginning with the second appointment, however, aggressive contouring of the appliance is begun in those patient who will benefit from increasing the vertical dimension during treatment (Fig. 15-27C).

The purpose of the acrylic contouring is to permit the mandibular first molars to erupt as the bite is opened. First, no acrylic of the lower appliance should touch the permanent molars, and the juxtaposition of the acrylic to the mandibular molars should be checked at the time of appliance delivery. At each recontouring appointment, the upper appliance is removed from the mouth, and an acrylic bur is used to remove acrylic so that there is 1–1.5 mm of interocclusal space between the posterior part of the bite block and the mandibular molars (Fig. 15-27C). Care should be taken not to remove acrylic excessively, as the tongue will posture in the

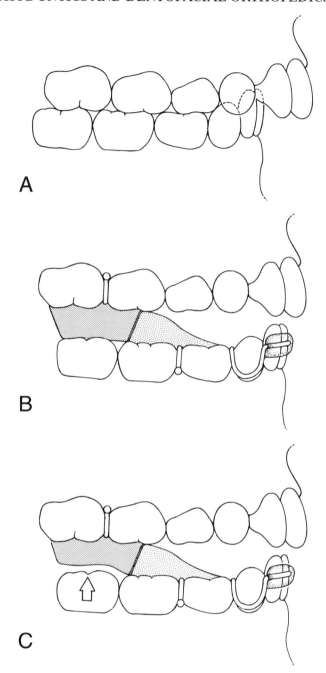

Figure 15-27. Initial contouring of the twin block appliance used in a mixed dentition patient. A, Bite in centric occlusion prior to treatment. B, Twin block appliance in place at the time of appliance delivery. The posterior bite block has positive contact against the opposing teeth. C, Initial contouring of the appliance in the mandibular molar region. Contact is maintained anteriorly between the upper block and the lower second deciduous molar. The molar is free to erupt (see arrow).

space, possibly preventing the eruption of the mandibular molars. During the trimming process, however, it is very important to maintain contact between the anterior portion of the posterior bite block and the mandibular second deciduous molars / premolars. Contouring is continued at subsequent appointments (Fig. 15-28),

TWIN BLOCK APPLIANCE

regardless of whether the appliance is in need of reactivation, so that often only a wedge of acrylic remains after the contouring is completed.

Reactivation of the Appliance

If the initial bite registration has been obtained using a "step-by-step" protocol, the appliance is reactivated 2–3 months after appliance delivery. Cold-cure acrylic can be used to activate the appliance, but we prefer to use a light-cure acrylic such as Triad™. Using such a product facilitates the activation of the appliance at chairside. The Triad™ material is available in soft acrylic sheets that are cut easily with a spatula. The material is removed from its protective light-tight wrapper, and two small squares or rectangles of acrylic are removed from the sheet (Fig. 15-29*AB*). The squares must be of appropriate bulk so that they can be rolled into balls (Fig. 15-29*C*) that approximate the size necessary to add sufficient material to the maxillary inclined planes.

The appliance is activated as follows. First, the maxillary appliance is removed from the mouth, the anterior surfaces of the inclined planes are roughened, and holes are drilled in the inclined plane to create undercuts. The soft acrylic balls are pressed into place and molded against the inclined planes (Fig. 15-29*D*). The Triad™ bonding agent is used to maximize acrylic adherence.

Petroleum jelly is applied to adjacent teeth and to the mandibular inclined plane to prevent the light-cured acrylic from adhering to any unwanted surfaces (Fig. 15-30*A*). The appliance then is placed in the mouth (Fig 15-30*B*), and the patient then is asked to close the two parts of the appliance together, with mandible postured sufficiently forward to allow for proper activation of the appliance (usually 3–5 mm).

The Triad™ material is activated using a curing light for approximately thirty seconds on each side (Fig. 15-31*A*). The maxillary appliance then is cured for an additional minute on each side (Fig. 15-31*B*), after which the excess acrylic is removed with an acrylic bur (Fig. 15-32), maintaining the 70° orientation of the inclined plane to the occlusal plane (Fig. 15-33). Reactivation is completed by finishing and polishing the acrylic and then checking the amount of bite advancement in the mouth. Minor adjustments in appliance fit can be made at that time.

The Support Phase

It has been our experience that the most critical part of twin block treatment may not be the achievement of the Class II correction, but rather the maintenance of this

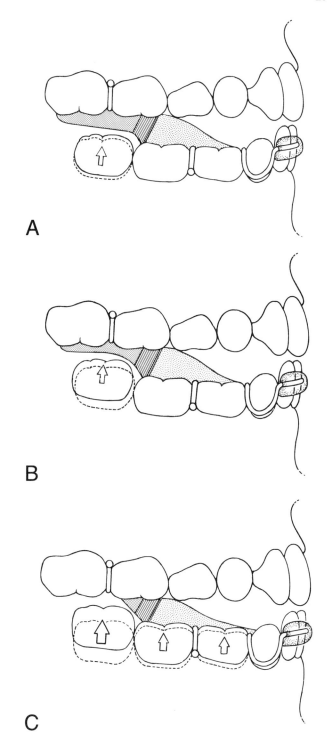

Figure 15-28. Appliance reactivation. The appliance is reactivated by adding acrylic to the maxillary inclined plane below the mesiobuccal cusp of the maxillary permanent first molar. *A* and *B*. Further acrylic contouring and molar eruption after reactivation of the appliance. *C*. At the end of the contouring process, most of the acrylic on the maxillary bite block has been removed. Acrylic also is removed from the superior aspect of the mandibular bite block, allowing for further tooth eruption (see arrows).

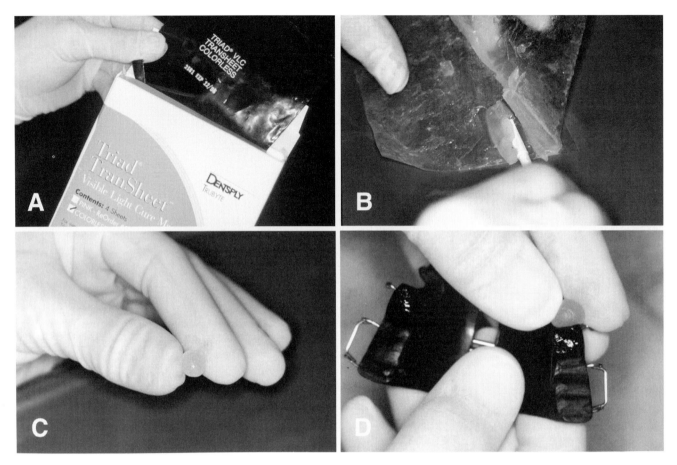

Figure 15-29. Reactivation of the appliance. *A*, The Triad™ acrylic is removed from its protective opaque plastic envelope. *B*, A small strip is cut from the soft acrylic sheet. *C*, The small strip is rolled into a ball. *D*, After the inclined plane has been roughened and after retention holes have been created, the soft acrylic ball is pushed against the inclined plane.

correction during the transition to the permanent dentition. Most of our experience with the twin block appliance has been in mixed dentition patients, and thus our recommendations deal primarily with children at this stage of dental development.

The active phase of twin block treatment should take 6–9 months if an edge-to-edge bite registration is used and 9–12 months if a "step-by-step" activation is used. At the end of active treatment, the Class II relationship should have been eliminated, and often the patient is left in a slightly overcorrected occlusal relation. By this time, the mandibular molars should be in contact with the maxillary molars, so that posterior support has been achieved. The next step is dependent on the type of overbite relationship the patient had prior to twin block treatment.

Deep Bite

In patients who had a deep bite and an accentuated curve of Spee at the beginning of treatment, the next part of the protocol is the fabrication of the support appliance and the discontinuation of the twin block. At the appointment prior to the end of twin block treatment, an impression is taken for what we term the "Clark support plate." This appliance consists of a simple maxillary palatal plate with ball clasps on either side of the maxillary second deciduous molar or second premolar. Alternatively, the appliance can be made with delta clasps anchored to the maxillary first molars (Fig. 15-34). Anteriorly, a modest incisal guide plane is added in the acrylic to stabilize the occlusion as the mandibular canines and deciduous molars or premolars erupt (Fig. 15-35). The inclined plane must be of sufficient width and height to prevent the mandible from dropping posteriorly after the twin block appliance has been discontinued.

Muscle splinting occasionally may lead to the erroneous conclusion that the mandible is in a stable position at the end of twin block treatment. An adequately-designed support plate worn on a full-time basis for at least six months, and at nighttime thereafter, usually will prevent or greatly reduce the tendency toward relapse of the Class II correction during the support phase of treatment.[5]

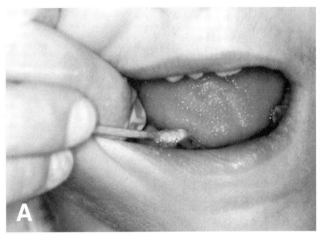
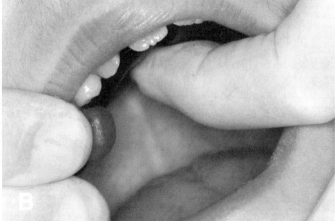

Figure 15-30. *A*. Petroleum jelly is smeared onto all surfaces not intended for bonding, including the mandibular appliance and the teeth. *B*. The maxillary appliance with the shaped acrylic balls anteriorly is placed in the mouth, and the patient closes into the new bite registration.

Open Bite

It has been our experience that in some patients, there has been a strong tendency toward relapse of the Class II correction during the support phase of treatment. This propensity to relapse has been most obvious in patients who started twin block treatment with an open bite or an open bite tendency. In such patients, the anterior guide plane of the Clark plate often is not sufficient to maintain the Class II correction, especially in patients who had a severe underlying skeletal discrepancy at the beginning of twin block treatment. In these patients, we recommend that the twin block appliance continue to be worn as a nighttime appliance, much in the same way that the FR-2 appliance of Fränkel[55,59] is worn at night after full-time wear has been discontinued. In this instance the bulk of the twin block appliance can be reduced further, especially the vertical dimension of the mandibular appliance. Part-time wear of the appliance should be encouraged until the posterior occlusion becomes stable and excellent interdigitation of the teeth is achieved.

EFFECTS OF TWIN BLOCK TREATMENT

Although the twin block appliance has been used for twenty years, there have been few published studies of the treatment effects of twin block therapy. Those papers that have been published consist primarily of case reports.[3,4,56]

Four clinical investigations have considered the treatment effects of the twin block appliance. In contrast to

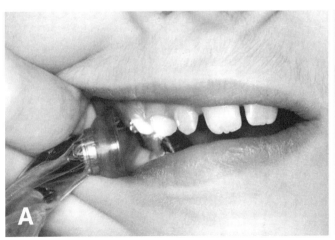
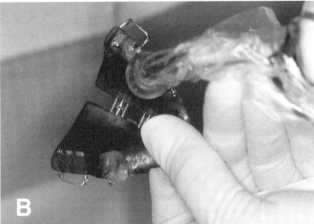

Figure 15-31. *A*, After the new bite registration has been attained, the soft acrylic is hardened intraorally with a curing light. *B*, Additional curing of the acrylic occurs extraorally.

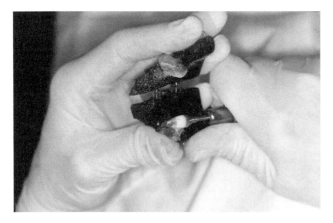

Figure 15-32. Excess acrylic is removed from the newly formed inclined planes by way of an acrylic bur in a low speed handpiece.

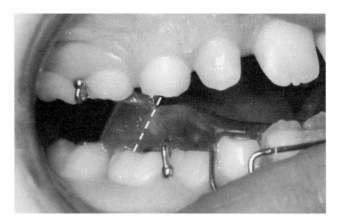

Figure 15-33. Intraoral view of the twin block appliance after reactivation has been completed. The dashed line indicates the new acrylic inclined plane on the maxillary appliance.

most previous studies of functional appliance therapy, these investigations compared the twin block patients to untreated Class II samples. Lund and Sandler[57] conducted a prospective clinical trial in which they compared 36 patients treated with the twin block to a control sample of 27 Class II patients who were on a waiting list to receive orthodontic treatment. In comparison to controls, the treated group demonstrated an increase in mandibular length. A difference in maxillary skeletal growth, however, could not be detected between the two groups. Lund and Sandler also noted distal movement of the maxillary molars, and the mandibular molars erupted in an anterior and superior direction in the twin block group. In addition, there was a significant amount of tipping of the anterior teeth in both arches in the treated group.

Mills and McCulloch[58] evaluated 28 consecutively treated patients from a private practice and compared them to a control group of 28 untreated Class II subjects from the *Burlington Growth Study*.[59] They noted an increase in mandibular length in the twin block group as well as significant increases in both anterior and posterior facial height, and a slight inhibition of forward maxillary growth. The maxillary molars were distalized in the twin block group, and some proclination of the mandibular incisors and lingual tipping of the maxillary incisors were noted as well.

Our group has completed a retrospective study of patients treated with twin block treatment.[60,61] In this study, the pre- and post-treatment cephalograms of 40 Class II patients treated with the twin block appliance were compared to those of 40 untreated Class II children from *The University of Michigan Growth Study*. In addition, the records of 40 patients treated with the

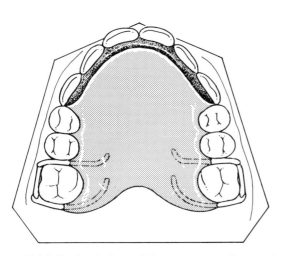

Figure 15-34. Occlusal view of the support appliance advocated by Clark.[5] The anterior bite plane is located just posterior to the incisors and canines.

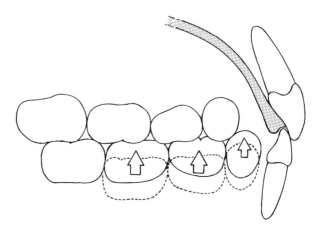

Figure 15-35. Sagittal view of the Clark support appliance. An inclined plane is present anteriorly to stabilize the bite as the canines and deciduous molars/premolars are allowed to erupt.

function regulator of Fränkel, from an earlier study of functional appliance therapy,[62] were used for comparisons. Compared with untreated subjects, the results of the study indicated that on an annualized basis the twin block appliance produced successful Class II correction through 2.5 mm of additional mandibular length, no inhibition of maxillary growth, and an increase in lower anterior facial height. In addition, dentoalveolar changes such as mandibular incisor proclination, maxillary incisor retrusion, distal movement of the maxillary molars, and extrusion of the mandibular posterior buccal segments were observed. In comparison, the Fränkel appliance produced similar effects, but to a smaller magnitude.

The results of this retrospective investigation indicated that the twin block appliance produced a mandibular response that was slightly greater in magnitude than that observed in our previous studies of functional appliance therapy.[44,62,63] It should be noted, however, that significant dentoalveolar responses also were noted in the twin block sample, including an inhibition of the normal downward and forward eruption of the maxillary posterior teeth and some mandibular incisor proclination. We anticipate that some of the dentoalveolar changes will rebound during a subsequent fixed appliance phase of treatment, as was observed in our previous study of two-phase treatment with the Herbst appliance.[63] The long-term results of twin block treatment remain unknown.

Finally, a recent cephalometric study by Baccetti and co-workers[64] evaluated skeletal and dentoalveolar changes induced by the twin block appliance in two groups of subjects with Class II malocclusion treated at different skeletal maturation stages in order to define the optimal timing for this type of therapy. Skeletal maturity in individual patients was assessed on the basis of the stages of cervical vertebrae maturation, as described in Chapter 5. The Early-Treated Group (ETG) was comprised of 21 subjects (11 females and 10 males). The mean age of ETG at Time 1 (T_1, immediately before treatment) was 9 years 0 months ±11 months, and at Time 2 (T_2, immediately after discontinuation of the twin block appliance) was 10 years 2 months ±11 months.

According to the cervical vertebrae maturation staging at T_1 and at T_2, the peak in growth velocity was not included in the treatment period for any of the subjects in the early group. The Late-Treated Group (LTG) consisted of 15 subjects (6 females and 9 males). Mean age of LTG was 12 years 11 months ±1 year 2 months at T_1 and 14 years 4 months ±1 year 3 months at T_2. In the LTG, treatment was performed during or slightly after the onset of the pubertal growth spurt. Both treated samples were compared with control samples consisting of subjects with untreated Class II malocclusions also selected on the basis of the stage in cervical vertebrae maturation.

The findings of this short-term cephalometric study indicate that optimal timing for twin block therapy of Class II disharmony is during or slightly after the onset of the pubertal peak in growth velocity. When compared with treatment performed before the peak, late twin block treatment produces more favorable effects that include: 1) greater skeletal contribution to molar correction, 2) larger increments in total mandibular length and in ramus height, 3) more posterior direction of condylar growth, leading to enhanced mandibular lengthening and to reduced forward displacement of the condyle in favor of effective skeletal changes.

CONCLUDING REMARKS

The purpose of this chapter has been to discuss the biological basis and clinical management of the twin block appliance, a functional jaw orthopedic appliance that has become increasingly popular with North American orthodontists. This appliance has many of the qualities of more traditional functional appliances and has been shown to increase the length of the mandible during the treatment period in comparison to untreated controls. This type of treatment has a sound biological basis, although the long-term effect of twin block treatment on craniofacial structures is not yet known.

One of the advantages of the twin block is the ability of the clinician to manipulate the vertical dimension in patients requiring bite opening during treatment. By judicious trimming of the posterior bite blocks, eruption of posterior teeth can be achieved in a controlled manner. The bite also can be advanced to an incisal "edge-to-edge" relationship or in a "step-by-step" manner, according to the protocol of choice.

Another perceived advantages of twin block treatment is improved patient cooperation in comparison to other removable functional appliances, such as the activator, bionator and FR-2 appliance of Fränkel. The appliance can be worn full-time, including while speaking and eating. Most patients have little difficulty in adapting to the appliance, especially if the bite has been opened sufficiently in the bite registration.

As with any new treatment approach, protocols are modified with time as more experience is gained in using the appliance and as both the short-term and long-term results of treatment become known. Our experience with the twin block appliance has been very encouraging thus far, and we expect that this treatment approach will find an appropriate place within the orthodontic and orthopedic appliance protocols available to the orthodontist.

REFERENCES CITED

1. Clark WJ. The twin block traction technique. Eur J Orthod 1982;4:129–138.
2. Clark WJ. The twin block technique. A functional orthopedic appliance system. Am J Orthod Dentofac Orthop 1988;93:1–18.
3. Clark WJ. The twin block technique. Part 1. Funct Orthod 1992;9:32–34, 36–37.
4. Clark WJ. The twin block technique. Part 2. Funct Orthod 1992;9:45–49.
5. Clark WJ. Twin block functional therapy. London: Mosby-Wolfe, 1995.
6. Clark WJ. The twin block technique. In: Graber TM, Rakosi T, Petrovic AG, eds. Dentofacial orthopedics with functional appliances. St. Louis: Mosby-Yearbook, 1997.
7. McNamara JA, Jr. Biological basis and clinical management of the twin block appliance. Rev d'Orthopéd Dento Faciale 1998;32:55–81.
8. McNamara JA, Jr. Aspectos práticos da utilização do "Twin Block." Ortodontia 1998;3:4–19.
9. Kingsley NW. A treatise on oral deformities as a branch of mechanical surgery. New York: D Appleton, 1880.
10. Rakosi T. The activator. In: Graber TM, Rakosi T, Petrovic AG, eds. Dentofacial orthopedics with functional appliances. St Louis: Mosby-Yearbook, 1997.
11. Schwarz AM, Gratzinger M. Removable orthodontic appliances. Philadelphia: WB Saunders, 1966.
12. Hotz RP. Application and appliance manipulation of functional forces. Am J Orthod 1970;58:459–478.
13. Oliver OA. A report of cases treated by use of lingual, labial appliances and guide plane. Int J Orthod 1932;18:1182–1190.
14. Oliver OA, Irish RE, Wood CR. Labio-lingual technik. St Louis: CV Mosby, 1940.
15. DeVincenzo JP, Huffer RA, Winn MW. A study in human subjects using a new device designed to mimic the protrusive functional appliances used previously in monkeys. Am J Orthod Dentofac Orthop 1987;91:213–224.
16. DeVincenzo JP, Winn MW. Orthopedic and orthodontic effects resulting from the use of a functional appliance with different amounts of protrusive activation. Am J Orthod Dentofac Orthop 1989;96:181–190.
17. DeVincenzo JP. Changes in mandibular length before, during, and after successful orthopedic correction of Class II malocclusions, using a functional appliance. Am J Orthod Dentofac Orthop 1991;99:241–257.
18. Breitner C. Experimentelle Veränderung der mesiodistalen Beziehungen der oberen und unteren Zahnreihen. Ztschr f Stomatol 1930;28:343–356.
19. Breitner C. Experimental change of the mesio-distal relations of the upper and lower dental arches. Angle Orthod. 1933;3:67–76.
20. Breitner C. The influence of moving deciduous teeth on permanent successors. Am J Orthod 1940;26:1152–1177.
21. Häupl K, Psansky R. Experimentelle Untersuchungen über Gelenktransformation bei Verwendung der Methoden der Funktionskieferorthopädie. Deutsche Zahn Mund Kieferheilkd 1939;6:439–448.
22. Hoffer O, Colico GL. Le modificazioni dell'A.T.M. conseguenti a spostamento mesiale della mandibola. Rass Int Stomatol Prat 1958;9 (Suppl 4):27–40.
23. Derichsweiler H. Experimentelle Tieruntersuchungen über Veränderungen des Kiefergelenkes bei Bisslageveränderung. Fortschr Kieferorthop 1958;19:30–44.
24. Baume LJ, Derichsweiler H. Is the condylar growth center responsive to orthodontic therapy? An experimental study in *Macaca mulatta*. Oral Surg Oral Med Oral Path 1961;14:347–362.
25. Hiniker J, Ramfjord S. Anterior displacement of the mandible in adult rhesus monkeys. J Pros Dent 1966;16:503–512.
26. Joho J-P. Changes in form and size of the mandible in the orthopaedically treated *Macacus Irus*: An experimental study. Trans Eur Orthod Soc 1968;44:161–173.
27. Stöckli PW, Willert HG. Tissue reactions in the temporomandibular joint resulting from anterior displacement of the mandible in the monkey. Am J Orthod 1971;60:142–155.
28. Lieb G. Application of the activator in rhesus monkey. Trans Europ Orthod Soc 1968;44:141–147.
29. Woodside DG, Metaxas A, Altuna G. The influence of functional appliance therapy on glenoid fossa remodeling. Am J Orthod Dentofac Orthop 1987;92:181–198.
30. Charlier JP, Petrovic AG. Recherches sur la mandibule de la rat en culture d'organs: le cartilage condylien a-t-il un potentiel de croissance indépendant? Orthod Franç 1967;38:165–175.
31. Charlier JP, Petrovic A, Herrmann-Stutzmann J. Effects of mandibular hyperpropulsion on the prechondroblastic zone of young rat condyle. Am J Orthod 1969;55:71–74.
32. Petrovic AG. Mechanisms and regulation of mandibular condylar growth. Acta Morphol Neerl Scand 1972;10:25–34.
33. Petrovic A. Experimental and cybernetic approaches to the mechanism of action of functional appliances on mandibular growth. In: McNamara JA, Jr, Ribbens KA, eds. Malocclusion and the periodontium. Ann Arbor: Monograph 15, Craniofacial Growth Series, Center for Human Growth and Development, University of Michigan, 1984.
34. Elgoyhen JC, Moyers RE, McNamara JA, Jr, Riolo ML. Craniofacial adaptation of protrusive function in young rhesus monkeys. Am J Orthod 1972;62:469–480.
35. McNamara JA, Jr. Neuromuscular and skeletal adaptations to altered function in the orofacial region. Am J Orthod 1973;64:578–606.
36. McNamara JA, Jr, Carlson DS. Quantitative analysis of temporomandibular joint adaptations to protrusive function. Am J Orthod 1979;76:593–611.
37. McNamara JA, Jr. Functional determinants of craniofacial size and shape. Eur J Orthod 1980;2:131–159.

38. McNamara JA, Jr, Bryan FA. Long-term mandibular adaptations to protrusive function: an experimental study in Macaca mulatta. Am J Orthod Dentofac Orthop 1987; 92:98–108.
39. Petrovic A, Stutzmann J, Gasson N. The final length of the mandible: Is it genetically determined? In: Carlson DS, ed. Craniofacial biology. Ann Arbor: Monograph 10, Craniofacial Growth Series, Center for Human Growth and Development, The University of Michigan, 1981.
40. Adams CP. The design and construction of removable orthodontic appliances. (3rd ed.) Bristol, England: John Wright and Sons, 1964.
41. Barrer HG. Protecting the integrity of mandibular incisor position through keystoning procedure and spring retainer appliance. J Clin Orthod 1975;9:486–494.
42. Howe RP. The bonded Herbst appliance. J Clin Orthod 1982;16:663–667.
43. McNamara JA, Jr, Howe RP. Clinical management of the acrylic splint Herbst appliance. Am J Orthod Dentofac Orthop 1988;94:142–149.
44. McNamara JA, Jr, Howe RP, Dischinger TG. A comparison of the Herbst and Fränkel appliances in the treatment of Class II malocclusion. Am J Orthod Dentofac Orthop 1990;98:134–144.
45. Spillane LM, McNamara JA, Jr. Maxillary adaptations following expansion in the mixed dentition. Semin Orthod 1995;1:176–187.
46. Brust EW, McNamara JA, Jr. Arch dimensional changes concurrent with expansion in mixed dentition patients. In: Trotman CA, McNamara JA, Jr, eds. Orthodontic treatment: Outcome and effectiveness. Ann Arbor: Monograph 30, Craniofacial Growth Series, Center for Human Growth and Development, The University of Michigan, 1995.
47. McNamara JA, Jr. Components of Class II malocclusion in children 8–10 years of age. Angle Orthod 1981;51: 177–202.
48. McNamara JA, Jr. Utility arches. J Clin Orthod 1986;20: 452–456.
49. Mulligan TF. Common sense mechanics. Phoenix: CSM, 1982.
50. Isaacson RJ, Lindauer SJ, Rubenstein LK. Activating a 2×4 appliance. Angle Orthod 1993;63:17–24.
51. Isaacson RJ, Lindauer SJ, Davidovitch M. The ground rules for archwire design. Semin Orthod 1995;1:3–11.
52. McNamara JA, Jr, Huge SA. The Fränkel appliance (FR-2): model preparation and appliance construction. Am J Orthod 1981;80:478–495.
53. Fränkel R, Fränkel C. Orofacial orthopedics with the function regulator. Munich: S Karger, 1989.
54. Leishman F. Personal communication, 1996.
55. Fränkel R. Lip seal training in the treatment of skeletal open bite. Eur J Orthod 1980;2:219–228.
56. Stangl D. A cephalometric analysis of six twin block patients—A study of mandibular (body and ramus) growth and development. Funct Orthod 1997;14:4,6,8,14,17–19, 21–22,24–25.
57. Lund DL, Sandler PJ. The effects of Twin Blocks: A prospective controlled study. Am J Orthod Dentofac Orthop 1998;113:104–110.
58. Mills C, McCulloch K. Treatment effects of the twin block appliance: A cephalometric study. Am J Orthod 1998;114: 15–24.
59. Popovich F, Thompson GW. Craniofacial templates for orthodontic case analysis. Am J Orthod 1977;71:406–420.
60. Ratner L. Treatment effects produced by the twin block appliance: A cephalometric investigation. Ann Arbor: Unpublished Master's thesis, Department of Orthodontics and Pediatric Dentistry, The University of Michigan, 1997.
61. Toth LR, McNamara JA, Jr. Treatment effects produced by the twin block appliance and the FR-2 appliance of Frankel compared to an untreated Class II sample. Am J Orthod Dentofac Orthop 1999;116:597–609.
62. McNamara JA, Jr., Bookstein FL, Shaughnessy TG. Skeletal and dental changes following functional regulator therapy on Class II patients. Am J Orthod 1985;88:91–110.
63. Lai M, McNamara JA, Jr. An evaluation of two-phase treatment with the Herbst appliance and preadjusted edgewise therapy. Semin Orthod 1998;4:46–58.
64. Baccetti T, Franchi L, Toth LR, McNamara JA, Jr. Treatment timing for twin block therapy. Am J Orthod Dentofac Orthop 2000;118:159-170.
65. McNamara JA, Jr. Fabrication of the acrylic splint Herbst appliance. Am J Orthod Dentofac Orthop 1988;94: 10–18.

Chapter 16

THE FUNCTION REGULATOR (FR-2) OF FRÄNKEL

The function regulator (FR) appliances (including the FR-2), developed by Rolf Fränkel of the former German Democratic Republic, are orthopedic exercise devices that aid in the maturation, training, and "reprogramming" of the orofacial neuromuscular system. This appliance system was developed according to the basic principles of Roux[1] concerning "functional orthopedics," principles that have been applied clinically in general orthopedics in medicine for many years. The FR appliances not only are constructed differently that other functional jaw orthopedic appliances (*e.g.*, the twin block, bionator, and activator that have much in common in their basic design), but more importantly the conceptual basis underlying the use of the FR appliances sets this treatment approach apart from other orthopedic and orthodontic philosophies and therapies.

Fränkel has based his treatment philosophy on the concept that the capacity to regulate growth resides in the soft tissue environment, and that adequate space must be available for the proper development of the hard tissues.[2–5] Thus, in contrast to most other removable appliances and all fixed appliances, all of which place forces directly on the hard tissues, treatment with the function regulator (Fig. 16-1) focuses primarily on the manipulation of the circumoral capsule. If there is inadequate development of the soft tissue capsule, the FR appliance acts to remove the restrictive forces that prevent the normal maturation of the maxilla and mandible from occurring in all three dimensions. This type of orthopedic exercise device has been designed to overcome functional disorders and reestablish physiologic conditions within the orofacial complex. Thus, the primary focus of treatment with this type of appliance is to establish a normal epigenetic milieu.[6–8]

Aberrant postural behavior of the orofacial musculature plays a primary role in the development of skeletal and dentoalveolar deformities. For example, in the treatment of patients with mandibular skeletal retrusion (Fig. 16-2), the major aim of functional orthopedics with the FR-2 is to overcome the poor postural performance of those muscles that determine the postural position of the mandible as well as mandibular movement. The vestibular shields and lower labial pads of the appliance (Figs. 16-1, 16-3) place gentle forces on the cheeks and lips. These parts of the appliance provide "sensory input" to the central nervous system (CNS), which in turn provokes neuromuscular changes to eliminate abnormal function and create an environment that will optimize normal growth processes.[4,5] The CNS acts to eliminate the pressure sensation by activation of the protractor musculature, and the mandible is carried in a downward and forward position.

Fränkel states that the creation of new space is essential for new growth to occur.[5] The change in the postural position of the mandible results in a number of positive treatment effects, with the displacement of the mandible the most important factor in the spontaneous development of the mandible. Further, one of the chief effects of FR therapy typically is expansion of the dental arches. Fränkel notes that the vestibular shields act directly on the circumoral capsule and only indirectly on the dentition, producing the typical broad arch form

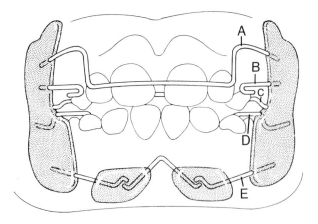

Figure 16-1. Frontal view of the FR-2 appliance. *A*, Upper labial wire. *B*, Canine extension. *C*, Upper lingual wire. *D*, Crossover wire to the lower lingual shield. *E*, Support wires to the lower labial pad. The vestibular shields and the lower labial pads also are visible.

that results from FR treatment.[4] Thus, treatment with the FR appliance promotes adaptations in the soft and hard tissues in all three dimensions.

Fränkel and Fränkel[4] stress that the FR appliances are not "orthodontic appliances" used for the correction of malocclusion. If movement of teeth through alveolar bone is desired, they state that the FR is inferior to other types of fixed or removable appliances in that precise tooth movement is not possible with the FR.

Fränkel and Fränkel[8] state that normal orofacial function can be achieved only when the training of the associated muscles, particularly those of the protractor group, begins slowly and is intensified gradually. Changes in mandibular postural position, and ultimately in the size and shape of the mandible, are not achieved through a mechanical advancement of the mandible but rather by modifications in the postural activity of the associated musculature, which before treatment demonstrates an "immature postural pattern."[8]

Fränkel and Fränkel[4] state that a training or retraining effect on the orofacial musculature can be achieved only if the appliance used for this purpose acts as a trainer. They make a sharp contrast between the FR and other so-called "functional appliances" such as the twin block, bionator, and Herbst appliances. The twin block and bionator, although thought to transmit "functional stimuli," constitutes a foreign body in the oral cavity. According to Fränkel and Fränkel:[4]

"Forces generated by muscles of the cheek, lip and tongue can only have the quality of "functional stimuli" if they are in natural and direct contact with the adjacent dentoalveolar structures and palate. The pressure exerted by any appliance, even if produced by muscular forces, is and remains an application of pressure and has nothing to do with a "functional stimulus." In terms of the orthodontic effect, there is, in principle, no difference whether forces press the appliances against the teeth and the supporting tissue as a result of a stretching of the muscular tissues or as a result of stretch-reflex contractions of the related muscles."[4]

Thus, Fränkel has developed a series of appliances designed according to the fundamental principle of oro-

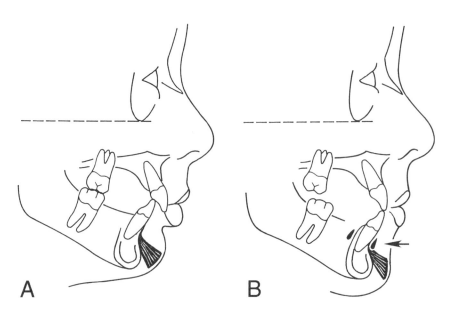

Figure 16-2. Alterations in the postural position of the mandible produced by the FR-2 appliance. *A*, Initial malocclusion. *B*, After the patient gradually has been brought forward to an end-to-end incisal position during treatment. Large bite advancements are avoided; the mandible is brought forward 2-3 mm in a step-by-step manner.

FUNCTION REGULATOR (FR-2) OF FRÄNKEL

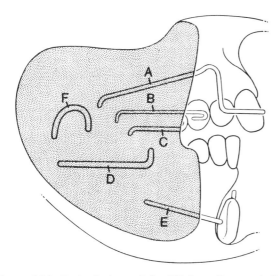

Figure 16-3. Sagittal view of the FR-2 appliance. *A*, Upper labial wire. *B*, Canine extension wire. *C*, Upper lingual wire. *D*, Extension of the crossover wire to the lower lingual shield. *E*, Support wire to the lower labial pads. *F*, Palatal/occlusal rest wire.

facial orthopedics, that is, optimizing the development of the orofacial structures, in part, by "removing restrictions or retardations in the accomplishment of growth patterns."[4] All Fränkel appliances are characterized not by large amounts of acrylic in the lingual and palatal areas (as the activator and bionator-type appliances) but rather by vestibular shields (Figs. 16-1, 16-3) that lie in the buccal vestibule outside of the dental arches. The appliances are constructed to act directly on the circumoral capsule, preventing faulty muscular functions and stimulating normal postural activity of all muscles that directly or indirectly help to establish a competent oral seal. The achievement of a competent lip seal is an essential aim of this type of functional orthopedic therapy. Lip seal training[6] (see Chapter 8) is used as an adjunct to orofacial orthopedics in the same way as physical therapy is used in general orthopedics.

TYPES OF APPLIANCES

Fränkel has described four main types of appliances.[2,4,9] The FR-1 and FR-2 appliances have been used most commonly in the treatment of Class II malocclusion, whereas the FR-3 appliance has been used in Class III patients, and the FR-1 and FR-4 appliances in patients with hyperdivergent facial patterns and anterior open bites.

Although Fränkel most often has described the use of the FR-1 appliance in the treatment of Class II malocclusion,[2,3,9–11] the FR-2 appliance is used most commonly today in the United States in the treatment of this type of problem. The FR-2 is similar in design to the FR-1 appliance except that a lingual wire has been added behind the upper incisors in the FR-2 appliance. A complete description of the FR-2 is provided in detail below.

PARTS OF THE APPLIANCE

The FR-2 appliance of Fränkel (Figs. 16-1 and 16-3) is composed of acrylic and wire. As mentioned earlier, the base of operation of the appliance is the buccal vestibule. The buccal (vestibular) shields and the lower labial pads act directly on the circumoral capsule to restrain and retrain any aberrant musculature and to remove restricting muscle forces from the dentition.

In the frontal view (Fig. 16-1), five wire components are visible. These wires include the upper labial wire, the canine extension, the upper lingual wire, the crossover wire to the lower lingual shield, and the support wires to the lower labial pads. Additionally, in sagittal view a portion of the palatal-occlusal rest wire also is seen, embedded in the vestibular shield (Fig. 16-3). Also apparent is the extension of the crossover wire to the lower lingual shield.

The maxillary view of the FR-2 appliance (Fig. 16-4) shows the orientation of the vestibular shields in their location 2.5–3.0 mm away from the maxillary alveolus. The upper lingual wire and the palatal wire are shown as well. The relationship of the lower labial pads to the lower lingual shield also can be seen in the mandibular view (Fig. 16-5), as can the lower lingual wires that lie on the cingula of the lower anterior teeth, presumably preventing these teeth from erupting during treatment.

TREATMENT EFFECTS PRODUCED BY THE FRÄNKEL APPLIANCE

As mentioned earlier, the wire and acrylic framework of the FR appliance is postulated to have several effects on the growing craniofacial region. These effects can be divided arbitrarily into two types: the effects on dentoalveolar development and the effects on skeletal development.

Dentoalveolar Development

The orientation of the teeth within a given dental arch can be viewed as being dependent, in part, on the interplay of the soft tissues (*e.g.*, lips, cheeks, tongue)

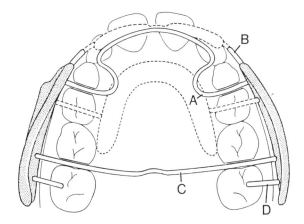

Figure 16-4. Maxillary occlusal view of the FR-2 appliance. *A*, Upper lingual wire. *B*, Canine extension. *C*, Palatal wire that is continuous with *D*, the occlusal rest on the upper first molars. The dashed lines indicate the outlines of the lower lingual shield and the crossover wires.

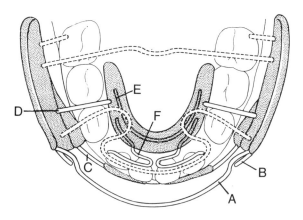

Figure 16-5. Mandibular occlusal view of the FR-2 appliance. *A*, Upper labial wire. *B*, Canine extension. *C*, Support wire to the lower labial pads. *D*, Crossover portion of support wire to the lower lingual shield that may be continuous with *E*, the base wire to the lower lingual shield. *F*, Lower lingual wires.

surrounding the arches. Fränkel[9] has stated that the developmental inhibition of the underlying skeletal structures that support the teeth is related causally to the circumoral soft tissue capsule, which determines the displacement of the teeth and bones.

The FR-2 appliance appears to have three effects on the dentition and the associated musculature that result in passive expansion of the dental arches (Fig. 16-6). First, the cheeks are held away from the dentition by the vestibular shields (Fig. 16-7); and, second, the tongue becomes relatively more of a force because the counterbalancing force of the cheek musculature is shielded. According to Fränkel,[10,12] the third effect of the FR-2 is produced by the vertical extensions of the vestibular shields. He hypothesizes that the vertical extensions of the shields cause a stretch on the alveolar mucosa, expanding the circumoral capsule, with subsequent tension produced on the periosteum. This tension results in new bone deposition occurring on the lateral borders of the alveolus, while at the same time inappropriate patterns of neuromuscular function are eliminated.

It is well known that applying tension on the periosteum can result in new bone deposition, as has been shown in animal studies[13-15] (Fig. 16-8). In addition, an investigation by Brieden and colleagues[16] of Fränkel patients in whom maxillary metallic implants had been placed has demonstrated that most of the widening of the maxilla associated with Fränkel treatment is due to deposition of new bone along the lateral border of the alveolus, rather than increased growth at the midpalatal suture.

A recent experimental study of the periosteal-pull hypothesis by Sotiriadou and Johnston,[17] however, cast doubt on this mechanism. These investigators concluded that, at least in their rat model, unbalanced tongue pressure, rather than periosteal traction, probably was responsible for the expansion produced by the buccal shields used in their experiment.

Typical findings in patients treated with the Fränkel appliance include a broadening of the arch form and relative increases in arch width, particularly in the posterior region. Fränkel explains that the mechanism by which arch expansion occurs is related to a change in the biomechanical forces produced by the circumoral capsule on the dentition. As a tooth erupts, it follows the path of least resistance.[18,19] If the biomechanical forces are altered during treatment by changing the circumoral capsule and the function of the CNS, the path of eruption of the tooth can be affected.

In the maxillary arch, eruption of the posterior dentition usually occurs buccally and inferiorly (Fig. 16-9). In contrast, the posterior teeth in the mandible normally tend to erupt not only vertically but also lingually.[20] Fränkel[9] postulates that removal of the buccal muscular forces by altering the circumoral capsule allows for an uprighting of the lower posterior teeth during eruption. Fränkel and co-workers[8] note that a different path of tooth eruption occurs in the lower arches in patients treated with the Fränkel appliance than normally occurs in untreated individuals, with a less lingually directed pattern of lower tooth eruption noted in the former.

Fränkel theorizes that his appliance system is especially valuable when treatment begins in the early mixed dentition. The appliance can utilize the ability of an erupting tooth to act as a "matrix" for alveolar growth.[12] Fränkel states that the developmental stage

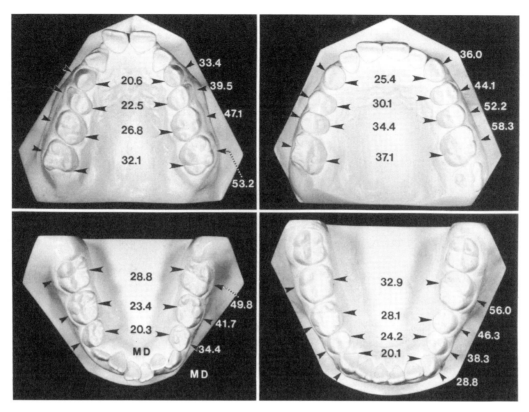

Figure 16-6. Typical arch changes seen during FR treatment. This female patient was treated with an FR-2 appliance for 36 months. Initial records (left) were taken when the patient was 9 years 9 months of age; the second set of records (right) was taken when the patient was 12 years 0 months of age. (From McDougall and co-workers.[21])

most amenable to arch expansion occurs before and during the time of eruption of the permanent canines and premolars.

Studies of Arch Expansion

Changes during Treatment

Statistical investigations of results of Fränkel therapy have been limited, particularly with regard to the development of the dental arches. Mosch (cited in Fränkel[10]) evaluated the treatment effects in 400 patients treated only with the Fränkel appliance. He observed that as a result of withholding cheek pressure through the use of the vestibular shields and the lower labial pads, a spontaneous widening of the dental arches occurred routinely. Mosch noted a mean increase in transpalatal width of over 4 mm in both the premolar and molar regions during a two-year treatment time. No data regarding mandibular arch expansion were published.

Our group also has published a study of arch width development in Class II patients treated with Fränkel's appliance.[21] Serial dental casts from 60 patients treated with the Fränkel appliance were compared to serial dental casts from 47 untreated individuals from the *University of Michigan Elementary and Secondary Growth Study*. The maxillary and mandibular dental arches expanded routinely when the FR-2 appliance was worn conscientiously. The expansion was not limited to a particular region of the dental arch. In absolute terms, the greatest amount of expansion occurred in the premolar and molar regions, whereas a lesser amount occurred in the canine region. The average amount of posterior expansion was 4–5 mm and 3–4 mm in the maxillary and mandibular arches, respectively.[21] These amounts of expansion of course are helpful in the treatment of borderline extraction cases, but will not resolve tooth-size/arch-size discrepancies characterized by severe crowding, particularly in the lower arch.

Post-Treatment Stability

Few long-term studies examining the stability of dental arch expansion following treatment with the Fränkel appliance have been published. Fränkel and Fränkel[4] report on a sample of 80 patients with severe tooth-

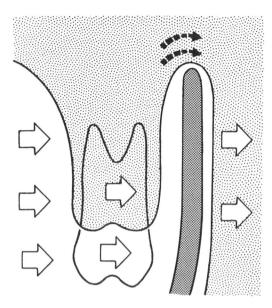

Figure 16-7. Schematic view of the vestibular shields of the FR appliance. Note that the cheek musculature is shielded from the teeth by the vestibular shield. The vestibular shield also extends superiorly, putting tension on the periosteum of the lateral alveolar region. In addition, the arrows on the left indicate the force of the tongue against the dentition (adapted from Fränkel[9]).

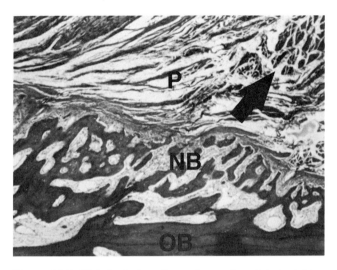

Figure 16-8. Histological section of experimental stretching of the periosteum, resulting in new bone deposition. P, periosteum; OB, older bone; NB, newly formed bone. The arrow indicates the direction of tension placed on the periosteum. (Photo courtesy of Ben Moffett.)

size/arch-size discrepancies and narrow arches. All patients were treated with either the FR-1 or FR-2 appliance and were deemed satisfactory cooperators. The treatment began at an average of eight years of age, and the appliance was worn for approximately 2½ years for at least 18 hours per day and then as a retainer for an additional two years, at which time a second set of records were taken. A third set of records was obtained at an average age of 18 years, with the patients at least 4½ years out of retention.

There was approximately 5 mm of expansion between the upper first premolars and upper first molars at the end of the retention period (Table 16-1). Four years and 8 months out of retention, there was a range of −0.8 mm to −1.6 mm change in intra-arch dimension, indicating approximately 75–80% long-term retention in maxillary arch width. In the mandible, a 3.3–4.0 mm increase in arch width was seen (Table 16-1). At the time of the third set of records, there was an average 1 mm loss of arch width in the premolar region and −0.3 to −0.8 mm in the molar region, indicating that, in general, the arch width increases obtained during FR treatment were stable over the long term.

In 1979, we had the opportunity to examine another sample of patients treated at Fränkel's clinic in Zwickau in the then German Democratic Republic. The serial dental casts of twenty randomly selected patients were analyzed, with three sets of study models available that were taken at approximately the same intervals as cited in the previous study[4] (pre-treatment, at the end of retention, and 4½ years out of post-retention). Both buccal and lingual measurements and width were obtained (Fig. 16-10). During the treatment period, the average expansion observed in the maxilla was 3.0 mm in the canine region, 5.7 mm in the first premolar region, and 4.6 mm in the first molar region (Table 16-2). The expansion occurring in the mandible was less than in the maxilla. The average values range from 2.1 mm in the canine area to 3.9 mm in the first premolar region to 2.9 mm in the first molar region (Table 16-2). Minimal changes in arch dimensions were observed during the four and one-half years post-retention period. (No change between the second set of dental casts and the third set of dental casts

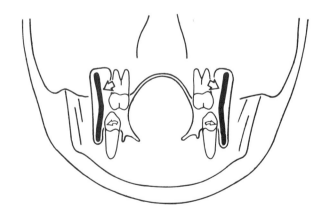

Figure 16-9. The effect of the vestibular shield in eliminating cheek pressure against the dentition, allowing for a spontaneous expansion to the upper and lower dental arches.

Table 16-1. Long-term post-retention stability of maxillary and mandibular expansion in millimeters (from Fränkel and Fränkel[4]).

Sex	Region	N	Expansion at the end of retention		Expansion at 4 yr, 8 mo out of retention		Post-retention relapse	
			Mean	S.D.	Mean	S.D.	Mean	S.D.
Maxillary								
F	4—4	37	5.3	1.7	3.7	1.5	−1.6	0.9
M	4—4	34	5.5	1.7	4.7	1.9	−0.8	1.4
F	6—6	45	5.0	1.7	3.7	1.6	−1.3	1.3
M	6—6	35	5.6	1.5	4.8	1.8	−0.8	1.0
Mandibular								
F	4—4	27	3.3	1.4	2.2	1.3	−1.1	0.7
M	4—4	23	4.0	2.0	2.9	2.4	−1.1	1.4
F	6—6	31	3.7	1.7	2.9	1.8	−0.8	0.9
M	6—6	28	3.9	1.5	3.6	2.1	−0.3	1.3

would be measured as 0.0 mm.) Although a few instances of decreases in arch dimensions were observed (Table 16-3), the average patient exhibited slight increases in arch dimensions during the post-retention period.

Cephalometric Studies

In the treatment of a Class II, division 1 malocclusion, the FR-2 appliance prompts a forward position of the lower jaw. This change in postural activity ultimately leads to a correction of the malocclusion, due in part to a change in the maxillo-mandibular relationship (Fig. 16-11). Both skeletal and dentoalveolar adaptations occur.

Falck[22] studied the long-term effect of FR treatment on the skeletal and dental structures of the craniofacial complex. The material of this study consisted of serial lateral cephalograms of 103 children with a Class II malocclusion associated with mandibular retrusion, 58 of whom were treated with either the FR-1 or FR-2 appliance. Forty-five untreated subjects monitored longitudinally served as controls. A comparison of pretreatment morphology indicated that the two groups were almost identical at the beginning of the study period. The patients were followed from 7 years, 6 months to 15 years, 5 months for the treated group, and 7 years 9 months to 15 years 1 month for the controls. Using the occipital reference system developed by Fränkel,[6,22] a 14 mm forward movement of pogonion in the treated group was measured. In the untreated Class II sample that was evaluated during the same time interval, an increase in mandibular length of 7.3 mm was observed, indicating that a statistically (and clinically) significant difference in mandibular growth increments was observed between the two groups.

Fränkel and Fränkel[4] reanalyzed a portion of the patients in Falck's study, using the cephalometric analysis described in Chapter 28.[23] They reported an increase in

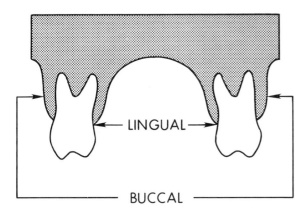

Figure 16-10. Buccal and lingual measurements of the study models. The buccal measurements were made 4 mm above the gingival margin.

Table 16-2. Changes in maxillary and mandibular arch widths during treatment.

	Lingual (N=20)				Buccal (N=16)			
	Mean	S.D.	Min	Max	Mean	S.D	Min	Max
Maxillary								
3—3	3.0	1.4	0.7	6.0	1.8	2.1	22.7	6.3
4—4	5.7	1.9	2.9	9.6	4.2	2.6	−2.4	7.4
6—6	4.6	2.1	0.9	8.8	4.2	2.4	−2.6	7.5
Mandibular								
3—3	2.1	1.8	−2.0	4.7	2.0	1.5	−0.9	4.4
4—4	3.9	1.8	1.2	7.8	3.3	1.3	1.3	6.3
6—6	2.9	1.5	−0.1	5.6	1.5	1.1	0	3.3

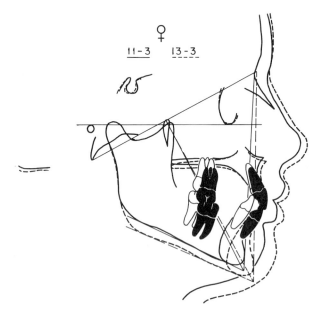

Figure 16-11. Typical skeletal changes produced by treatment of the FR-2 appliance. The superimposition of the tracings is along the basion-nasion line at the intersection of the pterygomaxillary suture.

Table 16-3. Adaptations in arch widths four and one-half years post-retention (in mm).

	Lingual (N=20)				Buccal (N=16)			
	Mean	S.D	Min	Max	Mean	S.D.	Min	Max
Maxillary								
3—3	0.7	1.4—	1.6	4.7	0.5	1.0	−0.4	3.2
4—4	−0.1	1.4—	2.0	3.1	0.3	1.2	−1.4	2.7
6—6	0.7	1.7—	0.9	5.1	0.3	0.8	−1.1	2.4
Mandibular								
3—3	0.1	1.0—	2.1	2.7	−0.01	1.1	−1.6	4.7
4—4	0.6	1.8—	1.7	5.0	0.01	1.4	−1.7	3.7
6—6	0.1	1.3—	1.4	2.9	−0.2	0.8	−2.1	1.4

mandibular length of 18.9 mm in the FR group as compared to 13.8 mm in the untreated group, a difference that again was statistically significant (Table 16-4). No statistically significant difference was noted in maxillary length or in lower anterior facial height between the two groups; however, posterior facial height (ramus length) was greater in the FR group, and the facial axis angle closed in the FR group, indicating a more horizontal vector of facial growth occurring in the FR patients. Fränkel[24] also states that *decreases* of lower facial height occur routinely if FR treatment is accompanied by an adequate regimen of lip seal training.

McNamara and co-workers[25] studied 100 patients treated with the Fränkel appliance. They divided the sample chronologically into a younger group (8.5 years of age at the beginning of treatment) and an older group (11.5 years at the beginning of treatment). These patients were compared to 41 untreated controls from the *University of Michigan Growth Study*, again divided by chronological age. Greater increases in mandibular growth increments were noted in the older treated group than in the younger treated group, and both treatment groups had larger mandibular growth increments than their respective matched control groups. Both treated groups showed an increase in lower anterior facial height, but no change in the mandibular plane angle or in maxillary position in comparison to controls.

A later study by McNamara and co-workers[26] compared patients treated with the Fränkel and with the acrylic splint Herbst appliance in comparison to untreated Class II controls. Greater dentoalveolar adaptation was produced by the acrylic splint Herbst appliance than by the Fränkel appliance. Similarly, a recent investigation by Toth and McNamara[27] that compared the FR-2 appliance with the twin block appliance of

Table 16-4. Cephalometric analysis using the method of McNamara (1984). Average changes of parameters in the FR group (n=36) and the comparison group (n=34) (from Fränkel and Fränkel[4])

Variables (in mm)	FR Group		Untreated		
	Mean	S.D.	Mean	S.D.	Sig.
Maxillary Length	9.5	3.3	8.5	2.4	NS
Mandibular Length	18.9	4.8	13.8	5.1	***
Maxillo-Mand. Differ.	9.4	2.6	5.3	3.9	***
N. Perp.-Point A	−0.1	1.6	0.4	1.6	NS
N. Perp.-Pogonion	6.1	3.8	2.6	3.8	***
Lower Ant. Facial Height	6.8	3.0	5.9	3.7	NS
Ramus Length	11.7	4.0	8.7	3.9	**
Facial Axis Angle (Ricketts)	1.8	2.4	0.2	2.7	**

**=p<0.01   ***=p<0.0001   NS = not significant

Clark also resulted in more dentoalveolar adaptations with the twin block appliance.

Only one study[28] has dealt with the use of the functional regulator in non-growing patients. A prospective clinical trial was initiated on five adult patients, three of whom completed at least one year of FR treatment. Although dentoalveolar adaptations were observed (including arch expansion, a lingual tipping of the upper incisors, and a labial tipping of the lower incisors), no significant increases in mandibular length were documented. The treatment effect in these adult patients was not great enough to resolve the underlying skeletal discrepancy, indicating the age-dependent response of this treatment. Thus, the use of FR appliances in adults with Class II malocclusion does not seem appropriate, unless relaxation of the buccal and perioral musculature is desired as a major part of the treatment.

CLINICAL MANAGEMENT OF THE FR-2 APPLIANCE

Dental Decompensation

As with other functional appliance therapy, many Class II patients require some decompensation of the dental arches before the onset of FR-2 treatment. For example, in instances of severe maxillary constriction, rapid maxillary expansion with a bonded or banded appliance is recommended. Schwarz appliances and lip bumpers also have been used before FR treatment to address underlying tooth-size/arch-size problems in the mandible and maxilla.

Further decompensation often is accomplished with fixed appliances to align the upper and lower anterior teeth. Following the banding of the molars, various types of utility arches (see Chapter 11) can procline and intrude the upper incisors as well as intrude and sometimes retract the lower anterior teeth. A transpalatal arch also can correct the position of severely rotated upper first molars.

The same care should be taken in managing dental decompensation before the use of an FR-2 appliance, as would be used in the presurgical management of an orthognathic surgical patient. Steps should be taken to avoid dental interferences, particularly when the lower jaw is postured forward. In a patient with a short lower anterior facial height, it is not necessary, and in fact not advisable, to intrude the lower incisors before treatment. In a patient who has a neutral or especially a long lower anterior facial height, however, it may be necessary to intrude the upper or lower anterior teeth (or both) prior to functional Jaw orthopedics (FJO) to avoid an unwanted opening of the vertical dimension. To optimize the anterior repositioning of the chin during FJO treatment, increases in the vertical dimension should be controlled. Fränkel[24] states that in patients with increased lower facial height (particularly open bites), the FR-1 should be used to provide "forward rotation," thus minimizing lower facial height increases.

After the dental arches have been decompensated appropriately, all upper and lower appliances are removed before impression-taking. In addition to the impressions obtained for the fabrication of the Fränkel appliance (to be described below), an additional set of impressions should be taken for the fabrication of invisible retainers (see Chapter 27). These thin plastic overlays are used to stabilize the occlusion during the time of appliance fabrication. Invisible retainers also are used during the appliance break-in period, during which time the patient becomes accustomed to wearing the FR-2 appliance. For the first month or so, the patient should wear the invisible retainers whenever the Fränkel appliance is not being worn.

Impression Technique

Successful Fränkel therapy depends on the fit and comfort of the appliance; thus, proper impression technique is of the utmost importance. When the appliance is in place, the edges of the vestibular shield and the lip pads should closely approximate the soft tissue. A properly fabricated appliance will have superior and inferior borders of the vestibular shields that will encroach slightly on the patient's resting vestibular sulcus, vertically and horizontally. Therefore, an impression tray that does not overextend or laterally distort the associated soft tissue should be used. Lateral distortion of the soft tissue prevents the proper extension of the flange of the impression tray deep into the vestibular sulcus and in the anterior lingual region.

The selection of the impression tray is critical. Every attempt should be made to adapt the tray as closely as possible to the facial and lingual surfaces of the dental arch. Ideally, custom trays should be made for each patient, particularly for the mandibular dental arch. Thermal-sensitive trays also have been used,[29-31] but such trays currently are not available commercially.

Many clinicians rely on the use of standard aluminum trays for taking FR-2 impressions. Care must be taken to ensure that the tray does not encroach on the soft tissue, particularly in the lower lingual region. The mucosa in this region can be distorted easily, if the edge of the tray presses against it. The aluminum tray is trimmed before impression-taking to ensure that no part of the tray touches the soft tissue. In addition, a bead of tray wax is placed along the posterior vestibular region to establish in wax the eventual lower border of the vestibular shield. Wax is placed along the lower lingual aspect of the impression tray as needed.

Impressions should be taken using alginate impression material. Because a close fitting tray is used in the impression-taking procedure, a lesser amount of impression material usually is required than for impressions for study models. An adequate mandibular impression (Fig. 16-12) is characterized by the reproduction of the dental and soft tissue anatomy of the region. The impression material in the lower anterior region should not be too thick; otherwise, an inadequate reproduction of the lower anterior region is maintained. The patient is instructed not to lift the tongue, as lifting the tongue may distort the lingual attachment, thus giving a faulty reading in a critical area of future acrylic application.[32]

Particular care must be taken with the fit of the tray in the lower anterior region of the vestibule. If the impression tray lies too far anterior to the labial alveolus, distortion of the vestibule will occur. In fact, it is nearly impossible to obtain an adequate impression of the lower labial vestibular region with virtually any type of impression tray. Thus, preparation of the work model is necessary to ensure proper fit of the lower labial pad (to be discussed later).

The accuracy of the maxillary impression (Fig. 16-13) is not as critical as that of the mandibular impression, although care must be taken to reproduce the soft tissue attachments, particularly in the canine/first premolar region. Because 2.5–3.0 mm of wax relief will be placed in the lateral aspect of the maxillary alveolus, the accuracy of the lateral extent of the impression is not as critical as in the lower anterior region. The depth of the maxillary vestibule, however, must be reproduced accurately so that the proper extent of the vestibular region is reproduced in the vestibular shields of the appliance. The clinician is cautioned against using "extended" trays because of the danger of distorting the soft tissue, and, thus, overextending the contours of the vestibular shields. Lateral overextension will reduce the depth of the vestibule.

Registration Bite

A proper construction bite is essential to good appliance fabrication. The construction bite, usually taken with horseshoe wafers of medium hard wax (Fig. 16-14A), must orient the upper and lower dental arches in all three planes of space. An incorrect spatial relationship of the upper and lower work models during appliance fabrication may result in a FR-2 appliance that will not fit the patient and may cause unwanted treatment results.

In the treatment of Class II malocclusions, Fränkel[4] recommends that the mandible be advanced no more than 2.0–2.5 mm at any one time, although other clinicians have advocated larger initial bite advancements. Fränkel[7] has emphasized the need for a "step-by-step" advancement of the lower jaw in order to stay within the physiological limits of the associated neuromuscular system. A 2.5–3.0 mm vertical clearance also is necessary in the premolar region to allow for the crossover wire to the lower lingual shield to pass through the interocclusal space.

The mandible may have to be advanced again one or more times in order to correct the underlying skeletal

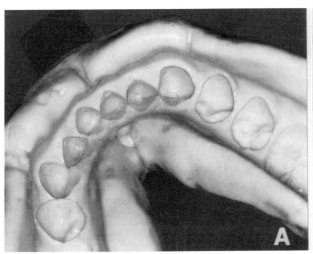
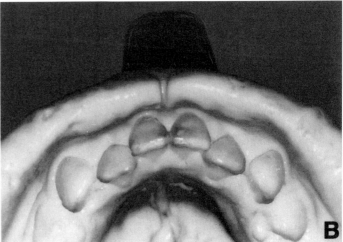

Figure 16-12. Typical mandibular impression. Note relative thickness of alginate in lower labial area. Excessive thickness of the alginate should be avoided. A, Overview. B, Close-up of anterior region of another impression.

FUNCTION REGULATOR (FR-2) OF FRÄNKEL

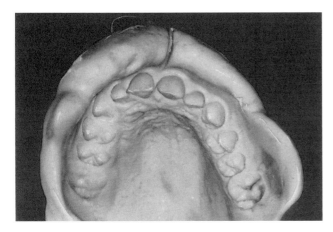

Figure 16-13. Typical maxillary impression. Note that the areas of soft tissue attachment, particularly in the first deciduous molar regions, have been reproduced.

discrepancy. The advancement usually is implemented three to four months following the achievement of full-time appliance wear. The technique of advancing the FR-2 will be discussed later in this chapter.

A number of techniques have been advocated for obtaining the proper bite advancement, including the Projet™ bite fork method described in the previous chapter. The following is a description of another method of bite registration that has been used successfully by us for over 25 years.

The patient is seated upright in the dental chair when the wax bite is taken. The patient is instructed to place his or her jaw in a forward position. The amount of bite advancement is determined by the clinician. A patient mirror may be useful in some instances in helping the patient visualize the desired mandibular position. The patient is told to align the upper and lower midlines in order to achieve symmetrical bite advancement, unless there is a dental asymmetry.

Three thicknesses of yellow wax (Great Lakes Orthodontic Products, Tonawanda NY) are softened and pressed together (Fig. 16-14A), and the wax horseshoe wafer is pressed against the maxillary teeth. The patient then brings the mandible forward to the desired position and closes into the wax (Fig. 16-14B and 16-15). After the proper bite registration is obtained, the lateral portions of the wax are compressed against the teeth to ensure an adequate bite registration in all three planes of space. The wax bite is removed and evaluated. If a current set of study models is available, the wax bite should be placed on the study models to check the amount of bite advancement.

In most instances, dental midlines are symmetrical and require equal bilateral advancement. If the dental midlines are asymmetrical (*e.g.,* early loss of a lower deciduous canine), however, the construction bite should reflect symmetrical mandibular advancement and a dental midline asymmetry. This dental asymmetry usually is corrected later with fixed appliances, although occasionally a spontaneous correction of dental asymmetry during Fränkel treatment is observed. If a skeletal mandibular asymmetry has no dental component, the bite registration is taken so that the dental midlines coincide. In effect, this construction bite corrects for the asymmetrical mandible by advancing one side of the mandible more than the other.

Preparation of Work Models

After the impressions have been obtained, they are poured in either plaster or stone with sufficient base to

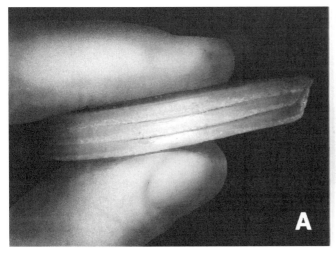
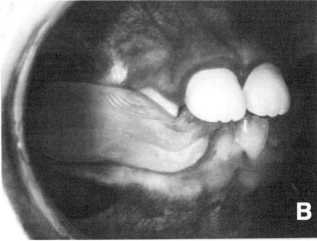

Figure 16-14. Construction bite registration for FR-2 appliance. Three thicknesses of yellow wax are compressed laterally after the bite registration has been achieved (from McNamara[30]).

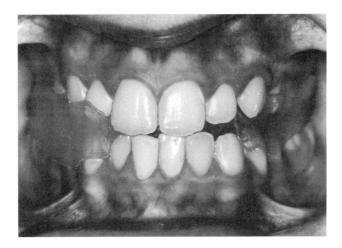

Figure 16-15. Intraoral view of wax bite registration. Note that no wax covers the incisors so that the clinician can monitor the midlines and the amount of bite opening easily. The wax is pressed against the teeth posteriorly.

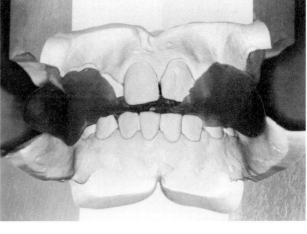

Figure 16-16. Trimmed work models used in the construction of the FR-2 appliance. Significant carving has been performed in the lower anterior region and in the region of the maxillary buccal segment.

allow for trimming in a manner similar to that used for orthodontic study models. An inadequate base can preclude the proper carving of the models at a later stage. The models then should be roughly trimmed with the construction bite in place. The wax bite is removed, and each model is prepared individually. As long as the basic trimming procedures are implemented properly, it is better to overtrim the work model slightly, because the borders of the shield can be shortened at the time of appliance delivery.[24]

The distance from the lateral extension of the base of the model to the alveolar surface should be at least 5 mm. This distance will allow for the proper application of wax relief and acrylic later. Also, the posterolateral corners of the model base should not be trimmed too closely, as doing so will make the placement of the wax relief in the region of the last molar difficult. The clinician also should evaluate the lower lingual region to ensure adequate extension for the fabrication of the lower lingual shield.

Mandibular Model

The first step in trimming the mandibular work model is to remove the flash with either a laboratory knife or a rotary instrument. No major changes should be made in the lateral sulcus areas that have been defined earlier by the impression. The removal of bubbles in this region usually is all the preparation that is necessary.

Carving will be needed in the lower anterior region so that the proper inferior and posterior extensions of the lower labial pads can be achieved (Fig. 16-16). The lower labial region is carved with a pear-shaped carbide bur and a laboratory knife, usually defining the inferior border of the lower labial region 3–4 mm in an inferior direction. The outline of the carving proceeds laterally and slightly inferiorly from the midline frenum.

Maxillary Model

Similarly, the removal of flash is necessary on the maxillary model. Some of the anatomical regions also must be defined, particularly in the area of the tuberosity that lies posterior to the muscle attachments located over the first premolar or first deciduous molar. In addition, the region superior to the canine and anterior to the area of soft tissue attachment is defined (Fig. 16-16).

Checking the Adequacy of the Bite Registration

After trimming, the adequacy of the wax bite is checked. The models are placed on a piece of paper (*e.g.,* the back of the laboratory prescription sheet), and the superior and inferior borders of the model are marked. The wax bite is removed from the work models, and the work models are placed back into the position indicated on the paper. The amount of vertical opening, both anteriorly and posteriorly, then can be assessed. As mentioned earlier, about three millimeters of vertical clearance is necessary in the posterior region to allow clearance for the crossover wires to the lower lingual shield. If the bite registration is inadequate, the wax bite should be retaken.

Laboratory Instructions

Prescription sheets for the FR-2 appliance vary from laboratory to laboratory, but there are specific parameters that must be described on any prescription sheet. The type of appliance (*e.g.*, FR-2) and the amount of wax relief needed is indicated. Usually, the standard amount of wax relief for the FR-2 appliance is 2.5–3.0 mm in the maxillary vestibular area and 0.5 mm in the mandibular vestibular area. In certain situations, however, other thicknesses of wax relief are desired. For example, only minimal wax relief is needed in the upper arch in an instance of a telescopic bite in which the lower teeth are trapped in a lingual orientation relative to the upper teeth.

The laboratory prescription sheet also indicates whether the teeth are to be notched. Notching is recommended strongly by Fränkel,[9] as well as by us, because the notches facilitate a positive seating of the appliance on the maxillary dental arch. The notching of the deciduous teeth helps prevent unwanted lingual tipping of the maxillary incisors during treatment. If notching is requested, the laboratory will place grooves along the distal surface of the upper canine, the mesial surface of the upper first deciduous molar, and the distal surface of the upper second deciduous molar (Fig. 16-17).

Obviously, the upper permanent first molars are not notched. If there are permanent premolars or canines present, these teeth could be notched on the model, though not in the mouth. In patients with a permanent dentition, the appliance usually seats spontaneously during the first few months of appliance wear. Elastomeric separators placed mesial to the upper first molars and distal to the canines are recommended to open the space before the placement of the appliance.[24]

FABRICATION OF THE APPLIANCE

The FR-2 appliance, as with other types of Fränkel appliances, usually is fabricated by a well-trained technician in a commercial laboratory rather than in an in-office laboratory. A step-by-step construction of the appliance is provided by Fränkel[4,9] and McNamara and Huge.[29]

After the FR-2 has been received from the laboratory, the appliance and work model should be checked to verify that they are delivered to the correct patient and that the proper type of Fränkel appliance has been constructed. The finished appliance should be placed on the work model, and all wires are checked for accuracy of placement, as wires can become distorted easily during the finishing process.

The acrylic borders also are checked on the models

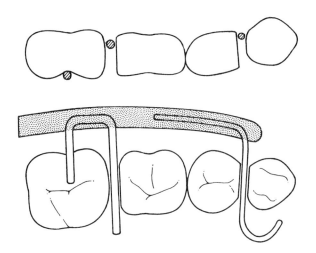

Figure 16-17. Notching the deciduous teeth. Fränkel and Fränkel[4,24] recommend disking the deciduous teeth to the depth of the gingival margin.

for accuracy. The anterior edge of the superior portion of the vestibular shield, when viewed from the side, extends forward in front of the maxillary buccal muscle attachment to approximate the middle of the canine. This portion of the shield should be well rounded. The anterior edge of the inferior portion of the vestibular shield extends anteriorly to the distal aspect of the maxillary canine.

In the posterior region, the appliance should extend beyond the last erupted tooth, usually the upper first molar. With the appliance seated on the work models, the heels should be checked again with a straight edge. By doing so, the accuracy of appliance fit can be assessed.

APPLIANCE DELIVERY

At the time of the appliance delivery, the patient is shown how to insert the FR-2 appliance by holding the cheek with one or two fingers and then inserting the appliance into the mouth with the other hand. The appliance should fit in all dimensions except for a slight vertical opening that will be eliminated when the deciduous teeth are notched.

Notching the Teeth

The clinician performs the notching of the deciduous teeth at the time of appliance delivery, by means of a 1.5 mm diameter diamond cylinder in a high-speed handpiece (Fig. 16-18*A*), or a #1156 carbide bur or a diamond disk in a low-speed handpiece (Fig. 16-18*B*) can be used to notch the appropriate teeth; this notching usually is performed without anesthesia. The notching should be

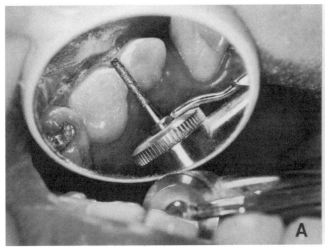 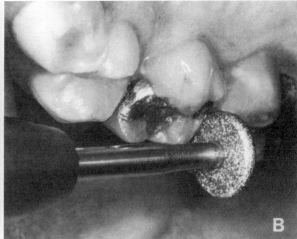

Figure 16-18. Notching of the deciduous teeth. *A*, Diamond cylinder in a high-speed handpiece. *B*, Diamond disk in a low-speed handpiece.

deep enough to provide a positive fit of the appliance on the maxillary teeth in order to avoid unwanted lingual tipping of the anterior teeth. Fränkel and Fränkel[24] recommend that the notching be made through the enamel of the deciduous teeth down to the level of the gingival margin (Fig. 16-17). The notching provides a posterior seat and keeps the appliance in a fixed reference position in the maxillary arch. If there is not an anteroposterior reference position for the appliance, the appliance may slip lingually, causing a retrusion of the upper incisors.

As mentioned earlier, the permanent teeth can be notched on the work model in order to facilitate spontaneous seating of the appliance between the permanent teeth. Separators can be used to provide initial spacing in this region. A transpalatal arch can also be used to rotate the molars distally, thus creating space distal to the upper second premolars.

Intraoral Evaluation of Appliance Fit

After the teeth have been notched, the fit of the appliance is checked (Figs. 16-19 and 16-20). The clinician should place the appliance in the mouth of the patient and evaluate the fit of the appliance on the maxillary dental arch, pushing firmly upward on the appliance with finger pressure. The palatal and upper lingual wires of the appliance should lie on either side of the deciduous molars in patients with grooves cut into the deciduous teeth during the notching procedure (Fig. 16-18 and 16-21*A*) or on either side of the premolars in patients in the permanent dentition (Fig. 16-21*B*). Sore

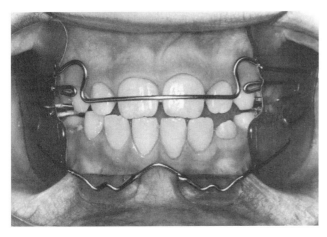 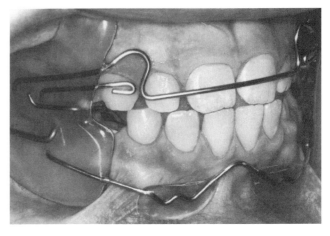

Figure 16-19. Frontal view of the intraoral fit of the FR-2 appliance.

Figure 16-20. Lateral view of the intraoral fit of the FR-2 appliance.

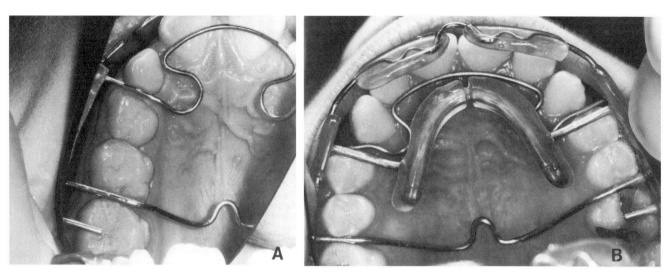

Figure 16-21. Fit of the wires of the FR-2 appliance on the maxilla. *A*, Mixed dentition patient after teeth have been notched. *B*, Permanent dentition patient.

spots produced by the pressure applied to the appliance are adjusted at this time. The appliance then should be pushed toward the mandible to verify that blanching of the soft tissue does not occur. Specific consideration should be given to insuring that the lower lingual shield does not impinge on the gingival margin (Fig. 16-22), a common cause of stripping of the lingual gingiva.

One of the most difficult areas of the appliance to adjust is the lower lingual shield. It is very common for patients to complain of sore spots in this region because the opaque acrylic of the lower lingual shield can obscure any blanching that may be present. Fränkel and Fränkel[24] recommend the use of transparent acrylic so that the blanching of the tissue can be observed directly by the clinician. Huge[32] suggests that in instances in which there is a problem with the lower lingual shield, the mandibular work model should be evaluated. Frequently, there will be an indentation on the model that will lead to a reverse imprint in the acrylic that was not obvious during the finishing of the appliance. Pressure-indicating paste also can be used to reveal areas of excessive pressure.

Pressure-indicating paste is applied to the lower lingual shield uniformly (Fig. 16-23*A*). The appliance then is placed back in the patient's mouth, and the patient is asked to close firmly on the appliance. Areas of excessive pressure can be identified easily (Fig. 16-23*B*) and subsequently adjusted.

Another common area of appliance adjustment is the region of the lower labial pads. The lower labial pads should be positioned so that the distance from the gingival margin of the lateral incisor to the top of the pad is the same distance as from the top of the pad to the bottom of the pad (see Fig. 16-20). Improper positioning of the lower labial pads can result if the work models are not carved in the lower anterior region before appliance fabrication. In addition, the lower labial pads should be teardrop shaped in sagittal view. If the pads are rectangular in cross-section (Fig. 16-24*A*), stripping of the gingiva again can occur. The proper shape of the pads (Fig. 16-24*B*) also allows for a closer fit of the pads against the labial surface of the mandibular symphysis.

The anteroposterior position of the lower labial pads is adjusted most easily using an acrylic bur and a low-speed handpiece. The position of the pads is altered by drilling out the ends of the support wire for the lower labial pads and then moving them anteriorly or posteriorly within the shield (Fig. 16-25). After the proper ad-

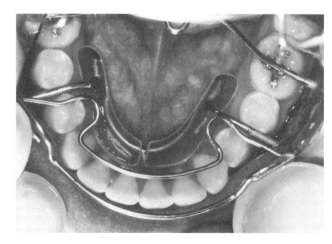

Figure 16-22. Fit of the FR-2 appliance on the mandible. The lower lingual shield does not touch the gingival margin.

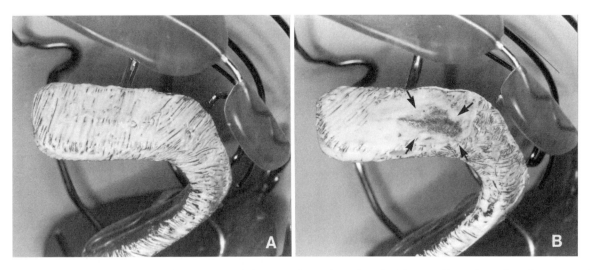

Figure 16-23. The use of pressure-indicating paste. A, Before appliance insertion. B, After appliance insertion. Note area of pressure (see arrows).

justment of the lower labial pads is completed, the holes in the vestibular shield should be filled with acrylic.

Other common areas of adjustment are in the upper canine region and the maxillary tuberosity region. These areas are adjusted most easily by trimming the vestibular shield with an acrylic bur. After the adjustment, the acrylic is smoothed and polished. If curvature of the canine extension is desired, the extension can be placed in warm or hot water and molded with finger pressure so that the acrylic is no more than 2.5–3.0 mm from the alveolar process.[34]

HOME CARE INSTRUCTIONS

The FR-2 is presented to the patient as a full-time appliance, with the expectation that the appliance should be worn 20–22 hours per day. The only time that the appliance is to be removed is during eating, tooth brushing, practicing a foreign language, and playing certain contact sports. The appliance also should be removed if the patient is swimming in a lake or river, but not when the patient is in a swimming pool, except during competitive swimming.

The break-in schedule for the appliance is gradual. Frankel[33] recommends that during the first four weeks, the function regulator is worn only in the afternoon. Unscheduled comfort adjustments during the first few weeks often are necessary. If the treatment continues to progress satisfactorily, the patient is told to increase the hours of wear by a few hours each day until the FR appliance is worn full-time during the day. If treatment is progressing satisfactorily, the patient then is told to wear the appliance on a full-time basis, including sleep-

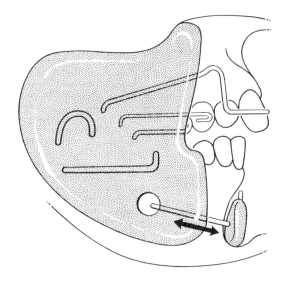

Figure 16-25. Comfort adjustments are made in the position of the lower labial pad by removing the acrylic around the ends of the support wires. The position of the lower labial pad then can be adjusted anteriorly or posteriorly.

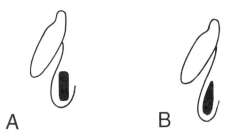

Figure 16-24. Shape of the lower labial pad. A, The pad should not be rectangular in shape. B, The pads should have a teardrop configuration in sagittal view.

ing hours. The delay in having the patient wear the appliance during sleep is to allow the training effect to occur during waking hours.

During the break-in period, the patient is asked to read aloud to his or her parents for 30 minutes per day, until the time that proper speech patterns are reestablished.[35] It is very important to reestablish speech patterns as soon as possible to ensure patient compliance with the desired amount of Fränkel wear. As soon as full-time wear is achieved, the patient usually is seen every five to seven weeks, depending on the level of patient cooperation. More frequent visits are necessary if the motivation of the patient is in question. These appointments involve checking for sore spots, evaluating the level of patient cooperation, and working on patient motivation.

When delivering the Fränkel appliance, it is essential to obtain parental and peer support. Parents and siblings should be told to avoid teasing the patient about wearing the appliance and to avoid commenting on changes in facial appearance. Fränkel and Fränkel[24] state that soft tissue distortion occurs only when the appliance is made incorrectly or if the amount of mandibular advancement is excessive.

As treatment progresses, there should be a gradual improvement in the facial appearance of the patient with the appliance in place, sometimes to an extent that it is difficult to determine quickly whether or not the patient is wearing the appliance. If soft tissue distortion occurs, the fit of the appliance should be checked thoroughly.

LIP SEAL EXERCISES

As mentioned earlier, the establishment of a competent oral seal is a major goal of function regulator therapy. Fränkel[6] has advocated a regimen of lip seal training that should occur not only during treatment with the FR appliance but also can be initiated as early as the initial examination appointment. According to Fränkel,[33] the intent of these exercises is to encourage "closure of the capsular matrix." The underlying goal of treatment is to establish normal neuromuscular function, particularly as it pertains to the perioral and masticatory musculature.

The patient is instructed to keep the lips together at all times. By doing so, normal nasal respiration is encouraged. Patients often are given some type of reminder sticker that should be placed on the desk at school and in the study area at home. These types of reminders are useful in encouraging lip closure. (See Chapter 8 for a more detailed discussion of lip seal exercises.)

CLINICAL EVALUATION OF APPLIANCE WEAR

Soft Tissue Adaptations

The most common problem associated with FR-2 wear is irritation of soft tissue. It is common to see areas of hyperemia of the tissue, particularly in the lower labial region. Areas of redness also may appear at any point at which the buccal shields touch the soft tissue of the vestibule. Ulceration or fibrous tissue build-up (Fig. 16-26) usually indicate that the lower labial pads or buccal shields are not positioned properly. Typically, keratinization or ulceration of the soft tissue is caused by an excessive lateral position of the buccal shields or by an excessive labial position of the lower labial pads. In certain instances, an ill-fitting appliance may produce significant soft tissue lesions, although such lesions can be asymptomatic to the patient. Such problems must be handled as soon as they are noticed, usually by adjusting the lower labial pads in an anteroposterior direction. Problems with the fit of the buccal shields are avoided through proper impression technique.

"Pterygoid Response"

After three or four months of appliance wear, a clinical sign of adaptation is the occurrence of the so-called "pterygoid response." This response is indicated by the inability of the patient to reposition the mandible in a posterior direction following full-time appliance wear. Although the patient can chew on the back teeth, there is a tendency for the patient to reposition the lower jaw anteriorly at rest. The term "pterygoid response" is, of course, a misnomer because the lateral pterygoid muscle is only one of the orofacial muscles that take part in determining mandibular posture and translation. This neu-

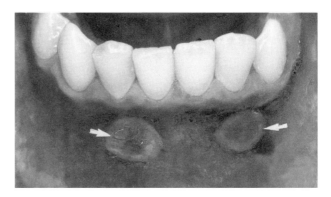

Figure 16-26. Areas of irritation and fibrous tissue build-up (see arrows).

romuscular activity observed in a clinical setting might be similar to that produced in experimental animals.[36,37]

The absence of the so-called "pterygoid response" may be a clinical indication that the patient is not wearing the appliance as expected. It is not, however, simply a matter of the number of hours per day that the patient wears the appliance but also the way the appliance is worn when it is in the mouth. In certain instances, the patient has the appliance in the mouth but does not position the mandible properly. For example, an appliance can be properly designed and fitted for a patient, and yet the patient may wear the appliance with the mandible out of the appliance and in a retruded position (Fig. 16-27). Thus, it is important that the patient understand why the appliance must be worn and that the jaw should be carried in a forward position at all times. Once again, a regimen of lip seal exercises[6] also will help prevent improper wearing of the appliance.

ADVANCEMENT OF THE APPLIANCE

In most instances, a small initial advancement in the construction bite, as recommended by Fränkel, is not adequate to resolve the entire Class II molar relationship. Therefore, a subsequent advancement of the appliance following three or four months of full-time wear is indicated (Fig. 16-28). With a crosscut fissure bur, a horizontal cut is made through the vestibular shields parallel to the occlusal plane above the crossover wire (Fig. 16-28A). A vertical cut then is made in the vestibular shield at its midpoint anteroposteriorly. Care should be taken not to damage the extension of the crossover wire.

A laboratory knife then is inserted into the cut in the vestibular shield and twisted, so that the lower anterior portion of the vestibular shields and the lower lingual shield is advanced anteriorly as a unit (Fig. 16-28B). This procedure is in contrast to the comfort adjustment shown in Figure 16-25, in which only the lower labial pads are advanced. The amount of advancement depends on the remaining problem but, according to Fränkel, should be no more than 2–3 mm at any one time.

After proper fit is obtained, acrylic is added to the vestibular shield to fill in the cut (Fig. 16-28C). Following rough trimming, the appliance is placed back in the mouth and the acrylic contours are checked. After the final adjustments in contour have been made, the appliance is polished and redelivered to the patient. If the appliance has been designed to allow for increased vertical opening with activation, the anterior part of the appliance is moved downward and forward.

Duration of Treatment

Fränkel states that his appliance can be used effectively in both mixed and permanent dentition patients, with tooth-size/arch-size problems before the eruption of the lower permanent canines. It has been our experience that the ideal time to use the Fränkel appliance is in the middle or late mixed dentition period. Our clinical studies have shown not only that a greater amount of mandibular growth occurs during this age period,[25] but that it is possible to follow Fränkel treatment directly with comprehensive orthodontic treatment, avoiding an intervening period of nighttime-only Fränkel wear, often a necessity when treatment is initiated in the early mixed dentition.

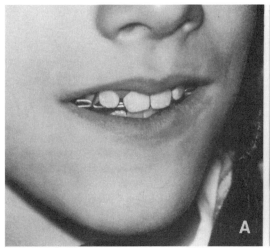
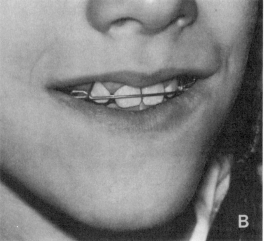

Figure 16-27. Improper wearing of the FR appliance. *A*, Upper labial wire lies behind the upper incisors. *B*, Proper appliance wear. Improper wear can prevent adequate mandibular repositioning from occurring.

FUNCTION REGULATOR (FR-2) OF FRÄNKEL

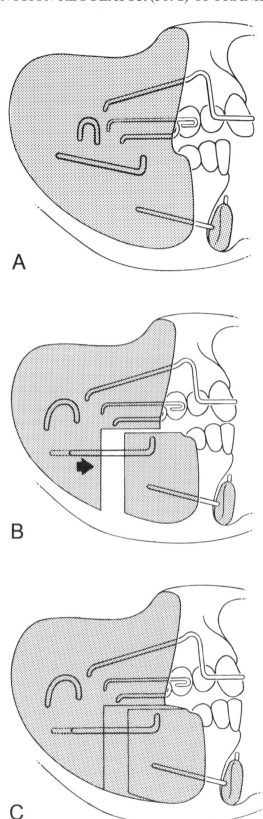

Figure 16-28. Advancement of the FR-2. *A*, A cut is made horizontally and vertically in the vestibular shield. *B*, The lower inferior part of the appliance is advanced in an anterior direction. *C*, The void is filled with acrylic to ensure a smooth contour.

If treatment is started during the late mixed dentition or during the early permanent dentition, the duration of treatment usually is 18–24 months of full-time appliance wear. After this time, a period of fixed appliances usually is required to align and detail the dentition.

CONCLUDING REMARKS

The purpose of this chapter has been to discuss the treatment effects produced by the Fränkel appliance and to provide, in detail, a description of the clinical management of the FR-2 appliance. This appliance differs from most other types of appliances in that it is primarily an orthopedic exercise device. Although typically the FR-2 is used today in Class II patients with obvious neuromuscular imbalances, this appliance has much broader applications in various types of malocclusion

The initial effect of the FR-2 is on the soft tissue, particularly the musculature, rather than on the teeth, in an attempt to modify the circum-oral capsule. The vestibular shields act to restrain and retrain the orofacial musculature, thus allowing a more unrestricted development of the dentition. In addition, the acrylic portions of the appliance produce anteroposterior changes in jaw position. Fränkel[33] maintains that the creation of space is essential for new growth to occur and that the displacement of the mandible is the most important factor in the spontaneous development of the lower face.

As the FR-2 appliance is essentially a tissue-borne appliance, except for the contact with the upper posterior teeth, proper management of the appliance requires a precise impression and bite registration technique, adequate carving of the work models (particularly in the lower anterior and upper posterior regions), and a knowledge of the proper clinical management techniques. If these procedures are followed, and if over-advancement of the mandible is avoided, predictable changes in the skeletal and dentoalveolar relationships may be achieved.

REFERENCES CITED

1. Roux W. Entwicklungsmechanik der Organismen, Bd. I und II. Leipzig: W Engelmann Verlag, 1895.
2. Fränkel R. The theoretical concept underlying the treatment with functional correctors. Trans Eur Orthod Soc 1966;42:233–254.
3. Fränkel R. The practical meaning of the functional matrix in orthodontics. Trans Eur Orthod Soc 1969;45:207–219.
4. Fränkel R, Fränkel C. Orofacial orthopedics with the function regulator. Munich: S Karger, 1989.

5. Fränkel R. Clinical implications of Roux's concept in orofacial orthopedics. In: McNamara JA, Jr, ed, The enigma of the vertical dimension. Ann Arbor: Monograph 36, Craniofacial Growth Monograph Series, Center for Human Growth and Development, The University of Michigan, 2000.
6. Fränkel R. Lip seal training in the treatment of skeletal open bite. Eur J Orthod 1980;2:219–228.
7. Fränkel R. Biomechanical aspects of the form/function relationship in craniofacial morphogenesis: A clinician's approach. In: McNamara JA, Jr, Ribbens KA, Howe RP, eds. Clinical alterations of the growing face. Ann Arbor: Monograph 14, Craniofacial Growth Series, Center for Human Growth and Development, University of Michigan, 1983.
8. Fränkel R, Fränkel C. A rejoinder. Am J Orthod Dentofac Orthop 1987;92:435-436.
9. Fränkel R. Technik und Handhabung der Funktionsregler. Berlin: VEB Verlag Volk and Gesundheit, 1976.
10. Fränkel R. Guidance of eruption without extraction. Trans Europ Orthod Soc 1971;47:303–315.
11. Fränkel R. The artificial translation of the mandible by function regulators. In: Cook JT, ed, Transaction of the Third International Orthodontic Congress. St Louis: CV Mosby, 1975.
12. Fränkel R. Decrowding during eruption under the screening influence of vestibular shields. Am J Orthod 1974;65:372–406.
13. Altmann K. Untersuchungen über Frakturheilung unter besonderen experimentellen Bedingungen. Z Anat Entwickl Gesch 1949;114:457.
14. Harvold EP. Neuromuscular and morphological adaptations in experimentally induced oral respiration. In: McNamara JA, Jr, ed. Naso-respiratory function and craniofacial growth. Ann Arbor: Monograph 9, Craniofacial Growth Series, Center for Human Growth and Development, The University of Michigan, 1979.
15. Harvold EP. Altering craniofacial growth: force application and neuromuscular-bone interaction. In: Clinical alteration of the growing face. McNamara, JA Jr, Ribbens KA, Howe RP, eds, Monograph 14, Craniofacial Growth Series, Center for Human Growth and Development, The University of Michigan, Ann Arbor, 1983.
16. Breiden CM, Pangrazio-Kulbersh V, Kulbersh R. Maxillary skeletal and dental change with Fränkel appliance therapy—an implant study. Angle Orthod 1984;54:232–66.
17. Sotiriadou AD, Johnston LE, Jr. Expansion with vestibular shields: An experimental test of the periosteal-pull hypothesis. Semin Orthod 1999;5:121–127.
18. Atkinson SR. Jaws out of balance. Part I. Am J Orthod 1966;52:47–55.
19. Atkinson SR. Jaws out of balance. Part II. Am J Orthod 1966;52:371–380.
20. Van der Linden FPGM, Duterloo H. The development of the human dentition: An atlas. Haggerstown: Harper and Row Publishers, 1976.
21. McDougall PD, McNamara JA, Jr, Dierkes JM. Arch width development in Class II patients treated with the Fränkel appliance. Am J Orthod 1982;82:10–22.
22. Falck F. Kephalometrische Längsschnittuntersuchung über Behandlungsergebnisse der mandibulären Retrognathie mit Funktionsreglen im Vergleich zu einer Controllgruppe. Berlin: Med Dissertation, 1985.
23. McNamara JA, Jr. A method of cephalometric evaluation. Am J Orthod 1984;86:449–469.
24. Fränkel R, Fränkel C. Personal communication, 1992.
25. McNamara JA, Jr, Bookstein FL, Shaughnessy TG. Skeletal and dental changes following functional regulator therapy on Class II patients. Am J Orthod 1985;88:91–110.
26. McNamara JA, Jr, Howe RP, Dischinger TG. A comparison of the Herbst and Fränkel appliances in the treatment of Class II malocclusion. Am J Orthod Dentofac Orthop 1990;98:134–144.
27. Toth LR, McNamara JA, Jr. Treatment effects produced by the twin block appliance and the FR-2 appliance of Frankel compared to an untreated Class II sample. Am J Orthod Dentofac Orthop 1999;116:597-609.
28. McNamara JA, Jr. Dentofacial adaptations in adult patients following functional regulator therapy. Am J Orthod 1984;85:57–71.
29. McNamara JA, Jr, Huge SA. The Fränkel appliance (FR-2): model preparation and appliance construction. Am J Orthod 1981;80:478–495.
30. McNamara JA, Jr. JCO interviews Dr James A McNamara, Jr on the Fränkel appliance. Part 1—Biological basis and appliance design. J Clin Orthod 1982;16:320–37.
31. McNamara JA, Jr. JCO interviews Dr James A McNamara, Jr on the Fränkel appliance. Part 2—Clinical management. J Clin Orthod 1982;16:390–407.
32. Huge SA. Personal communication, 1992.
33. Fränkel R. Personal communication, 1999.
34. Dierkes JM. Personal communication, 1992.
35. Kaufmann HJ. Personal communication, 1976.
36. McNamara JA, Jr. Neuromuscular and skeletal adaptations to altered orofacial function. Ann Arbor: Monograph 1, Craniofacial Growth Series, Center for Human Growth and Development, The University of Michigan, 1972.
37. McNamara JA, Jr. Neuromuscular and skeletal adaptations to altered function in the orofacial region. Am J Orthod 1973;64:578–606.

Chapter 17

THE HERBST APPLIANCE

With Donald R. Burkhardt and Scott A. Huge

Emil Herbst developed the Herbst bite-jumping mechanism in the early 1900s. This device was one of the early attempts to produce mechanically a "jumping of the bite," an idea that had been advocated earlier by Kingsley,[1] among others. This telescoping mechanism encourages forward repositioning of the lower jaw as the patient closes into occlusion.

The Herbst appliance has been compared to an artificial joint working between the maxilla and the mandible.[2] Common to all designs of the Herbst appliance is a bilateral telescopic mechanism, consisting of a tube and plunger apparatus (Fig. 17-1) that prompts closing of the mandible into a protruded orientation relative to the original mandibular position.

Tubes attached to the buccal surface of maxillary first molars extend anteroinferiorly toward the lower canines. Plungers (also termed rods) attached to the lower first premolars extend posterosuperiorly into tubes attached to the maxillary molars. When the appliance is adjusted properly, the presence of the plunger within the tube forces the mandible to be positioned anteriorly. Although the telescoping mechanism essentially is identical in all Herbst designs, many variations in overall composition are possible from one design to another.

HISTORICAL PERSPECTIVE

The original banded design of this appliance was introduced by Herbst at the International Dental Congress in Berlin in 1905. Herbst published very little on the appliance, except for a book written in 1910[3] (Figs. 17-2 and 17-3) and an article written in 1934.[4] Although achieving some initial popularity, there are very few references to Herbst's treatment technique in the orthodontic literature before its reintroduction in 1979 by Hans Pancherz, then of Malmö, Sweden. The only article written prior to Pancherz's reintroduction was an article by Held and co-workers[5] concerning an adult patient treated with this method. This case report described a 30-year-old woman who was treated with the Herbst bite-jumping mechanism fixed to a cast appliance. Held and co-workers reported that only dentoalveolar adaptations were observed.

Renewed interest in the Herbst appliance was due to the initial favorable reports of Pancherz.[6-8] In these early studies, Pancherz used a banded Herbst design (Fig. 17-4) that involved the placement of bands of thick material on the upper first molars and first premolars. The bands on each side were connected by sectional lingual wires. In the mandible, bands were placed on the lower first premolars, connected by a lower lingual arch. It should be noted that Pancherz used individually made bands that were pinched from heavy band material, formed on the work model. The indirect fabrication of the bands using thick band material is of significance, because breakage can occur using the banded design Herbst appliance if ordinary orthodontic bands are used during appliance fabrication.

Since 1995, Pancherz has used cast splints instead of bands on a regular basis on all Herbst patients.[9] Chrome-cobalt splints cover all erupted teeth in the maxillary and mandibular arches, including the mandibular canines. The lower splints are connected by a lin-

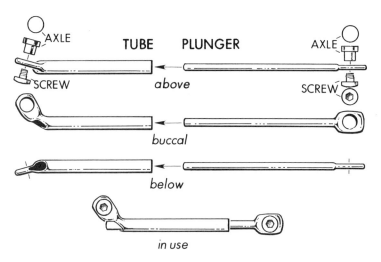

Figure 17-1. Components of the Herbst bite-jumping mechanism.[52]

gual archwire. In addition, the maxillary and mandibular anterior teeth are included in the anchorage system by way of labial archwires that are connected to the splints.

OVERVIEW OF TREATMENT EFFECTS

Perhaps more than any other type of functional appliance, whether fixed or removable, the treatment effects produced by the banded Herbst appliance have been well documented, especially by Pancherz and co-workers.[6–8,10–21] Other investigators have evaluated alternative designs, including the cast Herbst appliance by Wieslander,[22,23] the acrylic splint Herbst appliance by McNamara and co-workers,[24,25] and the stainless steel crown appliance by Burkhardt.[26]

A detailed discussion of the treatment effects produced by the various types of Herbst appliance designs is presented later in this chapter. One of the original articles that provides an overview of the treatment effects of the Herbst appliance was written by Pancherz in 1982,[10] a report that generally reflects the outcomes of most other studies conducted by his group and others. Pancherz evaluated 42 Class II, division 1 malocclusion patients. Twenty-two patients were treated with the Herbst appliance for six months, and the other 20 subjects served as controls. At the end of the six-month treatment period, all 22 treated patients had a Class I dental

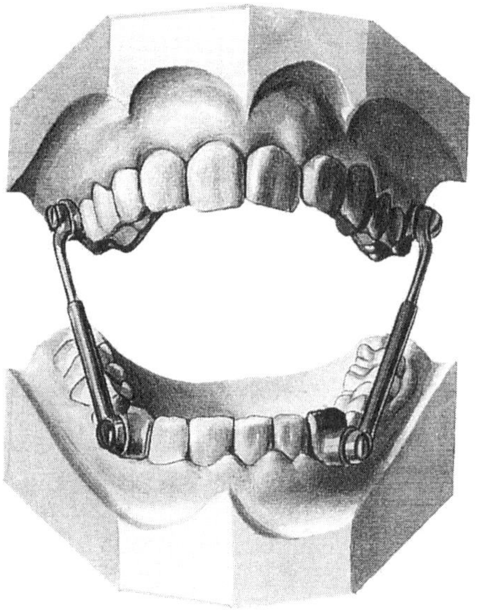

Figure 17-2. Frontal view if the original Herbst appliance as designed and published by Herbst[3] in 1910.

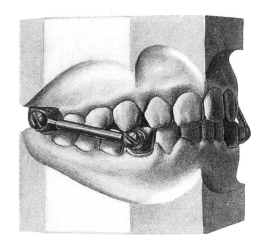

Figure 17-3. Lateral view if the original Herbst appliance as designed and published by Herbst[3] in 1910.

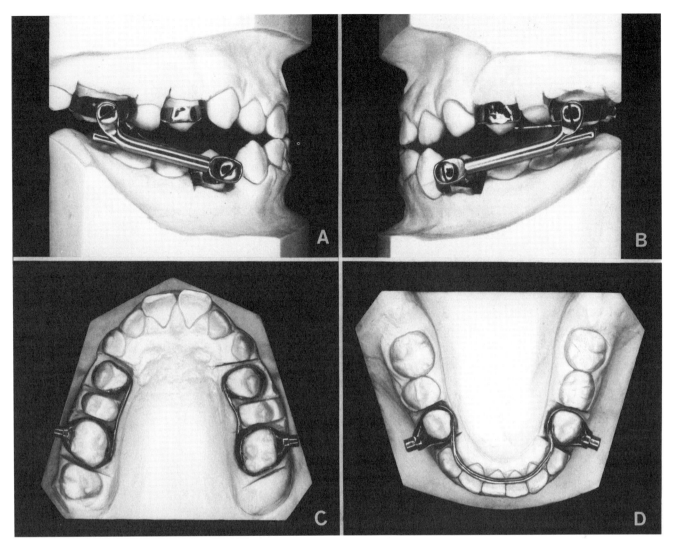

Figure 17-4. The banded design of the Herbst appliance originally used by Pancherz[6]. *A*, Right lateral view. *B*, Left lateral view. *C*, Maxillary occlusal view. *D*, Mandibular occlusal view. Note that heavy band material was used in the indirect fabrication of the bands on the molars and premolars. (Appliance courtesy of Hans Pancherz, Giessen, Germany.)

relationship. This change was almost equally a result of skeletal and dental adaptations. A molar correction of 6.7 mm typically was resolved by a relative posterior movement of the upper buccal segment as well as by increased mandibular growth. Little skeletal change was seen in the maxilla, regardless of whether change in molar relation (Fig. 17-5) or overjet (Fig. 17-6) was evaluated.

Thus, most clinical studies of Herbst appliance treatment, regardless of the design of the appliance used, have indicated that dental movements may be anticipated as part of the treatment effect produced by the Herbst appliance. Distalization of the maxillary buccal segment is similar to that which might occur following the use of extraoral traction (see Chapter 21). The upper first molar usually is in a position 2.5 mm posterior to that observed in untreated individuals. It should be noted, however, that distal movement of the upper molar movement is controllable, depending on the appliance design and clinical management. In the stainless steel crown design, when the molars are not connected with a transpalatal wire or expansion screw, the appliance can produce a force resulting in 5–6 mm of distalization. Conversely, when the first molars are consolidated with the rest of the arch (full brackets), only modest changes in the position of the upper molars may occur.

Variable proclination of the lower incisor also has been noted in both banded and acrylic splint Herbst treatment. The latter finding of incisor proclination has been shown to rebound during the fixed appliance treatment.[25,26] Patients who have proclined lower incisors at the beginning of treatment, however, are not well suited for this type of therapy.

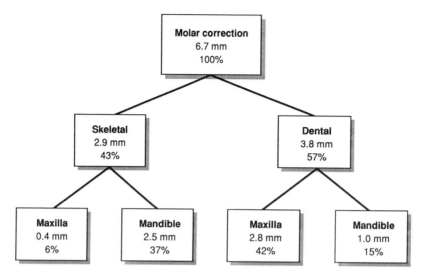

Figure 17-5. Maxillary and mandibular dental changes contributing to sagittal molar correction in 22 Class II, division 1 cases treated for six months with the Herbst appliance. (Adapted from Pancherz.[10])

ROLE OF EXPANSION IN HERBST TREATMENT

Another important issue regardless of the specifics of appliance design is the lateral movement of the mandible, allowed by the Herbst mechanisms, relative to arch width. Ideally, the mechanisms on each side should be free to open and close during jaw movement while simultaneously allowing lateral movements. Whenever the mechanisms are aligned improperly (*e.g.*, the pivots connecting the plungers and tubes to the attachments on the teeth are not parallel with the eyelets, the openings at one end of each part of the Herbst bite jumping mechanism that fit over the pivot), a binding can occur during wear. This restriction of free jaw movement will lead directly to stress and possible appliance breakage.

One of the most frequent situations in which this problem occurs is when the maxilla is too narrow in relationship to the lower arch. This condition, if not corrected (*i.e.*, with expansion of the maxilla), will result in the pivots on the upper appliance being located inside the ideal working angles of the mechanisms. On lateral movements, the mechanisms will contact the lower pos-

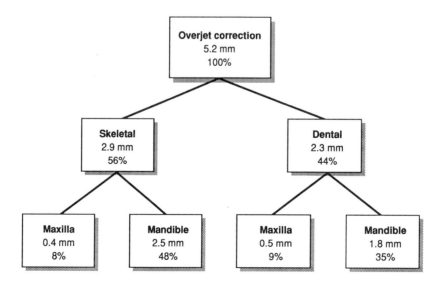

Figure 17-6. Maxillary and mandibular skeletal and dental changes contributing to overjet correction in 22 Class II, division 1 patients treated for six months with the Herbst appliance. (Adapted from Pancherz.[10])

terior teeth and set up undesirable occlusal forces throughout the appliance system.

In terms of clinical management, the upper arch can be expanded prior to Herbst therapy by way of a rapid maxillary expansion (RME) appliance. Alternatively, rapid palatal expansion can be combined with the Herbst, with expansion initiated before activating the Herbst. The upper member of the appliance is delivered without the tubes attached, although the Herbst screws typically are left in place to prevent debris from accumulating. Expansion is carried out along routine protocol as described in Chapter 13 in this text.

After upper expansion is complete, the previously fabricated lower Herbst is delivered and the plungers and tubes assembled. In a subsequent appointment, according to the clinician's preference, the RME screw may be removed from the crowns using a high-speed handpiece and diamond bur. The above sequence allows efficient arch expansion and Herbst therapy utilizing one appliance.

HERBST APPLIANCE DESIGNS

According to a recent unpublished survey of six major orthodontic laboratories,[27] the Herbst appliance is the most widely used type of appliance in the treatment of Class II malocclusions in the United States today. It should be noted that originally, the Herbst often was considered the appliance of "last resort" for the noncompliant patient. Today, in fact, patients who are deemed less than ideal cooperators still may be good Herbst candidates. The vast percentage of Herbst patients presenting with Class II malocclusions, however, do not require an in-depth evaluation concerning compliance. In this respect, many orthodontists now recognize that the Herbst offers a wide range of reasonably predictable treatment effects and at the same time insures patient compliance. The multiple benefits of this appliance system is why the Herbst has grown to become the most popular Class II functional appliance.

Many designs of the Herbst appliance have been developed over the last 20 years. We have chosen to discuss three types in detail: the banded, stainless steel crown, and acrylic splint designs. The reader is referred to the publications of Wieslander[22,28] and Pancherz[29] for the specifics of the clinical management of the cast Herbst design.

Banded Herbst Design

The Herbst appliance, as originally described by Herbst,[3,4] was intended to be worn 24 hours a day. The appliance consisted of gold crowns on the maxillary first molars and mandibular canines (Figs. 17-2 and 17-3). Herbst[3] referred to the gold crowns as thick rings around the teeth.

As mentioned above, Pancherz[6,10] modified the original Herbst design by using thick orthodontic bands (at least 0.15 mm) on the maxillary and mandibular first premolars and first molars (Fig. 17-4). A lingual bar extended from the first premolar band to the first molar band on each side of the maxillary arch. In the mandible, a lingual archwire interconnected the first premolars. Axles or pivots were soldered to the buccal surface of maxillary first molar bands, so that screws could secure the tubes in place. The plungers were secured to the buccal surface of the mandibular first premolars in a similar fashion.[9]

Pancherz has modified the banded design of the Herbst appliance as he has gained experience with this device.[9] In 1981, the maxillary teeth were included in the appliance by placing brackets on these teeth (Fig. 17-7). A labial archwire connected these brackets to the brackets on the upper first premolar bands. In the mandible, the lingual archwire was extended posteriorly to the molars, which also were banded. In 1983, the lower anterior teeth were included into anchorage by placing brackets on the teeth. A labial archwire was attached to the brackets and to tubes above the axels on the premolar bands (Fig. 17-7). Parallel to the design evolution Pancherz was undertaking, many early clinicians in the United States also began using fixed appliances on the anterior teeth with their banded and crown Herbst cases.[30–34]

The current banded version of the appliance (Fig. 17-8) incorporates additional anchorage units from the orig-

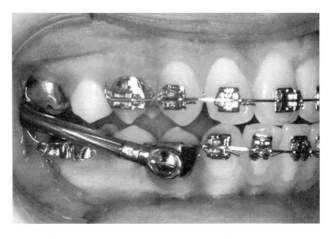

Figure 17-7. Intraoral view of a patient with brackets on the maxillary and mandibular anterior teeth. The incisors have been added as anchorage units for the banded Herbst appliance. (Photo courtesy of Hans Pancherz.)

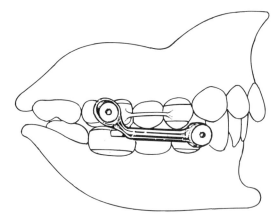

Figure 17-8. Lateral view of the banded Herbst appliance. Bands are placed on the lower first premolars and upper first molars and are connected sagittally by buccal and lingual support wires.

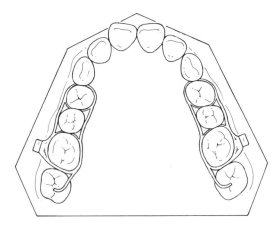

Figure 17-9. Occlusal view of the banded Herbst appliance. Occlusal rests extend to the upper second molars. The maxillary first premolars and first molars are connected by buccal and lingual support wires.

inal design of Pancherz. When used in the permanent dentition, bands are placed on all first premolars and all first molars, and both buccal and lingual wires connect the premolar and molar bands (Figs. 17-9 and 17-10).

An important design feature also calls for a reinforcement wire carefully adapted to the occlusal edge of each molar band (Fig. 17-11). This .040" or .051" wire, which ideally is part of the continuous connecting support wire, is soldered on the buccal and lingual and is adapted closely to the interproximal contacts between the teeth. With this design, the overall appliance is reinforced considerably and when fabricated correctly, does not interfere with the occlusion. The appliance also has been strengthened by the liberal addition of solder without annealing the band material (Fig. 17-12). In addition, occlusal rests were added to the second molars in both arches.

Manufacturers recently have introduced thicker (.010") preformed bands, which add to the strength of the banded Herbst. These blank bands can be adapted and fitted in the laboratory directly on the working model. The advantage to the orthodontist is the elimination of an appointment to fit bands and pour them into the impression. In the laboratory, there is the additional advantage of using a blank band (which many practices do not inventory), which means an orthodontic buccal attachment does not have to be removed from the buccal surface of the band. This process may lead to overheating of the band material.

One of the most significant problems encountered initially when we began to use the Herbst appliance in 1980 was band breakage (Fig. 17-13AB). We did not realize the importance of using individually fabricated bands from heavy band material, as recommended by

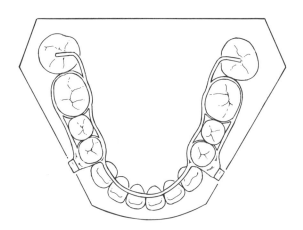

Figure 17-10. Occlusal view of the banded Herbst appliance. The lower lingual wire crosses the cingula of the lower incisors.

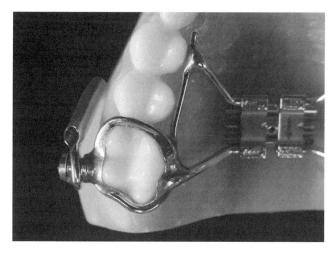

Figure 17-11. Banded Herbst design with a reinforcement wire carefully adapted to the occlusal edge of each molar band.

HERBST APPLIANCE

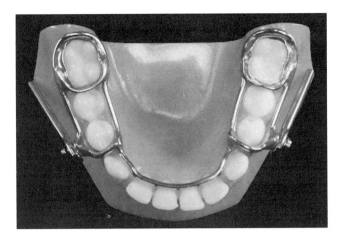

Figure 17-12. Banded Herbst design with reinforcement wires and liberal addition of solder to reinforce the appliance.

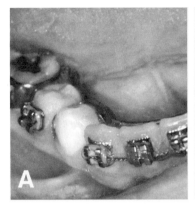
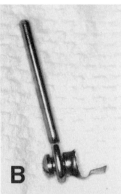
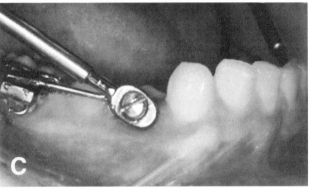

Figure 17-13. Appliance problems. *A* and *B*, appliance breakage, due to improper use of light band material. *C*, Undesirable vertical mobility and intrusion of the lower first premolars after several months of banded Herbst treatment.

Pancherz; thus, the same preformed bands that were available for routine orthodontic treatment were used. Initially we experienced significant band breakage, typically in the lower first premolar region. In retrospect, this breakage could have been avoided easily if band material of proper strength had been used. The band material also may have been annealed during appliance fabrication by the laboratory technician, weakening the band material further. Furthermore, by incorporating the lower first permanent molars in the overall anchorage unit (combined with a continuous lingual and buccal wire), the forces are distributed more widely, which we believe has reduced breakage.

Another significant discovery that greatly affected the reliability of the appliance was made during the time the commercial laboratories were gaining experience in fabricating the banded Herbst. As mentioned earlier, each plunger and tube has an "eyelet" (*i.e.*, opening) at one end that fits over the pivot or axle on each anchor tooth. The rods and tubes are secured to each pivot with the screws. There is a necessary amount of "travel" (*i.e.*, freedom for lateral movement) ideally built into the working motion of the entire system. When the mechanisms originally were made available in the United States, the mechanisms fit precisely over the pivots and subsequently if left unaltered, created a binding effect during jaw movement. This binding added considerable stress to the entire appliance and no doubt contributed to early failures with the banded Herbst.

With experience, we learned the Herbst bite jumping mechanisms required a routine laboratory (or clinical) procedure to enlarge the eyelets and "free up" the working action of the mechanisms. This discovery was made after we for the most part had moved away from the banded design. In retrospect, this relatively minor clinical problem probably was as much of a factor leading to the banded Herbst failure as the other fabrication problems.

Further, occasionally we noted undesirable intrusion and increased vertical mobility of the lower first premolars after a few months of treatment (Fig. 17-13*C*). Incorporating the lower anteriors and lower molars into the anchorage system (Fig. 17-7), again as advocated by Pancherz,[9,30] helps eliminate this problem.

Stainless Steel Crown Herbst Design

A number of clinicians, including Langford,[31-32] Goodman and McKenna,[33] Dischinger,[34] Smith,[35,36] Mayes,[37-40] Hilgers,[41] and Chastant[42] have advocated the use of stainless steel crowns as anchor units. The original design incorporated stainless steel crowns on the upper first molars to which were soldered the pivots that were used to secure the maxillary tubes of the Herbst bite-jumping mechanism (Fig. 17-14). It has been our experience that connecting the maxillary stainless steel crowns with a transpalatal arch or preferably, a Hyrax-type expansion screw (Fig. 17-15) makes the maxillary appliance more

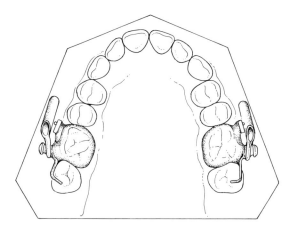

Figure 17-14. Occlusal view of the maxillary portion of the stainless steel crown Herbst without a midline expansion screw. Archwire tubes have been soldered anterior to the axles on the stainless steel crowns.

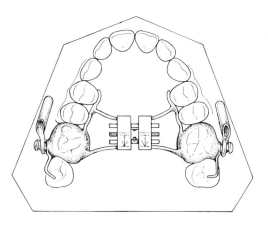

Figure 17-15. Preferred design of the maxillary stainless steel crown Herbst that incorporates a Hyrax-type midline expansion screw (Leone Co., Florence, Italy). Occlusal rests extend posteriorly to the upper second molars.

rigid and less likely to loosen. In addition, we estimate that at least half of Herbst patients benefit from expansion of the maxilla. With the advancement of the mandible and the subsequent fit of the lower teeth to the narrower upper dentition, expansion in many patients is critical to the success of the overall correction.[43]

Hilgers[44] has noted that often it is appropriate to use bands made from heavy band material on the upper molars to avoid the anterior open bite that can be created with a stainless steel crown type Herbst appliance. Proper overbite and overjet creation at the very outset of Herbst therapy is one of his main objectives. Although bringing the mandible forward will avoid creating anterior open bites in most patients (even when using a stainless steel crown on the upper molars), not having good incisal guidance and accompanying proprioception is a distinct possibility if the appliance is not fabricated specifically to the needs of the patient. Hilgers states that much of the favorable treatment changes attributed to the Herbst appliance occurs via lip competence and anterior vertical closure.

In the lower arch, we currently use one of two designs, both designs involving the placement of stainless steel crowns on the lower first premolars. The Type II design of Smith[35, 36] (Fig. 17-16) incorporates bands on the lower first molars that are connected to the stainless steel crowns and to each other by means of an .045" stainless steel lingual wire. Smith[35, 36] recommends that if simultaneous alignment of the lower anterior teeth is desired, rectangular archwire tubes can be soldered

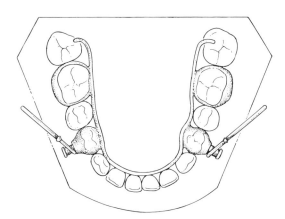

Figure 17-16. Mandibular occlusal view of the Smith Type II crown Herbst appliance. Stainless steel crowns are placed on the lower first premolars and bands are cemented on the lower first molars. A lingual wire extends from second molar to second molar.

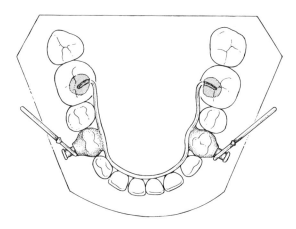

Figure 17-17. Mandibular occlusal view of the crown Herbst design that features bonded occlusal rests on the lower first molars. The ends of the lingual arch lie in the lingual grooves of the lower first molars, and these rests are bonded to the occlusal surfaces of these teeth.

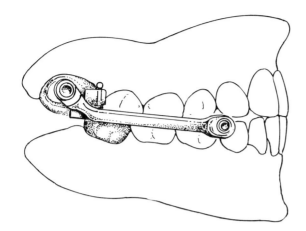

Figure 17-18. Lateral view of the cantilever Herbst appliance that is characterized by stainless steel crowns on the upper and lower first molars. An archwire tube and hook are visible anterior to the axle soldered to the upper first molar crown.

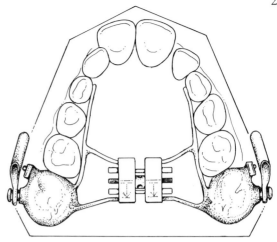

Figure 17-19. Occlusal view of the maxillary portion of the cantilever Herbst used in a mixed dentition patient. A midline expansion screw has been added. Optional archwire tubes have added anterior to the maxillary axels.

under the axle screw on the premolar crowns. An archwire can be used to connect the lower anterior teeth to the Herbst appliance, increasing anchorage in a manner similar to that advocated by Pancherz for the banded Herbst design.

The second design has been recommended by Hilgers.[45] This design (Fig. 17-17) is similar to the Type II design of Smith,[35,36] except that the lingual wire courses posteriorly and then curves laterally to lie in the lingual grooves of the lower first molars, where bilateral occlusal rests are formed. These occlusal rests are bonded to the lower first molars by means of light-cure or chemical-cure adhesive.

Another type of stainless steel crown Herbst, recommended by Dischinger[34,46] and Mayes[37–40] among others, has been termed the *cantilever* Herbst (Fig. 17-18), also known as the Smith Type I design,[35,36] because of the mandibular extension arms that are anchored to stainless steel crowns on the lower first molars. As the crowns are only on the permanent molars, this type of appliance design has been advocated for use in patients in both the mixed and early permanent dentitions.[35–37,46] Dischinger[46] also advocates this appliance design because it minimizes the anterior vector of force transferred to the mandibular incisors by moving the force vector from the mandibular premolars to the first molars.

The cantilever Herbst design incorporates stainless steel crowns on all upper and lower permanent first molars. The upper part of the appliance is essentially the same as described earlier for the crown-type Herbst (Fig. 17-19). The lower part of the appliance features heavy metal extension arms that are cantilevered off the lower first molars (Figs. 17-20 and 17-21). These arms extend anteriorly lateral to the dentition and terminate in the first premolar region. The Herbst axle is soldered to the cantilever arm adjacent to the buccal surface of the lower first premolar. In addition, support wires in the shape of occlusal rests to the lower second deciduous molars (Fig. 17-20) or permanent second molars (Fig. 17-21) may be added for additional stabilization of the appliance. Mayes[38,39] has taken the concept of the cantilever Herbst one step further by developing the Cantilever Bite-Jumper (CBJ; Ormco Corp., Orange CA) system of preformed components that are intended for single appointment delivery of the appliance.

Hilgers[44] for the most part has abandoned usage of the Herbst appliance in mixed dentition patients due to the tremendous tendency for relapse, which we have observed as well. The cantilever Herbst design still is used occasionally by Hilgers in extremely severe malocclusions where he feels it would be inappropriate to wait

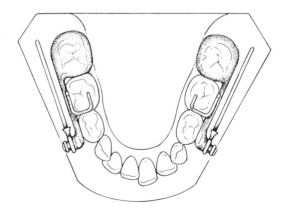

Figure 17-20. Occlusal view of a cantilever Herbst appliance in a mixed dentition patient. Occlusal rests have been placed on the lower second deciduous molars.

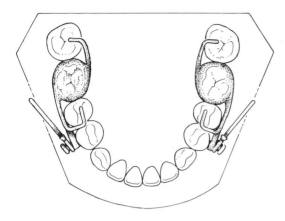

Figure 17-21. Occlusal view of the cantilever Herbst appliance in a patient in the early permanent dentition. Occlusal rests are placed on the lower deciduous second molars and the lower permanent second molars.

for the full dentition to begin treatment. In general, however, he feels that there are no major advantages to be gained starting Herbst therapy in a 7 or 8 year old that cannot be accomplished more easily in the 11 or 12 year old. Finishing the occlusion with good intercuspation of the permanent dentition appears to be important in avoiding unacceptable rebound. Hilgers[44] feels that the ideal starting time is after the lower first premolars have erupted, but before loss of the second deciduous molars, thereby maintaining the ability to save leeway space.

Clinical Management of the Crown-type Herbst

Although there are specific differences in the management of the various types of banded and stainless steel crown Herbst appliances, we will focus on the clinical management of the two types of crown Herbst appliances with which we are the most familiar (Smith Type II and Hilgers bonded occlusal rests). These clinical management comments generally apply to other types of Herbst appliances as well. The specifics of the management of the acrylic splint Herbst design will be discussed in a separate section.

Preparation of the Dentition before Herbst Treatment

As is the situation with a significant number of Class II malocclusions, some type of dental decompensation may be necessary before the initiation of Herbst treatment. As with other types of functional appliances, preparing a dental arch for a Herbst appliance should be no different conceptually than preparing a patient for orthognathic surgery. From an anteroposterior perspective, proclined lower incisors should be retracted, and significant spacing between lower incisors should be consolidated before impression taking.

Similarly, upper incisors that are tipped lingually should be proclined, usually with fixed appliance therapy before the onset of Herbst treatment. In patients with only mild lingual tipping of the upper incisors, this movement can be accomplished while the Herbst appliance is in place. Extruded upper incisors should be intruded using a utility arch or some other type of intrusion arch.

With regard to problems in the vertical dimension, the initial lower anterior facial height of the patient should be determined. In patients with normal or excessive lower anterior facial height and a pronounced curve of Spee, mechanics should be employed to intrude the lower incisors (*e.g.*, an intrusion utility arch). Only in patients with short lower anterior facial heights should lower incisor intrusion be avoided. Leaving an accentuated curve of Spee in some instances may result in a transient posterior open bite at the end of the Herbst phase of treatment and necessitate vertical space closure during the fixed appliance phase.

Most transverse problems of the maxilla can be handled adequately during the Herbst phase of treatment simply by adding a rapid maxillary expansion screw to the maxillary portion of the Herbst appliance (Fig. 17-15). The expander is activated one turn per day, as with any rapid maxillary expansion appliance.

If there is significant lingual tipping of the lower dentition, bonded brackets and arch wires can be used to upright the teeth. A removable Schwarz expansion appliance also can be used before Herbst appliance therapy to upright the buccal dentition in instances of lingual tipping of the posterior segments. The goal of the first phase of orthodontic treatment is to provide adequate dental decompensation so that there are no occlusal interferences that would inhibit the forward posturing of the lower jaw during Herbst therapy.

Impressions

Typically, the Herbst appliance is the first appliance received by the patient. Very often, the decision to use a Herbst appliance is made at the initial examination appointment, and impressions for the Herbst appliance are obtained at the records appointment.

If, on the other hand, dental decompensation has been undertaken previously with fixed appliances, the brackets on teeth not involved in the appliance may be left in place as long as the presence of the brackets does not interfere with the function of the Herbst appliance. When bands are used on the lower first molars, any buccal attachments must be removed (or new blank bands substituted) during fabrication. The Herbst mechanism will contact any buccal attachments on the lower first molars and cause interferences.

The orthodontist has a choice regarding the use of separators. He or she can choose to have the laboratory cut away the adjacent teeth on the work model, and thus no initial separation is necessary. On the other hand, if the clinician desires to create separation before the impressions are obtained, we recommend the use of elastomeric separators in most instances, placed on either side of the lower first premolars and the upper first molars. If the Smith Type II design is used, separators also should be placed adjacent to the lower first molars as well. In any case, adequate separation will be necessary at the time of appliance delivery.

At the next appointment, the separators are removed, if present. Accurate, bubble-free maxillary and mandibular alginate impressions are obtained using standard alginate impression material. Particular attention should be paid to the anatomy of the teeth, in that the stainless steel crowns will be fabricated indirectly from the work models made from these impressions.

In the laboratory, the teeth receiving crowns (molars and premolars) are prepared by defining the entire dental perimeter using a series of fine diamond burs. The crowns then are sized and fitted to the prepared teeth. Using this indirect technique, it is not necessary for the laboratory technician to see the space from the separators on the working model; it is estimated easily. Thus, as mentioned above, initial separation before impression taking is optional.

If desired, tight fitting bands are placed on the lower first molars before the impressions are taken. The bands then are removed from the mouth, are placed in the mandibular impression, and are secured in the impression with medium hard sticky wax. An optional technique is to fit the bands in the patient's mouth but not pour them in the impression. The loose bands are sent to the laboratory, where they are seated by the technician on the working casts. In many instances, this method is more accurate as it eliminates the possibility of the bands moving during the pour-up of the alginate impressions. The work models then are trimmed in a manner similar to study models (see Chapter 30).

Bite Registration

As discussed in detail in Chapter 15, there is no universal agreement as to the correct amount of mandibular advancement when fabricating a functional appliance. Many prominent clinicians, including Pancherz[29] and Clark,[47] have advocated an incisal edge-to-edge bite registration and have reported excellent treatment results. On the other hand, Fränkel[48, 49] has advocated a "step-by step" method of advancement where the bite is brought forward in 2–3 mm increments. Both methods are accommodated easily with this technique.

Hilgers[44] feels that the step-by-step advancement of the mandible has not resulted in a better overall response, or even improved patient comfort, and that the advantage of immediate functional closure of the anterior occlusion and its functional adaptation are lost. He states that one could argue that bringing the lower incisors up against the lingual of the upper incisors helps restrict forward movement of the lower arch (they are constrained by incisor engagement), a common negative response to Herbst therapy. In addition, Hilgers reports that he has not seen adverse temporomandibular joint responses to bringing the mandible fully forward, almost regardless of the amount of overjet.

Our current recommendation regarding the amount of bite advancement varies according to the severity of the original malocclusion. We recommend that in patients with an overjet of 7 mm or less, the bite registration be taken in an incisal end-to-end position. In those patients with overbites greater than 7 mm, the bite should be taken half way between centric relation and an incisal end-to-end position, with a subsequent advancement of the mandible to an edge-to-edge relationship 2–4 months later.

In Chapter 15, we discussed a precise methods of bite registration in which a Projet™ bite fork and medium hard pink wax are used to register the appropriate construction bite. The reader is referred to that chapter for the description of this technique that also may be used when fabricating a Herbst appliance.

There is a major difference, however, between the construction of a cemented stainless steel crown or banded Herbst appliance and a removable functional appliance such as a twin block, bionator, or FR-2 appliance of Fränkel. In the fabrication of a removable functional appliance, the vertical dimension is critical (e.g., the height of the posterior bite blocks of the twin block, the posterior vertical opening in the premolar region of a FR-2 appliance to allow for the crossover wires that support the lower lingual shield). In contrast, the fixed Herbst design can be fabricated without a precise vertical bite registration. The appliance is constructed and delivered, and the patient simply closes his or her mouth until contact is made between the upper and lower parts of the appliance.

In our practice, it is customary to order the fabrication of a fixed Herbst appliance simply by having the laboratory arbitrarily advance the bite according to our instructions. A centric occlusion bite registration is sent to the laboratory along with the work models. In patients with mild to moderated Class II relationships (7 mm overjet or less), the laboratory is instructed to advance the bite to an edge-to-edge position. In instances of larger overjet, the laboratory constructs the appliance with the bite registration midway between centric occlusion and an incisal edge-to-edge position. The appliance can be advanced again later during treatment by adding shims (*i.e.,* sleeves of tubing crimped or spot welded to the plunger) to the mandibular arms of the Herbst bite-jumping mechanism (to be discussed later).

Maintaining Space for Crowns

One of the major concerns during the time interval between impression taking and appliance delivery is the creation or maintenance of space interproximally to accommodate the stainless steel crown. Many orthodontists will schedule their patients about 10 days before Herbst delivery to place separators. Greenbaum[50] recommends the used of oversized elastomeric separators (#480-304, Ortho Technologies, Tampa FL). These thicker white separators are oversized relative to the usual elastomeric separators, and they create or maintain the interdental spaces adequately.

In our practice, we are more aggressive in creating interproximal space. We recommend the temporary cementation of bands on those teeth that will receive stainless steel crowns during the next appointment. Bands are cemented temporarily on the upper first molars and lower premolars. In addition, the clinician may choose to band the lower first molars in order to maintain space in these regions as well. The bands are cemented with Durelon™ (Premier Co., Frankfurt, Germany) or another easily removed adhesive. Elastomeric separators then can be replaced in the interproximal areas adjacent to the bands to open the interdental spaces further to accommodate the cementation of the thick stainless steel crowns at the next appointment.

Preparation and Delivery of the Appliance

Many of the details of the clinical management of the stainless steel crown Herbst appliance have been derived from conversations with a number of clinicians, including Dischinger,[34,46] Mayes,[37,38] Smith,[35,36] Hilgers,[41] and Chastant.[42] Many of their suggestions and recommendations are incorporated in the discussion that follows.

Preliminary Try-in

At the delivery appointment, all separators and temporary bands are removed and the patient is instructed to

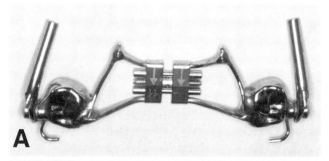
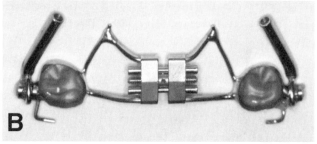

Figure 17-22. Maxillary stainless steel crown appliance with soldered midline expansion screw. *A*, Occlusal view. *B*, Palatal view. The inside surfaces of the crowns have been microetched to improve retention.

brush his or her teeth thoroughly. The maxillary and mandibular parts of the appliance are examined for proper construction (Figs. 17-22 and 17-23), making sure that the inside surfaces of the crowns and bands have been microetched. If the laboratory has not carried out this procedure, the crowns should be microetched in-office to facilitate the retention of the appliance during treatment. Note: Anytime a band or crown is microetched in the office, it should be placed in the ultrasonic for a few minutes in clean water to remove any particles from the etching process.

The parts of the appliance are placed in the mouth and seated in place. The upper and lower Herbst units typically are delivered from the laboratory with the mechanisms in place, secured by tightening the screws with finger pressure only. Tightening the screws in this manner allows the clinician to disassemble the mechanisms as necessary for the trial fit in the mouth. Typically, the upper member is seated with the tubes attached and temporarily secured to the crowns with elastics. Securing the tubes in this manner prevents the ends of the attached tubes from hitting tissue during the try-in process.

In the mandible, the plungers are removed from the appliance prior to delivery. It simply is not feasible to attempt to seat the lower appliance while simultaneously inserting the plungers in the tubes. Once both arches are seated fully, the lower rods are reinserted into the tubes, the lower jaw advanced, and the eyelets seated over the lower pivots. The rods either can be held

HERBST APPLIANCE

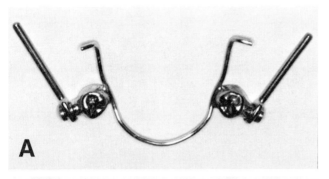
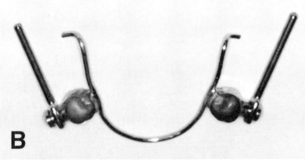

Figure 17-23. Mandibular stainless steel crown appliance with occlusal rests that will be bonded to the lower first molars. *A*, Occlusal view. *B*, Apical view. The inside surfaces of the crowns have been microetched.

in place over the pivots, or the screws are engaged but not tightened.

The next step is critical. The patient is instructed to open and close slowly and move the lower jaw from side to side. The clinician must assess the opening, closing, and lateral movements. The patient must be able to open and close with no binding of the mechanisms. In addition, there should be at least 4–5 mm of lateral freedom in each direction. Failure to detect problems at this stage in the appliance evaluation can lead directly to subsequent breakage. If there are restrictions in free movement of the mandible, the first area to check is the opening of the eyelets on the mechanisms. As necessary, these can be enlarged slightly with a bur to gain additional range of mandibular movement.

If difficulty is encountered in seating the stainless steel crowns, the patient can be instructed to bite firmly on cotton rolls that have been placed interocclusally. A band seater or bite stick also can be used to push the crowns in position. In some instances, it may be necessary to contour the crowns to gain a proper fit. The stainless steel crowns used for the Herbst are manufactured in eight sizes per quadrant as compared to well over thirty in some band series. In the laboratory, it sometimes is necessary to select a crown that is slightly larger than ideal to insure an adequate clinical fit. In this situation, the crowns must be contoured additionally for a secure fit.

Depending on the exact dental anatomy in the mouth, the crowns also may require minor adaptation during the try-in stage. One of the most important signs to note is excess blanching of the tissue, an indication of either too large of a crown or a lack of contouring of the side walls. This situation, if detected, must be corrected for health of the tissues during Herbst wear and to improve mechanical retention of the crowns to the teeth.

The Herbst bite jumping mechanism should be assembled to ensure that the desired amount of bite advancement has been achieved. If the amount of bite advancement is insufficient, preformed shims of varying lengths (Great Lakes Orthodontic Products, Tonawanda NY) can be added to the mandibular arms of the appliance. If the bite is advanced too much, the length of the maxillary tubes should be shortened appropriately. In addition, once the maxillary tubes have been shortened, the practitioner should make sure that the mandibular arms of the appliance are not too long. Arms that protrude more than 1–2 mm posteriorly out of the tube can lead to significant soft and hard tissue damage in the posterior ramal region.

Preparation of the Crowns

One of the most important steps in the delivery of the crown Herbst appliance is the preparation of the stainless steel crowns before cementation. This preparation is essential to facilitate the removal of the crowns at the end of the Herbst phase of treatment. During the preparation of the crowns, Mayes[51] has recommended creating small notches that extend from the gingival margin about 2–2.5 mm occlusally. These notches are used during the removal process as the crowns are cut prior to removal.

After the fit of the crown Herbst appliance has been verified and any necessary adjustments completed, the appliance is left in position. The orthodontist then makes a small nick in each stainless steel crown near the mesiobuccal line angle with a #557 crosscut fissure bur (Figs. 17-24 and 17-25). The marks on the crown should be made at the time of appliance delivery. These marks should be located at a logical point on each crown. Because active Herbst treatment usually lasts 9–12 months and because gingival hypertrophy often occurs during treatment, notching the crowns at delivery makes crown removal easier. Even if the gingival border of the crown is several millimeters away from the gingival margin at the time of delivery, notching the crowns is recommended strongly because the gingival margin of the crown typically becomes subgingival by the time Herbst treatment is completed.

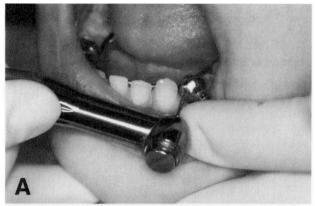
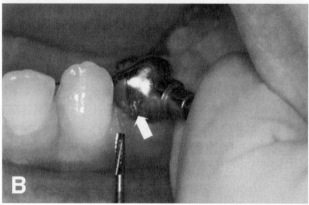

Figure 17-24. Preparing the mandibular crowns prior to cementation. *A*, A crosscut fissure bur in a highspeed handpiece is used to make a small mark in each crown along the mesiobuccal line angle. *B*, The position of the nick will indicate the location of the notch that will be placed in each crown before cementation.

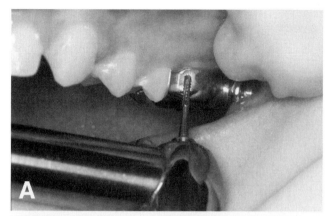
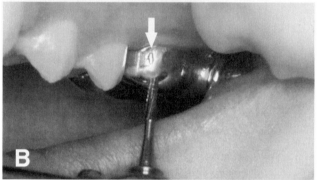

Figure 17-25. Preparation of maxillary crowns. *A*, the crosscut fissure bur is used to mark the stainless steel crown. *B*, The nick in the surface of the crown now is visible (see arrow).

After marking the crowns is completed, both parts of the appliance are removed from the mouth. The orthodontist then uses the #557 crosscut fissure bur to notch the crowns (Figs. 17-26). The notches are made about 1 mm thick and 2–2.5 mm in height. Care should be taken that the notches are not extended occlusally too much so that the integrity of the crown is not threatened (*e.g.*, crown tearing during normal function) but, on the other hand, the notches should be sufficient in height to allow their visualization at the time of appliance removal (Fig. 17-27).

The mesial and distal margins of the crowns also can be crimped at this point if retention of the appliance is in question.

Appliance Preparation

Once the clinical fit has been verified, the appliance is ready for cementation. Typically, the upper member is cemented with the Herbst tubes attached. As the working action of the Herbst has been checked in the previ-

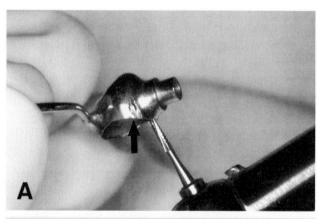
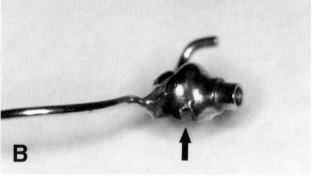

Figure 17-26. Notching the mandibular stainless steel crowns. *A*, Defining the extent of the notch with the crosscut fissure bur. *B*, Notching completed.

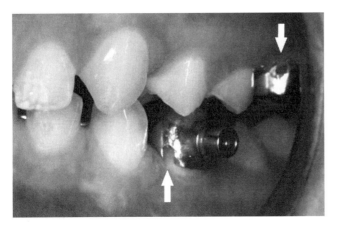

Figure 17-27. The crown Herbst appliance in place before cementation. The notches on each crown should be visible.

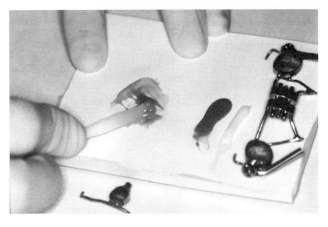

Figure 17-28. Cementation of the crown Herbst appliance with a chemical-cure adhesive that is not tooth-colored.

ous step, the screws holding the upper tubes to the crowns can be tightened completely at this time. Using the small Allen wrench, the screws are tightened with hand pressure. Care must be taken not to apply too much force as to strip the head of the screws. Some clinicians also elect to use a product called Ceka Bond™ (Preat Corp., San Mateo CA) to secure the screws. This liquid material, from the orthopedic industry, is applied to the ends of the screws and adds a chemical lock to the parts.

The maxillary tubes are held in place temporarily against the crowns with an elastic. Securing the tubes prevents tissue irritation from the ends of the tubes. The ends of the tubes also are filled with Chapstick™ or a similar medium to prevent adhesive from entering the holes in the tubes. This procedure also is performed on the lower pivots where the screws connect the Herbst mechanisms to the anchor unit.

The lower unit most often is cemented with the plungers disassembled. Once the lower appliance is delivered, the rods are fit into the upper tubes, the patient is asked to protrude the mandible, and the eyelets of the rods are slipped over the lower pivots. The lower screws are seated with the Allen wrench in the same manner as described above.

Appliance Cementation

A chemical cure adhesive (*e.g.*, Blue CrownLok™, Reliance Orthodontic Products, Itasca IL) is used to cement the parts of the appliance in place (Fig. 17-28). The two parts of the material are blended together on a mixing pad, and then the bonding material is placed in each crown. The maxillary and mandibular parts of the appliance are pushed to place, seated with occlusal biting force (*e.g.*, cotton rolls, bite stick, band seater), and the excess cementing material is removed. The use of cement that is not tooth colored is recommended so that the clinician can determine easily the location of the cement at the time of appliance removal.

When cementing crowns on molars, some clinicians advocate an additional step prior to delivery. A small amount of Vaseline™ is applied to the occlusal surface of each molar using a cotton applicator. The petroleum jelly prevents the adhesive from bonding in the deep occlusal pits of the tooth and greatly facilitates adhesive cleanup after crown removal. This procedure, when done judiciously, does not affect the adhesion strength of the crowns to the teeth as the cement is bonding the entire perimeter of the crown. In addition, there is the mechanical lock of the crown to the tooth that is produced from the correct anatomical fit and contouring.

Home Care Instructions

The patient is told that it will take several days to get used to the Herbst appliance. During this period, the jaw muscles may become tired and sore. With a few days, however, the patient will become increasingly comfortable. We have noted that the amount of patient discomfort has been minimized greatly by limiting the initial advancement to 4–7 mm, especially in patients with large overjets. Subsequent advancements are made easily.

Patients who have a Herbst with an RME screw are provided activation instructions and a key in accordance with the information in Chapter 13 covering rapid maxillary expansion appliances.

Some difficulty in chewing often is experienced, particularly during the first few weeks. A soft diet is suggested until the patient accommodates to the appliance and is able to chew. It has been our experience that once the break in period has passed, most patients encounter little difficulty when functioning with the cemented Herbst appliance.

The patient's responsibility in caring for the Herbst appliance and for oral hygiene includes attention to dietary intake, teeth cleaning, and fluoride rinsing. The patient is cautioned to avoid hard and sticky foods that may dislodge the appliance. It is especially important for the patient to restrict intake of foods containing sugar to avoid damage to the teeth from decalcification and dental caries. The patient is instructed to clean the teeth and the appliance by brushing carefully several times each day and to use a fluoride rinse at least twice each day.

The initial difficulty in wearing the Herbst appliance usually passes quickly. If the patient experiences pain that increases over time, or if hot or swollen cheeks and a bad taste or odor in the mouth accompanies this pain, an ulcerated area of mucosa may be infected, and the patient must be seen immediately. Discomfort also may be experienced if an attachment screw rubs against the cheeks, causing irritation. This condition is temporary and can be ameliorated by placing soft wax over the connections until the irritation passes. If any sharp edges are present on the attachment screws, the edges should be rounded and polished before delivery.

Patients and parents also may be given an Allen wrench in case a Herbst screw comes loose. In this instance, the screw simply is tightened, and unless further problems persist, the next regular appointment maintained.

Hilgers[44] has noted that patients and parents respond directly to the amount of confidence that the clinician has in the appliance. If they sense some hesitation (or even over-concern) on the part of the clinician, the number of negative responses seems to increase exponentially. For this one reason, clinicians with a great deal of experience using the appliance report far fewer negative patient responses than clinicians new to its use. It usually takes over a year for the orthodontist and staff to achieve a level of comfort/confidence that can be sensed by the apprehensive patient.[44]

Hilgers[44] has found that the patients who seem to have the most trouble with the appliance are smaller patients with relatively thin lip and cheek tissue thicknesses. Even though other diagnostic criteria may suggest Herbst therapy, the ability of these patients to handle the appliance comfortably appears to be diminished.

Subsequent Advancement

The appliance can be reactivated every other appointment as necessary after initial placement. This activation is accomplished either by substituting progressively longer maxillary tubes or by adding shims (sleeves of tubing) over the mandibular plunger. The latter is the method of choice in most instances.

A "Herbst advancement kit" (Great Lakes Orthodontic Products, Tonawanda NY) has pieces of tubing in 1–5 mm increments to facilitate accurate stepwise advancement. The lower rods are removed by unscrewing the hex head screws. Next, the tubing sleeves are crimped on to the mandibular plunger with heavy wire cutters (Figs. 17-29). The now "lengthened" lower rods then are reattached to the lower unit with the hex screws. Subsequent advancements can be performed at regular intervals until the desired amount of mandibular repositioning is obtained. The amount of advancement can differ bilaterally in instances in which a midline deviation needs correction.

Hilgers[44] has found that simply hand articulating the upper and lower models in the correct overbite-overjet and midline relationship and reporting this axle length to the laboratory is satisfactory. This method avoids having to take a check-bite altogether and it gives the clinician more control over exactly where they would like to see the mandible positioned.

Discontinuation of Herbst Appliance Therapy

It has been our customary practice to leave the Herbst appliance in place five to six months after the last activation. This recommendation concerning the time interval is made solely on the basis of clinical observation, not on the results of comparative clinical trials. The total

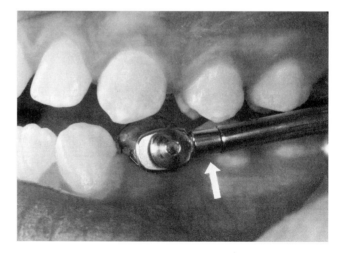

Figure 17-29. Advancement of the Herbst appliance with the addition of shims (small pieces of tubing) on the mandibular plunger. The shim can be crimped on the plunger with a heavy-duty wire cutter or it can be tack welded in place. (See also Fig. 17-40 later in this chapter.)

treatment time with the Herbst appliance usually is 9–12 months. Treatment time may be shorter if an edge-to-edge bite registration is used.* In contrast, Hilgers[44] believes in longer-term wear of the appliance (14–16 months is not unusual). He avoids placing brackets during Herbst appliance wear; the absence of brackets during this period aids in patient acceptance and avoids some of the common difficulties associated with early brackets and wires.

Although it has not been our practice, some clinicians advocate removing the RME screw once the expansion and stabilization phases of treatment are completed. Using a high-speed handpiece and a diamond or crosscut fissure bur, the screw is cut away from the crowns and the remaining surfaces smoothed. This procedure allows one appliance to be used throughout the entire expansion and Herbst phases of treatment. In our practice, however, the appliance remains intact with the screw in place throughout treatment.

Removal of the Crown Herbst

At the time of appliance removal, some clinicians prefer to remove the Herbst bite jumping mechanism as the first step, whereas other clinicians prefer to leave the plungers and/or tubes in place to aid in appliance removal. Routinely, we take out the plungers and tubes before beginning the removal process.

If there is a continuous archwire in either arch, from the Herbst archwire tubes to the brackets, it can either be removed or left in place during Herbst removal. Some clinicians prefer to leave the archwire intact, as the crowns (especially the upper first molars) cannot be lost (*i.e.*, swallowed) with this technique. In the lower arch, sectional archwires are left in place anterior to the connection points with the stainless steel crowns.

The first step in the sequence is to evaluate the appliance thoroughly, locating the notches in each crown, Frequently the gingival tissue has hypertrophied so that the notches are not immediately visible. In this instance, the notches can be palpated indirectly with a scaler or explorer.

At this point, a #557 crosscut fissure bur or a crown-removing bur (#H34-012, Brassler, Savannah GA) is used to cut each crown from the gingival margin to the center of the clinical crown (Fig. 17-30). The operator must be very careful not to cut the enamel of the underlying tooth. By using a colored cementing agent, the orthodontist usually can tell if s/he has penetrated the stainless steel crown or the cement surrounding the enamel. By taking advantage of the previously cut notch, the clinician typically avoids having to injure the hypertrophied gingiva that may have partially grown around the stainless steel crown, minimizing patient discomfort.

After a substantial groove has been made along the mesiobuccal line angle of the stainless steel crown, a Christiansen crown remover (Hu-Friedy Co., Chicago IL) is used to begin to remove the crown (Fig. 17-31). This type of crown removal instrument is intended for crown removal after the crown has been sectioned with a bur. It comes in two designs, a right-angled shank (#CRCH2; Fig. 17-31*A*) and a straight shank (#CRCH1; Fig. 17-31*B*). Two notches in the tip provide a secure grip on the crown as the instrument is turned, breaking the seal of the cement.

At this point, the crown usually becomes loosened. A specially made Herbst plier (Dentaurum, Newtown PA) then is used to remove the stainless steel crown from

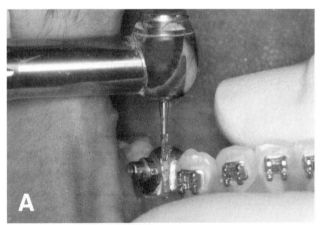

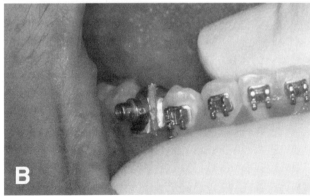

Figure 17-30. Removal of the stainless steel crowns. *A*, A crosscut fissure bur or a crown removing bur in a highspeed handpiece is used to cut the crown from the gingival margin to the center of the crown. Placing notches in the crown before cementation facilitates crown removal in instances of gingival hypertrophy, which often occurs during treatment. *B*, The completed cut.

---

*It should be noted that although Pancherz routinely has used a six-month treatment time in his clinical studies, he has stressed that this time interval was arrived at arbitrarily and that in clinical practice longer treatment intervals may be appropriate.

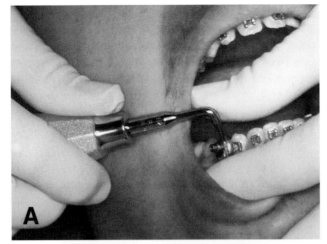

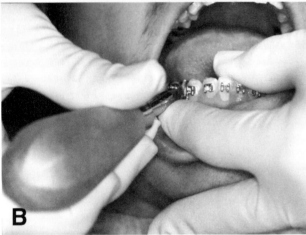

Figure 17-31. Removal of the stainless steel crowns (cont.) A, The tapered, notched end of a Christiansen crown remover (Hu-Friedy Co., Chicago, IL) is placed in the cut groove on the crown and rotated, splitting the crown and breaking the adhesive seal. Two designs of the crown remover are available. A, Right-angled shank. B, Straight shank.

the tooth. The contoured ends of the plier can be used to grip the axle soldered to the crown. The crown is rotated gently and the crown is lifted from the tooth. If a soldered mandibular lingual wire is present, occasionally it is advisable to section the wire before removing the lower stainless steel crowns. Alternatively, a Chastant crown-removing plier (Ormco Corp., Orange CA) can be used to dislodge the stainless steel crown after a hole has been made in its occlusal surface.[42]

As many clinicians use a cantilever type Herbst, crown removal from the molars is another clinical procedure to perform. There have been several methods proposed for removing molar crowns. One of the original (and still widely used) techniques involves strategically cutting the crown with a small diamond bur along the mesial line angle. Once this cut is completed, the crown simply is split and removed. With experience, this method works well, although there is the possibility of hitting enamel in areas where the inside of the crown is close to the tooth.

For this reason, another popular technique has been introduced which involves cutting the crown in a different manner. Also using a diamond bur with a "football" shape, the major portion of the occlusal surface of the crown is removed. Care is taken to avoid cutting the portions of the crowns directly adjacent to the lingual and buccal cusps of the molar. The occlusal area inside the crown is where the greatest thickness of adhesive exists, and there is a lesser chance for the bur to contact the enamel. With the center occlusal portion of the crown removed, the tip of crown-removing pliers can be located on the middle of the tooth and the opposing jaw under the edge of the crown. A direct vertical force is applied to the pliers to dislodge the crown. The advantage to using this technique is the avoidance of using the bur near the enamel, with an additional benefit that most of the adhesive will remain adhered to the inside of the crown instead of the tooth.

Following crown removal, the teeth should be cleaned thoroughly and checked for decalcification and decay, both of which occur extremely rarely if proper protocols have been followed.

Another method of dislodging the stainless crowns is the use of a spring-loaded crown remover, commonly called a "Thumper™" (Thumper Co., Lubbock TX), as recommended by Mayes[52] (Fig. 17-32). This device was developed to aid in the removal of gold crowns; the end of the attachment has been modified for the removal of stainless steel crowns as well. The end of the device can be placed against the axle soldered to the stainless steel crown (Fig. 17-33). The Thumper™ then is activated by pressing the release handle on the shaft of the appliance, and a strong but short-acting force is generated against the axle, dislodging the crown from the tooth.

We routinely obtain a lateral headfilm following

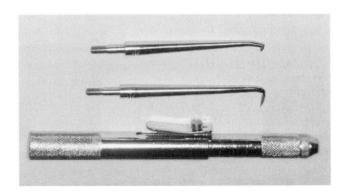

Figure 17-32. "Thumper" crown remover. This device is used to break the adhesive seal and loosen the stainless steel crown.

HERBST APPLIANCE

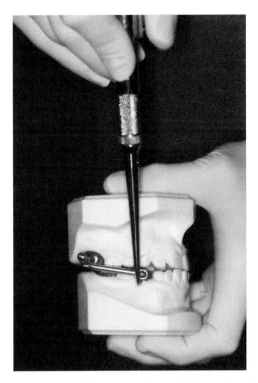

Figure 17-33. A set of Herbst study models is used to demonstrate the positioning of the Thumper crown remover against one of the soldered axles of the appliance after the spring-loaded device has been activated. The lever arm of the appliance is depressed by the clinician, and a strong but short-acting force is delivered to the stainless steel crown, braking the adhesive seal.

Herbst removal, either on the day of removal or during the next appointment. In that we choose to use the Herbst appliance almost exclusively in patients in the early permanent dentition, the patient proceeds directly into Phase II fixed appliance treatment, the details of which are described in Chapter 9.

ACRYLIC SPLINT HERBST APPLIANCE

Another design of the Herbst appliance is the acrylic splint Herbst, developed in the early 1980s by Howe, McNamara, and co-workers.[53–59] The treatment effects of this type of appliance have been studied by a number of investigators.[24,25,60–62]

Originally designed in an attempt to replace the breakage-prone banded Herbst, the acrylic splint now has several treatment applications. As an alternative Herbst design for Class II correction, the acrylic splint Herbst is very effective, especially when combined with an upper expansion screw. The acrylic splint design also has been used as a removable appliance in the treatment of temporomandibular disorders and sleep disorders.[63] Using the acrylic splint design in this way, while not specifically covered in this chapter, facilitates these non-orthodontic treatments, due to the ease of use by the patient and clinician. The removable acrylic splint Herbst enables the clinician to align the jaws precisely in all three planes of space to affect whatever dental or medical condition benefits from this jaw relationship.

Parts of the Appliance

The acrylic splint Herbst appliance is composed of a wire framework, over which has been adapted 2.5–3.0 mm thick splint Biocryl™. In lateral view (Fig. 17-34), the acrylic splints cover all of the lower teeth, except for the second molars. The design of the upper splint varies according to whether the splint is bonded or removable. If the splint is removable, the posterior teeth are covered from the canines through the first molars; if the maxillary splint is bonded, the labial surfaces of the canines are not covered with acrylic. The axles of the Herbst bite-jumping mechanism are soldered adjacent to the lower first premolars and the upper first molars (Fig. 17-34).

A frontal perspective is shown in Figure 17-35. In this example, the left side of the maxillary appliance is trimmed as if the splint were to be bonded, whereas the right side has been trimmed as if the splint were to be worn as a removable appliance (*i.e.*, full canine coverage). The lower splint, which always is removable, is trimmed so that one third to one half of the labial surfaces of the lower incisors are covered by the splint. This type of lower incisor coverage aids in the retention of the lower splint during treatment.

An occlusal view of the maxillary splint is shown in

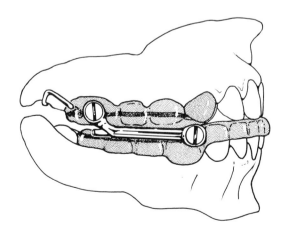

Figure 17-34. Right lateral view of the acrylic splint Herbst appliance. This drawing demonstrates full coverage of the maxillary canine, the design recommended when the maxillary splint is removable.

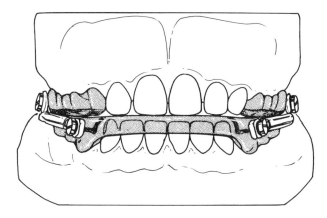

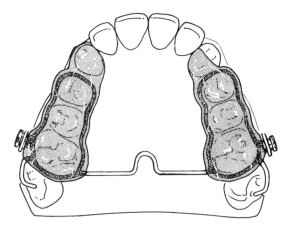

Figure 17-35. Frontal view of the acrylic splint Herbst appliance. Note that the lower splint covers at least one third of the labial surfaces of the lower incisors. Additional retention of the lower splint can be gained by extending the acrylic inferiorly on these teeth. Labial canine coverage is included when the splint is removable; the facial surface of the canine is not covered when the splint is bonded.

Figure 17-36. Maxillary portion of an acrylic splint Herbst appliance with a transpalatal wire connecting the two sides of the splint. The right side of the appliance demonstrates full canine coverage that is used when the splint is removable. On the left side, the acrylic extends only to the lingual aspect of the upper canine. This design is used when the upper splint is bonded.

Figure 17-36. In this example, the right side of the appliance is trimmed as a removable appliance, whereas the left side is trimmed for bonding. Only the lingual surface of the splint contacts the upper canine in the bonded design. The anterior extension of the splint is bonded to the lingual surface of the upper canine. If second molars are present, occlusal rests made from .036" wire are added to the splint to prevent extrusion of these teeth during treatment.

The maxillary splint shown in Figure 17-37 is our preferred design in that a rapid maxillary expansion screw connects the two sides of the splint together. We recommend including the expansion screw in most instances, in that transverse maxillary deficiency is a common finding in Class II patients.[43] The expansion screw also stabilizes the maxillary splint when the splint is worn as a removable appliance. The screw is activated once per week when the maxillary splint is removable and once per day when the maxillary splint is bonded. The maxillary splint also can be made without a midline screw if the patient has been expanded during an earlier phase of orthopedic treatment (Fig. 17-36).

The lower splint (Fig. 17-38) has full occlusal coverage that extends from lower first molar to lower first molar. If second molars are present, occlusal rests are provided as well. The axles that connect the Herbst bite jumping mechanism to the splint are soldered to the base archwire at the mesial aspect of the lower first premolar before the Biocryl™ is added. Ball clasps may be added to the removable design to aid in retention.

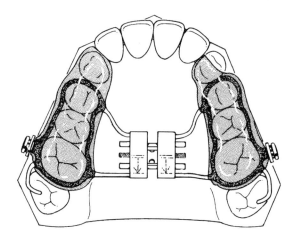

Figure 17-37. Maxillary view of the acrylic splint Herbst appliance with a midline expansion screw.

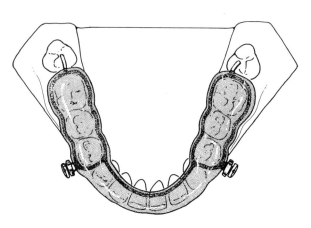

Figure 17-38. Mandibular acrylic splint Herbst appliance with full occlusal and incisal coverage.

Clinical Management of the Acrylic Splint Herbst

The lower portion of the acrylic splint Herbst always is removable. The maxillary portion, however, can be fixed or removable, depending on the choice of the orthodontist. In our practice, about 75% of patients who are given an acrylic splint Herbst wear it as a removable appliance. Many clinicians are uncomfortable having their patients wear a fixed functional appliance. On the other hand, some practitioners prefer 24-hour appliance wear and thus choose to bond the maxillary part of the appliance in place.

Impressions

Except for bonded brackets that may be left on the maxillary incisors at the discretion of the clinician, all initial phase appliances are removed before impression taking, and the teeth are pumiced. Accurate, bubble-free maxillary and mandibular alginate impressions are taken of the dentition and associated soft tissues according to standard impression-taking protocols. The impressions should be checked to make sure that adequate anatomic reproductions of the dentition and the immediate associated soft tissue are obtained.

If significant dental movement has been produced during an initial phase of dental decompensation, it is necessary to stabilize the dental arches during the time of Herbst fabrication. Thus, the use of a transitional retainer, such as an invisible retainer,[64,65] is used to stabilize the dentition during appliance fabrication. If a transitional retainer is not worn during the interval needed for appliance fabrication, unwanted tooth movement may occur that could prevent proper seating of the appliance at delivery.

Bite Registration

The recommended bite registration technique for the acrylic splint Herbst is essentially the same for the stainless steel Herbst described previously. The laboratory can be instructed to advance the work models a prescribed amount (*e.g.*, incisal edge-to-edge, midway) or the Projet™ bite fork (Great Lakes Orthodontic Products, Tonawanda NY) can be used, as described in detail in Chapter 15.

In the discussion of the clinical management of the Herbst presented previously, the point was made that an accurate reproduction of the vertical dimension was not critical for the fabrication for the stainless steel or banded types of Herbst appliance. This statement may or may not be correct for the fabrication of the acrylic splint Herbst. If the curve of Spee is relatively flat and the teeth generally are straight, a patient who will be receiving an acrylic splint appliance can have the appliance fabricated without a specific bite registration. Minor adjustments in occlusal contact can be made at the time of appliance delivery. If there are any concerns about the alignment of the teeth or the vertical relationship of the occlusion, however, the 2 or 4-mm Projet™ bite fork and medium hard pink wax can be used to obtain an accurate bite registration.

A horseshoe of medium hard pink wax is softened in warm water. While the wax is softening, the patient is instructed to practice positioning the mandible forward, according to the serrations on the bite fork. This practice session allows the clinician to inspect the molar relationships and to use the incisal overjet as an index of the amount of necessary forward repositioning. Care must be taken to align the skeletal midlines, using the dental midlines as reference points. Once the patient has practiced aligning the skeletal midlines and posturing the mandible forward, the wax bite registration can be made. Wax coverage of the anterior teeth is avoided, so that the overjet and midline relationship can be observed.

After the wax bite has been obtained, it is placed on the original study models. This procedure will allow the clinician to determine visually the amount of bite advancement in the bite registration by comparing the relationship of the backs of the dental casts that previously had been trimmed flush when the bite of the patient was recorded in centric occlusion. Of course, this procedure is not possible if initial fixed appliance therapy has been performed. In this instance, an additional wax bite taken in habitual occlusion is helpful in determining the amount of bite advancement by providing an initial reference position for the work models.

Preparation of Work Models

Before sending the appliance models to the laboratory, the impressions should be poured. After the stone has set, any bubbles or imperfections should be removed. The models then are oriented using the wax bite registration, and the backs of the models are trimmed flush. The models and wax bite are checked thoroughly to make sure that there is adequate vertical clearance for appliance fabrication and that the bite has not been advanced excessively.

Laboratory Prescriptions

Prescription forms for Herbst appliances vary greatly, depending on the individual commercial laboratory. In that the lower acrylic splint is always removable, full occlusal coverage (with the exception of the second molars) is recommended. If the maxillary splint is removable, full posterior coverage including the canines is desired; if the maxillary splint is to be bonded, only extensions of the appliance to the lingual surfaces of the upper canines are necessary.

Delivery of the Acrylic Splint Herbst Appliance

After the assembled appliance has been returned from the laboratory, the appliance is replaced on the construction models and tested for protrusive, opening, and lateral movements. If the appliance binds in any of these movements, the upper and lower parts of the bite-jumping mechanism are removed, keeping left and right sides separate, and each of the four connection holes are enlarged to permit more freedom of movement. The appliance is reassembled and rechecked on the construction models. Even though this procedure usually is performed at the laboratory, it is important for the clinician to recheck the freedom of movement as binding may dislodge the splints during function.

The upper and lower halves of the appliance are placed in the mouth separately to check the fit of each acrylic splint. The splints then are inserted with the plungers and sleeves engaged in order to check the length of the mandibular plungers as they exit the distal aspect of the maxillary tubes. Whenever the second molars are present, the distal end of the lower plunger can extend as far back as the distal end of the maxillary axle (Fig. 17-34). If second molars are not present, however, the distal ends of the plunger should be cut flush with the posterior opening of the upper tube.

The trimming is accomplished in this manner to prevent the plunger from impinging on and ulcerating the mucosa overlying the mandibular ramus that is repositioned forward by the appliance. If either the left or right plunger extends too far out of the distal end of its sleeve and impinges on the mucosa, it is marked, removed, and shortened to the desired length. Once rounded, it is replaced and checked. If this step is omitted, and the plungers impinge on the mucosa, ulcerations and serious infection may result.

Obviously, it is desirable to have the plunger as long as possible to allow the patient maximum opening. The clinician is cautioned against leaving the mandibular part of the bite-jumping mechanism excessively long, however, because of the potential for serious tissue damage. It has been noted that with a step-by-step bite registration, the incidence of tissue damage due to plunger impingement has been reduced greatly from that observed with an end-to-end bite registration.

If the entire appliance is removable, the parts of the appliance can be joined together before placement by the patient in his or her mouth. Alternatively, if the maxillary splint is bonded (to be discussed in detail below), the maxillary portions of the Herbst mechanism are left attached to the splint. The screws should have been tightened firmly to prevent loosening during appliance wear. The removable mandibular splint is placed in the mouth by the patient. In some instances, it is possible to assemble the Herbst mechanism after the appliance is in place; other times it is necessary to place the plungers of the lower splint into the tubes of the upper splint before seating the mandibular appliance. The patient is instructed to close, and the bite is checked. If "fulcruming" of the splints is detected, the occlusal contact is adjusted until even contact is established posteriorly.

With the telescoping mechanism in place, the patient is asked to move the mandible through all excursions, while the clinician explains that the appliance will limit the range of movement. The clinician then should show the patient how to avoid forceful lateral and retrusive movements of the lower jaw.

Next, the patient is given a mirror and asked to open the mouth as wide as possible. During wide opening, if the plunger and sleeve assemblies become disengaged, the patient is shown how to reinsert the lower plunger into the upper sleeves by holding the mouth wide open, aligning the lower plunger with the upper tubes, and then closing the mouth so that the plunger reinserts into the tube. In addition, the patient is instructed to keep the lower jaw postured forward, just avoiding contact with the tube-plunger mechanism at all times.

Bonding of the Maxillary Splint

In some instances, it may be advisable to bond the maxillary portion of the Herbst appliance. Obviously, this is indicated in patients in whom the anatomical shape of the teeth (e.g., conical) is such that the retention of the maxillary splint during normal jaw movements is either difficult or impossible. The bonding of the splint also may be advisable in instances of questionable patient cooperation. In addition, if any type of fixed orthodontic appliance (e.g., utility arch) is to be used in conjunction with the Herbst appliance, bonding of the maxillary portion of the splint, of course, is necessary. Bonding of the maxillary splint is optional when a rapid maxillary expansion screw is incorporated into the appliance. If the splint is bonded, the expander can be turned on a once-per-day basis; if the splint is removable, a once-per-week activation schedule is recommended.

Preparation of Splint for Bonding

Before the bonding procedure is initiated, the maxillary acrylic splint is prepared. A thin coat of acrylic primer (*i.e.*, the liquid monomer of methyl methacrylate, known as "plastic bracket primer") should be applied to the inside of the splint. The application of this liquid will enhance the bonding of the resin to the appliance.

Another procedure that will improve retention of the appliance to the teeth is microetching the inside of the acrylic. Microetching will produce a "frosted" appearance to the inside surface of the splint due to the etching. As mentioned previously, a recently microetched surface should be cleaned by placing the appliance in an ultrasonic with plain water to remove any particulates from the surfaces.

Pumicing the Teeth

The first step in preparing the patient for bonding is pumicing the teeth. Using a rotating rubber cup and non-fluoridated pumice, all of the teeth involved in the bonding procedure should be cleaned thoroughly. The maxillary dental arch is isolated with cheek retractors that have extensions into the buccal vestibule, but do not cross over the occlusal surface of the dental arches. Absorbent Dri-angles™ are placed in the buccal vestibule bilaterally to block secretion from the parotid gland.

Etching

Then the teeth are etched carefully with a diluted (37%) solution of phosphoric acid in either a liquid or a gel form. With the bonding of any large acrylic appliance, only the buccal and lingual surfaces of the teeth, as well as the mesial surface of the anterior tooth and the distal surface of the first molar are etched. *The occlusal surfaces are not etched*, thus facilitating the removal of the appliance. In instances of limited retention, the occlusal surface of deciduous teeth may be etched. The duration of etching usually is 30-60 seconds. Deciduous teeth may require 90 seconds. The etching solution is dabbed in place continuously, rather than rubbed on the tooth in a circular motion, to prevent fracturing of the fragile enamel rods that become exposed during etching.

Rinsing and Drying

After the etching material has been applied, the area is rinsed thoroughly with a continuous stream of water. This step is very important, as many bonding failures occur because the acid etch has not been removed adequately from the teeth. It is recommended that each tooth be rinsed for approximately 10–20 seconds. The teeth are dried with a clean, dry air source and inspected for a uniform chalky appearance. When a three-way syringe is used, it is recommended that the syringe be tested for dryness by blowing air into a patient napkin or into a facial tissue. Any contamination of the air supply with water or oil must be avoided.

Bonding

A bonding agent with low viscosity and long-working time that is well suited to the bonding of a large acrylic appliance is suggested. Two types of bonding material can be used in bonding the maxillary portion of the Herbst appliance: a two-part chemical mix and a light-cured resin. Both of these materials have proven satisfactory in the routine bonding of such an appliance.

A fourhanded approach is recommended during the bonding procedure. If a two-part chemical adhesive is used, usually the first step is to place a two-part sealant onto the teeth. This non-filled resin will seal all of the areas that have been exposed during the etching process. As the clinician is applying the sealant, an auxiliary paints the inside of the acrylic splints with another coat of plastic primer (mentioned earlier) and then begins to mix the two-part bonding agent.

When bonding a large acrylic appliance, one particular product is recommended (*i.e.*, Excel™, Reliance Orthodontic Products, Itasca IL). This material, which was formulated specifically for use with large bonded splints, has low viscosity and a long setting time that allows for adequate cleanup of the appliance. The auxiliary fills the maxillary splint with the bonding agent and passes it to the clinician, who places the loaded acrylic splint on the maxillary dental arch and holds it in place. Firm pressure is applied initially to force the excessive bonding material out of the splint, and the clinician can clean up the excess with cotton applicators (*i.e.*, Q-tips™), small cotton balls, and later a scaler.

When the material first is setting, it is not viscous. Cotton applicators are useful in removing the excess material from the appliance. The clinician also can use a gloved finger to clean around the outside of the splint. Then small cotton balls held in locking cotton forceps are used to clean under the lingual surface of the maxillary splint and under the arms of the expansion screw, if present.

As the gel phase of the setting bonding agent is approaching, the material becomes much more viscous and then is removed easily from the appliance with a universal scaler. Particular attention must be paid to the part of the appliance distal to the terminal molar. Once the bonding agent has set, the hardened bonding material is extremely difficult to remove. A bur and a handpiece may be necessary in these instances.

After the excess material has been cleared away, the splint then should be checked for any voids, particularly along the gingival margin. A second application of bonding agent can be used to fill any voids that are evident. Failure to fill a void can result in decalcification of the associated teeth during treatment.

Home Care Instructions

The patient and his or her parents are given the same information as was presented in the earlier section of the clinical management of the crown Herbst appliance. In addition, specific information is provided concerning the acrylic splints.

The appliance should be worn on a full-time basis, including at mealtime. The splints are removed only during brushing and flossing and when the appliance is being cleaned. The lower jaw should be held forward during the time that the appliance is not in place.

A soft diet is suggested until the patient accommodates to the appliance and is able to chew. Typically, patients wearing either fixed or removable splints accommodate to eating with the splints in place. Some clinicians, however, allow their patients to eat with the splints removed from the mouth. No comparative clinical studies to date have addressed this issue. Common sense dictates that the appliance should be worn full-time if possible, but both protocols have been used successfully for many years.

Subsequent Advancements

Advancement of the acrylic splint Herbst appliance is accomplished simply by adding shims to the mandibular plungers, as described previously (Figs. 17-39 and 17-40). If a less than incisal edge-to-edge advancement was chosen initially, the appliance is advanced in 2–3 mm increments every other appointment. Typically, the duration of treatment is 9–12 months after which a phase of fixed appliance therapy follows. The average total treatment time for acrylic splint Herbst therapy followed by fixed appliances is about two and one half years.[25]

TREATMENT EFFECTS

The Herbst appliance has been one of the most thoroughly studied orthodontic or orthopedic techniques, in large part due to the excellent clinical studies of Pan-

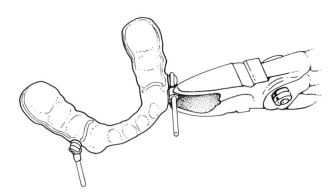

Figure 17-39. Advancement of the Herbst appliance. Heavy wire cutters are used to crimp the tubing sleeves on the mandibular plunger.

cherz and colleagues. In this section, the skeletal and dentoalveolar effects of Herbst treatment will be examined in detail. Treatment and post-treatment changes less than one millimeter or one degree in comparison to the growth of untreated subjects will be considered clinically insignificant.

Effects on the Maxilla

Treatment Changes

Even though the telescoping mechanism of the Herbst appliance produces a posterosuperiorly directed force on the maxillary bony base and dentition, in general, the Herbst appliance produces minimal short-term effects in the maxilla. Many studies[6,12,60,66] have shown that patients treated with the Herbst appliance over a period of six months or more undergo a slight reduction in the SNA angle, whereas no change or a slight increase in the SNA angle is observed in untreated controls. This slight reduction in the SNA angle commonly is seen following Herbst treatment, although significant differ-

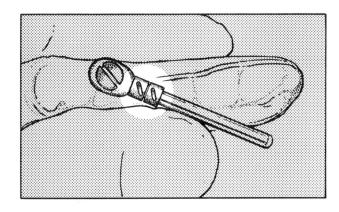

Figure 17-40. The mandibular plunger after two advancements with 2 mm pieces of tubing sleeves.

ences in maxillary length (relative to condylion or articulare) often are not found.[60,66]

McNamara and co-workers[24] compared the treatment effects of the acrylic-splint Herbst appliance to Class II untreated controls over a period of 12 months. Although a significant difference in SNA angle was not noted when the Herbst appliance was compared to untreated controls, a slight inhibition of midfacial length was detected. The 0.5 mm reduction in growth does not have a clinically meaningful effect on the growth and development of the maxillary complex.

Lai and McNamara[25] compared the treatment results of 40 subjects treated with the acrylic-splint Herbst appliance to normative values derived from the *University of Michigan Elementary and Secondary School Growth Study* and found a slight but statistically significant decrease in the SNA angle (−0.4° compared to controls) for treated patients. A significant difference in the size of the maxilla was not found for the measures of condylion-Point A or condylion-anterior nasal spine following Herbst treatment. None of these changes were clinically significant.

Posttreatment Changes

During the first twelve months after the Herbst appliance removal, the modest maxillary changes produced during treatment generally rebound. Pancherz[7] observed that the influence of bite jumping on maxillary growth appeared to be reversible or "temporary." Maxillary prognathism (*e.g.*, SNA angle) was reduced slightly during treatment (81.0° to 80.3°), but during a follow-up period of 12 months, maxillary growth increased, and the SNA angle rebounded to near pretreatment values (80.8°). Pancherz and Hansen[17] found that 12-month posttreatment angular measurements (81.8°, SNA angle) were similar to pretreatment values (81.9°).

Although the short-term treatment effects of the Herbst appliance on the maxilla have been found to rebound for the most part, modest long-term Herbst treatment effects on the maxilla have been described. In 1992, Hansen and Pancherz[67] reported that during a six months post-treatment interval, the Herbst treatment group underwent less sagittal maxillary change in position (0.6 mm difference in maxillary position measured parallel to the occlusal plane from sella to Point A) than did an untreated comparison group ("Bolton standards"[68]). In the six years that followed, anterior maxillary displacement in the Herbst sample was 1.3 mm less than that in the Bolton sample. Following the entire observation period, the average maxillary position of the Herbst patients was 1.9 mm posterior to that of the Bolton sample.

Pancherz and Anehus-Pancherz[69] followed patients treated with the Herbst appliance for 6.4 years following treatment. Lateral cephalograms taken before and after seven months of treatment, as well as six months post-treatment and 6.4 years post-treatment were analyzed. No statistical difference was seen when comparing displacement of the maxilla (Point A to occlusal line perpendicular through sella) during the treatment period to subjects in the Bolton control group. Interestingly, 6.4 years after treatment, the maxilla was positioned forward by 3.6 mm in the treated sample, which was about half of the amount seen in the Bolton control group. Although the headgear effect has been called "temporary" by Pancherz,[7,70] implying that the maxilla resumes normal growth following treatment, there is some evidence that a slight long-term treatment effect on the maxilla may exist.

In the period of fixed appliance therapy following the first phase of Herbst treatment, Lai and McNamara[25] found that the distance condylion-Point A increased less in the treatment group than was inferred from the control data, and there was a significant decrease in the SNA angle. These observations support Pancherz and Anehus-Pancherz's[69] finding of slight long-term reduced maxillary displacement following Herbst treatment.

In summary, slight inhibition of forward growth of the maxilla has been found during treatment, as well as during the post-treatment period. In general, the amount of inhibition, however, is not clinically relevant.

Effects on the Maxillary Dentition

Treatment Changes

Molars

The telescoping mechanism of the Herbst appliance places a upward and backward vector of force on the maxillary first molars. Subsequent molar distalization and intrusion have been shown with Herbst appliance therapy.[10] Following seven months of Herbst appliance therapy, Pancherz and Anehus-Pancherz[69] found that the upper first molars were distalized in 96% of the subjects, with the average first molar distalization of 2.1 mm (maximum 4.5 mm). Intrusion of the maxillary first molars also was observed in 69% of the subjects, resulting in an average intrusion of 0.7 mm during treatment (maximum 3.5 mm).

Other investigators have reported maxillary molar distalization as well.[24,25,61,62,66] Valant and Sinclair[66] observed 1.5 mm distal movement of the maxillary first molars (measured along the occlusal plane). The maxillary molars also exhibited 6.4° of distal crown tipping following treatment. Valant and Sinclair stated that, "A major advantage of this Herbst appliance is its ability to distalize molars, an effect not routinely seen with other functional appliances." Burkhardt[26] observed that the stainless steel crowned Herbst distalized molars 2.2 mm, whereas the acrylic-splint Herbst distalized molars 1.2 mm. These differences, however, were not statistically significant.

Pancherz[11] investigated the vertical dentofacial changes in 22 patients treated with the Herbst appliance for six months and found that the Herbst appliance had a pronounced effect on vertical tooth position. The maxillary first molars were intruded 1.0 mm relative to the same teeth in 20 untreated controls.

Studies of the acrylic-splint Herbst appliance have reported changes in horizontal and vertical molar position similar to those found in the banded Herbst appliance studies.[25,60,71] McNamara and co-workers'[24] evaluation of the acrylic-splint Herbst appliance showed significant maxillary dentoalveolar changes in patients treated with the acrylic-splint Herbst appliance when compared to untreated controls. When examining normal growth and development in the Class II untreated controls over the treatment period of 12 months, they found that the maxillary molar moved anteriorly 1.3 mm and extruded 1.6 mm. Posterior movement of the upper molar of 1.4 mm in the Herbst group was observed, resulting in a net horizontal difference of 2.7 mm in upper molar position. This change was considered clinically significant, in that the average change in molar position produced in Class II correction is approximately 6 mm. On average, the maxillary molar of the untreated control group erupted 1.6 mm over the observation period; however, the Herbst appliance allowed the upper molar to erupt only 0.5 mm during treatment, indicating a restrictive effect of the acrylic splints of the Herbst appliance on the eruption of the maxillary first molar.

Incisors

Most studies have found that the position of the maxillary incisors remains unchanged following Herbst therapy;[6,11,25,66] however, two of the acrylic-splint Herbst appliance studies have shown slight lingual movement of the upper incisors following Herbst treatment. Windmiller[60] observed that the maxillary incisors tipped lingually 4.3° and extruded 1.5 mm relative to the palatal plane. McNamara and co-workers[24] reported that upper incisor moved lingually 1.4 mm and extruded 0.8 mm relative to the untreated controls.

Posttreatment Changes

Molars

A short-term evaluation of the posttreatment period by Hansen and Pancherz[72] found distal molar movement was maintained following treatment. Six months following the cessation of Herbst treatment, molars were positioned distally by 1.2 mm when compared to their pretreatment positions. The maxillary molars in the untreated group moved mesially 0.6 mm during the same period, resulting in an overall 1.8 mm short-term treatment effect.

In a long-term study, Hansen and Pancherz[72] also found slight rebound in horizontal molar position six years following their first observation period. Throughout the posttreatment observation period, the maxillary first molars moved mesially only 0.2 mm more in the treated patients than in the untreated controls (1.4 mm compared to 1.2 mm). Relative to the maxilla, the molars of patients treated with the Herbst appliance were in essentially the same horizontal position in which they began. In comparison, the maxillary first molar in untreated subjects, on average, moved 1.8 mm mesially during growth and development.

Pancherz and Anehus-Pancherz[69] reported that the headgear effect of the Herbst appliance seen in the first phase of treatment generally seemed to be temporary in nature. Mesial molar movement (2.7 mm) was documented in the 6.5 years following during Herbst treatment, during which the molars moved distally 2.1 mm. The 0.6 mm of mesial molar movement seen over the seven years of observation was only 60% of that seen in matched controls from the Bolton study.[68]

Pancherz and Anehus-Pancherz[69] have analyzed changes in long-term vertical maxillary molar position as well. During Herbst treatment, the maxillary molars were intruded by an average of 0.7 mm. Over the following 6.5 years, maxillary molars extruded 4.6 mm. The total extrusion (3.9 mm) seen over the entire observation period was comparable to that in the Bolton control group.

During the years following Herbst treatment, normal growth and development appears to prevail, in that maxillary molars move mesially and extrude. Pancherz[69] compared the anterior and inferior maxillary molar movement in the six months following Herbst removal to the movement seen following headgear treatment. Although the Herbst appliance produces maxillary molar distalization, the long-term treatment effect appears to be temporary in nature (*i.e.,* the molars ultimately drift mesially); however, when comparing the long-term post-treatment molar position in subjects with those in untreated controls, evidence of a clinically significant treatment effect in the anteroposterior direction has been documented.

Incisors

As mentioned previously, most short-term Herbst studies have not shown a change in the anteroposterior position of the maxillary incisors.[6,11,25,66] Studies that have shown a retraction of the incisors have included the incisors in the Herbst appliance design.[24,60,72]

Currently, only one study has looked at the long-term change in position of the maxillary incisors following Herbst treatment. Hansen and Pancherz[72] measured the change in position of the maxillary incisors at the incisal edge 6.7 years following the completion of Herbst therapy. The maxillary incisors had moved 0.4 mm anteriorly in patients treated with the Herbst appliance and in patients in the Bolton control sample. The results of this study indicates that the change in maxillary incisor position following Herbst treatment is similar to that seen to occur during normal growth.

Effects on the Mandible

Treatment Changes in Mandibular Position

Clinically significant increases in the sella-nasion-Point B (SNB) angle and changes in mandibular position (mandibular displacement), consisting of measurements of mandibular length not involving the measurements condylion-gnathion (Co-Gn) or condylion-pogonion (Co-Pog), have been documented following Herbst appliance treatment.

Significant short-term increases in the length of the mandible also have been documented. In Pancherz's initial study of the Herbst appliance, he found that over a six-month period the SNB angle increased 1.2° in treated patients and remained constant in untreated individuals.[6] Mandibular length (condylion to pogonion) increased an average of 2.2 mm more in 10 patients treated with the Herbst appliance than in 10 untreated controls. In a subsequent study, Pancherz[10] found that mandibular displacement (condylion to pogonion measured parallel to the occlusal plane) increased an average of 2.2 mm more in 22 patients treated with the Herbst appliance when compared to 20 untreated Class II division 1 patients. The angle SNB in the Herbst appliance group increased 1.4° and remained constant in the untreated control group.

Other Herbst studies have supported Pancherz's findings. Over a twelve-month period, Windmiller[60] found that the treatment group experienced 3.4 mm of additional growth in length (Co-Gn) of the mandible and a 1.3° greater increase in SNB angle than in the untreated controls. Valant and Sinclair[66] found patients treated with the Herbst appliance over a ten month period experienced additional growth in mandibular length as measured by condylion to gnathion and articulare to gnathion (1.3 mm and 2.1 mm) than matched controls. They also reported a greater increase in the SNB angle (1.0°) in the treated patients than in the untreated controls.

In summary, most clinical studies have found that the mandibles of Herbst patients increase in length two to three millimeters more than do the mandibles of untreated controls.[23-25] The SNB angle in treated patients is found to be one to two degrees greater than in untreated controls.[12, 24, 25]

Long Term Changes in Mandibular Position

In general, it is common to see an accelerated growth of the mandible during the Herbst phase of treatment, followed by a decrease in the rate of mandibular growth in the follow-up phase (*i.e.*, fixed appliance treatment or retention). For example, Pancherz and Fackel[16] studied the growth pattern pre- and post-Herbst appliance treatment of Class II malocclusions. They examined the growth pattern of 17 patients for 31 months following seven months of active Herbst treatment. During the treatment phase, mandibular displacement increased (measured from articulare to pogonion), but in the follow-up phase, mandibular displacement was diminished. The authors concluded that, "Herbst treatment had a temporary impact on the existing skeletofacial growth pattern. After the orthopaedic interventive period, . . . mandibular growth seemed to strive to catch up with . . . earlier patterns."

Lai and McNamara[25] also found accelerated mandibular growth (2.2 mm greater than controls) during the Herbst phase of treatment, followed by a diminished rate of growth in subsequent edgewise treatment. During the fixed appliance phase, a decrease in the SNB angle was evident, resulting in no significant difference between the control and the Herbst groups for overall change in the SNB angle. Following the two phases, a small but mildly clinically significant difference (1.0 mm) between the two groups was seen for the overall change in mandibular length.[25]

The acceleration in growth of mandibular length during functional appliance therapy, followed by a less than normal growth rate thereafter, agrees with Pancherz,[7]

Wieslander,[28] and Pancherz and Fackel.[16] All showed a decrease in mandibular growth rate after Herbst appliances were removed. Pancherz[7] found a decreased rate in mandibular growth in the six months immediately following Herbst treatment. Wieslander[28] reported that significant increase in mandibular length, measured from condylion to gnathion, observed after five months of Herbst treatment was reduced to 1.2 mm after retention and was not statistically significant.

Burkhardt[26] compared the treatment changes of Herbst appliance treatment followed by fixed appliance therapy to the treatment changes of molar distalization using the Pendulum appliance followed by fixed appliance treatment. Differences is mandibular length (measured from condylion to gnathion) were not seen between the treatment groups. These results imply that the Herbst appliance does not produce a long-term increase in mandibular growth.

Temporomandibular Joint Adaptation During Herbst Treatment

Treatment Effects

Changes in condylar position relative to the cranial base have been documented in human and animal subjects following Herbst appliance therapy. Anterior condylar positioning as well as radiographic changes in the posterior aspect of the fossa in human subjects have been found in subjects following Herbst treatment.[6]

Woodside and co-workers[73] have shown that the position of the condyle relative to the cranial base changes in non-human primates because of treatment with the Herbst appliance. They found that anterior condylar displacement was accompanied by addition of new bone in the posterior aspect of the fossa as well as increased fibrous tissue mass in the posterior aspect of the disk. The accompanying changes surrounding the condyle were demonstrated functionally, cephalometrically, and histologically.

Condylar remodeling, glenoid fossa remodeling, and condylar positional changes within the fossa are all thought to contribute to the overall changes in mandibular position when correcting a Class II malocclusion using the Herbst appliance, at least in the short-term.

Ruf and Pancherz[74] analyzed these adaptive TMJ growth processes in a prospective magnetic resonance imaging (MRI) and cephalometric study. The results of this investigation indicate that condylar as well as glenoid fossa remodeling seem to contribute significantly to the increase in mandibular prognathism. The condyle-fossa relationship was unaffected, on average, by Herbst therapy and does not appear to contribute to the increase in mandibular prognathism.

Wieslander[23] reported that relative to the condylar base, the mandibular condyle was in a 1.3 mm more inferior-anterior position after active treatment; no significant difference in supracondylar space was registered. Windmiller[60] found that the most posterior aspect of the condyle did not change in sagittal position; however, the most superior aspect of the condyle moved inferiorly 0.7 mm.

Long-Term Temporomandibular Joint Adaptation

By way of lateral tomography with sections taken perpendicular to the long axis of the condyle, a clinical examination, and a questionnaire, Hansen[75] studied the long-term effects of the Herbst appliance on the temporomandibular joint. The relationship of the condyle within the fossa 7.5 years after Herbst treatment was evaluated. Measurements indicated that the condyle was on average slightly anteriorly positioned in the fossa following Herbst therapy. Hansen[75] suggested that the normal condylar position seen at follow-up probably is achieved by increased condylar growth during treatment and/or remodeling of the articular fossa.

From the clinical examination and questionnaire, Hansen[75] found that the prevalence of joint sounds within the treatment group (26 percent) was less than or equal to that found generally in children, adolescents, and young adults.[76-80] Furthermore, the prevalence of joint sounds in asymptomatic adults has been reported to be 65 percent[81] (see Chapter 29 for an in depth discussion of these issues).

In a clinical and MRI study, Ruf and Pancherz[74] evaluated the long-term effects of Herbst treatment on the temporomandibular joint in 20 patients who had completed treatment an average of four years previously. The incidence of anamnestic (i.e., from medical and dental history) and clinical signs and symptoms of temporomandibular disorders was within the normal range reported in the literature. The frequency of disk displacement was similar to that found in asymptomatic populations. The disk position relative to the condyle varied largely in the medial, central, and lateral MRI slices of the joints. A wide range in condylar position was seen throughout all MRI slices of the joints.

In summary, Herbst treatment does not appear to have an unfavorable long-term effect on the temporomandibular joint.

Effects on the Mandibular Dentition

Treatment Changes

Molars

Analysis of sagittal dentoalveolar changes has revealed that the lower first molars of treated subjects undergo increased mesial movement, usually one to two millimeters, as compared to untreated controls.[10,11,24,25,66]

Studies by McNamara and co-workers[24] and Lai and McNamara[25] indicate that occlusal coverage of the acrylic-splint Herbst inhibits the vertical movement of the mandibular molars in comparison to the banded design of the appliance.[11] In contrast, a study by Windmiller[60] found mandibular first molar extrusion in patients treated with the acrylic-splint Herbst appliance to be similar to that of the banded design.

Incisors

The telescoping mechanism of the Herbst appliance places an downward and forward vector of force on the mandibular dentition. Mesial movement of the mandibular incisors following Herbst treatment is consistent in patients treated with the acrylic-splint Herbst appliance and the banded Herbst appliance.

Studies of the banded Herbst have reported flaring of the mandibular incisors relative to the mandibular plane (IMPA) from 5.4°[66] to 10.8°,[82] whereas studies of the acrylic-splint Herbst appliance have reported IMPA increases from 2.5°[66] to 5.5°.[25] Burkhardt[26] found that the crown Herbst appliance produces greater proclination of the lower incisors (8.4°) than the acrylic splint Herbst appliance (5.0°).

Pancherz[11] compared 22 successfully treated Class II, division 1 malocclusion cases to 20 Class II, division 1 control subjects. He also found that the incisal edges of the mandibular incisors of patients treated with the Herbst appliance were intruded 1.8 mm relative to untreated controls. Pancherz[6,10,11] has noted that part of the vertical incisor changes are due to tooth proclination as a result of the mesially directed force vector of the appliance acting on the lower teeth. Referring to the increased eruption of the mandibular molars and the proclination of the mandibular incisors, Pancherz[11] stated, "Overbite changes in the Herbst treated cases were for the most part a result of mandibular dental changes."

Post-Treatment Changes

Molars

Posterior movement of the mandibular first molars following Herbst treatment has been observed in long-term follow-up studies.[75] Pancherz and Hansen[17] reported the majority of posterior movement (*i.e.,* rebound) of the mandibular molars occurred in the first six months following Herbst treatment. In the subsequent six months, the mandibular molars remained in a stable anteroposterior position relative to the mandible. Lai and McNamara[25] reported that posterior movement of the mandibular molars occurred in the 17 months following Herbst treatment, even in the presence of fixed appliances.

Incisors

Dentoalveolar rebound often is found in the period following Herbst treatment, as was shown earlier in the discussion of the treatment and post-treatment changes in the maxillary and mandibular first molar region. Similar findings have been described in the lower incisor region. For example, Hansen and co-workers[82] reported that the lower incisors were proclined by an average of 10.8° relative to the mandibular plane during active treatment, and the incisal edge of the lower incisor moved anteriorly by 3.2 mm. During the first six months following active treatment, the lower incisor position rebounded by uprighting 7.9° and moving posteriorly 2.5 mm. During the long-term posttreatment period, from six months after treatment to the end of the growth period, lower incisor inclination remained unchanged in relation to the mandibular plane, but the teeth retroclined in relation to the nasion-sella line.

Lai and McNamara[25] also reported dentoalveolar rebound in the mandibular incisor area following Herbst treatment. Although the fixed appliance phase following the acrylic-splint Herbst appliance treatment phase saw uprighting and posterior movement of the incisors relative to matched controls, these teeth still were located 1.4 mm anterior and flared 3.0° relative to the controls.

Burkhardt[26] found that proclination of the mandibular incisors during Herbst treatment was significantly greater in the crown Herbst treatment group than in the acrylic-splint Herbst treatment group. During fixed appliance treatment, however, the crown Herbst treatment group underwent greater rebound in incisor position than the acrylic-splint Herbst treatment group. Following fixed appliance therapy, the IMPA of the acrylic Herbst treatment group had increased less (3.4°) than that of the crown Herbst treatment group (5.2°); however, these differences were not statistically significant.

Pancherz[11] reported that the reduction in overbite following Herbst appliance therapy was due mostly to mandibular dental changes. When relapse of the overbite correction following Herbst therapy is observed,

Pancherz[7] found that retrusion and retroclination of the lower front teeth contributed to an increase in overbite. The tendency toward overbite relapse is greater when incisors are intruded.[83]

Effects on the Vertical Dimension

Short-Term Treatment Effects

Acrylic-Splint Herbst Appliance

Due to the potential for a bite-block effect during treatment, the acrylic-splint Herbst appliance, instead of the banded Herbst appliance has been advocated.[60] Following acrylic-splint Herbst treatment, many investigators have found increases in lower anterior face height (LAFH).[24,60] The findings of these studies, however, usually indicate that the mandibular plane angle does not increase when compared to untreated controls.[24,25,60] Increases in posterior face height were attributed to the maintenance of the mandibular plane angle.

Schiavoni and co-workers[84] compared the results of nine months of treatment of Class II malocclusion by way of two different designs of the Herbst appliance. The hyperdivergent group (eight patients) was treated with the Herbst appliance attached to acrylic splints; a high-pull headgear also was used. These patients had a mean Frankfort to mandibular plane angle (FMA) of 29.3°. The normohypodivergent group (11 patients) that had a mean FMA of 18.2° was treated with the Herbst appliance attached to bands. The results were compared between groups and to a control group matched for age and sex from the Bolton standards.[68]

In the normohypodivergent group, an increase in posterior face height and anterior face height did not lead to a significant change in the mandibular plane angle. In the hyperdivergent group, the posterior and anterior face heights increased differentially, leading to a significant decrease in the mandibular plane angle. The authors suggested that the acrylic-splint and high-pull headgear provided improved vertical control, allowing the full expression of the sagittal correction by preventing the chin from swinging backward and downward.

In summary, the acrylic-splint Herbst appliance often leads to increases in anterior and posterior face height; however, these increases routinely do not lead to increases in the mandibular plane angle. The acrylic-splint Herbst, in the absence of headgear, has not been shown to decrease the mandibular plane angle.

Banded Herbst

Pancherz[11] compared the vertical effects of 22 patients successfully treated with the Herbst appliance to 20 Class II untreated subjects. He noted that the banded Herbst appliance has a pronounced effect on the vertical dimension. Pancherz found that lower anterior face height increased by 1.8 mm; however, no significant difference in mandibular plane angle was noted following treatment.

Opening the bite and allowing the unimpeded eruption of the mandibular buccal segments leads to increases in both anterior and posterior face heights. Pancherz[11] cautioned that treatment of Class II patients with a long lower anterior face height might result in a further deterioration in facial esthetics.

Ruf and Pancherz[85] compared the skeletal and dentoalveolar effects contributing to Class II correction in subjects with small or large pretreatment mandibular plane angles. Lateral headfilms of 15 hypodivergent (mandibular plane to sella-nasion ≤26°) and 16 hyperdivergent (mandibular plane to nasion-sella >39°) Class II patients treated to a Class I occlusal relationship with the Herbst appliance for an average of seven months were analyzed. Except for increased overjet correction in the hyperdivergent group due to a larger pretreatment overjet, no significant group differences were present. Changes in mandibular plane angle were not observed. They concluded that the presence of a hyperdivergent jaw base relationship did not affect the mechanism of Class II correction unfavorably.

In summary, treatment changes in the vertical dimension seen with the banded Herbst are similar to changes seen with the acrylic-splint Herbst. Maxillary first molars are intruded and mandibular molars erupt freely. Lower anterior facial height increases during treatment, although changes in the mandibular plane angle are not observed, due to concomitant increases in posterior face height.

Crown Herbst

Burkhardt[26] compared the treatment effects of the crown Herbst appliance and the acrylic-splint Herbst appliance. He found that both Herbst appliances produced a slight increase in lower anterior face height (2 mm) and maintained the pretreatment mandibular plane angle. Evidence of a posterior bite-block effect from the stainless steel crown Herbst appliance was not observed.

Long-Term Treatment Effects

Many of the changes in the vertical dimension noted at the end of Herbst treatment remain at follow-up. Lai and McNamara[25] found significant treatment-related changes in vertical measures following Herbst treatment. Significant increases in upper facial height (nasion-anterior nasal spine or N-ANS), total anterior facial height (N-ME), lower posterior facial height (S-Go), and total posterior facial height (Co-Gn) noted following Herbst treatment remained larger in the Herbst group following fixed appliance therapy. No significant effects on lower anterior facial height or mandibular plane angle were found following fixed appliance therapy or at the end of two-phase treatment.

Ruf and Pancherz[86] evaluated the long-term effects of the Herbst appliance on the mandibular plane angle. They found that the mandibular plane on average was unaffected by Herbst treatment. Following treatment, a continuous decrease in the mandibular plane angle was observed. Patients were categorized based on vertical jaw base relationship (*i.e.*, hypodivergent, normodivergent, and hyperdivergent) at the beginning of treatment, and statistically significant differences were not found between groups.

Pancherz[70] summarized the long-term vertical changes following Herbst treatment as a continuous decrease in the mandibular plane angle. He interpreted these changes to occur "as a result of normalized function which permits normal growth and development." Although closing of the nasal plane angle and the mandibular plane angle have been observed following Herbst treatment, long-term increases in posterior and anterior face heights relative to untreated controls have been reported.

Class II Relapse Following Herbst Treatment

Relapse into a Class II relationship is a major concern following Herbst appliance treatment. A comparison was made between 15 relapse and 14 stable patients treated with the Herbst appliance at least five years following treatment.[14] Lateral cephalograms were taken just before and after treatment, six months after treatment, and five to ten years following Herbst treatment. No statistical significance was found between the stable and relapse groups at the beginning or end of treatment. Relapse in the overjet and sagittal molar position resulted mainly from posttreatment maxillary and mandibular dentoalveolar changes. The maxillary incisors and molars moved to an anterior position in the relapse group than in the stable group. Pancherz found that, "the interrelation between maxillary and mandibular posttreatment growth was favorable and did not contribute to occlusal relapse."

According to Pancherz,[14] a clinical examination and evaluation of the dental casts revealed two relapse-promoting factors. First, a lip-tongue dysfunction habit such as an atypical swallowing pattern was noted in 64% of the relapse patients but none of the stable patients. Additionally, an unstable Class I cuspal interdigitation existed in 57% of the relapse cases and 13 percent of the stable cases. Therefore, Pancherz[14] suggested than the main causes of the Class II relapse in-patient treated with the Herbst appliance were persisting lip-tongue dysfunction and an unstable cuspal interdigitation.

The Craniofacial Growth Pattern and the Herbst Appliance

Possible changes in the craniofacial growth pattern following Herbst treatment are an important consideration when deciding to use a Herbst appliance. Pancherz and Fackel[16] compared craniofacial growth changes during Herbst treatment to the changes before and after dentofacial orthopedics in 17 male patients treated with the Herbst appliance for an average of seven months. The pre- and post-treatment periods in each patient averaged 31 months each. When comparing the growth changes during Herbst treatment with those in the pretreatment control period, maxillary growth was inhibited and redirected; mandibular displacement was increased; anterior mandibular growth rotation was arrested; the sagittal intermaxillary jaw relationship was improved, and the skeletal profile straightened. During the post-treatment period, many of the treatment changes reverted. Pancherz and Fackel[16] noted that, "maxillary and mandibular growth seemed to strive to catch up with their earlier patterns" as the craniofacial growth pattern existing before treatment prevailed after treatment. Thus, dentofacial orthopedics using the Herbst appliance had only a temporary impact on the existing craniofacial growth pattern.

Lai and McNamara[25] reported a reduction in mandibular growth in the fixed appliance phase of treatment following Herbst treatment. They found that the increase in mandibular growth rate seen during the first phase of treatment was a transient phenomenon followed by a subnormal growth rate, that lead to a very minimal increase in final length of the mandible.

CONCLUDING REMARKS

This chapter has described the clinical management of two types of Herbst appliance design, the stainless steel crown Herbst and the acrylic splint Herbst. The Herbst appliance has been shown to be a device capable of producing rapid skeletodental changes leading to the correction of a Class II malocclusion.

As mentioned earlier, the Herbst appliance is the most widely used functional appliance in the United

States today, presumably because of excellent clinical success. This treatment approach has been studied more than any other functional appliance. It is somewhat surprising, therefore, that the long-term skeletal and dentoalveolar changes are not nearly as remarkable as the short-term Herbst results. Most of the well-documented short-term treatment effects tend to become more modest or disappear with further growth and development.

Why, then, is the Herbst appliance so popular, especially given its limited long-term effects? First, this treatment approach appears to "do no harm." There is no persuasive evidence that Herbst treatment leads to an increase in the prevalence of temporomandibular disorders or other functional problems. Further, Herbst treatment does not move the maxilla posteriorly, an undesirable effect in most Class II patients.

This approach requires relatively minimal patient cooperation, especially if the appliance is cemented or bonded in place, again a major concern of most clinicians. Finally, and perhaps most importantly, the occlusal results of Herbst treatment appear to be stable over the long-term. If a satisfactory interdigitation of the teeth is achieved at the end of treatment, and if there are no overriding functional concerns, excellent stablity of the treated results usually is observed.

REFERENCES CITED

1. Kingsley NW. A treatise on oral deformities as a branch of mechanical surgery. New York: D Appleton, 1880.
2. Pancherz H. The effect, limitations, and long-term dentofacial adaptations to treatment with the Herbst appliance. Semin Orthod 1997;3:232–243.
3. Herbst E. Atlas und Grundriss der Zahnärztlichen Orthopädie. Munich: JF Lehmann Verlag, 1910.
4. Herbst E. Dreissigjährige Erfahrungen mit dem Retentions-Scharnier. Zahnärztl Rundschau. 1934;42:151–1524, 1563–1568, 1611–1616.
5. Held AJ, Spirgi M, Cimasoni G. An orthopedically treated adult case of Class II malocclusion. Am J Orthod 1963;49:761–765.
6. Pancherz H. Treatment of Class II malocclusions by jumping the bite with the Herbst appliance. A cephalometric investigation. Am J Orthod 1979;76:423–442.
7. Pancherz H. The effect of continuous bite jumping on the dentofacial complex: a follow-up study after Herbst appliance treatment of Class II malocclusions. Eur J Orthod 1981;3:49–60.
8. Pancherz H, Anehus-Pancherz M. Muscle activity in Class II, division 1 malocclusions treated by bite jumping with the Herbst appliance. An electromyographic study. Am J Orthod 1980;78:321–329.
9. Pancherz H. Personal communication, 2000.
10. Pancherz H. The mechanism of Class II correction in Herbst appliance treatment. A cephalometric investigation. Am J Orthod 1982;82:104–113.
11. Pancherz H. Vertical dentofacial changes during Herbst appliance treatment: a cephalometric investigation. Swed Dent J Supp 1982;15:189–196.
12. Pancherz H. The Herbst appliance—Its biologic effects and clinical use. Am J Orthod 1985;87:1–20.
13. Pancherz H. Dentofacial orthopedics in relation to somatic maturation, an analysis of 70 consecutive cases treated with the Herbst appliance. Am J Orthod 1988;88:273–287.
14. Pancherz H. The nature of Class II relapse after Herbst appliance treatment: a cephalometric long-term investigation. Am J Orthod Dentofac Orthop 1991;100:220–233.
15. Pancherz H, Anehus-Pancherz M. The effect of continuous bite jumping with the Herbst appliance on the masticatory system: a functional analysis of treated Class II malocclusions. Eur J Orthod 1982;4:37–44.
16. Pancherz H, Fackel U. The skeletofacial growth pattern pre- and post-dentofacial orthopaedics. A long-term study of Class II malocclusions treated with the Herbst appliance. Eur J Orthod 1990;12:209–218.
17. Pancherz H, Hansen K. Occlusal changes during and after Herbst treatment: a cephalometric investigation. Eur J Orthod 1986;8:215–228.
18. Pancherz H, Hansen K. Mandibular anchorage in Herbst treatment. Eur J Orthod 1988;10:149–164.
19. Pancherz H, Hägg U. Dentofacial orthopedics in relation to somatic maturation. An analysis of 70 consecutive cases treated with the Herbst appliance. Am J Orthod 1985;88:273–287.
20. Pancherz H, Malmgren O, Hagg U, Omblus J, Hansen K. Class II correction in Herbst and Bass therapy. Eur J Orthod 1989;11:17–30.
21. Hagg U, Pancherz H. Dentofacial orthopaedics in relation to chronological age, growth period and skeletal development. An analysis of 72 male patients with Class II division 1 malocclusion treated with the Herbst appliance. Eur J Orthod 1988;10:169–176.
22. Wieslander L. JCO interviews Dr. Lennart Wieslander on dentofacial orthopedics. Headgear-Herbst treatment in the mixed dentition. J Clin Orthod 1984;18:551–564.
23. Wieslander L. Intensive treatment of severe Class II malocclusions with a headgear-Herbst appliance in the early mixed dentition. Am J Orthod 1984;86:1–13.
24. McNamara JA, Jr., Howe RP, Dischinger TG. A comparison of the Herbst and Fränkel appliances in the treatment of Class II malocclusion. Am J Orthod Dentofac Orthop 1990;98:134–44.
25. Lai M, McNamara JA, Jr. An evaluation of two-phase treatment with the Herbst appliance and preadjusted edgewise therapy. Semin Orthod 1998;4:46–58.
26. Burkhardt DR. A comparison of three non-extraction treatment modalities for the correction of Class II malocclusion. Ann Arbor: Unpublished Master's thesis, Department of Orthodontics and Pediatric Dentistry, The University of Michigan, 2000.
27. McNamara JA, Jr. Unpublished data, 1998.
28. Wieslander L. Long-term effect of treatment with the headgear-Herbst appliance in the early mixed dentition. Stability or relapse? Am J Orthod Dentofac Orthop 1993;104:319–329.
29. Pancherz H. The Herbst appliance. Seville: Editorial Aguiram, 1995.
30. Pancherz, H. Personal communication, 1990.

31. Langford NM, Jr. The Herbst appliance. J Clin Orthod 1981;15:558–561.
32. Langford NM, Jr. Updating fabrication of the Herbst appliance. J Clin Orthod 1982;16:173–174.
33. Goodman P, McKenna P. Modified Herbst appliance for the mixed dentition. J Clin Orthod 1985;19:811–814.
34. Dischinger TG. Edgewise bioprogressive Herbst appliance. J Clin Orthod 1989;23:608–617.
35. Smith JR. Matching the Herbst to the malocclusion. Clin Impressions 1998;7:6–12, 20–23.
36. Smith JR. Matching the Herbst to the malocclusion: Part II. Clin Impressions 1999;8:14–23.
37. Mayes JH. Improving appliance efficiency with the cantilever Herbst—A new answer to old problems. Clin Impressions 1994;3:2–5,17–19.
38. Mayes JH. The single appointment preattached cantilever bite jumper. Clin Impressions 1996;5:14–17.
39. Mayes JH. The cantilever bite-jumper system—exploring the possibilities. Clin Impressions 1996;5:14–17.
40. Mayes JH. The molar-moving bite jumper. Clin Impressions 1998;7:16–19.
41. Hilgers JJ. Hyper efficient orthodontic treatment using tandem mechanics. Semin Orthod 1998;4:17–25.
42. Chastant RB. Bite-jumpers: Effective strategies for streamlining crown placement and removal. Clin Impressions 1997;6:7–11, 26.
43. Tollaro I, Baccetti T, Franchi L, Tanasescu CD. Role of posterior transverse interarch discrepancy in Class II, Division 1 malocclusion during the mixed dentition phase. Am J Orthod Dentofac Orthop 1996;110:417–422.
44. Hilgers JJ. Personal communication, 2000.
45. Hilgers JJ. Personal communication, 1996.
46. Dischinger TG. Edgewise Herbst appliance. J Clin Orthod 1995;29:738–742.
47. Clark WJ. Twin block functional therapy. London: Mosby-Wolfe, 1995.
48. Fränkel R. Technik und Handhabung der Funktionsregler. Berlin: VEB Verlag Volk und Gesundheit, 1976.
49. Fränkel R, Fränkel C. Orofacial orthopedics with the function regulator. Munich: S Karger, 1989.
50. Greenbaum KR. Personal communication, 2000.
51. Mayes JH. Personal communication, 1998.
52. Mayes JH. Personal communication, 1999.
53. Howe RP. The bonded Herbst appliance. J Clin Orthod 1982;16:663–7.
54. Howe RP, McNamara JA, Jr. Clinical management of the bonded Herbst appliance. J Clin Orthod 1983;17:456–463.
55. Howe RP. Updating the bonded Herbst appliance. J Clin Orthod 1983;17:122–124.
56. Howe RP. The acrylic-splint Herbst. Problem solving. J Clin Orthod 1984;18:497–501.
57. Howe RP. Lower premolar extraction/removable plastic Herbst treatment for mandibular retrognathia. Am J Orthod Dentofac Orthop 1987;92:275–285.
58. McNamara JA, Jr. Fabrication of the acrylic splint Herbst appliance. Am J Orthod Dentofac Orthop 1988;94:10–8.
59. McNamara JA, Jr., Howe RP. Clinical management of the acrylic splint Herbst appliance. Am J Orthod Dentofac Orthop 1988;94:142–149.
60. Windmiller EC. The acrylic-splint Herbst appliance: a cephalometric evaluation. Am J Orthod Dentofac Orthop 1993;104:73–84.
61. Franchi L, Baccetti T, McNamara JA, Jr. Treatment and post-treatment effects of acrylic splint Herbst appliance therapy. Am J Orthod Dentofac Orthop 1999;115:429–438.
62. Lai M. Molar distalization with the Herbst appliance. Semin Orthod 2000;6:119–128.
63. Rider EA. Removable Herbst appliance for treatment of obstructive sleep apnea. J Clin Orthod 1988;22:256–257.
64. Ponitz RJ. Invisible retainers. Am J Orthod 1971;59:266–272.
65. McNamara JA, Kramer KL, Jeunker JP. Invisible retainers. J Clin Orthod 1985;19:570–578.
66. Valant JR, Sinclair PM. Treatment effects of the Herbst appliance. Am J Orthod Dentofac Orthop 1989;95:138–147.
67. Hansen K, Iemamnueisuk P, Pancherz H. Long-term effects of the Herbst appliance on the dental arches and arch relationships: a biometric study. Br J Orthod 1995;22:123–134.
68. Broadbent BH, Sr, Broadbent BH, Jr, Golden WH. Bolton standards of dentofacial developmental growth. St. Louis: CV Mosby, 1975.
69. Pancherz H, Anehus-Pancherz M. The headgear effect of the Herbst appliance: a cephalometric long-term study. Am J Orthod Dentofac Orthop 1993;103:510–520.
70. Clark GT, Tsukiyama Y, Baba K, Simmons M. The validity and utility of disease detection methods and occlusal therapy for temporomandibular disorders. J Orofacial Pain 1997;83: 101–106.
71. Sidhu MS, Kharbanda OP, Sidhu SS. Cephalometric analysis of changes produced by a modified Herbst appliance in the treatment of Class II division 1 malocclusion. Br J Orthod 1995;22:1–12.
72. Hansen K, Pancherz H. Long-term effects of Herbst treatment in relation to normal growth development: a cephalometric study. Eur J Orthod 1992;14:285–295.
73. Woodside DG, Metaxas A, Altuna G. The influence of functional appliance therapy on glenoid fossa remodeling. Am J Orthod Dentofac Orthop 1987;92:181–198.
74. Ruf S, Pancherz H. Long-term TMJ effects of Herbst treatment: A clinical and MRI study. Am J Orthod Dentofac Orthop 1998;114:475–483.
75. Hansen K, Pancherz H, Petersson A. Long-term effects of the Herbst appliance on the craniomandibular system with special reference to the TMJ. Eur J Orthod 1990;12:244–253.
76. Helkimo M. Studies on function and dysfunction of the masticatory system. Kungsbacka: Elanders boktryckeri AB, 1974.
77. Solberg WK, Woo MA, Houston J. Prevalence of mandibular dysfunction in young adults. J Am Dent Assoc 1979;98:25–34.
78. Nilner M, Lassing MA. Prevalence of functional disturbances and diseases of the stomatognathic system in 7–14 year olds. Swed Dent J 1981;5:173–187.
79. Egermark-Eriksson I, Carlsson GE, Ingervall B. Prevalence of mandibular dysfunction and orofacial parafunction in 7-, 11- and 15-year-old Swedish children. Eur J Orthod 1981;3:163–172.
80. Magnusson T. Five-year longitudinal study of signs and symptoms of mandibular dysfunction in adolescents. Cranio 1986;4:338–344.

81. Hansson T, Nilner M. A study of the occurrence of symptoms of diseases of the temporomandibular joint masticatory musculature and related structures. J Oral Rehabil 1975;2:313–324.
82. Hansen K, Koutsonas TG, Pancherz H. Long-term effects of Herbst treatment on the mandibular incisor segment: A cephalometric and biometric investigation. Am J Orthod Dentofac Orthop 1997;112:97–103.
83. Simons ME, Joondeph DR. Change in overbite: a ten-year postretention study. Am J Orthod 1973;64:349–367.
84. Schiavoni R, Grenga V, Macri V. Treatment of Class II high angle malocclusions with the Herbst appliance: a cephalometric investigation. Am J Orthod Dentofac Orthop 1992;102:393–409.
85. Ruf S, Pancherz H. The mechanism of Class II correction during Herbst therapy in relation to the vertical jaw base relationship: a cephalometric roentgenographic study. Angle Orthod 1997;67:271–276.
86. Ruf S, Pancherz H. The effect of Herbst appliance treatment on the mandibular plane angle: a cephalometric roentgenographic study. Am J Orthod Dentofac Orthop 1996;110:225–229.

Chapter 18

THE BIONATOR

With Valmy Pangrazio-Kulbersh and Scott A. Huge

The bionator is a generic term that refers to a family of tooth-borne appliances used to treat malocclusions characterized mainly by mandibular retrusion. The bionator produces a forward positioning of the lower jaw, promoting a new postural position of the mandible. The acrylic parts of the bionator contact the teeth and supporting structures, thus creating changes in the skeletal, dentoalveolar, and muscular environment of the craniofacial region.

The development of the bionator is credited to Wilhelm Balters.[1,2] The original Balters Bionator (Fig. 18-1) was constructed of acrylic and wire, with its base of operation lingual to the dentition. The labial wire extended posteriorly into the vestibular region to function as buccal shields. Due to the limited amount of acrylic used in its construction, speech is less impaired when compared to that of patients wearing the bulkier activator.[3-5] Since the introduction of the original bionator, many modifications have been made in appliance design, some of which are relatively minor in nature.[6-11] Major changes in the fabrication of the bionator have resulted in appliances on which published information is limited (*e.g.*, California bionator, orthopedic corrector) or nonexistent.

The increasing popularity of the bionator during the 1970s and 1980s was due, in part, to the overall increase in the use of functional appliances in the United States during that time.* This popularity was based on a number of factors, some real and some perceived. For example, the bionator was considered one of the easiest functional appliances to use. One of the main advantages of the bionator is the level of comfort it provides to the patient. Its reduced size makes it possible for it to be worn day and night. Due to the ability of the patient to wear the bionator comfortably nearly full time (except during meals, playing contact sports, etc.), the patient postures his or her mandible forward more constantly. The bionator, as with all functional appliances, is more effective when worn full-time rather than part-time.

Assuming a proper diagnosis and treatment plan, the bionator is a relatively simple appliance to implement clinically. The management of the appliance does not involve many of the time-consuming procedures necessary when using a Fränkel appliance (FR-2), such as detailed impression and model preparation techniques and complex laboratory instructions. Besides, as mentioned earlier, there is a perception among many clinicians that patients find the bionator more acceptable. Because of the relative ease in the clinical handling of the bionator, the clinician's positive attitude and confidence is conveyed to the patient, improving the chances for positive acceptance and compliance. An additional reason for the bionator's popularity is the fact that it often is used simultaneously with fixed appliance treatment. Such combined treatment is not typical with either the FR-2 or the acrylic splint Herbst appliance.

The correction of the Class II skeletal malocclusion is

---

* It should be noted that, according to unpublished data from six major orthodontic laboratories, the introduction of the twin block appliance has adversely affected the level of bionator use in recent years. Many clinicians now prefer the twin block to the bionator because the twin block appliance can be worn on a full-time basis, including when eating. Speaking with the twin block also is perceived to be easier than with the bionator.

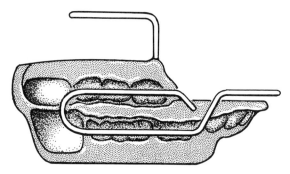

Figure 18-1. Lateral view of Balters bionator showing interocclusal acrylic in the area of the deciduous teeth. The acrylic has been relieved posteriorly to allow for the eruption of the maxillary and mandibular first permanent molars.

achieved with the bionator by the following dentoskeletal adjustments:

1. Headgear effect on the maxillary complex produced by the distal forces generated by the musculature as the mandible is advanced. A systematic advancement of the appliance is recommended to decrease the headgear effect on the maxilla when this effect is not indicated.
2. Mesial migration of the mandibular dentition and distal migration of the maxillary dentition, caused by the adjustments in the eruption facets. Some expansion also is observed as the result of the buccal and vertical eruption of the posterior teeth as guided by the eruption facets and adjustment of the transpalatal wire, as necessary.
3. Mandibular anterior repositioning, as an expression of condylar growth and glenoid fossa remodeling.
4. Neuromuscular adaptation due to forward mandibular repositioning. The principle of treatment with the bionator is not to activate the muscles, but to eliminate abnormal and potentially deforming muscle activity that would act deleteriously on the growth of the dentoskeletal facial framework.

The bionator is indicated for the correction of Class II mandibular retrognathism exhibiting all or some of the following dental characteristics:

1. Well-aligned dental arches.
2. Labially tipped maxillary incisors.
3. Upright or well positioned mandibular incisors.
4. Deep bite with accentuated curve of Spee.
5. Open bite with maxillary anterior alveolar deformation.

The correction of a skeletal vertical problem can be accomplished by proper manipulation of the interocclusal acrylic in the buccal segments (to be described later).

APPLIANCE TYPES

This chapter describes the clinical management of the bionator, including a detailed explanation of its components. A systematic method is proposed to aid the clinician in the selection of the proper appliance design according to the requirements of the patient. The concept of a "standard design" for a functional appliance such as the bionator should be questioned seriously, due to the complex needs of the individual orthodontic patient. Each patient presents with a unique malocclusion comprising several components; the bionator should be designed, constructed, and managed to influence each of these components optimally. By examining the parts of the appliance in a systematic fashion and relating them to the goals of treatment, the clinician can prescribe an exact design for more predictable treatment results. Thus, in contrast to most other chapters in this volume, appliance construction will be discussed in detail.

There are three general versions of the bionator, based on their effects on the vertical dimension (*i.e*, open, close, or maintain the bite). All bionators are fabricated so that the mandible is postured in a forward position.

The various versions of the bionator do not promote the generalized orthopedic training effect on the orofacial musculature produced by the FR-2 appliance of Fränkel. In patients with significant neuromuscular imbalances, the FR-2 appliance is indicated as the appliance of choice.

Bionators to Open the Bite

Most bionators that are in use today are designed not only to posture the mandible into a more forward position but also to facilitate the eruption of the posterior teeth in patients with decreased vertical dimension. The so-called "California bionator" (Fig. 18-2) is such an appliance. The wire and acrylic components of the appliance are constructed to allow vertical movement of the posterior teeth, while maintaining the anterior teeth in position. This design also can be used in patients in whom anteroposterior discrepancies do not exist but in whom vertical development of the face is desired by eruption of the maxillary and/or mandibular posterior teeth (*e.g.*, flattening of the curve of Spee). The eruption of these teeth can be controlled selectively by altering the interocclusal acrylic. Manipulation of this type of appliance is described in detail below.

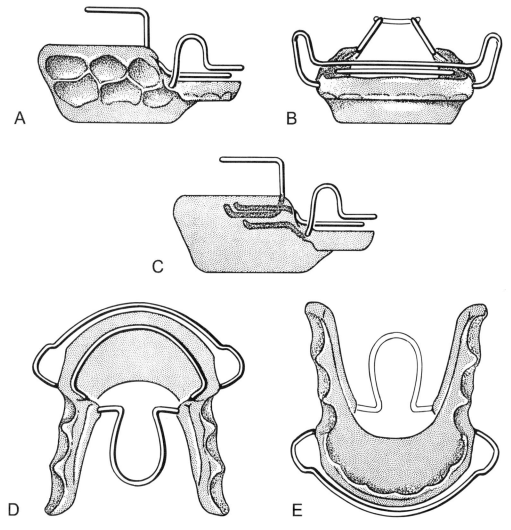

Figure 18-2. California bionator. *A*, Lateral view showing eruption facets. *B*, Frontal view showing incisal cap. *C*, Position of wires within the acrylic of the appliance. *D*, Maxillary occlusal view showing position of maxillary labial wire, maxillary lingual wire, and palatal wire. *E*, Mandibular view showing relief in the lower lingual region.

Bionator to Close the Bite

This type of bionator is constructed with posterior bite blocks and may or may not have anterior occlusal contact or coverage depending on the nature of the open bite.

When using this type of bionator, the clinician should differentiate between the presence of a dental open bite (alveolar deformation most likely caused by a thumb or tongue habit) and a skeletal open bite caused by vertical maxillary excess, a tipped up palatal plane, and/or a steep mandibular plane angle. In patients with a dentoalveolar anterior open bite, the occlusal acrylic is processed in full contact with the maxillary and mandibular posterior teeth to prevent vertical alveolar development in the buccal segments (Fig. 18-3). The wire and acrylic, however, do not contact the anterior teeth to allow for vertical eruption of the incisors and bite closure.

When a skeletal open bite exists, without an anterior alveolar deformation, and with a acceptable smile line, the bionator should be constructed with posterior bite blocks and acrylic lower incisor coverage. This anterior acrylic and lingual wire should contact the maxillary incisors to prevent their extrusion. When further control of the skeletal vertical problem is needed, facebow tubes can be added to the bionator to control maxillary vertical excess. Alternatively, a vertical pull chin cup can be used in conjunction with the appliance to allow for vertical ramus growth and mandibular remodeling in open bite patients characterized by a steep mandibular plane angle.

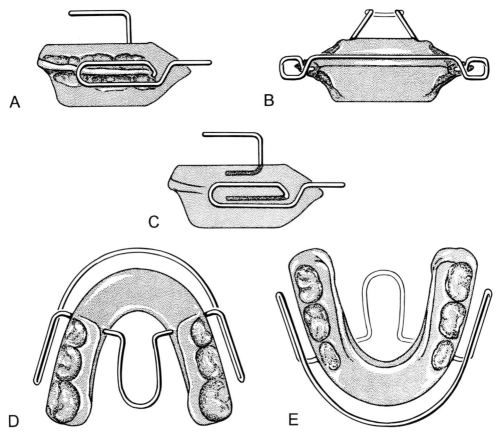

Figure 18-3. Bionator to close anterior dentoalveolar open bite (Balters design). *A*, Lateral view showing interocclusal acrylic. Acrylic does not touch either the maxillary or mandibular anterior teeth. *B*, Frontal view. *C*, Position of wires within acrylic. *D*, Maxillary occlusal view with interocclusal acrylic. *E*, Mandibular view showing relief in the lower lingual region.

Assuming the presence of an anteroposterior discrepancy, the mandible can be advanced with this design, since all posterior teeth lock into the interocclusal acrylic for orientation.

Bionator to Maintain the Bite

This type of bionator is used to reposition the mandible forward while maintaining the existing vertical dimension (Figs. 18-1 and 18-4). The acrylic and wire parts prevent vertical changes in both the anterior and posterior regions by providing full contact of the appliance against all teeth. As treatment progresses, the clinician can trim the interocclusal acrylic to allow for subsequent eruption of selected teeth (as, for example, in the first permanent molar region as shown in Figure 18-1). This sequence provides the most positive orientation for the bionator in the early stages of treatment, because all teeth in both arches contact the acrylic. It also places all vertical dentoalveolar changes under the control of the clinician, instead of the laboratory technician.

PREPARATION OF WORK MODELS

Impression Technique

In contrast to the FR-2 appliance of Fränkel, which is a tissue-borne appliance, the bionator has both tissue-borne and tooth-borne components. An accurate reproduction of the dentition and the associated soft tissue is essential for proper appliance fabrication. Of particular importance is the soft tissue in the lower lingual region.

Standard aluminum trays are adequate for most bionator impressions as long as there is no tissue impingement. Care should be taken to make sure that the tray is extended vertically an adequate amount in the lower lingual region; however, in no instance should the tray itself contact the lower lingual tissue.

Bite Registration

As stated throughout this text, differing opinions exist regarding the amount of bite advancement. The

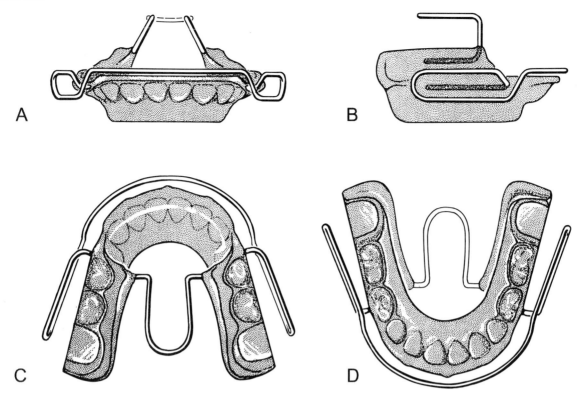

Figure 18-4. Balters bionator. *A*, Frontal view. The acrylic in the anterior part of the appliance lies against the mandibular anterior teeth. *B*, Position of wires in acrylic. *C*, Maxillary occlusal view, including the palatal ("Coffin spring") wire. *D*, Mandibular occlusal view.

greater the advancement, the stronger are the dislodging forces on the bionator created by the musculature, making the appliance more difficult to wear. An appliance worn incorrectly due to abnormal pull of the musculature may cause undesirable flaring of the lower incisors, an important point to consider when the bite registration is obtained. Therefore, the overall muscle pattern of the patient must be evaluated in addition to the dentoskeletal anteroposterior discrepancy.

One of the disadvantages of the bionator, in comparison to the twin block, FR-2, and Herbst appliance, is that typically the appliance cannot be advanced without remaking the appliance. An exception is the orthopedic corrector design of the bionator, which is characterized by sagittal screws that can advance the mandibular portion of the appliance. Thus, most clinicians obtain the construction bite with the patient biting in an end-to-end incisal relationship.

The technique for obtaining a wax construction bite by means of a Projet™ bite fork and a horseshoe of medium hard pink wax is described in detail in Chapter 15. This method is appropriate for the bionator as well. On the other hand, some clinicians obtain the bite registration either directly in the mouth without using a bite fork or from models mounted on an articulator (Fig. 18-5). A 5–10 mm thickness of medium-hard wax in either a tapered or horseshoe configuration is used to orient the maxillary and mandibular dental arches in all three planes of space. Adjustments of the bite registrations should not be performed in the laboratory, as the accuracy of the appliance may be compromised.

Because most bionators have an acrylic cap covering the mandibular incisors, a vertical opening of 2.0–2.5 mm between the incisors must be recorded in the wax bite. In place of a bite fork, a pair of tongue depressors can be used clinically to determine the proper amount of bite opening. A piece of wax, horseshoe-shaped or tapered in configuration and 5–10 mm in thickness, is placed in the mouth, the tongue depressors are added, and the wax is pressed into place. The wax bite is removed and trimmed so that the extent of the bite opening can be observed clearly. Depending on the amount of man-dibular advancement and the curve of Spee of the lower arch, the posterior opening typically will be 3–5 mm in patients with decreased vertical dimension.

When closure of an anterior dental open bite is desired, the thickness of the posterior acrylic should be 2–3 mm. Control of the increased vertical dimension requires a construction bite that will interfere with the freeway space. Therefore, the thickness of the wax bite in the posterior segment should be 5 mm or greater. For bionators to maintain the vertical dimension of the face,

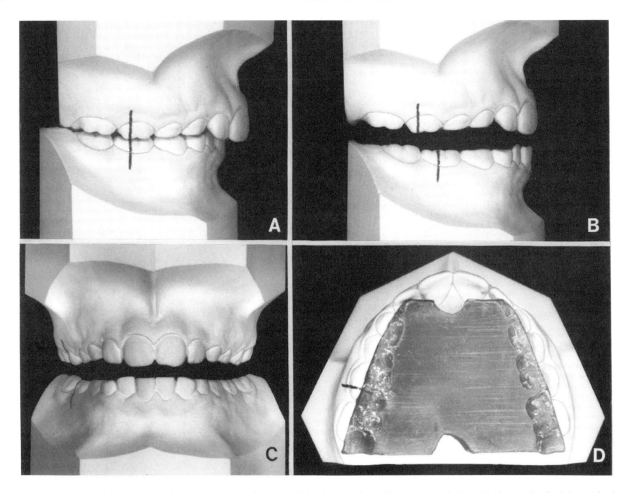

Figure 18-5. Wax bite construction. *A*, Sagittal view of original occlusion. The molar relationship is marked with vertical black line. *B*, Sagittal view of the downward and forward repositioning of the mandibular arch with wax bite in place. Note the change in molar relationship. *C*, Frontal view of the dental cast with the wax bite in place. Note that the maxillary and mandibular midlines are aligned. *D*, Occlusal view of maxillary cast with tapered wax bite in place.

the thickness of the wax registration should not exceed the dimension of the posterior freeway space. The dimension of the freeway space in patients with an increased or normal vertical dimension will dictate the anterior bite opening.

As the mandible is repositioned anteriorly, the maxillary and mandibular dental midlines should be aligned, if they coincide with the skeletal midlines. If the skeletal and dental midlines are not coincident, then the skeletal midlines should be aligned to avoid the creation of a skeletal asymmetry.

Fabrication of Work Models

The construction models are poured in stone or hard plaster. All bubbles and other artifacts are removed, and the models are carefully checked for distortion. Areas of prime concern include the palate, the lower lingual region, and the dentition. The models are trimmed with the wax bite in place and with their backs flush with each other. Trimming the models in this manner is important because it will allow the laboratory to check the wax bite when the work models are received, and it will allow the clinician to check the wax bite registration when the appliance is returned from the laboratory.

SEQUENCE OF CONSTRUCTION

The type of bionator we have used most commonly is the California bionator (Fig. 18-2). The mechanism of action of this type of bionator is described most easily by providing a discussion of the fabrication of the appliance.

Mounting the Work Models

The laboratory technician first checks the work models and bite for accuracy. The wax construction bite is seated firmly on the maxillary and mandibular models, and the technician checks to ensure that the midline re-

BIONATOR

lationship correspond to the prescription sheet filled out by the clinician (any midline deviations present in the models and wax bite should be noted by the clinician on the prescription sheet to avoid confusion).

With the wax bite in place, the models are mounted on a model holder (*e.g.,* fixator) using laboratory plaster. Once the plaster securing the models has hardened, the wax bite is removed, and the interocclusal space is checked in all dimensions. If the interocclusal space is inadequate, a new wax bite will be needed. Accurate mountings of the working models without altering the vertical dimension established by the wax bite is essential for proper appliance fit. If this dimension is altered during the mounting, the arc of closure of the mandible will not coincide with that of the appliance and the lower incisors will not rotate into their cap.

Application of Wax Relief

Lead pencil outlines are drawn on the maxillary and mandibular work models to indicate the final edges of all acrylic parts of the bionator (Fig. 18-6). The pencil lines serve as a guide for the application of the acrylic.

The clinician initially must determine the extensions of the lower lingual flanges. Typically, the acrylic flanges extend into the lingual alveolar process about 5 mm in the posterior region. This extension produces an acrylic flange that does not lock into the undercut area of the mandible but rather guides the mandible into a proper orientation. Because the mandible is not locked into position, the patient actively postures the mandible forward to seat the bionator between the dental arches.

An alternative design used by some clinicians is to extend the lower lingual acrylic into the undercut regions in a method similar to that used in the construction of some activator appliances. The bionator snaps into place with a definitive lock on the mandible.

Wax relief is applied lingually to the lower incisors. This wax relief will prevent direct acrylic contact with the lower anterior teeth. Acrylic contact on these teeth may cause undesirable labial pressure due to the forces of the retractor muscles on the advanced mandible. This is particularly important in the early stages of treatment, when the patient is adapting to the appliance. If wax relief is used in the lower lingual anterior area (Fig. 18-6), the pressure originating from the pull of the retractor muscles is transferred to the posterior aspect of the lingual alveolar area, rather than directly to the incisors, thus avoiding flaring.

Wire Fabrication

Maxillary Labial Wire

The maxillary labial wire is bent in a Hawley configuration from .040" stainless steel wire (Fig. 18-7). The adjustment loops of this wire are about the same width as the canines and extend upward approximately 7–8 mm above the gingival margin (Fig. 18-7*AB*). The labial bow traverses the anterior teeth at their middle one third.

A critical area in the construction of the labial wire is the 90° bend at the point where the wire enters the interocclusal acrylic. This bend must be well rounded to avoid stress points that can lead to breakage of the appliance during treatment.

If the retracting forces of the mandible pull the bionator in a posterior direction during treatment, the labial wire can cause lingual tipping of the maxillary in-

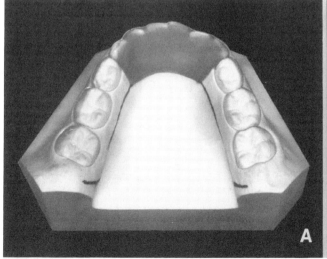
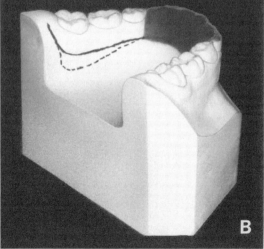

Figure 18-6. Placement of wax relief. *A.* Occlusal view of mandibular dental cast. Note the application of wax on the lingual surface of the anterior region. The pencil lines indicate the eventual outline of the acrylic. *B.* Oblique view.

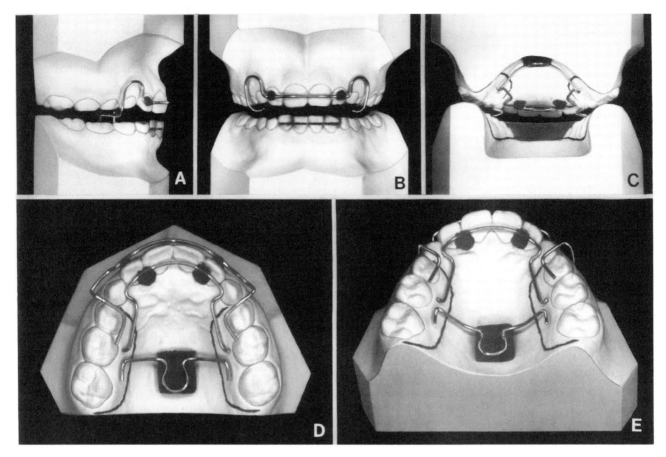

Figure 18-7. Wire fabrication. *A*, Right maxillary view of dental cast showing maxillary labial wire. *B*, Frontal view of dental cast showing maxillary labial wire. *C*, Posterior view showing maxillary lingual wire and palatal wire. *D*, Maxillary occlusal view. *E*, Maxillary oblique-occlusal view. Note wax spacer supporting the palatal wire. The pencil lines indicate the eventual acrylic outlines.

cisors. Therefore, in the laboratory construction and clinical management of this part of the appliance, the wire usually is positioned slightly away from the teeth (approximately 0.5 mm).

Maxillary Lingual Wire

The maxillary lingual wire is bent from .036" stainless steel wire. This wire provides support for the bionator by using the lingual surfaces of the maxillary anterior teeth for anchorage (Fig. 18-7*DE*). The wire is constructed in an ideal arch form at the level of the cingula of these teeth. When a midline expansion screw is incorporated (to be discussed later), this wire is cut between the central incisors to avoid pressure on the appliance as the screw is expanded. The bionator used to close a dentoalveolar open bite may lack this wire.

Palatal Wire

The palatal wire (the so-called "Coffin spring") is constructed from .045" stainless steel wire (Fig. 18-7*DE*). The loop of the palatal wire is much smaller than the original version described by Balters (Fig. 18-4). A wax spacer, 2–3 mm in thickness, is used to support the loop in the palate to ensure adequate clearance for tissue comfort. This wire design can be activated in conjunction with the midline expansion screw (if included) for lateral arch development.

Acrylic Fabrication

After all the wires have been bent and secured to the construction models, the acrylic is processed using a "salt and pepper" method. Typically, the bionator is fabricated as a single unit, made from clear acrylic for maximum esthetics (Fig. 18-8). After the acrylic block has been formed, the appliance is removed from the construction models, and a rough trim is accomplished with large burs and sandpaper arbor bands. For optimum patient comfort, the acrylic should be kept as thin as possible in all areas. Important considerations in the final trim of the bionator are described below.

BIONATOR

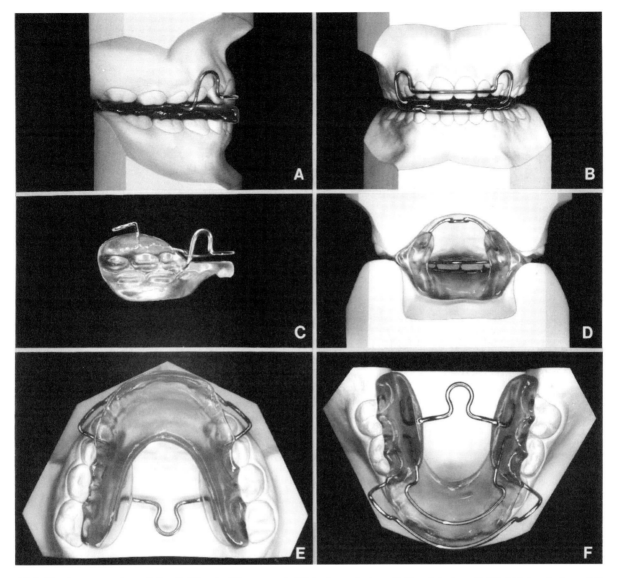

Figure 18-8. Final construction of the California Bionator. *A*, Right lateral view. *B*, Frontal view. *C*, Right lateral view of the appliance showing the eruption facets, the palatal wire, the maxillary labial wire and the incisal cap. *D*, Posterior view. *E*, Maxillary-occlusal view. Note the placement of the wax relief has eliminated contact of the acrylic with the lingual surfaces of the mandibular incisors. *F*, Mandibular view. Note the contours of the eruption facets.

Control of Posterior Eruption

The clinician must determine whether the patient requires eruption of the posterior teeth. The interocclusal acrylic can be adjusted in several ways, depending on the dentoalveolar effect desired.

Eruption Facets

One of the mechanisms postulated for the correction of Class II malocclusion is the differential eruption of the posterior teeth. If eruption of both maxillary and mandibular posterior teeth is needed, eruption facets can be fabricated from the interocclusal acrylic (Figs. 18-2 and 18-8*C,F*). These channels, which contact the teeth (Fig. 18-9), allow for vertical and slight distal eruption of the maxillary posterior teeth and vertical and mesial eruption of the mandibular posterior teeth (Fig. 18-10*A*). If expansion of both arches is desired, additional interocclusal acrylic is removed (Fig. 18-10*B*).

Occlusal Table

According to Harvold,[12] Class II correction can be achieved by preventing the normal downward and forward movement of the maxillary posterior teeth while allowing vertical eruption of the mandibular posterior teeth. This particular mechanism can be used in biona-

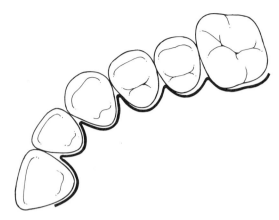

Figure 18-9. Maxillary view of the trimmed acrylic. Note that the eruption facets are contoured so that each facet touches the premolar or molar mesially while allowing space distally.

tor therapy through the fabrication of an occlusal table from the interocclusal acrylic.

An occlusal table (Fig. 18-11A) is fabricated so that the maxillary posterior teeth remain in contact with the interocclusal acrylic. The acrylic adjacent to the mandibular posterior teeth is removed, allowing for their unrestricted differential eruption.

Interocclusal Acrylic

If vertical or lateral eruption of the posterior teeth is not desired, no modification is made in the interocclusal acrylic (Fig. 18-11B; see also Figs. 18-1, 18-3, and 18-4). Thus, vertical and lateral tooth movement is prevented.

Control of Incisor Eruption

The bionator typically is constructed so that the mandibular incisors are covered with an acrylic incisal cap Figs. 18-1 and 18-2). The covering of the lower incisors presumably prevents the vertical eruption of these teeth and stabilizes the bionator in the mouth. The thickness of the acrylic cap can be reduced for increased patient acceptance.

The maxillary incisors are restricted anteroposteriorly by the upper labial and lingual wires (Figs. 18-2 and 18-8). The incisal edges of the maxillary incisors usually contact the top of the lower incisal cap, preventing vertical eruption of the incisors.

Lower Lingual Region

As described earlier, the lower lingual flanges of the bionator can be constructed according to many specifications. When additional anchorage and support is required from dentoalveolar segments, the acrylic flanges are extended in a design similar to that used in constructing the activator.

AUXILIARIES

In the fabrication of the bionator, several types of auxiliaries can be added to the basic design.

Expansion Screws

Expansion screws can be added during the fabrication of the acrylic parts of the appliance. A midline screw is

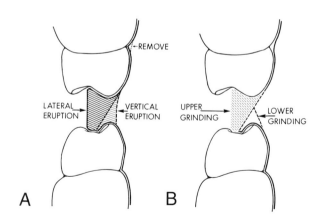

Figure 18-10. A, Eruption facets. If lateral eruption is desired, the acrylic is removed at an angle. If vertical eruption is desired, additional acrylic is removed. B, Guidance of mandibular eruption. If eruption and lateral expansion of the mandibular dentition are desired, additional interocclusal acrylic is removed.

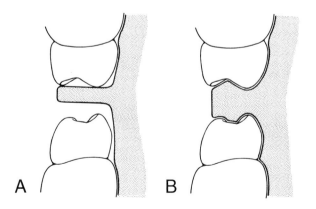

Figure 18-11. A, Occlusal table. The interocclusal acrylic is trimmed so that the maxillary posterior teeth touch the acrylic. The mandibular teeth remain free of the acrylic. B, Interocclusal acrylic. If no change in vertical eruption is desired, the interocclusal acrylic is left between the maxillary and mandibular posterior teeth.

BIONATOR

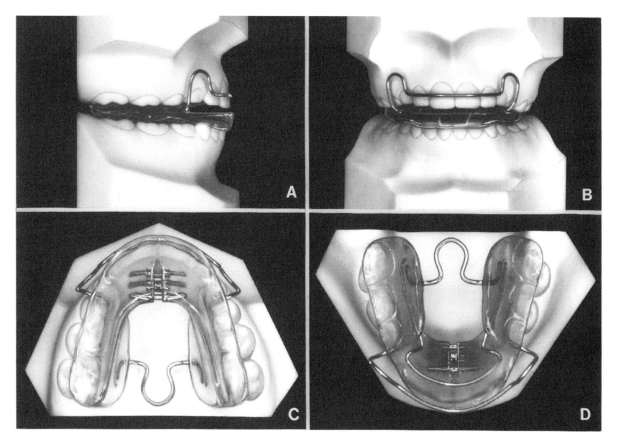

Figure 18-12. Expansion bionator. *A*, Right lateral view. *B*, Frontal view. *C*, Maxillary-occlusal view. Note position of expansion screw. *D*, Mandibular occlusal view. Note that the maxillary lingual wire has been cut in the midline to allows expansion.

placed to encourage lateral expansion of the dental arches (Fig. 18-12). This type of effect is biomechanical in nature, because the appliance has direct contact with the teeth. This type of expansion can be contrasted with that produced by the FR-2 appliance of Fränkel, the latter type of expansion being passive rather than active.

Expansion screws also can be inserted sagittally in the posterior area. Many clinicians advocate the use of these screws to increase arch length posteriorly, again by biomechanical application of pressure to the dentition. These expansion screws also can be used to advance the bite registration of the bionator in a systematic fashion, if the acrylic touching the posterior teeth is removed.

Facebow Tubes

Extraoral traction can be used in association with bionator therapy either to distalize or control the vertical growth of the maxillary complex or to stabilize the appliance in the mouth. One example of this type of approach is the appliance advocated by Teuscher[13] (Fig. 18-13). A high-pull facebow can be used to restrict the downward and forward movement of the maxilla as the Teuscher appliance is worn.

Lower Labial Pads

One of the major criticisms of the bionator is the lack of direct muscle training, particularly of the perioral musculature. Teuscher[13] has advocated the addition of lower labial pads (Fig. 18-13) similar to those present in the FR-2 appliance of Fränkel.[14] If lower labial pads are to be incorporated into the basic bionator design, a careful reproduction of the lower anterior vestibular region is necessary as it is for the fabrication of the FR-2 appliance.

DELIVERY OF THE APPLIANCE

At the time of appliance insertion, the bionator should be checked thoroughly on the work models to make sure that it has been constructed according to the specifications of the clinician.

The patient should be instructed that the appliance is

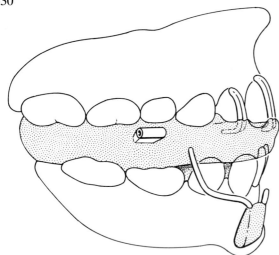

Figure 18-13. Lateral view of the Teuscher appliance. Note the facebow tube and the maxillary incisor uprighting springs.

a full-time appliance, and that eventually the appliance will be worn at all times except during meals, toothbrushing, language lessons, contact sports, and when playing certain musical instruments. As with the FR-2 appliance, there usually is some speech difficulty associated with wearing the bionator, particularly during the early phases of treatment. The patient is instructed to read aloud for one half hour per day until normal speech can be accomplished while wearing the appliance.[14] If speech competence is not regained quickly, the patient will have a tendency to remove the appliance during conversation. Increased salivation also is present for the first few days after insertion.

Some soreness of the lower incisors also is to be expected due to the pressure of the acrylic. The patient should be instructed that if this occurs, it is only temporary and that appliance wear should not be discontinued. If necessary, a pain medication could be prescribed to alleviate the experienced soreness.

During the break-in period, the patient is instructed to wear the appliance an increased amount of hours each day, starting with 3–4 hours during the day and gradually increasing to fulltime wear, including sleeping. The appliance should be worn full-time during the day for a few weeks before night-time wear is allowed, permitting the establishment of the neuromuscular reflex that will help maintain the mandible in a forward position.

The patient should be seen approximately every six to eight weeks until the desired treatment outcome is obtained. At each appointment, the eruption facets should be checked with an explorer to make sure that the maxillary and mandibular posterior teeth are free to erupt distally and mesially, if so desired. In addition, the overjet should be measured in centric relation to determine the amount of correction obtained as well as to check the level of patient compliance. If further advancement of the mandible is necessary, a new appliance should be made. Alternatively, the advancement screws previously described can be adjusted to accomplish the rest of the mandibular repositioning. Advancement should be considered only after there is good muscle response or when the mandible could not be repositioned distally when checking centric occlusion. For patients demonstrating good compliance, the advancement of the bionator (or the fabrication of a new appliance) may be necessary after 3–6 months.

CONCLUDING REMARKS

This chapter has described an approach for design and clinical management of the bionator. One of the difficulties in dealing with bionator therapy is the fact that, as with activators, there is no recognized standard bionator. This chapter has attempted to divide the bionator into its component parts, so that the clinician can understand better the effect that each part of the appliance has on the overall treatment result. If the clinician gains a thorough understanding of the component parts of the appliance, he or she can design a bionator that is adapted to the specific needs of each patient.

Perhaps one of the chief advantages to the bionator in comparison to other functional appliances is its use during the late mixed dentition. The appliance can be worn effectively, even during the transition from the deciduous molars to the premolars. This appliance provides the clinician the ability to treat a patient orthopedically in spite of a relatively unstable occlusion.

REFERENCES CITED

1. Balters W. Die Technik und Übung der allgemeinen und speziellen Bionator-therapie. Quintessenz, Heft 5: 77, IV Kieferorthopädie, 1964.
2. Balters W. Die Einführung in die Bionator Heilmethode. Ausgewählte, Schriften und Vortrange. Heidelberg: Druckerei Holzer, 1973.
3. Andresen V. The Norwegian system of gnatho-orthopedics. Acta Gnathol 1936;1:4–36.
4. Pancherz H. Long-term effects of activator treatment: a cephalometric roentgenographic investigation. Odont Revy 1976;27:31–42.
5. Graber TM, Neumann B. Removable orthodontic appliances. Philadelphia: WB Saunders, 1984.
6. Ascher F. Hemmung bei Anwendung moderner Aktivatoren. Fortschr. Kieferorthop 1964;25:490–501.
7. Ascher F. Praktische Kieferorthopädie. Munich: Urban and Schwarzenberg, 1968.
8. Ascher F. Kontrollierte Ergebnisse der Rückbissbehand-

lung mit funktionskieferorthopädischen Geräten. Fortschr Kieferorthop 1971;32:149–159.
9. Ascher F. Der Diagonalwinkel als Richtwert für Diagnose, Prognose und Therapie in der Kieferorthopädie. Handlexikon der Zahnäzlichen Praxis. Stuttgart: Medica Verlag, 1973.
10. Janson I. Bionator-Modifikationen in der kieferorthopädischen Therapie. Verlag, Munich: Karl Hanser, 1987.
11. Rudzki-Janson I, Noachtar R. Functional appliance therapy with the bionator. Semin Orthod 1998;4:33–45.
12. Harvold EP. The activator in interceptive orthodontics. St Louis: CV Mosby, 1974.
13. Teuscher U. A growth-related concept for skeletal Class II treatment. Am J Orthod 1978;74:258–275.
14. Fränkel R. Technik und Handhabung der Funktionsregler. Berlin: VEB Verlag Volk and Gesundheit, 1976.

Chapter 19
THE JASPER JUMPER

This chapter* describes the basic components of the jumper mechanism (Jasper Jumper™),[1] which can be viewed as a modification of the Herbst bite jumping mechanism.[2] This interarch flexible force module allows the patient greater freedom of mandibular movement than is possible with the original bite jumping mechanism of Herbst.

One of the major advantages of the Herbst appliance, and of any other fixed intermaxillary appliance, is the relative speed at which treatment effects are achieved. Traditional approaches to treating a Class II malocclusion (e.g., extraoral traction, Class II elastics) often are hampered by problems with patient compliance. By anchoring the device intraorally, the need for patient cooperation is reduced substantially.

One of the disadvantages of the Herbst appliance is the rigidity of the Herbst bite jumping mechanism itself. Although every attempt is made to allow freedom of movement by having the orthodontist or laboratory technician enlarge the attachment holes of the tube and plunger to the axles, the bite jumping mechanism can restrict lateral movements of the mandible.

In an attempt to overcome these problems, in 1987 Jasper[3] developed a new pushing device that is flexible (Figs. 19-1 and 19-2). This appliance produces both sagittal and intrusive forces, as does the Herbst bite jumping mechanism, but affords the patient much more freedom of mandibular movement. These force mod-

ules also can be used in other applications and in other types of malocclusions, as will be discussed later.

Another significant advantage of this auxiliary appliance system is that it can be added to existing appliances virtually at any point after initial arch alignment is completed. The modules can be used as a primary method of treatment or can be added later after alternative treatments have proven unsuccessful (e.g., extraoral traction, functional jaw orthopedics). There is no need to remove the entire fixed appliance setup before the force modules are placed, nor is there additional laboratory cost or lost time during treatment.

PARTS OF THE APPLIANCE

The Jasper Jumper™ modular system can be used with most types of fixed appliances. The system is composed of two parts: the force module and the anchor units.

Force Module

The force module, analogous to the tube and plunger parts of the Herbst bite jumping mechanism, is flexible (Fig. 19-3). The force module is constructed of a stainless steel coil or spring (see inset in Fig. 19-3) that is attached at both ends to stainless steel endcaps, in which holes have been drilled in the flanges to accommodate the anchoring unit. This module is surrounded by an opaque polyurethane covering for hygiene and comfort. The modules are available (American Orthodontics, Sheboygan WI) in seven lengths, ranging from 26 mm to

---

*This chapter is based, in part, on an article[1] by Jasper and McNamara that appeared in the *American Journal of Orthodontics and Dentofacial Orthopedics* in 1995 that has been updated for this volume.

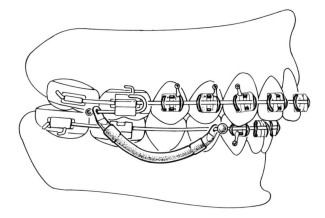

Figure 19-1. The Jasper Jumper™ force module. Note that the maxillary and mandibular archwires extend to the second molars and are cinched back posteriorly. Tie backs also can be used.

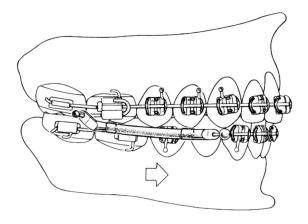

Figure 19-2. The Jasper Jumper™ force module. As the module straightens, the module becomes passive, in that all stored energy is released. The mandible is brought into a forward position.

38 mm in 2 mm increments. They are designed for use on either side of the dental arch.

When the force module is straight, it remains passive (Fig. 19-2). As the teeth come into occlusion, the spring of the force module is curved axially as the muscles of mastication elevate the mandible, producing a range of forces from one to sixteen ounces. This kinetic energy then is captured when the force module is curved, and the force is converted to potential energy to be used for a variety of clinical effects.

If properly installed to produce mandibular advancement, the spring mechanism will be curved or activated 4 mm relative to its resting length, thus storing about eight ounces (250 gm) of potential energy for force delivery (Fig. 19-1). If less force is desired (*e.g.,* force levels that produce tooth movement alone), the Jumper is not activated fully. Increasing the activation beyond 4 mm does not yield more force from the module, but only builds excessive internal stress in the module. The tendency to increase the force for faster treatment results is to be avoided.

Anchor Units

A number of methods are available to anchor the force modules to both the permanent and mixed dentitions.

Attachment to the Main Archwire

The most common method of attachment of the force module to the dental arches in patients in the permanent dentition is with previously placed fixed orthodontic appliances. When the Jumper mechanism is used to correct a Class II malocclusion, the force module is attached posteriorly to the maxillary arch by a ball pin that is placed through the distal attachment of the force module and then extends anteriorly through the facebow tube on the maxillary first molar band (Fig. 19-3). The ball pin is anchored in position by having the clinician place a return bend in the ball pin at its mesial end.

Anteriorly, the module is anchored to the mandibular archwire. Bayonet bends are placed distal to the mandibular canines, and small Lexan™ beads are slipped over the archwire to provide an anterior stop. The mandibular archwire is threaded through the hole in the anterior endcap, and then the archwire is ligated in place. The removal of the brackets on the mandibular second premolars in addition to the mandibular first

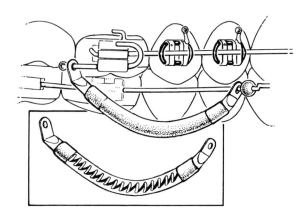

Figure 19-3. The attachment of the distal end of the force module to the maxillary dental arch with a ball pin. Moving the ball pin anteriorly can activate the appliance. The alignment of the spring within the Jumper mechanism is shown in the inset.

premolars (as advocated originally) allows the patient greater freedom of movement.

Attachment to Auxiliary Archwires

An alternative design incorporates the use of "outriggers"[4] (Fig. 19-4). This .016 x .022" (.018" slot) or .018 x .025" (.022" slot) auxiliary sectional wire allows the clinician to leave the premolar brackets or bands in place by attaching the force module to a sectional wire that is anchored anteriorly to the main archwire between the first premolar and canine (Fig 19-4A). Additionally, because the modules have greater freedom to slide, there is a greater range of jaw movement. Repairs and replacement of the Jumper components are simplified with this outrigger modification.

The segmental archwire is attached posteriorly through an auxiliary tube located on the mandibular first molar band (Fig. 19-4A). The auxiliary wire can be bent so that the vestibular section is parallel to the occlusal plane (as shown in Figure 19-4). A shorter vertical step also can be placed posteriorly so that the inclination of the outrigger more closely approximates the downward and forward growth direction of the patient's face. The posterior part of the Jumper module is attached to the ball pin placed through the maxillary molar tube (Fig. 19-4B), as described previously.

If outriggers are used to anchor the module to the mandibular dentition, care must be taken to assure that the sectional archwire provides adequate space between the alveolus and the gingiva to allow the module to slide without tissue impingement. Contouring the sectional archwire and placing first order step out bends in the archwire may be helpful. Once the module has been placed, the module should slide smoothly along the sectional outrigger wire.

Attachment in the Mixed Dentition

The force module also can be used in mixed dentition patients whose premolars have not yet erupted (Fig. 19-5). The maxillary attachment is similar to that previously described, in that the ball pin is used to connect the force module to maxillary first molars. The mandibular attachment of the force module is through an archwire that extends from the brackets on the mandibular incisors posteriorly to the first permanent molars, bypassing the region of the deciduous canines and molars (Fig. 19-5). In a mixed dentition patient, the use of a transpalatal arch and fixed lower lingual arch is mandatory to control potential unfavorable side effects produced by the appliance (*e.g.*, molar and incisor tipping and flaring).

TREATMENT EFFECTS

Although a number of case reports have appeared in the literature,[5-9] only a few clinical studies have considered the treatment effects of the Jasper Jumper™. The findings of these studies are somewhat conflicting regarding the treatment effects produced by this force module on the growth of the craniofacial complex.

The first published statistical study of the Jasper Jumper™ was by Cope and colleagues[10] in 1994. These investigators evaluated a sample of 31 consecutively treated growing Class II patients. Lateral cephalograms were taken immediately before appliance placement and immediately after appliance removal (mean interval of approximately five months). The sample was matched to untreated controls based on age, sex, and mandibular plane angle. Cope and co-workers found that the majority of Class II correction was due to dentoalveolar rather than skeletal change. The maxilla un-

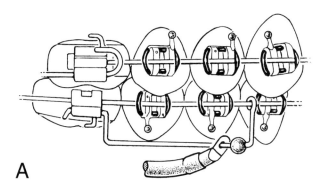
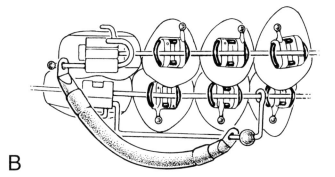

Figure 19-4. The use of "outriggers" for anchoring the force module. *A*, The rectangular auxiliary archwire is looped over the main archwire anteriorly and is cinched back through the auxiliary tube posteriorly. *B*, A ball pin is inserted through the distal hole in the Jumper module, is placed anteriorly through the facebow tube on the maxillary first molar band and is cinched forward to activate the module.

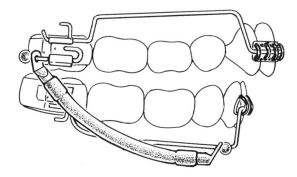

Figure 19-5. The use of the force module in a mixed dentition patient. In this instance, a bayonet bend is placed distal to the lateral incisor, and a Lexan™ ball acts as a stop for the force module anteriorly. In this example, maxillary and mandibular rectangular utility arches connect the anterior and posterior teeth.

derwent significant posterior displacement, the maxillary incisors became retroclined, and the maxillary molars tipped distally. Downward and backward mandibular rotation also was evident. The mandibular incisors also proclined significantly, and the mandibular molars moved forward and tipped mesially.

Covell and co-workers[11] evaluated a sample of 36 growing patients treated with the Jasper Jumper™ appliance. The sample was divided into two groups, 24 patients with records obtained at the start and completion of orthodontic treatment, and an additional 12 patients with records available at the beginning and end of the Jumper phase of treatment. Treatment effects were determined by statistical comparisons of cephalometric changes in the patients relative to age-adjusted cephalometric standards, and from structural superimpositions. While the modules were in place, the maxillary incisors were retroclined and the molars were moved distally, tipped back, and intruded. The mandibular incisors were proclined and intruded, and the mandibular molars were translated mesially, tipped forward, and extruded. Skeletal measures showed reduced forward maxillary displacement, but no significant increase in sagittal mandibular growth. During orthodontic finishing, molar tipping and maxillary incisor retroclination were corrected, although the mandibular incisors remained proclined. Thus, Covell and co-workers[32] concluded that the Jasper Jumper™ appliance corrected Class II discrepancies largely through maxillary and mandibular dentoalveolar effects and, to a limited extent, by restraint of forward maxillary growth. The rate of mandibular growth, however, remained unaffected.

Somewhat different findings regarding mandibular growth were reported by Stucki and Ingervall,[12] who studied the effect of the Jasper Jumper™ in 26 consecutive 13–25-year-old Class II patients. The median treatment time was five months, followed by a seven-month observation or retention period. Cephalometric records were obtained at each treatment interval. The Jumpers brought about a slight retrusion of the maxilla, and, in contrast to the two previously mentioned studies,[10,11] increased growth of the mandible also was noted. The maxillary incisors and molars were retruded, and the mandibular incisors and molars protruded. The median correction of the overjet and molar relationship was almost 5 mm and 3 mm, respectively. Stucki and Ingervall[12] noted that the intrusive forces of the Jumper also resulted in a transient intrusion of the maxillary molars and the mandibular incisors. After the period of retention and observation, however, the dentoalveolar effects had partially or totally relapsed. At the end of observation, about 60 per cent of the overjet reduction and 75 per cent of the molar correction remained. The authors concluded that key factor contributing most to the correction was the skeletal effect on the mandible, *i.e.,* increase mandibular growth.

The only comparative study of appliance systems involving the Jasper Jumper™ was published by Weiland and colleagues,[13] who evaluated the initial effects of treatment of Class II, Division 1 malocclusion with the Herren activator (27 patients), the activator-headgear combination (20 patients), and the Jasper Jumper™ appliance (25 patients). The patients' ages ranged from 9 to 12 years. Treatment effects were evaluated by analyzing serial lateral headfilms obtained before and after 6–8 months of treatment. The investigators found that the correction in overjet and molar relationship was more complete in the patients with the Jasper Jumper™ than in the patients with the activator. Whereas all the patients with the Jasper Jumper™ achieved a Class I occlusion, such a correction was achieved in only 20 of the 47 patients treated with the activator. The Class II correction occurred through a combination of skeletal and dentoalveolar adaptations. Skeletal changes accounted for 42%, 35%, and 48% of the overjet correction by the Herren-type activator, the headgear-activator, and the Jasper Jumper™, respectively. Similarly, the skeletal component of molar correction was 55%, 46%, and 38% in the respective groups. Dentoalveolar compensation (distal movement of the maxillary molars, mesial movement of the mandibular molars) appeared to be inversely related to skeletal adaptation. The patients with the Jasper Jumper™ also showed a marked intrusion of the mandibular incisors with a consequent reduction in overbite.

Thus, the few clinical studies to date report universal agreement that a major component of Class II correction with the Jumper force modules is maxillary and mandibular dentoalveolar adaptation. Conflicting findings exist, however, as to the extent of the contribution of skeletal sagittal changes in the mandible or maxilla.

CLINICAL MANAGEMENT

Preparation of Anchorage

The most important aspect of the clinical management of this appliance system is the preparation of mandibular anchorage and the control of mandibular mesial tooth movement. As stated earlier, mesial movement of the mandibular incisors has been reported using this appliance system.[10,12,14,15] Unfavorable dentoalveolar adaptations can be minimized in the mandible through proper anchorage preparation.

Alignment of the maxillary and mandibular anterior teeth during the initial phases of orthodontic treatment must be completed. Full-sized (or nearly full-sized) archwires should be inserted into the brackets in both arches before the placement of the force modules. The archwires should be tied or cinched back posteriorly to increase anchorage (Fig. 19-1), including second molars whenever possible. In addition, the clinician can place posterior tip-back bends in the mandibular archwire to enhance anchorage.

When jumpers are anticipated in the treatment plan, anterior lingual crown torque can be placed in the archwire. Alternatively, mandibular incisor brackets with five degrees of lingual crown torque incorporated into the slot of the bracket also can be used to prepare anchorage. Lingually torqued mandibular incisor brackets are used in addition to, not as a substitute for, anchorage in the mandible.

Stabilization Wires

Two types of auxiliary archwires can be used to enhance anchorage: the transpalatal arch and the lower lingual arch. A transpalatal arch (Fig. 19-6A) can be used in those instances in which distal maxillary molar movement is to be minimized and mandibular adaptations are to be maximized. A transpalatal arch is not incorporated into the appliance system if maxillary dentoalveolar movement is desired.

The use of a fixed lower lingual arch (Fig. 19-6B) is encouraged strongly in most instances. This type of anchorage preparation is used routinely except when significant mandibular incisor proclination is desired as part of the overall treatment plan (*e.g.*, patients with mandibular dentoalveolar retrusion).

Preparation of the Arches

As noted above, the Jumper mechanisms are not placed until the initial leveling and alignment of the dentition has been completed and full-sized or nearly full-sized archwires have been placed in both arches. After the archwires have become passive, the mandibular archwire is disengaged, and the brackets on the first and second premolars are removed bilaterally (Fig. 19-1, 19-6). Unless outriggers are used, bayonet bends are placed in the archwire distal to the mandibular canine bracket. Three millimeter Lexan™ beads are slipped over the ends of the archwire and moved forward to rest against the bayonet bends bilaterally (Figs. 19-1, 19-6).

Installation of the Modules

In order to determine the proper length of the module, the distance from the the mesial surface of the maxillary

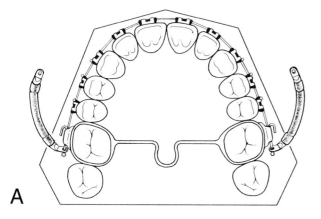
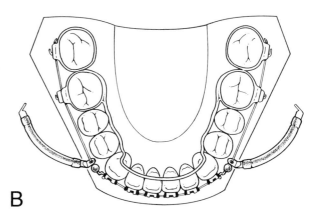

Figure 19-6. *A*, The use of the transpalatal arch combined with fixed appliances to enhance maxillary anchorage. *B*, The use of a lower lingual arch in conjunction with fixed appliances to enhance mandibular anchorage.

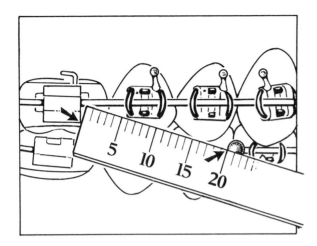

Figure 19-7. The determination of proper length of the force module. Twelve millimeters are added to the measurement of the distance between the mesial aspect of the facebow tube and the distal aspect of the Lexan™ ball. In this example, the distance from the ball to the facebow tube is 20 mm. Thus, a 32 mm module should be selected.

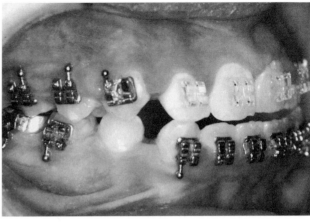

Figure 19-8. Intraoral photograph of a patient who wore a Jasper Jumper™ but did not have the mandibular archwire cinched back. Note the interdental spacing mesial to the mandibular first premolars and the flaring of the mandibular incisors. Currently, the brackets on both the mandibular first and second premolars typically are removed when the Jumper is installed.

molar tube to the distal of the lower Lexan™ bead is determined by way of a flexible millimeter ruler (Fig. 19-7). Adding 12 mm to this measurement will give the appropriate length for the module. The archwire is threaded through the hole in the anterior endcap of the force modules. The mandibular archwire is ligated in place, and the ends of the archwire are cinched or tied back firmly to prevent proclination of the mandibular anterior teeth during treatment (Fig. 19-8). Thus, the force generated by the module theoretically is distributed throughout the mandibular dentition. Then the ball pin is placed through the distal hole in the force module and inserted anteriorly into the facebow tube on the maxillary first molar band and cinched forward, as described previously (Fig. 19-3).

In high mandibular plane angle patients, the pin is cinched to achieve approximately 2 mm of module deflection (150 gms per side). In normal or low mandibular plane angle patients, the ball pin is cinched forward to achieve 4 mm of module deflection (300 gms of force per side). The patient should be coached to practice opening and closing movements slowly at first and told to avoid excessively wide opening during eating and yawning. The patient is cautioned to note any sticking of the module and is taught how to move the modules forward with his or her fingers to "unlock" them. The clinician must warn the patient against biting on the jumpers or "popping" them as this will result in breakage. Stucki and Ingervall[33] report that the incidence of breakage in their clinical study was 9%.

Activation of the Module

The protocol advocated here is based primarily on clinical experience. As described above, the Jumper modules initially are selected and placed so that the module assumes a mildly curved contour when the patient is holding his or her jaw in a comfortably retruded position. If molar distalization is desired, as can be accomplished in an adult patient, a transpalatal arch will not be placed, and the maxillary archwire will not be tied or cinched back. The Jumpers are placed in this instance so that the modules produce only two to four ounces of force (a measuring gauge can be used to determine the precise amount of activation). In a growing individual in whom an orthopedic repositioning of the mandible is desired, higher force levels (*e.g.,* 6–8 oz.) are used continuously.

Reactivation of the Module

If the Class II molar relationship is not corrected completely by the initial activation of the appliance, the modules should be reactivated 2–3 months after initial placement. Shortening the attachment to the maxillary first molar bands activates the modular system most easily. The pin extending through the facebow tube is pulled anteriorly 1–2 mm on each side to reactivate the module (higher mandibular plane angle cases are activated 1 mm per side). One should avoid shortening the ball pin excessively, so that the Jumper

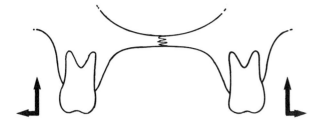

Figure 19-9. Expansive forces are a positive side effect produced by the intrusive forces of the Jumper mechanism.

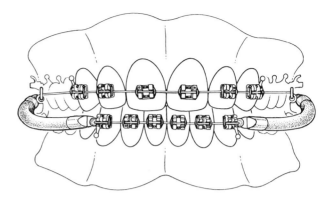

Figure 19-10. The force module curves to the buccal, producing a shielding effect on the dentition. The offset bends in the main archwire are not observable in this view.

will not bind against the distal aspect of the facebow tube and prevent its rotation. Two to four millimeters of the pin should extend distally when the pin is activated maximally.

Activation of the force module also can be made through adjustments in the mandibular arch. Crimpable stops (*e.g.,* 1 mm, 2 mm) placed mesial to the Lexan™ ball can be used to produce a precise, controlled activation of the modules. Activation of the appliance in this manner is more accurate and easier to perform. It also avoids unintentional restriction of the ball pin/molar tube relationship as well as the necessity to replace the module with a larger size.

At each appointment, the clinician should check to be certain that none of the anchoring bands or tiebacks have become loosened. Additionally, the distal extensions of the ball pin often must be re-straightened so that it is parallel with the occlusal plane. If outriggers are used, the anterior portion must be adjusted so as not to contact the distal of the mandibular canine bracket. Observance of increasing interdental spacing in the anterior segment (Fig. 19-8) indicates a breakdown of appliance integrity.

TYPES OF FORCES PRODUCED

Directions of force generated by the modules bilaterally include sagittal as well as intrusive and expansive forces. The sagittal forces will distalize the posterior anchor unit (*e.g.,* maxillary first molars or maxillary first and second molars) and will apply an anterior force to the mandible and mandibular dentition. In addition, an intrusive force is produced in the maxillary posterior region as well as the mandibular anterior region.

The modules also produce forces that are directed buccally (Fig. 19-9). An intrusive force applied along the buccal surface of a tooth will produce maxillary arch expansion, a treatment response typically observed using the Jumper mechanism in combination with fixed appliances. In addition, the modules curve toward the buccal, producing a modest vestibular shielding effect (Fig. 19-10).

Expansive forces can be minimized or eliminated using a transpalatal arch (Fig. 19-6A) and/or a heavy archwire that has been narrowed and to which buccal root torque has been applied. Indeed, clinicians are encouraged to add buccal root torque if arch expansion, not molar tipping, is desired. The expansive forces produced by the module can be contrasted to the lingual crown torque that is produced by extrusive pulling mechanics (*e.g.,* Class II elastics).

MECHANISM OF ACTION

After the dental arches have been prepared properly, the modules can be used to produce numerous treatment effects.

Maxillary Adaptations

"Headgear Effect"

One of the treatment effects produced most easily by the force modules is the distalization of the maxillary posterior segment (*i.e.,* the "headgear effect"). This type of movement is achieved by not cinching or tying back the maxillary archwire but rather by allowing the archwire to remain straight and slightly extended past the buccal tubes. Light forces (*e.g.,* 2–4 oz.) then can be expressed by the modules to distalize the maxillary molars. Because the forces are resisted by the entire mandibular dentition, modest changes in the mandibular dentition are noted. The headgear effect can be produced not only in actively growing patients, but also in some adult patients in whom maxillary molar distalization is desired. There is no clinical evidence to support the hypothesis that the Jasper Jumper™ or any similar type of jaw ad-

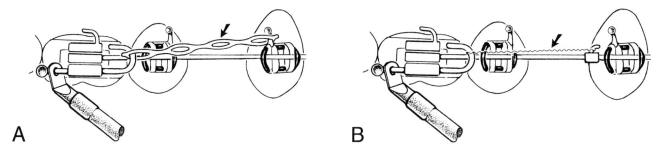

Figure 19-11. The retraction of the maxillary canine using the ball pin and the force module. A NiTi spring or an elastomeric chain can be attached from the ball pin anteriorly to either *A,* the canine bracket or *B,* the maxillary archwire. In this manner, forces generated against the mandibular dentition rather than the maxillary dentition anchor anterior retraction posteriorly.

vancing appliance can be used to promote mandibular growth in adult patients.

Once the desired distal movement has been achieved, the module can be left in place to support the retraction of the premolars and canines. Segmental or continuous arch mechanics can be used to retract these teeth while maintaining molar anchorage. Alternatively, the force module can be left in place to support the molars while the premolar and canine teeth spontaneously move posteriorly due to the pull of the gingival transseptal fibers between the teeth (the so-called "driftodontic effect"). A transpalatal arch or Nance holding arch also may be used to maintain the correction.

Retraction of Anterior Teeth

Canines can be retracted in both extraction and non-extraction patients with the posterior maxillary dentition supported by the force module (Fig. 19-11*A*). In addition, a NiTi coil or intramaxillary elastic attached to the pin through the facebow tube can be used to retract maxillary canines or the six anterior teeth *en masse.* The pull on the pin is resisted by the modules and the mandibular dentition (Fig. 19-11*B*).

Dental Asymmetries

The force module system also can be used in patients who have sagittal dental asymmetries. In a Class II subdivision type patient, the maxillary archwire can be tied back on the side of the existing Class I molar relationship. Asymmetrical orthopedic effects may be developed as well.

Mandibular Adaptations

As stated previously, every effort should be made to incorporate maximum anchorage techniques when preparing the mandibular arch for this appliance system (Fig. 19-1). In growing individuals, changes in mandibular position and, at least theoretically, changes in mandibular length are achieved after force module application. As mentioned earlier, however, the clinical studies of treatment effects to date are equivocal regarding the effect of the Jumper modules on the growth of the mandible.[10–12,15]

When attempting to produce mandibular advancement, the major variation in clinical management is the preparation of the maxillary anchor unit. To maximize mandibular change, the movement of the maxillary posterior dentition must be minimized. The archwire should be cinched or tied back, as is accomplished routinely in the mandibular dentition. In addition, a transpalatal arch (Fig. 19-6*A*) should be used to obtain intraarch anchorage and minimize posterior tooth movement. A fixed lower lingual arch also is recommended (Fig. 19-6*B*).

As discussed above, when mandibular advancement is desired, generally the level of force generated by the module is greater (*i.e.,* 6–8 oz.) than that when maxillary molar distalization is intended (2–4 oz.). By maximizing the force values produced by the module, patients tend to posture their jaw in a forward position. In contrast to the Herbst bite jumping mechanism, however, the spring mechanism allows more freedom in both sagittal and lateral movements.

ADDITIONAL APPLICATIONS

This chapter thus far has considered the use of the Jumper mechanism primarily in the treatment of Class II malocclusion, the typical application of this type of appliance. This system of modules also has been used to support anchorage for the retraction of maxillary anterior teeth (described previously) in Class I patients.

Jumper modules also can be used in the Class III individual.[16] In contrast to the rigid bite jumping mechanism of the Herbst appliance, the flexibility of the Jumper mechanism allows its use in Class III individuals. It is recommended that this appliance be used in patients who are characterized by maxillary skeletal retrusion rather than mandibular prognathism.

When using this system in a Class III patient, the mandibular anchor points are mesial to the permanent first molars. Bands that have auxiliary headgear tubes or lip bumper tubes are used to anchor the ball pin of the distal endcap of the force module. Anteriorly, the Lexan™ ball is placed distal to a bayonet bend just behind the bracket on the maxillary canine (or in an appropriate place on the maxillary archwire if the canines are not yet erupted). This appliance in Class III individuals can be used in conjunction with rapid maxillary expansion. Forces generated when the modules are used in this manner typically are light (*e.g.,* 2–4 gms.). This type of treatment should be discontinued immediately if any signs or symptoms of temporomandibular disorders develop.

Other potential applications may include the correction of anterior crossbites in functional (pseudo) Class III patients, the post-surgical stabilization of Class II or Class III patients, and pre-surgical muscle conditioning of Class II patients.

CONCLUDING REMARKS

This chapter has described the use of a flexible force module (the Jasper Jumper™) that can be incorporated into existing fixed appliances to correct various types of sagittal malocclusion. The flexible spring module provides greater freedom of mandibular movement than is possible with a more rigid bite jumping mechanism, such as that of the Herbst appliance. The facial musculature applies force via these modules to the anchor points to produce a variety of treatment effects.

One of the major criticisms of this appliance system has been breakage. The manufacturer has improved the modules over the last fifteen years; the current iteration is more resistant to fracture during appliance wear. Patients should be instructed not to chew on the appliance and not to perform wide-open movements. Strict dietary controls are mandatory. The patient should be cautioned repeatedly not to "pop" the modules after yawning or excessive wide opening.

As mentioned earlier, it is critical that the clinician must prepare anchorage before the force module is placed against the mandibular arch. If the archwire is full-sized (or nearly so) and is properly anchored posteriorly, forward movement of the mandibular dentition can be minimized. The placement of lingual crown torque anteriorly and tip-back bends posteriorly will further enhance anchorage. If the clinician is concerned about the mesial movement of the mandibular dentition, use of lighter forces with the module is advocated.

As is usual with the incorporation of a new technique or appliance into an established regimen, clinical experience is necessary before the practitioner becomes comfortable with the manipulation and handling of the new adjunct. Thus, initial case selection is important for first-time users of the appliance. For example, a seemingly cooperative patient presenting with mild Class II diagnostic features and minimal anchorage requirements is ideal. The treatment of non-cooperative patients, "bail-out" patients, or patients who have severe skeletal Class II problems initially should be avoided or should be left to practitioners who have had considerable experience in manipulation of the modules.

REFERENCES CITED

1. Jasper JJ, McNamara JA, Jr. The correction of interarch malocclusions using a fixed force module. Am J Orthod Dentofac Orthop 1995;108:641–50.
2. Herbst E. Atlas und Grundriss der Zahnärztlichen Orthopädie. Munich: JF Lehmann Verlag, 1910.
3. Jasper JJ. The Jasper Jumper—A fixed functional appliance. Sheybogan: American Orthodontics, 1987.
4. Blackwood HO. Clinical management of the Jasper Jumper. J Clin Orthod 1991;25:755–760.
5. Cash RG. Adult nonextraction treatment with a Jasper Jumper. J Clin Orthod 1991;25:43–47.
6. Weiland FJ, Bantleon HP. Treatment of Class II malocclusions with the Jasper Jumper appliance—a preliminary report. Am J Orthod Dentofac Orthop 1995;108: 341–350.
7. Weiland FJ, Droschl H. Treatment of a Class II, Division 1 malocclusion with the Jasper Jumper: a case report. Am J Orthod Dentofacial Orthop 1996;109:1–7.
8. Mills C, McCulloch KJ. Case report: Modified use of the Jasper Jumper appliance in as skeletal Class II mixed dentition case requiring palatal expansion. Angle Orthod 1997;67:277–282.
9. Schwindling FP. Improving dentofacial esthetics while paying attention to the anterior facial height index. J Orofac Orthop 1996;57:372–381.
10. Cope JB, Buschang PH, Cope DD, Parker J, Blackwood HO. Quantitative evaluation of craniofacial changes with Jasper Jumper therapy. Angle Orthod 1994;64: 113–122.
11. Covell DD, Jr., Trammell DW, Boero RP, West R. A cephalometric study of Class II Division 1 malocclusions treated with the Jasper Jumper appliance. Angle Orthod 1999;69:311–320.
12. Stucki N, Ingervall B. The use of the Jasper Jumper for the correction of Class II malocclusion in the young permanent dentition. Eur J Orthod 1998;20:271–281.
13. Weiland FJ, Ingervall B, Bantleon HP, Droschl H. Initial

effects of treatment of Class II malocclusion with the Herren activator, activator-headgear combination, and Jasper Jumper. Am J Orthod Dentofac Orthop 1997;112:19-27.
14. Fraser ED. A pilot study on the evaluation of short-term effects of Jasper Jumper therap. Loma Linda: Unpublished Master's thesis, Loma Linda University, 1992.
15. May TW, Chada J, Ledoux WR, Wineberg R, Block MS, McMinn RW. Skeletal and dental changes using a Jasper Jumper appliance. J Dent Res, IADR Suppl 1992;71.
16. Pham T, Goz G, Bacher M, Alfter G. New clinical applications for the Jasper Jumper. J Orofac Orthop 1996;57:366-371.

Chapter 20

THE PENDULUM AND OTHER MOLAR DISTALIZING APPLIANCES

With James J. Hilgers

The use of so-called "distalization" mechanics to correct Class II malocclusions is a common treatment modality. This type of mechanotherapy typically is used in patients with maxillary skeletal and/or dentoalveolar protrusion. Molar distalization also can be initiated when extraction of maxillary teeth is not indicated and the mandibular tooth-size/arch-perimeter relationship does not permit mesial movement of the lower molars.

In a survey by Sinclair,[1] all responding orthodontists reported utilizing molar distalization; however, nearly all indicated that patient cooperation was the most significant problem encountered in distalizing maxillary molars.

Most traditional approaches to molar distalization, including extraoral traction, Wilson distalizing arches, removable spring appliances, and intermaxillary elastics with sliding jigs, require considerable patient compliance to be successful. More recently, the subjectivity and problems of predicting patient behavior have led many clinicians to devise appliances that minimized reliance on the patient and which are under the control of the clinician.[2-4] Relying on the patient's willingness to wear an appliance consistently may result in increased treatment time, a change of treatment plans, or both.

An assortment of molar distalizing appliances requiring varying degrees of patient compliance are reviewed in this chapter, most of which require minimal patient cooperation. Extraoral traction appliances are considered separately in the next chapter.

PENDULUM AND PENDEX APPLIANCES

A popular method of molar distalization that requires no patient cooperation is the so-called "Pendulum" appliance system. In 1992, Hilgers described the development of two hybrid appliances, the Pendulum and Pendex. Modifications in appliance design and clinical management also have been described by Hilgers and Bennett[5-7] and Snodgrass.[8]

Types of Appliances

Pendulum

The Pendulum appliance (Fig. 20-1) consists of a large acrylic Nance button that covers the midportion of the palate. The acrylic pad is connected to the dentition by means of occlusal rests that extend from the lateral aspect of the pad and are bonded to the occlusal surfaces of the upper first and second premolars. Posteriorly directed springs, made of .032″ TMA™ wire, extend from the distal aspect of the palatal acrylic to form a helical loop near the midline and then extend laterally to insert into lingual sheaths on bands cemented on the maxillary first molars.

When in a passive state, the springs extend posteriorly, approaching the midpalatal raphe. When activated and inserted into the lingual sheaths, they produce a distalizing force against the maxillary first molars that

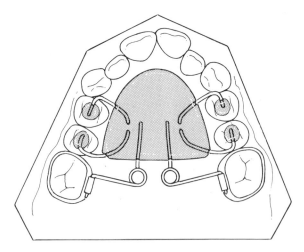

Figure 20-1. The Pendulum appliance of Hilgers that has been bonded in place after cementing the molar bands. The distalizing springs are activated after the occlusal rests have been bonded to the premolars by placing the ends of the springs into the lingual sheaths on the maxillary first molars.

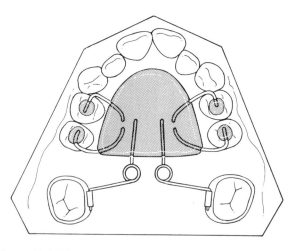

Figure 20-2. The Pendulum appliance after distalization of the maxillary first molars. The "Pendulum effect" is observed in that the maxillary first molars move distally and medially along the arc produced by the TMA™ springs. If the maxillary arch is too narrow, the Pendex version is indicated.

move the molars distally and medially (Fig. 20-2). Hilgers[9] estimates that these springs deliver approximately two hundred and thirty grams per side to the maxillary molars. The springs also may have adjustment loops that can be manipulated to increase molar expansion, molar rotation, or distal root tip.[10]

Pendex

The design of the Pendex appliance (Fig. 20-3) is essentially the same as the Pendulum, except for the addition of a palatal expansion screw in the midline (hence the name "Pendex"). In most instances, we use the Pendex design because of the tendency toward transverse maxillary constriction in patients with Class II malocclusion.[11,12]

The so-called "T-Rex" configuration of the Pendex is our design of choice (Fig. 20-3). This design features two wires that extend from the palatal acrylic and are soldered to the lingual aspect of the maxillary first molars. These wires provide addition stability to the Pendex appliance during the expansion phase of treatment; they are severed or removed when the molar distalization phase is initiated.

Another appliance in the Pendulum "family" is termed the Phd appliance. This version features an all-metal design with no acrylic palate, the primary advantage being comfort and improved hygiene for the patient. Anchorage consists of banded first premolars with stabilizing wires from the premolars to the molar bands. This appliance allows for phasing the treatment if desired, with palatal expansion first, followed by sectioning of the holding wires and distalizing of the molars.

The pendulum springs in the Phd appliance insert into sheaths welded or soldered to the palatal side of the expansion screw housing. This configuration allows the clinician to remove the springs, either before the palatal expansion is started or for adjustment/re-activation of the springs during the molar distalizing phase.

Clinical Management of the Pendex

In this section, the specifics of the management of the Pendex appliance are described, because the Pendex is the standard design used by us routinely and because the Pendulum is a simplified version of the Pendex. We

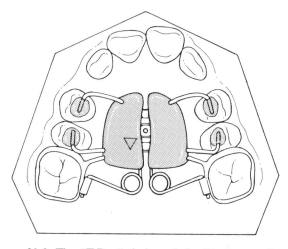

Figure 20-3. The "T-Rex" design of the Pendex appliance. Locking wires connect the bands on the maxillary first molars to the acrylic button. These connecting wires are removed after the desired expansion has been achieved.

choose the Pendex design because of the potential for expansion, even in those patients who may have undergone RME during Phase I treatment. As mentioned above, the action of the distalizing spring not only moves the maxillary molars posteriorly, but also moves them toward the midline. The need for maxillary expansion often is not obvious at the beginning of treatment, but may become apparent as treatment progresses.

The first step in the management of the Pendex is banding the maxillary first molars. It is assumed that adequate separation has been achieved. Tight-fitting bands are placed on the molars, and an alginate impression is obtained in the usual manner. The bands are removed, placed in the impression, and secured in place with sticky wax. The model is poured in stone and trimmed, and the positions of the bands on the maxillary first molars are checked for accuracy. The work model then is sent to the laboratory with an accompanying prescription sheet indicating the fabrication of the "T-Rex version" of the Pendex appliance.

An alternative approach is to have the bands fit indirectly in the laboratory. This procedure can save a clinical appointment as the initial working model is obtained without first having to create space to fit the bands. In instances in which the Pendulum is the first appliance used at the outset of treatment, the construction model can be made from the "first pour" of the alginate taken for the study models. Separators, however, need to be placed prior to delivering the appliance.

After the Pendex has been returned from the laboratory, the patient is prepared for appliance delivery. The separators are removed, and compomer band cement (*e.g.*, BandLok™, Reliance Orthodontic Products, Itasca IL) is used when the bands are placed on the

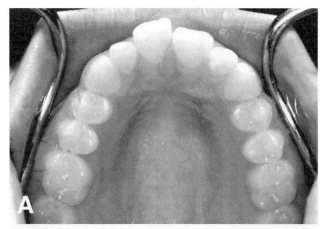

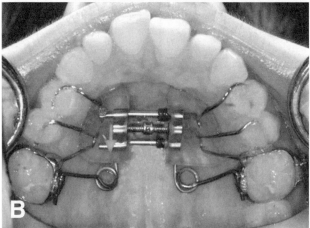

Figure 20-5. Intraoral view of the Pendex appliance. *A*, Initial photograph before expansion. *B*, After the desired expansion is achieved (37 days of active expansion). A modest midline diastema opened during the expansion process, but the diastema had closed before this photograph was taken.

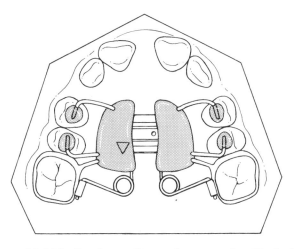

Figure 20-4. The Pendex appliance after expansion. The locking wires still connect the molar bands to the acrylic Nance button.

maxillary first molars (Fig. 20-3.). The occlusal rests of the Pendex now should lay passively in the central grooves of the maxillary first and second premolars. These rests are bonded to the premolars with a bracket adhesive such as Phase II™ (Reliance Orthodontic Products). Light-cured adhesive also can be used (*e.g.*, Light-Bond™, Reliance; Enlight™, Ormco).

If the midline expansion screw is to be activated (Fig. 20-4), a one-turn-per-day protocol is followed, as is described for RME appliances in Chapter 13. Usually the Pendex is expanded initially for 28 days. At the next appointment, additional turns of the expansion screw are prescribed, as needed, so that the desired expansion is attained (Fig. 20-5). If desired, the expander can be sealed or tied off at this point.

The next step in the Pendex protocol is to activate the distalizing function of the appliance. Because of anchorage considerations, we have chosen to activate the distalizing springs one side at a time (Fig. 20-6), so the

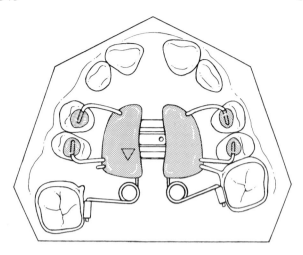

Figure 20-6. Unilateral activation of the Pendex by cutting and removing the locking wire on the side that is more Class II. Alternatively, both locking wires can be removed at the same appointment to initiate bilateral distalization.

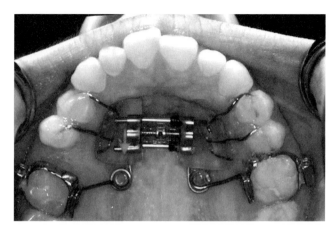

Figure 20-7. Subsequent activation of the Pendex. The locking wire on the right side, the side that originally was more Class II, was cut and removed eight weeks earlier, resulting in molar distalization. The locking wire on the left side was cut and removed just prior to taking this photograph.

locking wire on the side that is more Class II is removed first by means of a crosscut fissure bur in a highspeed handpiece. The locking wire either should be removed entirely or the remaining wire should be curved out of the way to allow for adequate tissue clearance. In that the locking wire is made from .028" stainless steel, the wire also can be severed with a heavy pin cutter or heavy distal end cutter.

The locking wire securing the other molar band is cut at the next appointment (Fig. 20-7). The rationale for this sequence is based on the concept that the initial movement of one molar is supported by all the other teeth including the opposite molar, thus maximizing anchorage. Hilgers[9] states that it is common to see approximately 5 mm of distal molar movement in a three to four-month period.

After the desired molar distalization has been realized (Fig. 20-8), the next step is to remove the occlusal rests on the maxillary second premolars (Fig. 20-9), much in the same manner the locking wires were removed. The maxillary second premolars will drift posteriorly, due to the pull of the transseptal fibers (Fig. 20-10). This spontaneous movement improves the Class II correction with minimal anchorage loss.

Maxillary anchorage can be increased appreciably by bracketing the maxillary arch at the time of Pendex

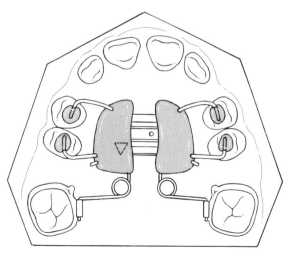

Figure 20-8. Full activation of the Pendex appliance. The maxillary first molars now are in an overcorrected ("super Class I") relationship with the mandibular first molars. The molars have been rotated distolingually as well.

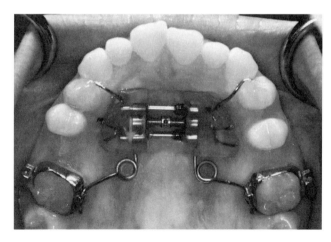

Figure 20-9. Removal of the occlusal rests to the maxillary second premolars. The rest to the left second premolar was removed at the previous appointment; the right rest was removed just before this photograph was obtained.

MOLAR DISTALIZATION

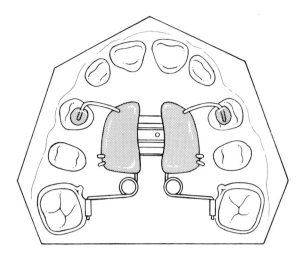

Figure 20-10. The spontaneous movement of the maxillary second premolars distally due to the pull of the transseptal fibers. The occlusal rests of these teeth have been removed.

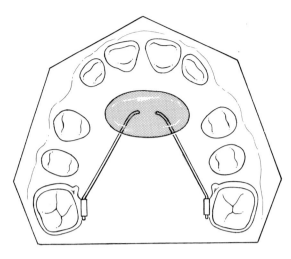

Figure 20-11. Placement of a Nance holding arch following molar distalization. The arch shown here is removable; the distal ends of the Nance arch extend into the lingual sheaths.

placement. Hilgers has found less tissue impingement of the large Nance button when the maxillary arch is bracketed early. Sectional leveling wires (.014″ NiTi) are extended from the second premolar (or second deciduous molar) to the midline, thereby allowing midpalatal separation without tying the two parts of the maxilla together with a continuous archwire. Early bracket placement also allows for alignment of the maxillary arch during the molar distalization process.

Two or three appointments later, the Pendex appliance is removed, and a so-called "Quick Nance"[13] is inserted (Figs. 20-11 and 20-12). A preformed Nance crib, made from .032″ stainless steel and available in various sizes, (Ormco Corp., Orange CA), the ends of which have been doubled over to fit into the .036″ lingual sheaths on the maxillary first molar bands, is used to make the Quick-Nance. Hilgers and Bennett[13] recommend taking a maxillary impression during the appointment before the Pendulum appliance is to be removed to allow for preselection of the proper sized Nance button.

The Nance holding arch is useful in maintaining molar distalization and saving maxillary leeway space in mixed dentition treatment. In addition, it serves to help maintain the expansion of the molars. Hilgers, on the other hand, usually does not use the Nance holding arch in patients in the permanent dentition due to difficulty in fabrication, cleanliness, and patient comfort (see utility arch stabilization below).

After the Pendulum has been removed and the crib adjusted for proper fit, the acrylic pad can be fabricated directly in the mouth (Fig. 20-12). Light-cured acrylic (e.g., Triad™, Dentsply Corp., York PA) can be applied in the anterior part of the palate in the form of a Nance button. Alternatively, if an in-office laboratory is available, an impression is taken, the molar bands are removed and placed in the impression, a work model is poured and trimmed, and a conventional Nance appliance (see Fig. 5-18 in Chapter 5) is fabricated. If the palatal tissue is inflamed, an invisible retainer[14,15] can be given to the patient temporarily until the inflammation has subsided.

Hilgers suggests the immediate placement of a .016 × .016″ stainless steel maxillary utility archwire (or alternatively a .016 × .022″ blue Elgiloy™ archwire) with the posterior vertical legs abutting the maxillary molar tubes. This process is especially useful when continuation of treatment is anticipated and torque or advance-

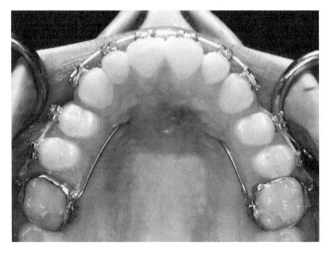

Figure 20-12. Intraoral view of a "Quick Nance" appliance that was fabricated from two sections of .036″ wire, to which was applied a button of light-cured acrylic.

ment of the maxillary incisors is indicated (*e.g.*, Class II, division 2 malocclusion). The maxillary utility arch serves to initiate maxillary molar uprighting and rotation. Its anterior vertical step also can be used as an anchor point for Class II elastics, freeing the maxillary buccal segments to drift distally or to be free floated with light elastomeric chain.[16]

It is critical that once the Pendex appliance is removed, a method of molar stabilization should be placed the same day (maximum 24 hours after Pendex removal) to prevent unwanted mesial movement of the previously distalized molars. Hilgers and Bennett[5,7,9] recommend maintaining the overcorrection with various techniques, including Nance buttons, short-term headgear wear, utility arches, or stopped continuous archwires. Regardless of the appliance selected, molar anchorage should be maintained until the premolars and canines have been retracted.

Final distalization of the premolars and canines is accomplished by placing brackets on these teeth and using elastomeric chain (Fig. 20-12) sequentially to move these teeth distally one at a time per side (*i.e.*, moving "beads on a string"). Anterior space closure can be achieved by way of a retraction utility arch or an anterior closing loop arch. Typically, space closure also is supported by Class II elastics.

Treatment Effects of the Pendulum Appliance

There have been only a few clinical studies of the treatment effects produced by the Pendulum/Pendex appliance. Ghosh and Nanda[17] evaluated forty-one patients treated with the Pendulum appliance and found fifty-seven percent of the average Class II correction was molar distalization and forty-three percent maxillary first premolar and anterior anchorage loss. The patients in this sample also demonstrated a 2.8 mm average increase in lower anterior facial height. The investigators also noted that the presence of the maxillary second molars had minimal effect on distalization of the first molars.

Joseph and Butchart[18] evaluated the treatment results of the Pendulum appliance in seven patients. They noted an average of 5.1 mm of molar distalization and 3.7 mm anterior movement of the maxillary incisors. They also reported an average distal tipping of the maxillary first molar of 15.7° and an average flaring of the maxillary incisor of 4.9°.

Byloff and Darendeliler[19] studied 13 patients in whom a Pendex version of the appliance was used. In a companion study, the same team[10] examined another group of 20 patients, 12 of whom wore a Pendulum appliance and eight of whom underwent slow expansion (one turn per week) with the Pendex version of the appliance. Each appliance had been modified following molar distalization (after about 16 weeks) by incorporating an uprighting bend into the molar distalizing spring during the second phase of treatment (an additional 11 weeks of treatment) to eliminate excessive distal tipping of the maxillary molars. In comparison to the results of their initial study,[19] the uprighting bends reduced molar tipping with minimal anteroposterior effects, except for a slight increase in the flaring of the maxillary incisal edge. Treatment time was increased as well. There was no significant difference in anchorage loss between the patients with and without expansion.

Bussick and McNamara[20] examined the dentoalveolar and skeletal effects of the Pendulum appliance in 101 Class II patients at varying stages of dental development and with varying facial patterns (high, neutral and low mandibular plane angles). Specifically, the amount and nature of the distalization of the maxillary first molars and the reciprocal effects on the anchoring maxillary first premolars and incisors were studied, as were skeletal changes in the sagittal and vertical dimensions of the face.

Pre-treatment (T_1) and post-treatment (T_2) cephalometric radiographs obtained from thirteen practitioners were used to document the treatment of one-hundred-and-one patients (forty-five boys and fifty-six girls). The average maxillary first molar distalization was 5.7 millimeters, with a distal tipping of 10.6°. The anchoring anterior teeth moved mesially, as indicated by the 1.8-mm anterior movement of the maxillary first premolars; with a mesial tipping of 1.5°. The maxillary first molars intruded 0.7 mm, and the first premolars extruded 1.0 mm. Lower anterior facial height increased 2.2 mm, with no significant difference in lower anterior facial height increase between patients of high, neutral, or low mandibular plane angles. In patients with erupted maxillary second molars, there was a slightly greater increase in lower anterior face height and in the mandibular plane angle and a slightly greater decrease in overbite in comparison to patients with unerupted second molars. Similar findings were observed in patients with second premolar anchorage versus those with second deciduous molar anchorage.

The results of the Bussick and McNamara study[20] suggest that the Pendulum appliance is effective in moving maxillary molars posteriorly during orthodontic treatment. For maximum maxillary first molar distalization with minimal increase in lower anterior facial height, this appliance is used most effectively in patients

MOLAR DISTALIZATION

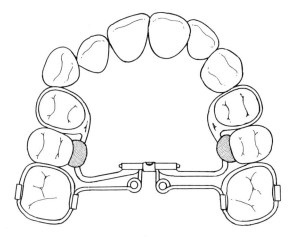

Figure 20-13. The Mini-Distalizing Appliance (MDA) of Hilgers. The lingual arms of the spindle-type expansion screw are soldered to bands on the maxillary first premolars and bonded to the lingual aspect of the maxillary second premolars. Distalizing springs made from .027″ TMA™ wire extend from the expansion screw and insert into lingual sheaths on the maxillary first molar bands. This distalizing appliance is easier for the patient to keep clean than is the Pendulum or Pendex, because there is no palatal acrylic.

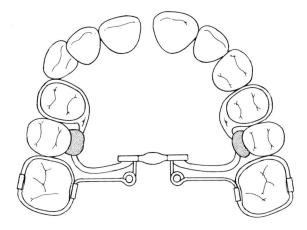

Figure 20-14. The MDA appliance after palatal expansion has been completed. The midline expansion has been stabilized by way of light cure acrylic covering the screw and housing.

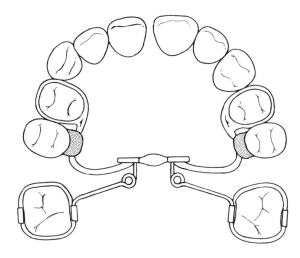

Figure 20-15. The MDA appliance after completion of molar distalization. At this stage, the bonds from the lingual wire to the second premolars can be removed to allow spontaneous distal movement of these teeth due to the pull of the transseptal fibers.

with deciduous maxillary second molars for anchorage and unerupted permanent maxillary second molars. Clinically significant bite opening, however, was not a concern in any patient in this study.

MINI-DISTALIZATION APPLIANCE

Hilgers also recommends the use of a smaller, tooth borne distalizing/expansion appliance that he refers to as the Mini-distalizing appliance (MDA; Fig. 20-13). This appliance is comprised of a small, spindle-type expander (Ormco Corp.) that is soldered to bands on the maxillary first premolars. Distalizing springs that are made from .032″ TMA wire are secured to the palatal side of the spindle with a flattened recurved loop fitted into a braised .036″ lingual sheath.

Once the appliance is cemented, the lingual arms are bonded to the second premolars or second deciduous molars to enhance anchorage and to aid in maxillary expansion (Fig. 20-13). Instead of using an acrylic Nance button for anchorage, the maxillary arch is bracketed at the time of appliance placement, and sectional leveling wires are placed from the second premolar to the midline, allowing for maxillary expansion.

Hilgers favors this appliance for its cleanliness and rigidity for expansion, as well as for the fact that it is not occlusally borne (like the Pendulum appliances), which helps avoid some of the bite opening that can occur with occlusally bonded rests. The expansion screw is activated slowly (one turn per day), and usually a maxillary utility arch is placed at appliance removal to stabilize molar position.

After the desired amount of palatal expansion has been achieved, the midline expansion screw is sealed with light cure acrylic (Fig, 20-14). Molar distalization then occurs at about the same rate as described previously for the Pendulum appliance (Fig. 20-15). The bond on the lingual aspect of the second premolars can be removed after maxillary expansion is completed to allow these teeth to drift distally along with the maxillary first molars.

Hilgers cautions that the MDA should be used in patients with stronger masticatory muscular patterns (*e.g.*, brachyfacial Class II, division 2) and in patients in whom some forward movement of the anterior dentition is acceptable or even desirable. He stresses that appropriate appliance selection when using the Pendulum family of appliances is necessary to gain maximum molar distalization and maxillary expansion without unwanted negative sequelae.

DISTAL JET APPLIANCE

A distant relative of the Pendulum appliance is the Distal Jet, developed by Carano and Testa of Italy[21, 22] as another method of distalizing molars without active patient compliance.

This lingual appliance has many features in common with the Pendulum appliance, but it has three distinct advantages. First, the maxillary molars are distalized without the lingual movement that occurs with the Pendulum appliance. Second, the Distal Jet can be converted to a Nance holding arch easily after molar distalization is completed. Third, less molar tipping and more bodily movement has been reported compared to the Pendulum appliance and the Jones Jig.[23,24]

Appliance Design

The basic design is similar to the Pendulum appliance in that an acrylic Nance button anchors the appliance against the palatal mucosa. The appliance is anchored to the maxillary dentition by placing bands on the maxillary second premolars (Fig. 20-16). Alternatively, the appliance can be anchored on the maxillary first premolars (Fig. 20-17), the maxillary second deciduous molars, or the maxillary first and second premolars (like the Pendulum).[25,26] Not surprisingly, more anchorage loss was reported when anchorage was from the first premolars, rather than the second premolars.[24]

The premolar bands are connected to the palatal acrylic by way of a .036″ wire that is soldered to the lingual aspect of the bands, courses anteriorly along the lingual surface of the premolars and canines, and then becomes imbedded in the Nance button.

Bilateral tubes, with an internal diameter of .036″, are imbedded in the palatal acrylic. A stainless steel wire "piston" lies within the lumen of the tube and extends posteriorly, making a lateral bayonet bend, and inserting into the lingual sheath on the maxillary first molar band (Figs. 20-16 and 20-17). A coil spring and an activation collar (locking ring with two set screws[27]) are placed over each tube. In addition, an acrylic ball, that is similar to the Lexan™ ball of the Jasper Jumper™ appliance[28] is placed at the more anterior bayonet bend, facing the lingual tube. A push-coil spring is placed between the acrylic ball and the adjustment collar. Carano and Testa[21,25] recommend using nickel titanium springs that generate 240 gms of force in adults and 180 gms in children, although they state that stainless steel springs may be used as well.

Bowman[27] has modified the original design of the Distal Jet by incorporating helical loops in the bayonet

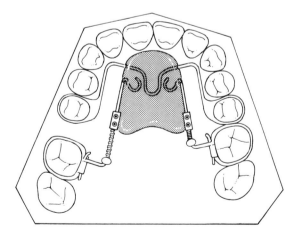

Figure 20-16. The Distal Jet appliance that is anchored to the maxillary second premolars. The locking collars have a pair of setscrews. Only the mesial setscrew is used during the activation or compression of the springs for distalization. Both setscrews are locked when converting the Distal Jet to a Nance holding arch after completion of distalization.

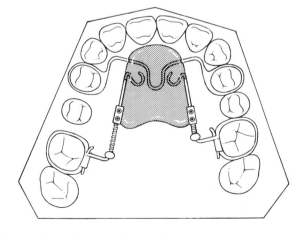

Figure 20-17. The Distal Jet appliance anchored to the maxillary first premolars. This design can be used if the maxillary second premolars are in the process of erupting or if the second deciduous molars are in the process of exfoliation. The coil springs are activated every six weeks by adjusting the position of the activation collar.

MOLAR DISTALIZATION

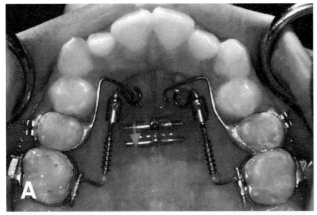

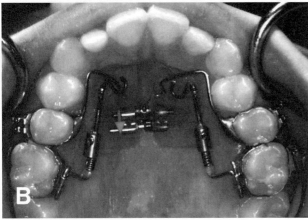

Figure 20-18. Occlusal views of the original design of the Distal Jet with single setscrews in the activation collars. *A.* Before activation of the coil springs. *B.* After compression of the springs and tightening of the activation collar.

bands are removed from the teeth, placed in the impression, and secured in proper position in the impression with sticky wax. The laboratory prescription form is completed; an optional RME screw may be added, if necessary (Fig. 20-18).

The original design of Carano and Testa had a single setscrew in each sliding activation collar (Fig. 20-18). Bowman[27] has modified the appliance by incorporating an additional setscrew in each collar (Fig. 20-19) to simplify the later conversion of the Distal Jet into a molar holding arch at the end of distalization.

At the time of appliance delivery, the Distal Jet may be cemented as one piece. Compomer cement (*e.g.*, BandLok™, Reliance Orthodontic Products, Itasca IL) is placed in the molar and premolar bands, and the appliance is seated in place. At this point, the springs have not been activated (Fig. 20-18*A*).

The activation collar is moved posteriorly with a ligature director, and the mesial setscrew is tightened with a small Allen wrench held in a pair of hemostats (Fig. 20-20). Bowman[27] suggests the use of an autoclavable hex key handle to hold the Allen wrench (AOA/Pro, Sturtevant WI). The coil now is compressed, producing a distalizing force on the molars (Fig. 20-18*B* and 20-19*A*). Thus, only the mesial setscrew is used during the activation process. Both screws are used only during the conversion of the Distal Jet to a Nance molar holding arch.[26]

wires just anterior to the lingual sheaths. The adjustment of these loops can produce distal molar rotation or upright mesially tipped maxillary molars. The helical loops are not a necessity to produce molar rotation. Simply bending the double-back of the bayonet with utility pliers (much like activating a transpalatal arch) is sufficient.

If expansion of the molars is desired, Carano and Testa[22] suggest that the appliance should be constructed parallel to the line of the occlusion (*i.e.*, the line formed by the central grooves of the posterior teeth). If molar expansion is not necessary, the appliance should be constructed with the distalizing mechanism 5° inward to the line of occlusion. The details of appliance construction have been provided by Carano and Testa.[22]

Clinical Management of the Distal Jet

The first step in the Distal Jet protocol is obtaining an impression, after having placed bands on the maxillary first molars and the maxillary second premolars. The

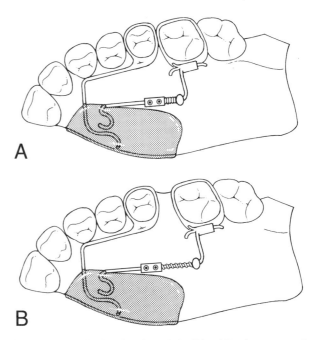

Figure 20-19. Initial activation of the Distal Jet (two screw design). *A*, After compression and tightening the mesial setscrews in the activation collar. *B*, Several appointments later.

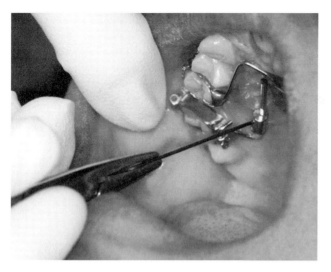

Figure 20-20. Tightening of the mesial setscrew with an Allen wrench held in locking hemostats. An autoclavable hex key handle[27] also can be used to hold the Allen wrench.

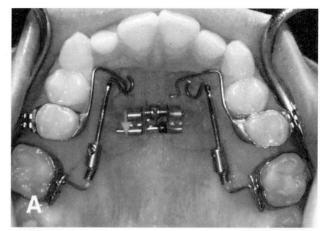

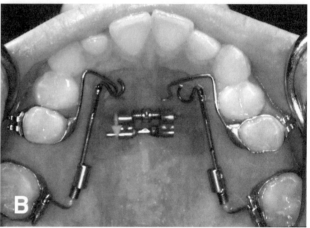

Figure 20-21. Distalization of the maxillary molars with the Distal Jet appliance. *A*, After two months. *B*, After five months.

Carano and Testa[21] and Bowman[26] recommend activating the appliance once every six weeks. Carano[25] states that the Distal Jet is activated bilaterally from the beginning, in contrast to the unilateral sequence recommended earlier in this chapter for the Pendex appliance. As treatment progresses, spaces will open distal to the bands on the maxillary second premolars as the springs lengthen (Figs. 20-19*B* and 20-21).

The appliance is reactivated by compressing the springs again in the same manner (Fig. 20-22) until molar distalization is complete. As with all distalizing mechanics, we recommend that the maxillary molars be overcorrected to a "super-Class I" position to allow for some rebound in molar relationship that may occur during the next phase of treatment; on average, seven months of molar distalization with four activations is required.[23,24]

Once the desired amount of distal movement of the maxillary molars has been achieved, Carano and Testa[21] suggest converting the appliance into a Nance holding arch by covering the activation collar and the spring assembly with cold-cure or light-cure acrylic. The arms to the premolars then are removed.

The double setscrew design is useful when converting the Distal Jet into a Nance holding arch. The activation collar is loosened and moved anteriorly, gaining access to the coil spring. Bowman[27] recommends removing the spring by grasping a free end of the coil with pliers (*e.g.*, small Weingart) and peeling the spring outward from the bayonet wire. The distal end of the tube, into which the bayonet wire enters, can be seen. The collar with the double setscrew can be slid over this junction; the mesial setscrew can be tightened against the tube while the dis-

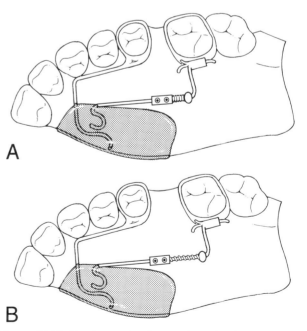

Figure 20-22. Further activation of the Distal Jet. *A*, After compression and tightening the mesial setscrews in the activation collar. *B*, Several appointments later, the desired distal movement of the maxillary first molars has been achieved.

tal setscrew is secured against the bayonet wire. This action locks the tube and the wire together to prevent molar movement. Bowman then suggests removing the wires that connect the premolars to the palatal acrylic by means of a diamond bur in a highspeed handpiece.

If there is any mobility of the double-back wire within the lingual sheath, the Nance acrylic may lift away from the palatal mucosa. Bowman[27] suggests that to avoid this problem, the lingual sheath can be crimped with utility pliers. In addition, the bayonet wire can be bent with three-prong pliers to adjust the pressure of the acrylic against the palatal mucosa. It is critical to position this activation collar accurately.

One of the challenges that arises in any treatment that involves intentional molar distalization is the consolidation of the arches after posterior molar movement has been completed. In some instances, in addition to the Nance button, Bowman[29] has suggested the use of fixed appliances combined with the simultaneous use of a Jasper Jumper™ appliance. This fixed force module is added to maintain the distalization of the maxillary molars, to provide anchorage during anterior retraction with closing-loop or sliding mechanics, and to encourage a more favorable pattern of craniofacial growth. Carano,[25] however, states that the Jumpers should be used only in non-compliant patients, raising concerns about lower arch stability.

Another difference between the approaches of Carano[25] and Bowman is with regard to the use of fixed appliances in conjunction with Distal Jet treatment. Carano[25] states that he never uses maxillary brackets, maintaining that the best dental anchorage are teeth that have not been moved orthodontically.

For patients in the mixed dentition, Carano's[25] sequence includes conversion of the Distal Jet into a retainer after molar distalization is complete. He then uses utility archwires in both arches combined with Class II elastics to "gently retract" the maxillary incisors. A final phase of fixed appliance therapy is needed to detail the occlusion after the transition to the permanent dentition is complete. After stabilization of the Distal Jet and placement of fixed appliances in permanent dentition patients, omega stops are placed mesial to the distalized molars. *En mass* retraction of the canines and premolars is accomplished with Class II elastics, followed by fine detailing of the occlusion.

Treatment Effects of the Distal Jet

In addition to the unpublished Master's theses cited previously,[23,24] the only other study of the treatment effects of the Distal Jet appliance is that of Carano and Testa.[21] The treatment effects were studied through the analysis of intraoral photographs on 25 patients. The investigators stated that they relied on these photographs because of the difficulty in obtaining progress models due to the bulk and complexity of the appliance. Direct clinical measurements were obtained as well. They reported an average space opening mesial to the maxillary first molar of 0.9 mm per month. They found that 80% of the increased space was due to distal movement of the maxillary first molars and 20% due to anchorage loss anteriorly. Carano and Testa[21] also noted other occlusal changes, including distolingual molar rotation and variable amounts of molar expansion.

WILSON DISTALIZING ARCH

Another method of molar distalization that we have found surprisingly useful is the Wilson distalizing arch, one component of a system of removable orthodontic appliances developed by Wilson and Wilson[30-33] that can be used as adjuncts to virtually any fixed appliance system. Although this auxiliary can be used as a primary method of molar distalization, typically we use this adjunct toward the end of fixed appliance treatment when a 2–3 mm Class II occlusal discrepancy remains either unilaterally or bilaterally.

Parts of the Appliance

The Bimetric Distalizing Arch™ (Rocky Mountain Orthodontics, Denver CO) is used to produce distal movement of maxillary molars. This arch is "bimetric" in that the anterior segment is made from .022″ stainless steel, whereas the posterior part of the arch is made from .040″ stainless steel (Fig. 20-23). To the posterior segment are attached elastic hooks in the region of the maxillary canines. An omega-shaped stop is located in the premolar region. A .010 × .045″ open-wound coil

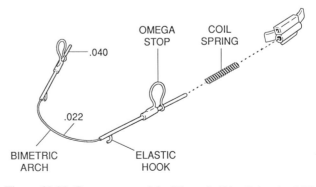

Figure 20-23. Components of the Bimetric Distalizing Arch™ (after Wilson and Wilson[33]).

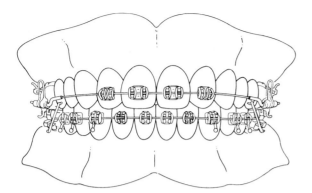

Figure 20-24. Frontal view of the Wilson arch used as a primary distalizing appliance. Brackets are placed on the maxillary anterior teeth, and full appliances are placed on the mandibular arch. Class II elastics are worn from the hooks on the arch in the region of the canines to the hooks on the mandibular first or second molar bands.

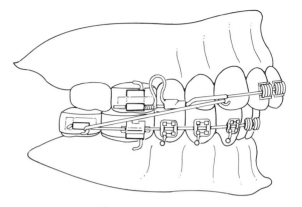

Figure 20-25. Lateral view of the Wilson distalizing arch at the beginning of treatment. The ends of the lower arch are cinched back posteriorly to prevent lower anchorage loss. Elastomeric chain also can be placed around the mandibular arch from molar to molar to increase anchorage.

spring is placed between the distal leg of the omega stop and the facebow tube.

The distalizing force on the molars is produced by the compression of the push coil spring anchored by the pull of Class II elastics (Figs. 20-24 and 20-25). The force of the elastics counteracts the force of the push coil springs so that the anterior segment of the Wilson arch approximates the incisor brackets before ligation to the anterior teeth.

Clinical Management of the Wilson Arch

Regardless of whether the Wilson arch is used as a primary treatment appliance or as a secondary appliance near the end of the active phase of treatment, a prerequisite is making sure that the buccal surfaces of the maxillary first molars are parallel to each other and to the midline of the palate before the Wilson arch is inserted into the buccal tubes. As has been discussed previously in Chapter 12, a transpalatal arch (TPA) can align the molars in three dimensions in a few appointments.

Before inserting the Wilson arch, the TPA is removed and stored for use later. The proper size arch then is selected. Each Wilson Bimetric Distalizing Arch™ kit comes with an "arch selector guide," a flexible ruler that can be used to determine the appropriate size of the arch. This measurement can be made on the pretreatment study models. Alternatively, the distance around the arch from facebow tube to facebow tube can be measured with a brass wire and this distance transferred to the arch selector guide.[33] Seven sizes of the Wilson arch are available.

Before fitting the distalizing arch, we routinely modify each arch to fit the specifics of our fixed appliance prescription. Specifically, we use molar bands with gingivally located auxiliary tubes and occlusal facebow tubes. In order for the anterior segment of the arch to fit over the bracket slots anteriorly at the proper vertical height (we use an .018″ appliance, so the .022″ Wilson anterior wire is tied with stainless steel ligature on top of the bracket slots, not in the slots), a vertical bayonet bend must be placed bilaterally in each arch (Fig. 20-25). Using #142 Tweed arch-forming pliers, a vertical step is made just anterior to the omega loop and posterior to the hook in the canine region. These bayonet bends can be made in each arch in the distalizing arch kit before selecting an arch for a specific patient.

We have found that an easy way to size the arch is simply to fit a size 5 or 6 Wilson arch into the facebow tubes with the omega loops open. The posterior ends of the omega loops should contact the facebow tubes on the maxillary first molars, and the anterior section of the arch should approximate the brackets on the maxillary anterior teeth. When the Wilson arch is activated, the omega loops are compressed with a pair of Weingart pliers, and a precut 5 mm section of .010 x .045″ open wound coil spring is placed over the end of the Wilson arch bilaterally. To facilitate insertion of the springs, a small amount of wax can be placed at the ends of the Wilson arch to prevent the coil springs from falling off during insertion. In addition, the Wilson arch should be sized so that the ends of the arch protrude posteriorly beyond the facebow tubes, in order to compensate for the anticipated distal movement of the upper first molars.

Wilson and Wilson[33] suggest modifying the distalizing arch so that it fits any irregularities present in the alignment of the anterior teeth. We usually align the maxil-

MOLAR DISTALIZATION

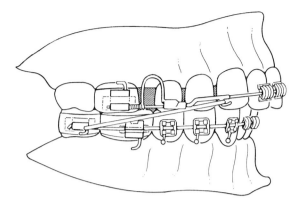

Figure 20-26. Lateral view of Wilson distalizing arch after molar correction has been achieved. Space has opened distal to the maxillary second premolars and also anteriorly.

lary incisors before inserting the distalizing arch, so there is no need for us to modify the contour of the anterior segment.

Wilson and Wilson[33] have advocated the sequential use of elastics with decreasing force values over time. They recommend the use of a 5/16″, 6-oz. elastic during the first week of treatment, a similar-sized 4-oz. elastic during the second week of treatment, and a similar sized 2-oz. elastic the third and subsequent weeks of treatment. Elastic force is reduced gradually because the force of the spring dissipates with tooth movement. When using the Wilson arch near the end of fixed appliance treatment, however, we have found that the continuous used of heavy elastic force (*e.g.*, 6 oz.) throughout treatment with the Wilson arch is satisfactory.

At subsequent activation appointments, the appliance is activated by placing loop-forming pliers (#881, Masel Corporation, Bristol PA) into the omega loop. The loop is crimped, forcing the posterior leg distally. The elastic sequence begins again, whenever the appliance is activated.

After four to six months of activation and with full compliance of the patient in wearing the elastics, a distalization of the maxillary molars usually is observed (Fig. 20-26). This movement is similar to that produced by other distalizing methods, except that the mandibular arch is used as anchorage. The lower arch should have a stiff rectangular archwire or lingual arch in place, and the clinician should monitor the lower arch routinely for anchorage loss.

Figure 20-27 illustrates the fit of the Wilson distalizing arch when it is ligated into position. Note that no brackets are placed on the maxillary canines or premolars. These teeth are free to drift posteriorly as the molars are retracted. Occasionally, interdental spacing will develop between the premolars (Fig. 20-28).

After the molar position has been corrected (or overcorrected into a Class III relationship) the distalizing arch is removed. The transpalatal arch (removed previously) is replaced, and a passive utility arch is used to stabilize molar and incisor position while the premolars and canines are allowed to drift posteriorly due to the pull of the transseptal fibers. As the molars may have been distalized into a wider part of the arch, the TPA may need expansion or other adjustments before cementation. After the retraction of these teeth is completed, a retrusive utility arch is used to retract and intrude the maxillary incisors. Class II elastics usually are worn during the retraction of the anterior teeth.

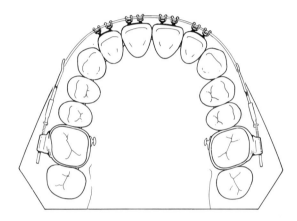

Figure 20-27. Maxillary occlusal view of Wilson distalizing arch at the beginning of treatment. The transpalatal arch that was used to align the buccal surfaces of the maxillary molars has been removed.

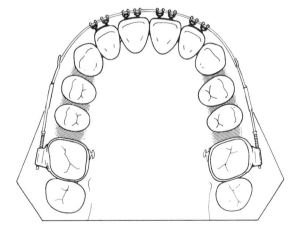

Figure 20-28. Maxillary occlusal view of Wilson distalizing arch after molar distalization has been completed. Interdental spacing is observed in the premolar region. The transpalatal arch that was used to align the buccal surfaces of the maxillary molars has been removed.

Treatment Effects

There have been only two studies in the literature that have considered the treatment effects produced by the Wilson distalizing arch. Muse and co-workers[34] investigated the magnitude and direction of maxillary and mandibular first molar and incisor changes that occur during Class II molar correction with Wilson mechanics. Nineteen patients received maxillary bimetric distalizing arches and either a mandibular three-dimensional lingual arch, with or without a passive .016 x .016″ utility arch, or a traditional edgewise full banded and bonded arch. The appliance was activated a maximum of five times or until visual inspection revealed a Class I molar relationship had been attained. Initial and progress lateral cephalograms were taken with molar bands cemented. The mean change in molar relation measured at the occlusal plane was 4.1 mm. The mean maxillary molar distalization was 2.2 mm, with 8° of tip. The mean mandibular molar mesial movement was 1.4 mm. The maxillary incisors protruded 0.3 mm, and extruded 1.6 mm.

A recent study by Rana and Becher[35] also considered the treatment effects of the Wilson distalizing arch in 18 predominantly adolescent patients. Contrary to Wilson's recommendations,[30-32] the maxillary molar bands had facebow tubes placed occlusally, not gingivally. All patients were fitted with a Wilson three-dimensional lingual arch in the mandible. Nickel titanium coil springs, not stainless steel springs (again as recommended by Wilson[32]), were used. Rana and Becher[35] reported that the maxillary molars moved distally about 1 mm and tipped posteriorly 2°. They also reported greater flaring of the maxillary anterior teeth (3.5°) and greater incisor extrusion (2.7 mm) than did Muse and co-workers.[34] Rana and Becher[35] also found very little change in the lower molars, whereas Muse and colleagues[34] reported that the lower molars moved mesially 1.4 mm.

When comparing the results of these studies to those of the Pendulum appliance, it appears that the Wilson distalizing arch is less effective in moving molars distally. Patient compliance obviously is an issue with the Wilson arch, as is the reliance on mandibular anchorage. Modest mesial movement of the lower has been noted when Class II elastics have been worn as part of the protocol.

One of the major advantages of the Wilson arch, in comparison to the Pendex or Distal Jet, is the speed and ease of insertion. After the decision has been made to actively distalize the molars, the appliance can be placed at the same appointment with no laboratory involvement. Although not as efficient as the Pendulum appliance as a primary method of molar distalization, the Wilson Bimetric Distalizing Arch™ has a place in routine orthodontic therapy, especially in those patients nearing the end of treatment with residual Class II occlusal problems remaining.

OTHER METHODS OF DISTALIZATION

A number of other methods of molar distalization are available to the orthodontic practitioner. Several remaining methods will be mentioned briefly.

Compressed Springs

Springs made from compressed stainless steel or nickel titanium also have been used in conjunction with various non-cooperation-based appliances to produce maxillary molar movement[36-41] (Figs. 20-29 and 20-30). Gianelly and co-workers[36,42] described the use of one hundred-gram superelastic nickel titanium coils developed by Miura[43] to move maxillary molars distally.

The NiTi coils are placed on a sectional wire made from .016 x .022″ stainless steel that extends from the first premolar to the first molar (the second premolar remains unbracketed). The NiTi coil is activated about 10 mm to produce 100 grams of continuously acting

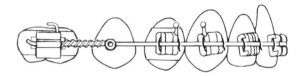

Figure 20-29. Lateral view of the distalization of the maxillary first molar by way of NiTi coils and a Nance acrylic palatal button. A movable Gurin lock is used to activate the compression spring (after Gianelly[42]).

force. The first premolars are anchored by a Nance holding arch (Fig. 20–30). Gianelly[36] also states that the coil springs can be compressed by placing a sliding Gurin lock. The archwire must extend at least 5 mm past the end of the molar bracket to allow the molar to move distally along the archwire.

Deflection of Straight Wires

The deflection of straight wires also has been used to produce distal molar movement (Fig. 20-31). Gianelly and associates[44,45] have demonstrated distalization of maxillary molars with a one hundred-gram nickel tita-

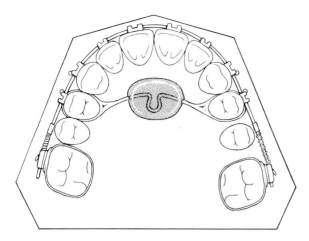

Figure 20-30. Occlusal view of NiTi coils used to distalize the maxillary molars. Bands on the maxillary first premolars are connected to palatal acrylic (Nance button). The size and shape of the palatal acrylic depends on the anchorage requirements of the patient. The spring is compressed on the right side of the arch; molar distalization has occurred on the left side. (After Gianelly.[42])

nium wire (.018 × .025″ NeoSentalloy™ wire, GAC International, Central Islip NY) compressed between the maxillary first premolars and maxillary first molars with crimpable stops. A Nance holding arch cemented to the first premolars is used for anchorage.

In addition, Kalra[46] has developed a titanium molybdenum alloy (TMA™) archwire compressed between the maxillary first premolars and maxillary first molars. This design, combined with the anchorage of a Nance button, has been shown to effectively move molars distally.

Gianelly[36] recommends the use of sectional archwires, not a continuous archwire in this protocol. To facilitate distal molar movement, two stops are placed on the archwire, one distal to the bracket on the maxillary first premolar and the second at the terminal part of the facebow tube of the first molar bracket. Gianelly recommends that the distance between the stops should be 5–6 mm longer than the space between the bracket and the molar tube. The archwire then is inserted into the molar tube, and finger pressure is deflected into the buccal vestibule. Gianelly[36] suggests that ice be used to cool the archwire (*e.g.*, ice, Endoice™; Hygienic Corp., Akron OH) before insertion to facilitate insertion. Cooling the archwire makes the wire soft and pliable.

Repelling Magnetic Appliances

Repelling magnets combined with a Nance anchorage appliance also have been used to distalize maxillary molars.[47-54] This procedure has been used both in the late mixed dentition after the eruption of the maxillary premolars has occurred and as a permanent dentition appliance that can be used successfully in adult patients.

After the maxillary first molars have been rotated using a transpalatal arch, the first premolars or second premolars are banded, and an impression is made. A palatal stabilization plate (Fig. 20-32) is fabricated and cemented in place. The transpalatal arch is removed, and the maxillary first molars are rebanded. An assembly containing the repelling magnets is placed into the molar tube on the maxillary first molars, and the magnets are placed in a repelling position by ligating a sliding yoke to an eyelet on the premolar.

The sequential activation of the magnets (every 2 or 4 weeks) produces a distalizing force that ultimately results in a posterior movement of the maxillary first molars. According to Gianelly,[55] approximately 25% of the total tooth movement is a forward positioning of the anchoring premolar teeth, indicating a mild loss of anchorage. Within four or five months, a space equivalent to the width of a premolar can be produced anterior to the maxillary first molars (Fig. 20-32).

These magnetic forces unquestionably can produce tooth movement; the use of this approach, however, has not gained wide acceptance because the magnets tend to be expensive and bulky (although Blechman and Alexander[54] developed a more compact magnetic molar distalization system in 1995), their force dissipates rapidly with increasing intermagnet distance, and their biologic systemic effects still are a subject of spec-

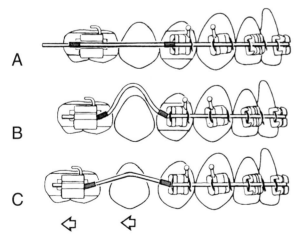

Figure 20-31. Deflection of straight NiTi wires to distalize molars. *A*, Two stops are placed on the archwire, one at the distal of the first premolar bracket and one at the distal of the bracket on the first molar. The archwire is not engaged in the molar tube. *B*, The archwire is inserted in the molar tube and deflected gingivally into the vestibular area. The wire can be cooled before insertion to make the wire more flexible.[42] *C*, Distalization of the maxillary molar.

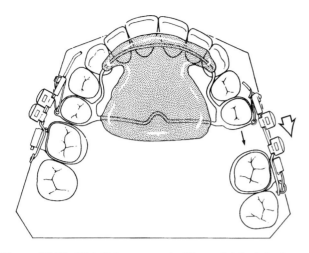

Figure 20-32. Distalizing magnets. The palatal plate is anchored to the second premolars. On the right side of the arch, the magnets are in a repelling configuration. On the left side of the arch, distalization of the maxillary molars has occurred.

ulation. Because of these drawbacks, along with the necessity of frequent recall reactivation, Darendeliler[56] has concluded that magnets offer no advantage over conventional systems in molar distalization.

CONCLUDING REMARKS

This chapter has considered a number of options for intentional molar distalization, an effective method of treatment for Class II malocclusions characterized by maxillary dentoalveolar protrusion. Recent clinical studies have shown that the Pendulum and Pendex appliances efficiently produce predictable posterior movement of the maxillary molars without the need for a high level of patient compliance, as is necessary with extraoral traction. Although a slight amount of bite opening often is seen with this type of treatment mechanics, the amount usually is not clinically significant.

The Wilson arch has proven to be effective as a primary treatment appliance, especially in the management of borderline Class II, division 2 patients, in whom some forward movement of the lower dentition is desired or allowable. We also have found the Wilson arch useful toward the end of treatment when only a few millimeters of Class II correction remain unilaterally or bilaterally. NiTi coils also have been shown to move molars distally during various stages of treatment.

The Distal Jet appliance is presented as new technology. Ongoing clinical studies will determine the effectiveness of this technique in comparison to other available appliances.

In conclusion, the treatment approaches described in this chapter generally produce excellent results with minimal reliance on patient cooperation, thus reducing the importance one of the major variables in orthodontic treatment.

REFERENCES CITED

1. Sinclair PM. The reader's corner. J Clin Orthod 1994;28: 361–363.
2. White LW. A new paradigm of motivation. Pac Coast Soc Orthod Bull 1988:44–45.
3. White LW. A new paradigm of motivation. In: Trotman CA, McNamara JA, Jr, eds. Creating the compliant patient. Ann Arbor: Monograph 33, Craniofacial Growth Series, Center for Human Growth and Development, The University of Michigan, 1997.
4. Alexander RG. Creating the compliant patient. In: Trotman CA, McNamara JA, Jr, eds. Creating the compliant patient. Ann Arbor: Monograph 33, Craniofacial Growth Series, Center for Human Growth and Development, The University of Michigan, 1997.
5. Hilgers JJ. The Pendulum appliance...An update. Clin Impressions 1993:15–17.
6. Bennett RK, Hilgers JJ. The Pendulum appliance: Creating the gain. Clin Impressions 1994;3:14–18.
7. Bennett RK, Hilgers JJ. The Pendulum appliance: Maintaining the gain. Clin Impressions 1994;3:6–9, 14–8, 22.
8. Snodgrass DJ. A fixed appliance for maxillary expansion, molar rotation, and molar distalization. J Clin Orthod 1996;30:156–159.
9. Hilgers JJ. The Pendulum appliance for Class II noncompliance therapy. J Clin Orthod 1992;26:706–714.
10. Byloff FK, Darendeliler MA, Clar E, Darendeliler A. Distal molar movement using the Pendulum appliance. Part 2: The effects of maxillary molar root uprighting bends. Angle Orthod 1997;67:261–270.
11. Tollaro I, Baccetti T, Franchi L, Tanasescu CD. Role of posterior transverse interarch discrepancy in Class II, Division 1 malocclusion during the mixed dentition phase. Am J Orthod Dentofac Orthop 1996;110:417–422.
12. McNamara JA, Jr. Maxillary transverse deficiency. Am J Orthod Dentofac Orthop 2000;117:567–570.
13. Hilgers JJ, Bennett RK. The Pendulum appliance, Part II: Maintaining the gain. Clin Impressions 1994;3:5–9, 14–18, 22.
14. Ponitz RJ. Invisible retainers. Am J Orthod 1971;59: 266–272.
15. McNamara JA, Jr, Kramer KL, Jeunker JP. Invisible retainers. J Clin Orthod 1985;19:570–578.
16. Hilgers JJ, Tracey S. Hyperefficient orthodontic treatment employing Bioprogressive principles. Clin Impressions 2000;9:18–27.
17. Ghosh J, Nanda RS. Evaluation of an intraoral maxillary molar distalization technique. Am J Orthod Dentofac Orthop 1996;110:639–646.
18. Joseph AA, Butchart CJ. An evaluation of the Pendulum distalizing appliance. Semin Orthod 2000;6:129–135.
19. Byloff FK, Darendeliler MA. Distal molar movement using the Pendulum appliance. Part 1: Clinical and radiological evaluation. Angle Orthod 1997;67:249–260.

20. Bussick TJ, McNamara JA, Jr. Dentoalveolar and skeletal changes associated with the pendulum appliance. Am J Orthod Dentofac Orthop 2000;117:333–343.
21. Carano A, Testa M. The distal jet for upper molar distalization. J Clin Orthod 1996;30:374–380.
22. Carano A, Testa M. Clinical applications of the distal jet. Genova: RS Editore, 1997.
23. Huerter GW, Jr. A retrospective evaluation of maxillary molar distalization with the distal jet appliance. St Louis: Unpublished Master's thesis, Department of Orthodontics, St Louis University, 1999.
24. Patel A. Analysis of the distal jet appliance for maxillary molar distalization. Oklahoma City: Unpublished Master's thesis, Department of Orthodontics, University of Oklahoma, 1999.
25. Carano A. Personal communication, 2000.
26. Bowman SJ. Personal communication, 2000.
27. Bowman SJ. Modifications of the distal jet. J Clin Orthod 1998;32:549–556.
28. Jasper JJ, McNamara JA, Jr. The correction of interarch malocclusions using a fixed force module. Am J Orthod Dentofac Orthop 1995;108:641–650.
29. Bowman SJ. Combination Class II therapy. J Clin Orthod 1998;32:611–620.
30. Wilson WL. Modular orthodontic systems. Part 1. J Clin Orthod 1978;12:259–67, 270–278.
31. Wilson WL. Modular orthodontic systems. Part 2. J Clin Orthod 1978;12:358–375.
32. Wilson WL, Wilson RC. New treatment dimensions with first phase sectional and progressive edgewise mechanics. J Clin Orthod 1980;14:607–627.
33. Wilson RC, Wilson WL. Enhanced orthodontics. Denver: Rocky Mountain Orthodontics, 1988.
34. Muse DS, Fillman MJ, Emmerson WJ, Mitchell RD. Molar and incisor changes with Wilson rapid molar distalization. Am J Orthod Dentofac Orthop 1993;104:556–565.
35. Rana R, Becher MK. Class II correction using the bimetric distalizing arch. Semin Orthod 2000;6:106–118.
36. Gianelly AA, Bednar J, Dietz VS. Japanese NiTi coils used to move molars distally. Am J Orthod Dentofac Orthop 1991;99:564–566.
37. Jones RD, White JM. Rapid Class II molar correction with an open-coil jig. J Clin Orthod 1992;26:661–664.
38. Reiner TJ. Modified Nance appliance for unilateral molar distalization. J Clin Orthod 1992;26:402–404.
39. Greenfield RL. Fixed piston appliance for rapid Class II correction. J Clin Orthod 1995;29:174–183.
40. Carano A, Testa M, Siciliani G. The lingual distalizer system. Eur J Orthod 1996;18:445–448.
41. Puente M. Class II Correction with an edgewise-modified Nance appliance. J Clin Orthod 1997;31:178–182.
42. Gianelly AA. Bidimensional technique theory and practice. Central Islip: GAC International, 2000.
43. Miura F, Mogi M, Ohura Y, Karibe M. The super-elastic Japanese NiTi alloy wire for use in orthodontics. Part III. Studies on the Japanese NiTi alloy coil springs. Am J Orthod Dentofac Orthop 1988;94:89–96.
44. Gianelly AA, Bednar J, Dietz VS, Locatelli R. Molar distalization with superelastic NiTi wire. J Clin Orthod 1992;26:277–279.
45. Gianelly AA. Distal movement of maxillary molars. Am J Orthod Dentofac Orthop 1998;114:66–72.
46. Kalra V. The K-loop molar distalizing appliance. J Clin Orthod 1995;29:298–301.
47. Blechman AM, Smiley H. Magnetic force in orthodontics. Am J Orthod 1978;74:435–443.
48. Blechman AM. Magnetic force systems in orthodontics. Clinical results of a pilot study. Am J Orthod 1985;87:201–210.
49. Itoh T, Tokuda T, Kiyosue S, Hirose T, Matsumoto M, Chaconas SJ. Molar distalization with repelling magnets. J Clin Orthod 1991;25:611–617.
50. Bondemark L, Kurol J. Distalization of maxillary first and second molars simultaneously with repelling magnets. Eur J Orthod 1992;14:264–272.
51. Steger ER, Blechman AM. Case reports: molar distalization with static repelling magnets. Part II. Am J Orthod Dentofac Orthop 1995;108:547–555.
52. Gianelly AA, Vaitas AS, Thomas WM, Berger DG. Distalization of molars with repelling magnets. J Clin Orthod 1988;22:40–44.
53. Gianelly AA, Vaitas AS, Thomas WM. The use of magnets to move molars distally. Am J Orthod Dentofac Orthop 1989;96:161–167.
54. Blechman AM, Alexander C. New miniaturized magnets for molar distalization. Clin Orthod Res 1995;4:14–19.
55. Gianelly AA. Personal communication, 1992.
56. Darendeliler MA. Contemporary mechanics: magnets and constant forces. Pac Coast Soc Orthod Bull 1995;67:43–45.

Chapter 21
EXTRAORAL TRACTION

Perhaps the most common adjunct traditionally used in the treatment of Class II malocclusion has been extraoral traction. This family of appliances typically is used to restrict the normal downward and forward growth of the maxilla. The forces produced affect the normal craniofacial growth of the patient, allowing for the correction of the Class II occlusal condition. Maxillary growth is restrained and/or redirected so that basal bones become more harmoniously related to one another as the unimpeded mandible "catches up" during normal growth.[1]

The frequency of use of this methodology varies widely among clinicians because of a number of factors, including educational background, treatment philosophy, and more recently the availability of other treatment methods that have become available which do not depend on patient compliance (*e.g.*, Pendulum, Distal Jet, NiTi coils).

HISTORICAL PERSPECTIVE

Use of extraoral forces to modify the growth of the maxilla has a long history, dating back to Kingsley[2,3] and Angle[4] in the nineteenth century. Both used occipital headgears to retract and intrude maxillary incisors. Interest in extraoral traction diminished in the first half of the 20th century, especially with the increased popularity of intermaxillary elastics. Interest in headgear was revived by Oppenheim[5] and later by Kloehn[6–8] who recommended the application of extra-oral forces for the mass distal movement of teeth.

Kloehn made many modifications in headgear design, until he began to use only the neck strap as the basis for traction (Fig. 21-1).[9] To obtain adequate molar control required specific manipulation of the outer arms of the facebow (Fig. 21-2), which cannot be obtained when a facebow with short outer arms is used. The use of this appliance system is described in detail below, in that his technique forms the basis of contemporary facebow treatment.

Kloehn's original facebow design featured a .045″ inner bow soldered to a .052″ outer bow (Fig. 21-2), with the inner bow fitting into .045″ tubes on the maxillary first molar bands.[9] The original neck straps were constructed of several layers of heavy canvas and were covered with carpet binding tape. By necessity, the neck straps had to be thick, because the force from the rubber bands was 3.0–3.5 pounds. The cervical strap reached to 1.0–1.5″ from the corners of the mouth (as close to the mouth as possible without saliva contamination that may cause skin irritation). At the end of the strap, a slot was formed in the padding through which passed the outer bow[9] (Fig. 21-1).

Each end of the outer bow connected by way of heavy elastics to dress hooks sewn to the middle of the neck strap. The outer bow was bent away from the cheeks, so that it would not push against them when the elastics were attached. The inner bow was adjusted to produce distal molar rotation, which typically is needed during Class II treatment. The inner bow was compressed by the patient's fingers when inserted into the facebow tubes.[9]

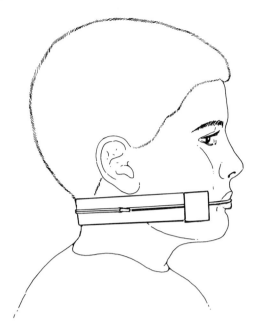

Figure 21-1. Original design of the Kloehn cervical facebow.[9] The neck strap extended anteriorly to within 1.0–1.5 inches of the corners of the mouth. The outer bow of the facebow passed through a sleeve on the anterior aspect of the neck strap and connected posteriorly to elastics attached to hooks sewn to the middle of the neck strap.

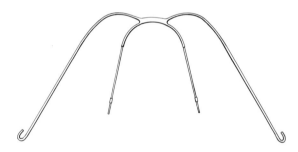

Figure 21-2. Kloehn facebow with soldered stops on the inner bow.

The initial direction of force used by Kloehn was straight, because this type of force was least likely to cause molar tenderness and helped the patient adjust to the appliance. Lighter elastics were worn during this period, and the patient was instructed to wear the appliance 14 hours per day. After 4–6 weeks, the inner and outer bows were adjusted to impart a distal crown tip to the maxillary first molars, and the inner bow was adjusted to expand the molars (Fig. 21-3). With this adjustment, spaces typically appeared interdentally between the molars and premolars.

If the results of the previous adjustments were satisfactory, the inner and outer bows were adjusted to

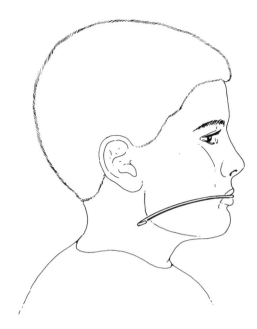

Figure 21-3. Adjustment of the outer bow of the facebow made to impart distal crown tip to the maxillary first molars.[9] The inner bow was adjusted to expand the molars.

create distal root tip and molar depressing forces (Fig. 21-4); expansion was continued. When the distal root tip became excessive, the crowns were tipped distally again and the process repeated until the maxillary molars were over-treated relative to the mandibular molars. If no other appliances were used except for the cervical

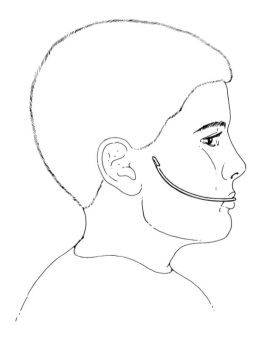

Figure 21-4. Adjustment of the outer bow of the facebow made to impart distal root tip and intrusion to the maxillary first molars.[9]

EXTRAORAL TRACTION

traction, expansion of the mandibular arch occurred frequently.[9]

Extraoral traction therapy has evolved since the pioneering work of Oppenheim[10] and Kloehn,[6–9] but the principles established during this early treatment are relevant today. In one of the few clinical studies conducted on a facebow sample treated by Silas and John Kloehn, Hubbard and co-workers[11] did not find tipping of the palatal plane or the mandibular plane, and the downward growth of the maxillary first molars essentially was similar to that observed in an untreated individual. As we will see later in this chapter, conflicting results have been reported concerning the treatment effects produced by various types of extraoral traction.

FACEBOWS

Extraoral traction devices can be divided arbitrarily into two types: facebows and J-hook headgears. Facebows attach to tubes on the maxillary first molars. Headgears, on the other hand, attach anteriorly to the archwire or to an auxiliary on the archwire.

Most extraoral traction devices used today have some version of a safety release mechanism.[12,13] A few reports of severe eye injuries caused by facebows have been published.[14–17] Although rare, the potentially high morbidity of such injuries has led manufacturers to develop a wide variety of safety devices that have become part of this type of appliance system.[13]

Types of Facebows

The facebow (Figs. 21-2 and 21-5) consists of two parts, an inner bow that attaches to the facebow tubes and a longer outer bow that is bent upward so that the point of force application and the direction of force lie above the center of resistance of the maxillary molar.

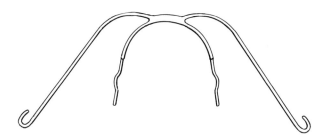

Figure 21-5. Cervical facebow. The inner bow has adjustment loops that also act as stops against the facebow tubes on the maxillary first molar bands. The outer bow is longer than the inner bow and typically is connected to an elastic neck strap or to elastics that attach to hooks on a cervical pad.

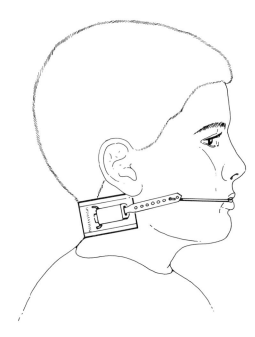

Figure 21-6. Sagittal view of Kloehn-type facebow with cervical neck strap and safety release.

Cervical-pull Facebow

The cervical (low-pull or "Kloehn") facebow, the type of facebow seen most frequently in clinical practice worldwide today (Figs. 21-6 and 21-7), typically is used in patients with decreased vertical skeletal dimensions. The purpose of the facebow is to restrict the forward growth of the maxilla and/or to prevent the forward movement of the maxillary posterior teeth. The force of

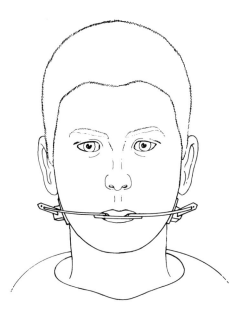

Figure 21-7. Frontal view of Kloehn-type facebow with cervical neck strap.

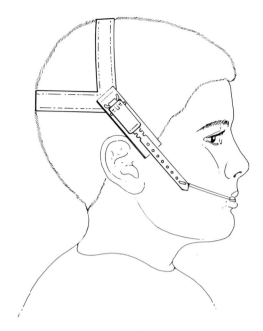

Figure 21-8. Sagittal view of high-pull (occipital) facebow.

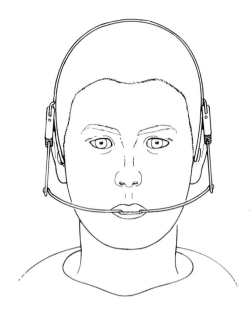

Figure 21-9. Frontal view of high-pull (occipital) facebow.

the cervical facebow is exerted below the occlusal plane, producing both extrusive and distalizing effects. This type of extraoral traction is selected when molar extrusion is a desirable treatment outcome.

High-pull Facebow

The force generated by a high-pull (occipital) facebow (Figs. 21-8 and 21-9) has both distalizing and intrusive effects, in that the force is exerted above the occlusal plane. Such force is used in all instances in which vertical control of the molars is important, as for example in patients with a skeletal or dentoalveolar open bite pattern and/or a steep mandibular plane angle.

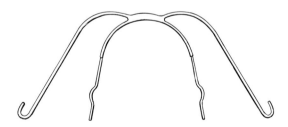

Figure 21-10. High-pull facebow. The inner bow and outer bow are the same length.

The high-pull facebow (Fig. 21-10) is attached to the maxillary first molars by way of an inner bow that is the same length as the outer bow. The outer bow is bent upward so that the point of force application and the direction of force lie above the center of resistance of the maxillary first molars. The inner bow lies passively in the molar tubes, or it can be expanded if an increase in transpalatal width is desired.

A high-pull facebow is used in individuals in whom increases in vertical dimension are to be minimized or avoided. The outer bow is attached to the occipital anchoring unit (headcap) to produce a more vertically directed force. As a growth guidance appliance, a high pull facebow can decrease the vertical development of the maxilla, thereby allowing for autorotation of the mandible and maximizing the horizontal expression of mandibular growth.[18]

Combi Facebow

The cervical facebow and the high-pull facebow can be used in combination (hence the term "combi facebow") to alter the direction of force more along the plane of the occlusion (Fig. 21-11).

Asymmetrical Facebow

The basic facebow design also can be modified (Fig. 21-12) to manage sagittal asymmetries within the dental arch (*e.g.*, Class II molar relationship on one side, Class I on the other.) The inner bow is shortened on the Class I side, and the outer bow is bent away from the cheek.[19] The center of attachment to the inner bow is moved laterally, thus producing asymmetrical forces against the

EXTRAORAL TRACTION

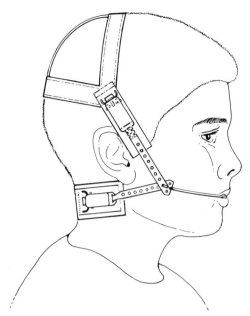

Figure 21-11. Lateral view of Combi headgear.

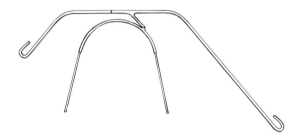

Figure 21-12. Asymmetrical facebow with a flexible connection between the inner and outer bows.

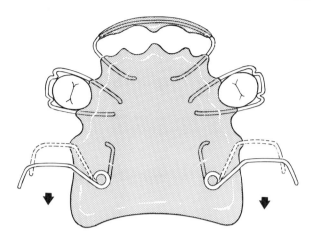

Figure 21-13. Distalizing plate of Margolis and Cetlin (ACCO appliance). This plate can be used to help move the maxillary molars posteriorly.

two sides of the dental arches. Extended use of this device will tend to skew the arch to one side.[20]

Current Uses of Facebows

Extraoral traction is an integral part of some treatment philosophies. For example Cetlin and co-workers[15,16] advocate the use of extraoral traction as part of their non-extraction treatment protocol. During the space-gaining phase, the maxillary molars first are rotated with a transpalatal arch, and then extraoral traction is applied. In addition, a removable plate (Fig. 21-13) is used to distalize the maxillary molars bodily. During the second phase, during which space consolidation occurs, extraoral forces help maintain anchorage posteriorly. The forces of occlusion may counteract the extrusive forces and favorable condylar growth can compensate for molar extrusion.

The facebow often is part of what has been referred to as a "2×4 hook-up."[23-26] Patients who undergo this type of treatment typically are characterized by a Class II molar relationship, flared maxillary incisors, and a decreased lower anterior facial height. Such patients can be treated with four brackets on the maxillary incisors that are connected by means of an archwire to the maxillary first molars. An elastic can be stretched between hooks that are attached to the anterior part of the inner bow to assist in incisor retraction.

HEADGEARS

Types of Headgears

J-Hook Headgear

The forces produced by extraoral traction also can be attached anteriorly by means of J-hooks to the archwire or to hooks soldered to the archwire. Flared maxillary incisors can be retracted using either a high-pull (Figs. 21-14 and 21-15) or a straight-pull headgear (Figs. 21-16 and 21-17) combined with J-hooks that are attached to the archwire anteriorly or by using a closing arch supported by headgear. Headgears with J-hooks also are used to potentiate archwire mechanics by helping control forces incorporated into the archwire (*e.g.,* torque, intrusion).

Variable-Pull Headgears

The use of the variable-pull headgear (Figs. 21-18 and 21-19) provides additional treatment options with a variable direction of force. The original Interlandi[27] headgear actually was designed for use with facebows.

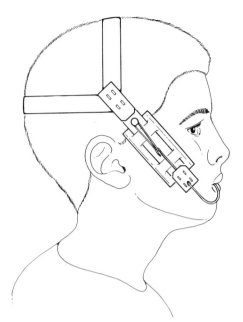

Figure 21-14. Sagittal view of high-pull headgear with J-hooks.

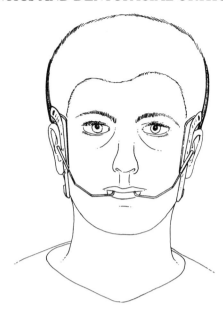

Figure 21-15. Frontal view of high-pull headgear with J-hooks.

The "C"-shaped anchor unit provided the opportunity for varying the force vector of the facebow.

Later, Hickham[14,22,23] modified the Interlandi headgear by adding metal tubes to accommodate J-hooks and cheek pads to resist the lateral forces produced by the J-hooks.[20] A third strap also was added to stabilize the headcap for variable force application.

J hooks can be applied to the maxillary teeth in a variety of force vectors to retract and intrude the maxillary incisor teeth. A similar type of retraction-stabilization of the mandibular dental arch also can be achieved. In addition, it is possible to attach J-hooks to the maxillary arch and the mandibular arch simultaneously (Fig. 21-20).

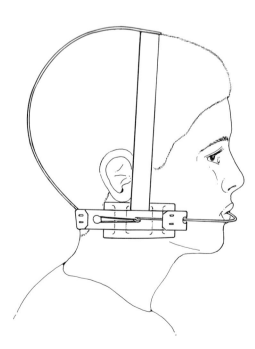

Figure 21-16. Sagittal view of straight-pull headgear with J-hooks.

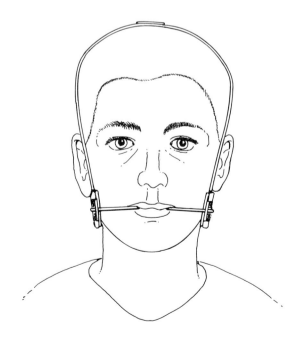

Figure 21-17. Frontal view of straight-pull headgear with J-hooks.

EXTRAORAL TRACTION

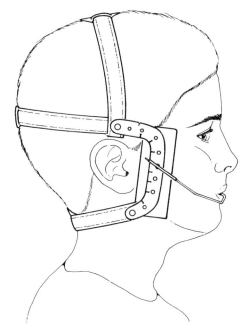

Figure 21-18. Sagittal view of the variable-pull headgear with J-hooks to the maxilla. The angle of pull of the J-hooks is adjustable.

Current Uses of J-Hook Headgears

One treatment approach that incorporates headgear use is the Tweed-Merrifield Edgewise philosophy,[12,24–26] a superb method of conserving anchorage and preventing "gummy smiles."[20] A cornerstone of current Tweed-Merrifield treatment is the application of "directional forces"[27,28] to move teeth. Vaden and co-workers[32] define directional forces as "controlled forces that place the teeth in the most harmonious relationship with the environment." Practitioners of this technique place emphasis on controlling the positions of the mandibular posterior teeth and the maxillary anterior teeth, with the resultant vector of all forces directed forward and upward.

Current Tweed-Merrifield treatment is divided into four steps: denture preparation, denture correction, denture completion, and denture recovery. Maxillary and mandibular J-hooks are used routinely in Tweed-Merrifield premolar extraction treatment, sometimes combined with elastomeric chain, to retract the maxillary and mandibular canines during the denture preparation stage. It should be remembered that all the steps in the protocol are utilized only when the clinician is presented with a difficult maximum anchorage high angle case.[20]

During the denture correction stage, vertical support to the maxillary arch is achieved with J-hook headgear attached to hooks soldered to the maxillary archwire between the maxillary central and lateral incisors. Vertical support of the mandibular anterior teeth is facilitated by way of anterior vertical elastics. Later during mandibular anchorage preparation, gingivally directed hooks are soldered on the archwire distal to the mandibular central incisors, and the headgear is used to support the placement of tipbacks in the mandibular dentition. At this stage in treatment, usually nighttime wear of the headgear is sufficient.

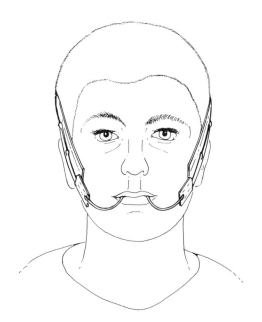

Figure 21-19. Frontal view of the variable-pull headgear with J-hooks to the maxilla. The J-hooks attach to the archwire or to hooks on the archwire.

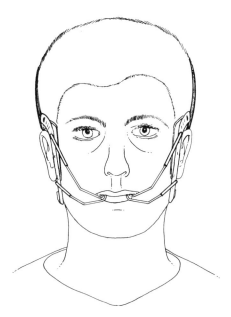

Figure 21-20. Frontal view of the variable-pull headgear with J-hooks to the maxillary and mandibular archwires. The direction of pull of the J-hooks is adjustable.

In the stage of denture completion, maxillary and mandibular stabilizing wires along with the appropriate elastic and headgear forces are used to detail the dentition. First, second and third order bends are placed in the finishing archwires. The maxillary archwire also has hooks for the high-pull headgear, anterior vertical elastics, and Class II elastics.

Headgear forces are not used during the denture recovery phase. All appliances are removed and the patient is given removable retainers to allow for a settling or "recovery" of the dentition. Recovery, based on the concept of overcorrection, is predicated on the known rebound phenomena that occur following appliance removal.

Directional forces also are incorporated into Tweed-Merrifield non-extraction treatment. Typically, a J-hook headgear is attached to the mandibular anterior teeth to prevent mandibular incisor proclination during the resolution of lower incisor crowding and the preparation of mandibular anchorage. Headgear forces later are applied to the maxillary archwire in a manner similar to that described previously for extraction treatment.

Virtually all of the extraoral traction appliances described above restrict the normal downward and forward movement of the maxilla and may help retract the maxillary and mandibular dentitions. These types of appliances are indicated in instances of maxillary skeletal protrusion, maxillary dentolaveolar protrusion, and mandibular dentoalveolar protrusion. The direction of force (*i.e.,* low-pull, straight-pull, high-pull) is determined by the pretreatment vertical dimensions of the patient.

TREATMENT EFFECTS

Extraoral traction has been shown to produce a variety of skeletal and dentoalveolar effects in Class II patients. Even though there is some agreement among investigators as to the effects produced, the clinical management of the appliance, the direction of force applied and the amount of force used may explain some of the differences among investigations.

Anteroposterior Dimension

Maxillary Skeletal Position

A primary treatment effect of extraoral traction is the restriction of maxillary skeletal growth. There is virtually universal agreement that because of treatment, Point A is repositioned posteriorly relative to the remainder of the face,[8,29–36] resulting in a reduction in maxillary prognathism.[6–8,12,29,30,37–45] Wieslander[40] has shown that this technique also influences the cranial base by producing a counterclockwise tilting of the spheno-ethmoid plane during 3–4 years of treatment with a headgear.

Maxillary Dentoalveolar Position

Distal movement of the maxillary molars is a typical treatment effect produced by cervical headgear therapy.[6,30,33,35,42,46–52] In contrast, Hubbard and co-workers,[11] who studied a sample of patients treated by Silas and John Kloehn, reported a mesial movement of the first molar. Extrusion of the maxillary molars also has been observed,[25,30,32,43,53–56] with two[11] to three[60] times as much extrusion reported as would be expected during normal growth. On the other hand, Hubbard and colleagues[11] did not observe molar extrusion.

Melsen and Egemark,[57] using the implant method of Björk,[63] studied the effect of cervical-pull headgear on the craniofacial complex, in part to determine whether the specific angulation of the outer bow relative to the occlusal plane was clinically significant. In one group of children, the outer bow was tilted 20° above the occlusal plane; in the second group, the outer bow was angled 20° below the occlusal plane. In the first group with the outer bow angled upward, only slight tooth movement was observed, but the entire maxillary complex moved posteriorly and inferiorly relative to the anterior cranial base.

Melsen and Egemark[57] stated that this method of facebow adjustment is appropriate for those patients with true maxillary skeletal protrusion. In the second group, more tooth movement was observed, particularly a distal tipping of the maxillary first molar. The extraoral traction had no appreciable influence on the maxillary complex. Melsen and Egemark[57] stated that orienting the outer bow of the facebow below the occlusal plane may be appropriate in patients with mesially migrating or tipped maxillary first molars, or both.

Mandibular Dentoalveolar Position

There is virtually no literature that addresses the effect of the cervical-pull facebow on the mandibular dentition other than the treatment effects that are produced in association with fixed appliance treatment. There appears to be no effect.[19]

Mandibular Skeletal Position

The anteroposterior relationship of the chin has been correlated to the amount of vertical opening produced during treatment. A downward and backward rotation of the mandible and a similar movement of Point B and pogonion have been reported, as has an opening of the mandibular plane angle.[25,40,53,54] Kloehn[6] and Ringenberg and Butts[39] report no change in the SNB angle, but other investigators note either a posterior[25,44,53,54] or anterior[32,36] movement of Point B.

Vertical Dimension

There is no universal agreement as to the effect of cervical headgear treatment on the vertical dimension, as investigators have differed in describing the effect of this type of therapy on the various aspects of vertical facial measures.

Mandibular Plane Angle and Lower Anterior Facial Height

An increase in the mandibular plane angle as the mandible is hinged open has been reported by many investigators.[25,34,49,53,54,56] An opening of the bite and an increase in lower anterior facial height also has been a frequent finding.[30,45,53,58-62] Klein[36] and Ricketts[50] report that extraoral force tends to open the Y axis angle and lengthen the face more than would occur with normal growth. A high-pull headgear has been recommended to reduce the extrusion of the maxillary first molars. In contrast, Ringenberg and Butts,[39] Baumrind,[67] and Hubbard and co-workers[11] report a closure of the mandibular plane angle with treatment, whereas others reported no change.[6,32,36,43,62,63]

Occlusal Plane Angle

Investigators have differed as to the effect of extraoral traction on the orientation of the occlusal plane relative to the cranial base. The anatomic occlusal plane normally closes with age.[70] Klein,[36] King,[49] and Hubbard and colleagues[11] reported that the angle of the occlusal plane remains relatively unchanged during treatment, while Sandusky,[38] Merrifield and Cross,[31] and Cangialosi and colleagues[42] report an increase in the angle of the occlusal plane relative to the cranial base. Hubbard and associates[11] noted a slight downward tipping of the anterior part of the palatal plane. The functional occlusal plane closed slightly with treatment as well.

Palatal Plane Angle

The palatal plane has been shown to tip anteriorly with an uneven descent, resulting in the anterior nasal spine tipping more inferiorly than the posterior nasal spine.[11,25,30,32-34,36,48,56] On the other hand, Kloehn[8] and Boecler and co-workers[69] noted no change in the angulation of the palatal plane.

Transverse Dimension

Most clinical studies of extraoral traction have used cephalometrics as the primary analytical tool. Thus, consideration in the literature of changes in the transverse dimension with extraoral traction has been minimal. The only investigation to consider transverse changes is that of Ghafari and co-workers,[71] who conducted a comparative study of the straight-pull headgear and FR-2 appliance of Fränkel. The inner bow of the facebow was adjusted at every appointment "to avoid any constriction or major expansion of the intermolar distance," resulting in a total expansion of the inner bow of 1.5–2.0 mm.[71] Ghafari and colleagues noted increases not only in intermolar distance, but in intercanine distance as well. These investigators hypothesized that the change in intercanine distance, a region not directly affected by the facebow, may have been a result of a shielding effect by the inner bow on the lip and cheek musculature, an indication of the influence of the buccal and labial musculature on tooth position.

COMPARISON WITH FUNCTIONAL JAW ORTHOPEDICS

In the orthodontic and facial orthopedic literature, a number of studies have contrasted extraoral traction to various types of functional appliances. For example, Meach,[72] Baumrind and co-workers,[68] and Derringer[67,68] have compared extraoral traction to the activator. Other studies have compared the function regulator and extraoral traction directly.[75-78]

A direct comparison of facebow therapy versus functional jaw orthopedics in mixed dentition patients was conducted by McNamara and co-workers,[25] who evaluated the cephalometric radiographs of three groups of Class II, division 1 subjects. This study will be discussed in detail because the findings demonstrate pronounced differences in treatment effects, at least over the short-term. The comparison of starting forms also indicates morphological differences pretreatment among patients according to the protocol selected by the clinician.

Records from patients treated with the function regulator (FR-2) of Fränkel[79] were compared with records of patients treated with a cervical-pull facebow combined with incisor bracketing and archwires, and with longitudinal cephalograms of untreated children with Class II malocclusion form the *University of Michigan Growth Study*.[70]

After each group of records was assembled, specific exclusionary rules were applied,[25] including absence of Class II malocclusion, inadequate timing of radiographs, poor radiographic quality, or obvious errors in mandibular positioning. The application of these exclusionary rules reduced each sample substantially. One additional selection criterion was added, chronological age. The groups were defined further by excluding patients and subjects who were younger that 7 years 6 months or older than 11 years 0 months at the beginning of the treatment/observation period. The application of this last criterion to the Fränkel sample reduced the size of the sample to 26. Similarly, the facebow group was composed of 34 patients and the control group was composed of 20 subjects. At the end of the selection process, the groups were well matched according to chronological age, with an average age of about nine years initially for all groups.

An evaluation of starting form (*i.e.*, facial morphology before treatment) revealed that the Fränkel and control groups were reasonably well matched according to the 28 variables considered. In spite of these efforts to match the groups, however, some significant differences existed between the facebow group and the other sample groups. Specifically, both the maxilla and the mandible were slightly more retruded in the control sample, and lower anterior facial height was less in the facebow group than in the control. In addition, both the maxillary incisors and molars were more anterior in the facebow group before treatment than in the control.

The results of this retrospective study indicated that the FR-2 appliance of Fränkel, and the cervical-pull facebow combined with anterior brackets and archwire, produce significant treatment effects on the craniofacial structures of Class II mixed dentition patients. These treatment approaches, however, affect the skeletal and dentoalveolar structures in differing ways. For example, there was a 3 mm difference between the change in position of Point A between the facebow group and control during the treatment period. Similar changes were observed in the SNA angle and in the increments of midfacial length increase, as measured from condylion to Point A. In contrast, the Fränkel appliance had minimal effect on midfacial development.

One of the most striking differences between the two treatments was with regard to the anteroposterior position of the maxillary incisors and molars. The FR-2 appliance tipped the maxillary incisor posteriorly and did not affect the position of the maxillary molar in comparison to the controls. In contrast, the facebow, combined with partial anterior appliances, produced a significant posterior relocation of the maxillary incisor, a *six millimeter difference* in comparison to control values. Similarly, the maxillary molar was relocated almost 4 mm posteriorly in comparison to the untreated group. Thus, the facebow and fixed appliance combination had a profound effect on the position of the maxillary dentition in comparison to controls.

One explanation for the difference in maxillary incisor movement is that often in Class II, division 1 patients, the maxillary incisors were spaced and flared before treatment. One of the objectives of so-called "2×4 treatment" is to close the spaces and to reduce the flaring of the maxillary incisors through the application of lingual crown torque. Such movement, of course, is appropriate in these types of patients.

The two appliances had opposite effects on the movement of the mandibular dentition, but to a much less extent than in the maxilla. Modest mandibular incisor proclination was observed following FR-2 treatment, whereas modest incisor retroclination was noted in the facebow group. In addition, increased molar eruption was noted in the FR-2 group compared to the other groups.

As has been demonstrated in this sample, as well as in other such samples,[69,73,74] increased increments of mandibular length were noted following FR-2 treatment. A statistically significant increase in mandibular length also was measured in the facebow sample in comparison to the untreated Class II sample. This increase in mandibular length lends support to the concept of "mandibular response" during therapy with extraoral traction. Although this concept has been part of the "conventional wisdom" of many orthodontic practitioners and has been mentioned in passing in papers dealing with the Tweed-Merrifield edgewise philosophy,[26,75,76] few data have been presented previously to support or refute this concept.

Similar findings concerning increased rates of mandibular growth with extraoral traction treatment have been reported by other investigators. For example, Jenkins,[83] in an unpublished Master's thesis, evaluated a group of 48 patients treated for 18 months with a cervical-pull headgear. The cervical-pull headgear-anterior bite plane group demonstrated an increase in mandibular length (Co-Gn) that was 1.7 mm greater than was seen in untreated controls. Baumrind and colleagues[78,79] and Derringer[74] also found increased levels of mandibular growth in headgear patients that were similar to that seen with functional appliance therapy. Tulloch and co-workers,[86] in a large, federally-funded prospective study, noted that the annualized increment of change in mandibular length was greater in children treated with straight-pull headgear than in a group of untreated Class II controls.

Chu[87] evaluated the serial lateral headfilms of 30 patients treated with a maxillary traction splint and 25 patients treated with a bionator. The analysis of Phase I records resulted in significantly more maxillary skeletal and dentoalveolar changes in the traction group and greater mandibular growth in the bionator group. During the fixed appliance phase, headgear patients experienced considerable relapse of maxillary growth restriction and maxillary molar distalization was lost. The increased rate of mandibular growth in the bionator group also was not maintained during Phase II treatment. Chu[87] concluded that the overall changes (T_1-T_3) were remarkably similar between groups, and the choice treatment (headgear *vs.* functional appliance) should be based on other factors such as treatment efficiency or a patient's preference/acceptance of one appliance over the other.

LONG-TERM STUDIES OF EXTRAORAL TRACTION

Only a few investigations[40,88–91] have evaluated the long-term effect of extraoral traction. Wieslander and Buck[40] evaluated the stability of cervical traction therapy six years post-treatment. They reported that maxillary downward and forward growth continued equally in both the treated and untreated groups. They noted only a minor tendency toward relapse.

Melsen[88] also evaluated patients treated with cervical traction by means of metallic implants, but her findings were different from those of Wieslander and Buck.[40] She reported maxillary growth that was greater in the treatment group than what would be expected during normal growth. Melsen suggested that the effect of headgear treatment might be temporary, with a subsequent relapse of the earlier changes. Evaluating her sample 7–8 years following treatment, it appeared that the effect of the headgear therapy was reversed, with pronounced anterior maxillary growth occurring in almost all patients.

Glenn and co-workers[89] evaluated 28 subjects treated with a non-extraction approach and cervical facebow therapy. Serial lateral cephalograms and dental casts taken pretreatment, post-treatment and eight years post-treatment were examined. During treatment, the SNA angle decreased 2.0°. The investigators judged the overall long-term stability to be good. Overbite and overjet remained relatively stable following treatment. Class II malocclusions with large ANB values and short mandibular lengths were associated with increased incisor irregularity, shorter arch lengths and deeper overbites at the post retention stage.

Elm and colleagues[84,85] evaluated the effects of facebow therapy in conjunction with comprehensive edgewise orthodontics in 42 patients. Serial study models[90] and lateral cephalograms[91] were examined before treatment, after treatment, and eight years post-treatment. The ANB angle decreased 2.0° during treatment and the mandibular plane angle did not open. The investigators concluded that the treatment effects produced were relatively stable, with the major long-term changes related to those patients who had excessive amounts of tooth movement during treatment.

CONCLUDING REMARKS

Extraoral traction has proved to be a dependable method of Class II correction for over 100 years, and this treatment adjunct is used with varying frequency worldwide. The major "Achilles heel" of this method, as with other methods that involve participation of the patient in the treatment process, is patient cooperation. When the correct type of extraoral traction appliance is prescribed for a patient who is compliant, effective and efficient treatment is the result. In non-cooperative patients, however, alternative methods of Class II correction are indicated.

REFERENCES CITED

1. Bernstein M, Rosol ML, Jr, Gianelly AA. A biometric study of orthopedically directed treatment of Class II malocclusion. Am J Orthod 1976;70:683–689.
2. Kingsley NW. Report of discussion of the Society of Dental Surgeons of the City of New York. Dent Cosmos 1866; 8:90–91.
3. Kingsley NW. A treatise on oral deformities as a branch of mechanical surgery. New York: D Appleton, 1880.
4. Angle EH. The Angle system of regulation and retention of the teeth and treatment of fractures of the maxillae. Philadelphia: SS White, 1897.
5. Oppenheim A. Biologic orthodontic therapy and reality. Angle Orthod 1936;6:153–183.
6. Kloehn SJ. Guiding alveolar growth and eruption of teeth to reduce treatment time and produce a more balanced denture and face. Angle Orthod 1947;17:10–23.
7. Kloehn SJ. Orthodontics—force or persuasion. Angle Orthod 1953;23:56–65.
8. Kloehn SJ. Evaluation of cervical anchorage force in treatment. Angle Orthod 1961;31:91–104.

9. Kloehn JS. Personal communication, 2000.
10. Oppenheim A. A possibility for physiologic orthodontic movement. Am J Orthod 1944;30:345-368.
11. Hubbard GW, Nanda RS, Currier GF. A cephalometric evaluation of nonextraction cervical headgear treatment in Class II malocclusions. Angle Orthod 1994;64:359-370.
12. Samuels RH, Evans SM, Wigglesworth SW. Safety catch for a Kloehn facebow. J Clin Orthod 1993;27:138-141.
13. Stafford GD, Caputo AA, Turley PK. Characteristics of headgear release mechanisms: Safety implications. Angle Orthod 1998;68:319-326.
14. Seel D. Extra oral hazards of extra oral traction. Br J Orthod 1980;7:53.
15. Booth-Mason S, Birnie D. Penetrating eye injury from orthodontic headgear—a case report. Eur J Orthod 1988;10:111-114.
16. Samuels RH, Jones ML. Orthodontic facebow injuries and safety equipment. Eur J Orthod 1994;16:385-94.
17. Holland GN, Wallace DA, Mondino BJ, Cole SH, Ryan SJ. Severe ocular injuries form orthodontic headgear. Arch Opthamol 1985;103:649-651.
18. Tweed CH. Clinical orthodontics. St Louis: CV Mosby, 1966.
19. Alexander RG. Personal communication, 2000.
20. Hickham JH. Personal communication, 2000.
21. Cetlin NM, Ten Hoeve A. Nonextraction treatment. J Clin Orthod 1983;17:396-413.
22. Cetlin NM, Spena R, Vanarsdall RL, Jr. Nonextraction treatment. In: Graber TM, Vanarsdall RL, Jr, eds. Orthodontics: Current principles and practices. St Louis: CV Mosby, 2000.
23. Alexander RG. The vari-simplex discipline. Part 1. Concept and appliance design. J Clin Orthod 1983;17:380-92.
24. Alexander RG. The vari-simplex discipline. Part 2. Nonextraction treatment. J Clin Orthod 1983;17:474-82.
25. McNamara JA, Jr, Peterson JE, Jr, Alexander RG. Three-dimensional diagnosis and management of Class II malocclusion in the mixed dentition. Semin Orthod 1996;2:114-137.
26. Alexander RG. The Alexander discipline: Contemporary concepts and philosophies. Glendora: Ormco Corp, 1986.
27. Interlandi S. Ortodontia: Basespara a iniciação. Sao Paulo: Artes Medicas, 1994.
28. Hickham JH. Directional edgewise orthodontic approach. J Clin Orthod 1974;8:617-33.
29. Hickham JH. Directional forces revisited. J Clin Orthod 1986;20:626-637.
30. Tweed CH. A philosophy of orthodontic treatment. Am J Orthod Oral Surg 1945;31:74-103.
31. Merrifield LL, Cross JJ. Directional forces. Am J Orthod 1970;57:435-464.
32. Vaden JL, Dale JG, Klontz HA. The Tweed-Merrifield edgewise appliance: Philosophy, diagnosis, and treatment. In: Graber TM, Vanarsdall RL, Jr, eds. Orthodontics: Current principles and practices. St Louis: CV Mosby, 2000.
33. Merrifield LL. Edgewise sequential directional force technology. J Charles Tweed Found 1986;14:22-37.
34. Klontz HA. Tweed-Merrifield sequential directional force treatment. Semin Orthod 1996;2:254-267.
35. Holdaway R. Changes in relationship of points A and B during orthodontic treatment. Am J Orthod 1956;42:176-193.
36. Klein PL. An evaluation of cervical traction on the maxilla and the upper first permanent molar. Angle Orthod 1957;27:61-68.
37. Moore AW. Orthodontic treatment factors in Class II malocclusion. Am J Orthod 1959;45:323-352.
38. Sandusky WS. The cephalometric evaluation of the effects of the Kloehn type of cervical traction used as an auxiliary with the edgewise mechanism following Tweed's principles for correction of Class II division 1 malocclusion. Am J Orthod 1965;51:262-287.
39. Ringenberg QM, Butts WC. A controlled cephalometric evaluation of single-arch cervical traction therapy. Am J Orthod 1970;57:179-185.
40. Wieslander L, Buck DL. Physiologic recovery after cervical traction therapy. Am J Orthod 1974;66:294-301.
41. Mills CM, Holman RG, Graber TM. Heavy intermittent cervical traction in Class II treatment: a longitudinal cephalometric assessment. Am J Orthod 1978;74:361-79.
42. Cangialosi TJ, Meistrell ME, Jr, Leung MA, Ko JY. A cephalometric appraisal of edgewise Class II nonextraction treatment with extraoral force. Am J Orthod Dentofac Orthop 1988;93:315-324.
43. Closson DA. Extraoral anchorage, its indications, use and application. Am J Orthod 1950;36:265-280.
44. Gould E. Mechanical principles in extraoral anchorage. Am J Orthod 1957;43:319-333.
45. Parker WS. A technique for treatment with cervical gear. Angle Orthod 1958;28:198-209.
46. Poulton DR. Changes in Class II malocclusion with and without occipital headgear therapy. Angle Orthod 1959;29:234-250.
47. Nelson BG. Extraoral anchorage in the treatment of Class II division 1 malocclusions—its possibilities and limitations. Angle Orthod 1953;23:121-133.
48. Graber TM. Extra-oral force—facts and fallacies. Am J Orthod 1955;41:490-505.
49. King EW. Cervical anchorage in Class II division 1 treatment, a cephalometric appraisal. Angle Orthod 1957;27:98-104.
50. Ricketts RM. The influence of orthodontic treatment on facial growth and development. Angle Orthod 1960;30:103-133.
51. Poulton DR. The influence of extraoral traction. Am J Orthod 1967;53:8-18.
52. Epstein W. Analysis of change in molar relationships by means of extraoral anchorage (head-cap) in treatment of malocclusion. Angle Orthod 1948;18:63-70.
53. Graber TM. Appliances at the crossroads. Am J Orthod 1956;42:683-701.
54. Newcomb MR. Some observations on extraoral treatment. Angle Orthod 1958;28:131-148.
55. Wieslander L. The effect of orthodontic treatment on the concurrent development of the craniofacial complex. Am J Orthod 1963;62:15-27.
56. Funk AC. Mandibular response to headgear therapy and its clinical significance. Am J Orthod 1967;53:182-216.
57. Melsen B, Enemark H. Effect of cervical anchorage studied by the implant method. Trans Europ Orthod Soc 1969;45:435-447.
58. Cangialosi TJ, Meistrell ME, Jr. A cephalometric evaluation of hard- and soft-tissue changes during the third stage of Begg treatment. Am J Orthod 1982;81:124-129.

59. Hanes RA. Bony profile changes resulting from cervical traction compared to those resulting from intermaxillary elastics. Am J Orthod 1959;45:353–364.
60. Mays RA. A cephalometric comparison of two types of extraoral appliance used with the edgewise mechanism. Am J Orthod 1969;55:195–196.
61. Barton JJ. High-pull headgear versus cervical traction: a cephalometric comparison. Am J Orthod 1972;62:517–29.
62. Brown P. A cephalometric evaluation of high-pull molar headgear and face-bow neck strap therapy. Am J Orthod 1978;74:621–632.
63. Björk A. The use of metallic implants in the study of facial growth in children: Method and application. Am J Phys Anthrop 1968;29:243–254.
64. Schudy F. Vertical growth versus anteroposterior growth as related to function and treatment. Angle Orthod 1964;34:75-93.
65. Schudy FF. The rotation of the mandible resulting from growth: its implications in orthodontic treatment. Angle Orthod 1965;35:36–50.
66. Salzmann JA. Limitations of roentgenographic cephalometrics. Am J Orthod 1964;50:169–188.
67. Baumrind S. Facial changes associated with the use of headgear. In: Cook JT, ed. Transactions of the Third International Orthodontic Congress. London: Staples, 1975.
68. Baumrind S, Molthen R, West EE, Miller DM. Mandibular plane changes during maxillary retraction. Am J Orthod 1978;74:32–40.
69. Boecler PR, Riolo ML, Keeling SD, TenHave TR. Skeletal changes associated with extraoral appliance therapy: an evaluation of 200 consecutively treated cases. Angle Orthod 1989;59:263–270.
70. Riolo ML, Moyers RE, McNamara JA, Jr, Hunter WS. An atlas of craniofacial growth: Cephalometric standards from The University School Growth Study, The University of Michigan. Ann Arbor: Monograph 2, Craniofacial Growth Series, Center for Human Growth and Development, The University of Michigan, 1974.
71. Ghafari J, Jacobsson-Hunt U, Markowitz DL, Shofer FS, Laster LL. Changes of arch width in the early treatment of Class II, division 1 malocclusions. Am J Orthod Dentofac Orthop 1994;106:496–502.
72. Meach CL. A cephalometric comparison of bony profile changes in Class II, division 1 patients treated with extraoral force and functional jaw orthopedics. Am J Orthod 1966;52:353–70.
73. Derringer K. A cephalometric study to compare the effects of cervical traction and Andresen therapy in the treatment of Class II division 1 malocclusion. Part 1—Skeletal changes. Br J Orthod 1990;17:33–46.
74. Derringer K. A cephalometric study to compare the effects of cervical traction and Andresen therapy in the treatment of Class II division 1 malocclusion. Part 2—Dentoalveolar changes. Br J Orthod 1990;17:89–99.
75. Righellis EG. Treatment effects of Fränkel, activator and extraoral traction appliances. Angle Orthod 1983;53:107–121.
76. Creekmore TD, Radney LJ. Fränkel appliance therapy: orthopedic or orthodontic? Am J Orthod 1983;83:89–108.
77. Battagel JM. The relationship between hard and soft tissue changes following treatment of Class II division 1 malocclusions using Edgewise and Fränkel appliance techniques. Eur J Orthod 1990;12:154–165.
78. Gianelly AA, Arena SA, Bernstein L. A comparison of Class II treatment changes noted with the light wire, edgewise, and Fränkel appliances. Am J Orthod 1986;86:269–276.
79. Fränkel R, Fränkel C. Orofacial orthopedics with the function regulator. Munich: S Karger, 1989.
80. Falck F. Kephalometrische Längsschnittuntersuchung über Behandlungsergebnisse der mandibulären Retrognathie mit Funktionsreglen im Vergleich zu einer Lontrollgruppe. Berlin: Med Dissertation, 1985.
81. Gebeck TR, Merrifield LL. Orthodontic diagnosis and treatment analysis—concepts and values. Part I. Am J Orthod Dentofac Orthop 1995;107:434–443.
82. Gebeck TR, Merrifield LL. Orthodontic diagnosis and treatment analysis—concepts and values: Part II. Am J Orthod Dentofac Orthop 1995;107:541–547.
83. Jenkins D. A cephalometric evaluation of early headgear therapy in the correction of Class II, division 1 malocclusion. St Louis: Unpublished Master's thesis, Department of Orthodontics, St Louis Univ, 1988.
84. Baumrind S, Korn EL, Molthen R, West EE. Changes in facial dimensions associated with the use of forces to retract the maxilla. Am J Orthod 1981;80:17–30.
85. Baumrind S, Korn EL, Isaacson RJ, West EE, Molthen R. Quantitative analysis of the orthodontic and orthopedic effects of maxillary traction. Am J Orthod 1983;84:384–98.
86. Tulloch JFC, Proffit WR, Phillips C. Influences on the outcome of early treatment for Class II malocclusion. Am J Orthod Dentofac Orthop 1997;111:533–542.
87. Chu JW. A comparison of two non-extraction Class II treatment strategies. Ann Arbor: Unpublished Master's thesis, Department of Orthodontics and Pediatric Dentistry, The University of Michigan, 1997.
88. Melsen B. Effects of cervical anchorage during and after treatment: An implant study. Am J Orthod 1978;73:526–40.
89. Glenn G, Sinclair PM, Alexander RG. Nonextraction orthodontic therapy: posttreatment dental and skeletal stability. Am J Orthod Dentofac Orthop 1987;92:321–328.
90. Elms TN, Buschang PH, Alexander RG. Long-term stability of Class II, Division 1, nonextraction cervical face-bow therapy: I. Model analysis. Am J Orthod Dentofac Orthop 1996;109:271–276.
91. Elms TN, Buschang PH, Alexander RG. Long-term stability of Class II, Division 1, nonextraction cervical face-bow therapy: II. Cephalometric analysis. Am J Orthod Dentofac Orthop 1996;109:386–392.

Chapter 22

THE FACIAL MASK

With Lorenzo Franchi and Tiziano Baccetti

Of all the options available for the treatment of Class III malocclusion in children, the orthopedic facial mask (Fig. 22-1) may provide the greatest opportunity to correct this problem, whether identified during the late deciduous or early transitional dentition. As the craniofacial complex in juveniles still is malleable, significant changes in all three planes of space may be produced by this type of therapy, especially when combined with rapid maxillary expansion. Limited success has been reported in some young permanent dentition patients as well.

Although the facial mask was developed over 100 years ago,[1-3] this approach was used infrequently until reintroduced by Delaire[4-6] in the late 1960s for the treatment of cleft patients. Interest in the facial mask in the United States later was stimulated by Petit[7-9] through his studies conducted at Baylor University.

As discussed in detail in Chapter 6, there is no question that a wide variety of skeletal and dental configurations can lead to the clinical manifestation of a Class III malocclusion. From a theoretical perspective, it would seem appropriate to select a treatment modality that would fit the needs of an individual (*e.g.*, the FR-3 of Fränkel in patients with maxillary skeletal retrusion, a chin cup in patients with mandibular prognathism). The nature of the treatment response produced by the facial mask (Fig. 22-2) and the age at which this therapy is initiated, however, indicate the appropriateness of this appliance in a wide range of Class III problems.

TREATMENT EFFECTS PRODUCED BY FACIAL MASK THERAPY

Even though this methodology has been available for over a century, surprisingly few studies have dealt with the treatment effects produced with the facial mask. Most studies dealing with facial mask therapy published before the last decade have been anecdotal in nature.[8,10-18] During the last few years, however, a number of cephalometric studies have analyzed the treatment outcome of facial mask therapy in larger samples.[19-28] It appears that the facial mask, especially when combined with a maxillary anchorage unit (*e.g.*, bonded acrylic splint expander) can produce one or more of the following treatment effects:

1. Correction of CO-CR discrepancy. This correction is immediate and usually is observed in pseudo-Class III patients.
2. Maxillary skeletal protraction. Usually 1–3 mm of forward movement of the maxilla is observed.
3. Forward movement of the maxillary dentition.
4. Lingual tipping of the lower incisors. This tipping often occurs as a pre-existing anterior crossbite is being corrected.
5. Backward rotation of the mandible in relation to the cranial base. In instances in which the patient begins treatment with a short or neutral lower an-

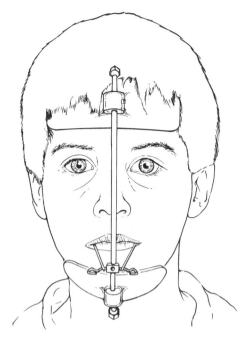

Figure 22-1. Frontal view of the Petit facial mask. Note that the elastics converge on and attach to the crossbow immediately adjacent to the central support bar. The positions of the forehead and chin pads are adjustable.

duces a significant forward displacement of the maxillary tuberosity from the pterygoid process of the sphenoid bone only when treatment is performed in the early mixed dentition. This finding supports, from a clinical perspective, the observations of Melsen and Melsen[29] on human autopsy material. According to these investigators, disarticulation of the palatal bone from the pterygoid process is possible only on skulls representing the infantile and juvenile (early mixed dentition) periods. Attempted disarticulation in the late juvenile (late mixed dentition) and adolescent periods always is accompanied by fracture of the heavily interdigitated osseous surfaces.

Figure 22-3 illustrates the anatomy of the pterygomaxillary suture in dry skulls belonging to a 6-year-old (early mixed dentition) subject and to a 12-year-old (late mixed dentition) subject, respectively. There is a dramatic difference in the appearance of the sutures that can be recognized and appreciated easily.

In the studies conducted by our group,[25,28,30] the mean annualized forward growth of the maxilla registered at Point A was about 1 mm in both early and late control groups with untreated Class III malocclusion, as reported in Chapter 6. In the early-treated group, the annual increment in sagittal maxillary growth at Point A

terior facial height, this change obviously is advantageous. In instances in which a patient has a long lower anterior facial height at the beginning of treatment, this treatment effect may be undesirable.

6. Favorable changes in mandibular growth, at least over the short-term. Condylar growth in a forward direction can be associated with reduced increments in mandibular length.[25,28]

TREATMENT TIMING FOR ORTHOPEDIC FACIAL MASK THERAPY

In recent cephalometric and morphometric studies,[25,28] we have seen evidence that treatment of Class III malocclusion with the facial mask in the early mixed dentition results in more favorable craniofacial changes than treatment beginning in the late mixed dentition. The most notable change is the forward displacement of maxillary structures that is achieved as an outcome of early treatment, whereas patients treated in the late mixed dentition do not show any significant improvement in maxillary growth with respect to matched untreated Class III controls.

Additionally, posteroanterior orthopedic traction in-

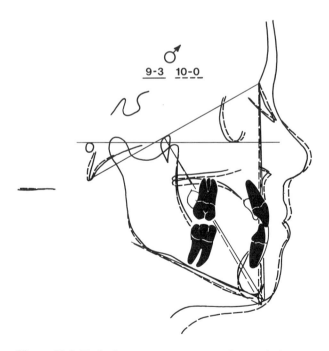

Figure 22-2. Typical treatment response observed after seven months of orthopedic facial mask therapy. Superimposition of the two tracings is along the basion-nasion line at the pterygomaxillary fissure. Note the changes in both hard tissue and soft tissue facial contours.

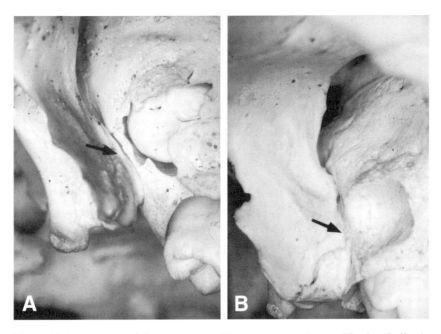

Figure 22-3. Anatomy of the pterygomaxillary suture as observed in dry skulls. *A*, 6-year-old subject in the early mixed dentition. *B*, 12-year-old subject in the late mixed dentition.

was four times greater (4.1 mm) than in corresponding controls, whereas the late-treated group showed no statistically significant increments, which were only two times greater (2.1 mm) than in corresponding controls.

As for the effects of facial mask therapy on the mandible, mandibular length (Co-Gn) showed significantly smaller increments only in the early-treated group when compared to controls, whereas overall mandibular dimensions were not affected significantly by treatment in the treated late-mixed dentition group. In both early and late untreated groups, the increment in the Co-Gn measurement was about 4.5 mm per year. In the group treated in the late mixed dentition, the increment was about 3.5 mm per year, whereas in the early-treated group the increment was only 2 mm per year. The favorable change in total mandibular length was associated with a more upward and forward direction of condylar growth in the early-treated subjects. According to Lavergne and Gasson,[31] this mechanism, namely "anterior morphogenetic rotation" of the mandible, is a biological process that is able to dissipate excess of mandibular growth relative to the maxilla, and it has been reported as a major effect of early functional treatment of Class III malocclusion.[32]

All these observations suggest that the early mixed dentition phase of dental development is the most appropriate period to perform treatment of Class III malocclusion with the orthopedic facial mask. A bonded maxillary expander can be used in conjunction with the facial mask to further enhance the positive effect of early treatment.

An analysis of the skeletal changes that occur in the post-treatment period of facial mask therapy is an issue of further interest when performing an appraisal of ideal treatment timing. Regardless of the retention protocol following active orthopedic treatment of Class III skeletal disharmony, most clinical studies[20,21,33–35] seem to agree on the observation that maxillary and mandibular growth rates are similar in treated and untreated Class III subjects in the post-protraction period. In particular, we have found that a Class III craniofacial growth pattern is re-established within one year of post-treatment observation in absence of any retention appliance.[35] When considering combined outcomes of both active treatment and post-treatment periods, however, orthopedic treatment of Class III malocclusion in the early mixed dentition still appears to induce more favorable overall craniofacial changes than treatment in the late mixed dentition.

COMPONENTS OF ORTHOPEDIC FACIAL MASK THERAPY

The standard technique involves a facial mask, a bonded maxillary expansion splint, and heavy elastics.

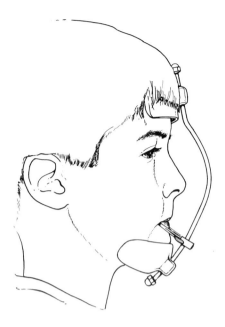

Figure 22-4. The lateral view of the orthopedic facial mask. Note the downward direction of pull of the elastics. The direction of pull can be adjusted by raising or lowering the crossbar; however, the elastics must not interfere with the function of the lips.

The Facial Mask

The individual most responsible for reviving interest in this orthopedic technique is Jean Delaire of Nantes, France.[4-6] Delaire's approach involves applying traction to the maxillary sutures, while reciprocally pushing on the mandible and the forehead through the anchorage provided by the facial mask. This approach provides a repositioning of the bones of the craniofacial complex to a greater extent than that which could be carried out by traditional orthodontic methods. Other clinicians, including Irie and Nakamura,[12] also have used this basic treatment technique.

Major changes in facial mask design have been prompted by Henri Petit, formerly of Baylor Dental College and now of Paris.[7-9,36] Petit has advocated the use of the facial mask for a relatively short period (4-6 months); however, during this treatment period very heavy forces are applied to the craniofacial complex. The Petit facial mask originally was constructed on a patient-by-patient basis, using 0.25″ round lengths of stainless steel, to which pads for the forehead and chin were attached. This initial approach was not practical on a routine basis, because several hours were required to fabricate each appliance. Later, the design of the facial mask was simplified and made available commercially (Great Lakes Orthodontic Products, Tonawanda NY; Ormco Corp., Orange CA). This latter design was relatively simple in that it contained a single midline rod connected to a chin pad and forehead pad (Figs. 22-1 and 22-4). In addition, heavy elastics were connected to an adjustable crossbow.

The current version of the Petit facial mask (Fig. 22-5) is made of two pads that contact the soft tissue in the forehead and chin regions. The pads are made from acrylic and are lined with soft closed-cell foam that is non-absorbent, easily cleaned, and replaceable. The pads are connected by a midline framework made from a round, contoured length of .25″ stainless steel with acorn nuts on each end. The positions of the pads are adjustable through the loosening and tightening of a setscrew. The midline framework also can be bent to conform better to the outline of the face of the individual patient (Fig. 22-4).

In the center of the midline framework is a crossbar made from 0.075″ stainless steel that is secured to the main framework by a setscrew, thus allowing the position of the crossbar to be adjusted vertically. The ends of the crossbar are contoured for patient safety (Fig. 22-1).

Bonded Maxillary Splint

The second component of this appliance system is the maxillary splint (Figs. 22-6 and 22-7), an acrylic and wire maxillary expansion appliance that is bonded to

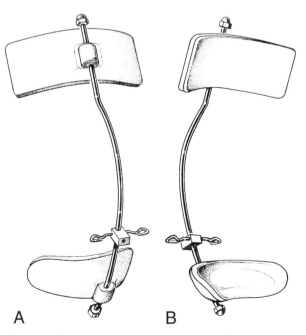

Figure 22-5. The orthopedic facial mask of Petit. *A*, Anterior oblique view. *B*, Posterior oblique view.

FACIAL MASK

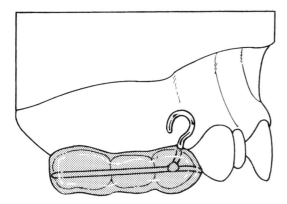

Figure 22-6. Lateral view of a bonded maxillary expansion appliance used in a mixed-dentition patient. Note the position of the facial mask hooks.

the posterior dentition. This splint is of the same design as the acrylic splint expander described elsewhere in this text. Facial mask hooks are added to the appliance.

In mixed dentition patients, the splint usually covers the first and second deciduous molars and the permanent first molars. The hooks for the elastics arise at the anterior aspect of the appliance in the region of the maxillary first deciduous molar (Fig. 22-6). In instances in which only a deciduous dentition is present, the splint can be constructed so that the maxillary canines as well as the deciduous molars are included. In these instances, the hooks for the elastic are fabricated adjacent to the maxillary deciduous canines.

If a bonded maxillary splint is used in patients in the late mixed or early permanent dentition, modification of the appliance design often is necessary. If permanent second molars are erupted, it is necessary to place an occlusal rest against these teeth to prevent supraeruption of these teeth during appliance wear. The framework should not be extended to encompass the second molars posteriorly because of the danger of opening the bite due to placement of the acrylic on the occlusal surfaces of the maxillary second molars.

Modifications also can be made in the position of the facial mask hooks, depending on the direction of force desired. If a more downward direction of force on the maxilla is desired, the facial mask hooks are placed at varying heights within the maxillary vestibule. If a more horizontal pull is desired, the hooks are placed adjacent to the acrylic near the occlusal surface. The limiting factor with regard to the direction of pull is the relative positions of the upper and lower lip.

The maxillary splint is made of a framework of .045" round stainless steel wire to which an expansion screw has been soldered. The hooks for elastics and any occlusal rests are made from the same size wire. A sheet of 3 mm thick splint Biocryl™ is heated and adapted to the framework and associated teeth using a Biostar™ thermal pressure machine (Great Lakes Orthodontic Products, Tonawanda NY). The use of splint Biocryl™ less than 3 mm thick can lead to problems in occlusal decalcification in some patients because of the abrasion of the appliance by the opposing dentition and the subsequent contact of tissue fluids with the occlusal surfaces of the involved teeth. In instances of severe bruxism, a lower invisible retainer can be used at night to reduce the occlusal abrasion due to bruxism.

The maxillary splint also can be fabricated using methyl methacrylate orthodontic resin and a "salt and pepper" application method, but this fabrication technique is not recommended. One disadvantage of using cold cure acrylic is that often a flat plane is created on the occlusal surface of the appliance, making mastication initially difficult. The use of a Biostar™ allows for the general approximation of the original occlusal configuration in the Biocryl™. More importantly, splints made from Biocryl™ also are generally easier to remove than are splints made from cold-cure acrylic, because the Biocryl™ tends to be more flexible and resilient.

Midfacial orthopedic expansion, in itself, has been shown to be beneficial in the treatment of certain types of Class III malocclusion. Oppenheim[10] was one of the first to discuss this possibility. Haas[37–39] has demonstrated that rapid palatal expansion can produce a slightly forward movement of Point A and a slightly downward and forward movement of the maxilla, and Dellinger[40] has shown this phenomenon in non-human primates. Haas also has shown that increased maxillary movement can be enhanced by the use of Class III traction from a chin cup to the distal aspect of the palatal appliance.[38]

Within the context of facial mask therapy, the presumed effect of such expansion is to disrupt the maxil-

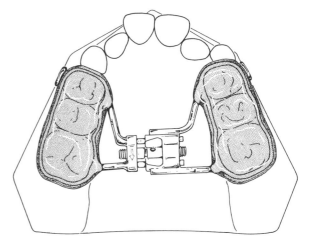

Figure 22-7. Occlusal view of the bonded rapid palatal expansion appliance used on a mixed-dentition patient.

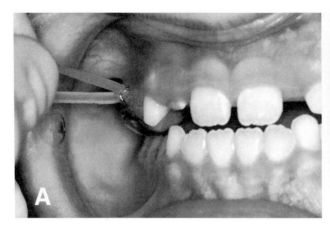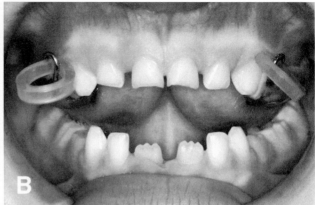

Figure 22-8. Attachment of elastics to the hooks on the bonded expander. *A*, Oblique frontal view. *B*, Frontal view.

lary sutural system, thus enhancing the effect of the orthopedic facial mask by making sutural adjustments occur more readily. The bite-opening effect of the maxillary splint also may reduce the tendency toward extrusion of posterior teeth, which has been observed using the banded design of the appliance.[41] In controlled clinical trials, however, the bonded RME appliance has not yet been shown to be superior to other means of intraoral anchorage.[19-24,33]

Elastic Traction

The facial mask is secured to the face by stretching elastics from the hooks on the maxillary splint to the crossbow of the facial mask (Fig. 22-8). Heavy forces are generated, usually with a sequence of elastics, beginning with 8 oz. of force being generated by 1/2" elastics and ultimately resulting in the use of 14 oz. 5/16" elastics.[8] Lighter forces are used during the break-in period, but forces increase as the patient adjusts to the appliance.

CLINICAL MANAGEMENT OF THE FACIAL MASK

The procedures used in bonding the maxillary splint are the same as those described in detail in Chapter 13 that concerned the bonding of the acrylic splint rapid maxillary expansion appliance. These procedures will be summarized below. The overall clinical management of this treatment approach has been described previously in the orthodontic literature.[14]

Impressions

A standard aluminum tray can be used effectively when making an impression for the maxillary splint. The impression should be checked for proper reproduction of the teeth and associated soft tissue. The work models then are poured and trimmed.

Splint Fabrication and Delivery

The wire framework is formed from .045" round stainless steel wire that is contoured to the posterior teeth. Hooks facing posteriorly are soldered to the framework in the desired position (Fig. 22-6). Usually the hooks attach to the framework in the region of the maxillary first deciduous molar or the deciduous canine. A Hyrax-type expansion screw (Leone Co., Florence, Italy) is placed in the middle of the palate and soldered to the base wire. Then a sheet of splint Biocryl™ is softened and formed over the framework and the work model using a Biostar™. After cooling, the appliance is trimmed and polished with the acrylic extending to the gingival margins of the involved teeth. The splint is bonded into place, following the protocol described in a systematic fashion in Chapter 13.

At the time of appliance placement, the clinician, using dental floss, should check to make sure that the facial mask hooks are free from excessive bonding agent. As the bonding agent is transparent, excess bonding material within the hooks occasionally is not detected at the time of bonding and only is discovered on the day that the elastics are first attached to the appliance. The hooks should be free of excessive bonding material and should not contact the underlying gingival tissue.

Activation of the Splint

The patient is instructed to turn the midline expansion screw of the appliance once per day, generally before bedtime. In the majority of Class III individuals for whom the use of an orthopedic facial mask is indicated,

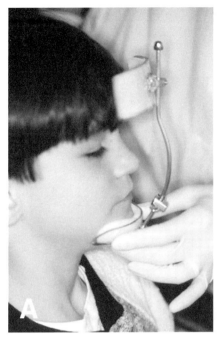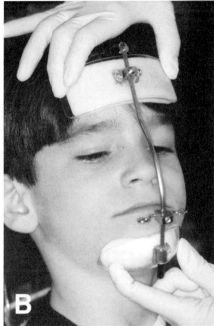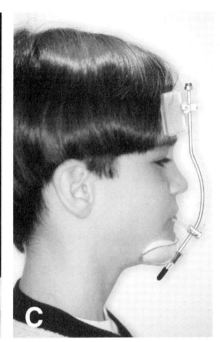

Figure 22-9. Fitting the facial mask. *A*, The mask should be placed first on the chin to check the shape of the center support bar. If the forehead pad lies away from the forehead, the center support should be adjusted (see Figure 22-10). *B*, The forehead pad now lies against the forehead without the edge of the chin cup impinging on the soft tissue of the chin. *C*, Proper fit of the facial mask after adjustment.

some maxillary expansion is beneficial. In such instances, the maxillary splint is expanded until the desired change in the transverse dimension is achieved. In instances in which no transverse change is necessary, the maxillary splint still is activated, usually once a day for eight to ten days to produce a disruption in the sutural system that in some patients may facilitate the action of the facial mask.

In borderline cases, the placement and expansion of the bonded RME appliance and the associated change in the vertical and transverse dimension may produce the desired change in the occlusal relationship, thus either eliminating the need for facial mask wear entirely, or allowing the patient to wear the mask only after school and during nighttime hours.

Delivery of the Facial Mask

The facial mask usually is delivered two to six weeks after placement of the splint. The current version of the Petit facial mask is available in two sizes and can be adjusted to fit the facial contours of most patients. When delivering the facial mask, the appliance first is placed on the chin of the patient (Fig. 22-9*A*), and the position of the forehead pad is evaluated. The forehead pad lies away from the forehead when the chin cup fits the chin in a balanced fashion. Thus, some adjustment must be made in the contour of the central support bar, and this adjustment can be made by way of strong hand pressure (Figs. 22-9*B* and 22-10).

The position of the forehead pad is adjusted vertically by loosening the setscrew holding the forehead pad to the center support wire. Then the forehead pad can be centered between the eyebrows and the hairline (Fig. 22-9*B*).

The position of the crossbar is adjusted in the vertical dimension in a similar manner by loosening the setscrew. The final position of the crossbar is determined first by placing the appropriate elastic intraorally on the hooks of the maxillary splint (Fig. 22-8). The elastics are stretched anteriorly and are attached to the crossbar near the midline, not on the hooks at the lateral aspects of the crossbar, as is intuitive. The vertical position of the crossbar then is adjusted so that the elastic extends anteriorly from the appliance, crossing at the point of contact of the upper and lower lip (Fig. 22-9*C*). Any impingement on upper or lower lip function should be avoided. Care must be taken that the elastics do not cause irritation to the corners of the mouth.

Aggressive customizing of the facial mask is recommended in those instances in which the center support bar is too long for the size of the patient's face. If the center support extends too far superiorly or inferiorly, a pipe cutter (purchased at a local hardware store; Fig.

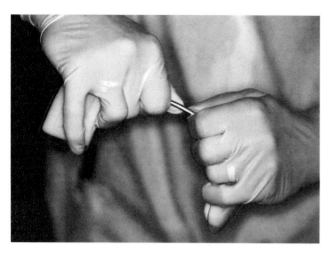

Figure 22-10. Adjustment of the center support bar by way of heavy hand pressure.

22-11) can be used to shorten the length of the center support. By doing so, the overall height of the facemask is minimized.

Sequential Use of Elastics

At the time of the delivery of the facial mask, the use of bilateral 3/8″, 8 oz. elastics (*e.g.*, Tiger™ elastics, Ormco

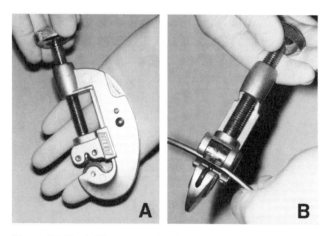

Figure 22-11. *A*, Pipe cutter. *B*, Tightening the pipe cutter can lead to the shortening of the center support bar.

Corp., Orange CA) for the first two weeks is recommended. After that time, the force on the mask is increased by using 1/2″, 14 oz. elastics (*e.g.*, Whale™ elastics). Maximum force is delivered by 5/16″ elastics (*e.g.*, Walrus™ elastics) that are rated at 14 oz. of force. If a patient develops redness or other problems with the soft tissue, the amount of elastic force can be lessened or the duration of appliance wear can be reduced.

Care should be taken to make sure that excess pressure is not applied to the soft tissue. Such heavy pressure can lead to reddening and irritation of the skin and to gingival problems intraorally. Figure 22-12 shows a patient with two different problems concerning irritation of the soft tissue in the chin area. The irritation at the point of the chin indicates heavy contact of the chin cup against the skin. The curved line under the lower lip indicates that the superior border of the chin cup is impinging on the soft tissue. If this latter condition persists, stripping of the gingiva underlying the lower incisors may occur. The encroachment of the chin cup on the tissue under the lip may be corrected by adjusting the angle of the center support (Fig. 22-10). The irritation of the chin point may be improved by adding additional padding to the inside surface of the chin cup.

Optimally, the patient is instructed to wear the facial mask on a full-time basis, except during meals. Young (5–9 years old) patients usually can follow this regimen, particularly if the patient is told that full-time wear (including to school) will last only 4–6 months. In older patients, full-time wear may not be feasible. The appliance should be worn at all times except when the patient is in school or participating in contact sports. Some patients find the facial mask ideally is worn during the summer rather than during the school year, whereas other patients find the summer the most difficult time to wear

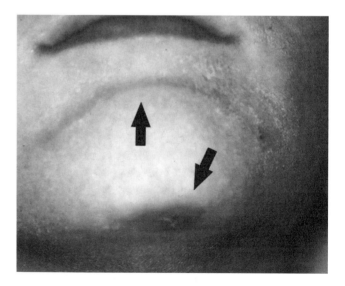

Figure 22-12. Chin irritation produced by a chin cup that does not fit correctly. The chin point irritation (inferior arrow) is due to excessive localized pressure from the chin cup. The line of irritation under the lip (superior arrow) is caused by pressure from the acrylic edge of the chin cup.

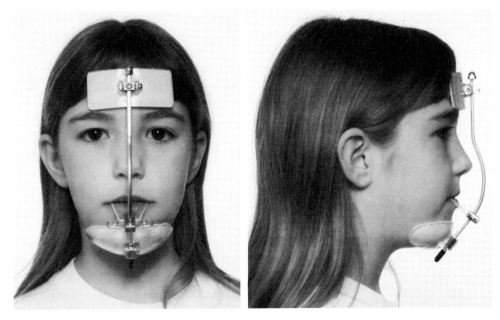

Figure 22-13. Proper fit of the facial mask after all adjustments have been made.

the appliance because of swimming, soccer, baseball, and other summer activities.

Patients must be instructed to maintain a high level of oral hygiene and to report immediately any indications that the bonded splint might become loosened in any area. The patient should be seen every four to eight weeks to check the condition of the splint and to evaluate hard and soft tissue changes. The proper fit of the facial mask after all adjustments have been made is illustrated in Figure 22-13.

Discontinuation of Treatment

One question that often arises concerns the indications for the discontinuance of treatment. The facial mask usually is worn until a positive overjet of 2–5 mm is achieved interincisally. Substantial vertical overlap (overbite) of the maxillary and mandibular incisors should have been achieved as well. At this time, part time or nighttime wear is recommended for an additional three to six month period. The maxillary splint is then removed, using anterior bracket-removing pliers with a sharp edge (*e.g.*, ETM 349 pliers, Ormco Corp., Orange CA). A removable palatal stabilization plate with ball clasps between the first and second deciduous molars is worn full time (Fig. 22-14).

Another viable option for retention after RME and facial mask therapy is represented by the removable mandibular retractor.[32] The appliance consists of a palatal plate with a labial arch that extends to the cervical edge of the mandibular incisors. In order to be activated, the labial arch should be placed 2 mm in front of the mandibular incisors when the mandible is forced into maximum retrusion. The intention is to have the labial arch work merely as a functional stop for the sagittal movement of the mandible. The plate may bear auxiliary devices such as expansion screws or springs for the proclination of the maxillary incisors, when required. The patient is instructed to wear the appliance on a full-time basis for the first six months of the retention period, and then appliance wearing is discontinued progressively.

In patients with initially severe skeletal imbalances and/or severe neuromuscular imbalances, the FR-3 appliance of Fränkel[42-44] should be worn as an active retainer following correction of the Class III relationship with the facial mask. A chin cup (see Chapter 6) can be worn as a retainer in patients with residual mandibular prognathism.

The facial mask should be discontinued immediately if the patient complains of any symptoms of temporomandibular (TM) disorders. Although rare, signs and symptoms of TM disorder have been observed in patients wearing the facial mask, and immediate discontinuance of the appliance usually results in a reversal of the symptomatology.

CONCLUDING REMARKS

Most clinical studies demonstrate that the optimal time to intervene in an early Class III patient is in the early mixed dentition, *e.g.* at the time of initial eruption of the maxillary central incisors. Usually the mandibular in-

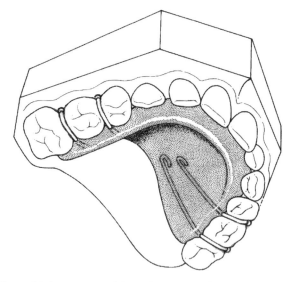

Figure 22-14. A removable maintenance plate with ball clasps between maxillary posterior teeth is worn full time after the facial mask is removed.

cisors have erupted as well. By timing facial mask therapy to coincide with the eruption of the maxillary incisors, a positive vertical and horizontal overlap of the permanent incisors can be achieved and maintained. It appears that the establishment of a positive overbite and overjet relationship perhaps is the most important factor in maintaining the Class III correction over the long-term.

As with all types of orthodontic treatment, not every Class III malocclusion can be intercepted and treated successfully. Obviously, the older the patient at the time of the onset of treatment and the more severe the malocclusion, the less is the likelihood of successful treatment without surgery. In addition, a strong family history of mandibular prognathism or other Class III problems lessens the prognosis for a stable outcome.

Further, a few dentoskeletal features already present at the start of treatment may have a role in predicting an unsuccessful treatment outcome in Class III malocclusion. These early features include excessive intermaxillary vertical relationships (skeletal open bite), posterior inclination of the mandibular condyle, and large mandibular intermolar width.[45]

In many of the mild to moderate and some rather severe Class III problems, however, this type of therapy produces a pronounced occlusal change within a relatively short period. When used with caution and with the appropriate disclaimers to the parents regarding the lack of guarantees of long-term stability, this type of treatment has proven extremely rewarding in a wide variety of Class III conditions.

It also must be noted that in approximately 50% of those patients in whom facial mask therapy is initiated in the mixed dentition, a second intervention is necessary before the placement of fixed appliances after the eruption of the permanent teeth has occurred. This type of treatment simply may involve the placement of a bonded or banded rapid maxillary expansion appliance. It also may require the reintroduction of facial mask therapy, either on a full-time or part-time basis. No guarantees should be given to the patient or the parents regarding the long-term outcome of this type of treatment program because of the varied etiologies of Class III malocclusion that include both hereditary and environmental factors.

This type of treatment provides a means of actively intervening in the patient with the developing Class III malocclusion. The results of this treatment are dramatic, usually occurring within a four to six month period, and if a positive vertical overlap of the maxillary and mandibular incisors is achieved, there is a reasonable chance of maintaining the corrected result during the transition to the permanent dentition.

REFERENCES CITED

1. Potpeschenigg R. Deutsche Viertel Jahrschrift für Zahnheilkunde,. Monthly Review of Dental Surgery III, 1974–1975 1885:464–465.
2. Jackson VH. Orthodontia and orthopedia of the face. Philadelphia: JB Lippincott, 1904.
3. Sutcliffe HW. Correction of a case of prognathism by the retraction of the mandible and the lower teeth. Trans Sixth Inter Congress, London, 1914.
4. Delaire J. Confection du masque orthopedique. Rev Stomat Paris 1971;72:579–584.
5. Delaire J, Verson P, Lumineau JP, Ghega-Negrea A, Talmant J, Boisson M. Quelques resultats des tractions extraorales a appui fronto-mentonnier dans le traitement orthopedique des maloformations maxillo mandibulaires de Class III et des sequelles osseuses des fente labio-maxillaires. Rev Stomat Paris 1972;73:633–642.
6. Delaire J. L'articulation fronto-maxillaire: Bases theoretiques et principles generaux d'application de forces extraorales postero-anterieures sur masque orthopedique. Rev Stomat Paris 1976;77:921–930.
7. Petit HP. Syndromes prognathiques: schemas de traitement "global" autour de masques faciaux. Rev Orthop Dento Faciale 1982;16:381–411.
8. Petit HP. Adaptation following accelerated facial mask therapy. In: McNamara JA, Jr, Ribbens KA, Howe RP, eds. Clinical alterations of the growing face. Ann Arbor: Monograph 14, Craniofacial Growth Series, Center for Human Growth and Development, The University of Michigan, 1983.
9. Petit H. Orthopadie et/ou orthodontie. Orthod Fr 1984; 55:527–533.
10. Oppenheim A. A possibility for physiologic orthodontic movement. Am J Orthod 1944;30:345–368.
11. Cozzani G. Extraoral traction and Class III treatment. Am J Orthod 1981;80:638–650.

12. Irie M, Nakamura S. Orthopedic approach to severe skeletal Class III malocclusion. Am J Orthod 1975;67: 377–392.
13. Cooke MS, Wreakes G. The face mask: a new form of reverse head-gear. Br J Orthod 1977;4:163–168.
14. McNamara JA, Jr. An orthopedic approach to the treatment of Class III malocclusion in young patients. J Clin Orthod 1987;21:598-608.
15. Roberts CA, Subtelny JD. Use of the face mask in the treatment of maxillary skeletal retrusion. Am J Orthod Dentofac Orthop 1988;93:388–394.
16. Turley PK. Orthopedic correction of Class III malocclusion with palatal expansion and custom protraction headgear. J Clin Orthod 1988;22:314–325.
17. Navarro CF, Arcoria C. Early management of maxillary dentofacial deficiency: three case reports. Compend Cont Educ Dent 1991;12:708–716.
18. Tanne K, Sakuda M. Biomechanical and clinical changes of the craniofacial complex from orthopedic maxillary protraction. Angle Orthod 1991;61:145–152.
19. Baik HS. Clinical results of the maxillary protraction in Korean children. Am J Orthod Dentofac Orthop 1995; 108:583–592.
20. Shanker S, Ngan P, Wade D, Beck M, Yiu C, Hagg U, Wei SH. Cephalometric A point changes during and after maxillary protraction and expansion. Am J Orthod Dentofac Orthop 1996;110:423–430.
21. Ngan P, Hagg U, Yiu C, Wei H. Treatment response and long-term dentofacial adaptations to maxillary expansion and protraction. Semin Orthod 1997;3:255–264.
22. Williams MD, Sarver DM, Sadowsky PL, Bradley E. Combined rapid maxillary expansion and protraction facemask in the treatment of Class III malocclusion in growing children: a prospective study. Semin Orthod 1997;3: 265–274.
23. Ngan P, Yiu C, Hu A, Hägg U, Wei SH, Gunel E. Cephalometric and occlusal changes following maxillary expansion and protraction. Eur J Orthod 1998;20:237–254.
24. Kapust AJ, Sinclair PM, Turley PK. Cephalometric effects of face mask/expansion therapy in Class III children: a comparison of three age groups. Am J Orthod Dentofac Orthop 1998;113:204–212.
25. Baccetti T, McGill JS, Franchi L, McNamara JA Jr, Tollaro I. Skeletal effects of early treatment of Class III malocclusion with maxillary expansion and face-mask therapy. Am J Orthod Dentofac Orthop 1998;113:333–343.
26. Pangrazio-Kulbersh V, Berger J, Kersten G. Effects of protraction mechanics on the midface. Am J Orthod Dentofac Orthop 1998;114:484–491.
27. da Silva Filho OG, Magro AC, Capelozza Filho L. Early treatment of the Class III malocclusion with rapid maxillary expansion and maxillary protraction. Am J Orthod Dentofac Orthop 1998;113:196–203.
28. Baccetti T, Franchi L. Updating cephalometrics through morphometrics: Thin-plate spline analysis of craniofacial growth/treatment changes. In: McNamara JA Jr, ed. Growth modification: What works, what doesn't, and why. Ann Arbor: Monograph No 35, Craniofacial Growth Series, Center for Human Growth and Development, The University of Michigan, 1999.
29. Melsen B, Melsen F. The postnatal development of the palatomaxillary region studied on human autopsy material. Am J Orthod 1982;82:329–342.
30. Franchi L, Baccetti T, McNamara JA Jr. Shape-coordinate analysis of skeletal changes induced by rapid maxillary expansion and facial mask therapy. Am J Orthod Dentofac Orthop 1998;114:418–442.
31. Lavergne J, Gasson N. Operational definitions of mandibular morphogenetic and positional rotations. Scand J Dent Res 1977;85:185–192.
32. Tollaro I, Baccetti T, Franchi L. Craniofacial changes induced by early functional treatment of Class III malocclusion. Am J Orthod Dentofac Orthop 1996;109: 310–318.
33. McGill JS, McNamara JA Jr. Treatment and post-treatment effects of rapid maxillary expansion and facial mask therapy. In: McNamara JA, Jr, ed. Growth modification: What works, what doesn't and why. Ann Arbor: Monograph 36, Craniofacial Growth Series, Center for Human Growth and Development, University of Michigan, 1999.
34. Macdonald KE, Kapust AJ, Turley PK. Cephalometric changes after correction of Class III malocclusion with maxillary expansion/facemask therapy. Am J Orthod Dentofac Orthop 1999;116:13–24.
35. Franchi L, Baccetti T, McNamara JA Jr. Treatment and post-treatment craniofacial changes following rapid maxillary expansion and facial mask therapy. Am J Orthod Dentofac Orthop 2000;118:404-413.
36. Petit H. Normalisation morphogenetique, apport de l'orthopadie. Orthod Fr 1991;62:549–557.
37. Haas AJ. Rapid expansion of the maxillary dental arch and nasal cavity by opening the mid-palatal suture. Angle Orthod 1961;31:73–90.
38. Haas AJ. Palatal expansion: just the beginning of dentofacial orthopedics. Am J Orthod 1970;57:219–255.
39. Haas AJ. Rapid palatal expansion: A recommended prerequisite to Class III treatment. Trans Eur Orthod Soc 1973:311–318.
40. Dellinger EL. A preliminary study of anterior maxillary displacement. Am J Orthod 1973;63:509–516.
41. Wertz RA. Skeletal and dental changes accompanying rapid midpalatal suture opening. Am J Orthod 1970;58: 41–66.
42. Fränkel R. Technik und Handhabung der Funktionsregler. Berlin: VEB Verlag Volk and Gesundheit, 1976.
43. Fränkel R, Fränkel C. Orofacial orthopedics with the function regulator. Munich: S Karger, 1989.
44. McNamara JA Jr, Huge SA. The functional regulator (FR-3) of Fränkel. Am J Orthod 1985;88:409–424.
45. Franchi L, Baccetti T, Tollaro I. Predictive variables for the outcome of early functional treatment of Class III malocclusion. Am J Orthod Dentofac Orthop 1997;112: 80–86.

Chapter 23

THE FUNCTION REGULATOR (FR-3) OF FRÄNKEL

The FR-3 version of the function regulator of Fränkel has been used during the deciduous, mixed, and early permanent dentitions to correct Class III malocclusion. The FR-3 can serve as a primary treatment appliance in Class III patients with mild, moderate, or severe dentoalveolar, skeletal, and/or neuromuscular imbalances. In addition, this appliance can function as a nighttime retainer following orthopedic facial mask therapy, as described in the previous chapter.

Of all methods of correcting Class III malocclusion, the FR-3 appliance perhaps is the most physiologic, in that this removable intraoral appliance not only affects the skeletal and dentoalveolar components of the malocclusion, but also the associated soft tissue. The vestibular shields and the upper labial pads redirect the forces generated against the maxilla by the perioral musculature and associated soft tissues to the mandible, producing treatment effects similar to that described previously for the facial mask. In comparison to the facial mask, the FR-3 is more "patient friendly," in that it is worn entirely intraorally, often improving the soft tissue profile of the patient with maxillary skeletal retrusion. The duration of treatment, however, generally is longer with the FR-3 (typically 12–24 months of full-time wear).

A primary indication for the FR-3 is the presence of maxillary skeletal retrusion. According to Fränkel,[1-3] the vestibular shields and upper labial pads function to counteract the forces of the surrounding musculature that restrict forward maxillary skeletal development and cause a retrusion in maxillary tooth position. Fränkel[4] also has stated that vestibular shields should stand away from the alveolar process of the maxilla, but they should fit closely to the tissue of the mandible, thus stimulating maxillary alveolar development and restricting mandibular alveolar development.

PARTS OF THE APPLIANCE

The FR-3 appliance (Figs. 23-1 and 23-2) is composed of wire and acrylic. As with the FR-2 appliance, the base of operation is the buccal and labial vestibule. In contrast to the FR-2, there is no need to prompt a forward functional position of the mandible, and thus in the FR-3 appliance there is no lingual shield.

Acrylic Components

The vestibular shields extend from the depth of the mandibular vestibule to the height of the maxillary vestibule. These shields act to remove the restrictive forces created by the buccinator and associated facial muscles against the lateral surface of the alveoli and buccal dentition (Fig. 23-3). These forces are transmitted through the appliance to the mandible, on which a backward and downward force is produced.

As with the FR-2, the FR-3 appliance also has labial pads. The labial pads are located above the maxillary incisors and lie about three millimeters anterior to the maxillary mucosa (Fig. 23-4). These pads function to eliminate the restrictive pressure of the upper lip on the

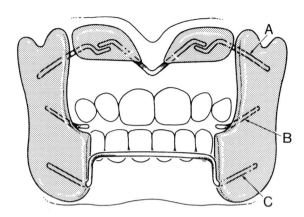

Figure 23-1. Schematic illustration of the FR-3 appliance of Fränkel, frontal view. The wire components of the appliance are: *A*, Upper labial wires (three-wire design). *B*, Upper lingual wires. *C*, Lower labial support wire. The vestibular shields allow for the passive expansion of the maxillary dental arch. (from McNamara and Huge.[8])

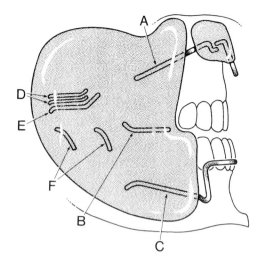

Figure 23-2. Schematic illustration of FR-3 appliance of Fränkel in lateral view. *A*, Upper labial wire. *B*, Upper lingual wire. *C*, Lower labial support wire. *D*, Upper occlusal rest. *E*, Palatal wire. *F*, Lower occlusal rest (from McNamara and Huge.[8])

presumably "underdeveloped" maxilla. The upper labial pads are larger and more extended than the corresponding lower pads of the FR-2 and are tolerated more easily by the patient, despite their greater size. According to Fränkel,[1,4] these pads also provide a stretching of the adjacent periosteum, stimulating bone apposition on the labial alveolar surface.

The upper labial pads of the FR-3 are fabricated in an inverted teardrop shape in sagittal view (Fig. 23-3). They should lie in the height of the vestibular sulcus with a contour parallel to that of the alveolus (Fig. 23-5*A*). If the pads are placed with a vertical orientation (Fig. 23-5*B*), the pads will lie too close to the alveolus and may produce gingival irritation or stripping during function.

External palpation should verify that the superior border of the upper labial pad is near the base of the nose (see Figure 23-12 later in the text). This placement of the appliance presumably causes a stretching of the upper lip as it is displaced anterior to its normal position by the upper labial pads. The upper labial pads transfer the force of the upper lip to the vestibular shields (Fig. 23-3). Because the vestibular shields lie in close approximation to the mandibular alveolus, the force of the associated tissue is transmitted through the appliance to the mandible. It can be hypothesized that this force either may restrict the growth of the mandible

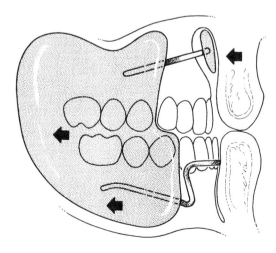

Figure 23-3. The method of action of the FR-3 as proposed by Fränkel.[2] The distracting forces of the upper lip are removed from the maxilla by the upper labial pads. The force of the upper lip is transmitted through the appliance to the mandible because of the close fit of the appliance to that arch.

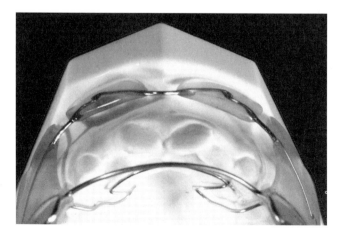

Fig. 23-4. Fit of the upper labial pads. The pads should lie three millimeters anterior to the maxillary alveolus.

THE FUNCTION REGULATOR (FR-3) OF FRÄNKEL

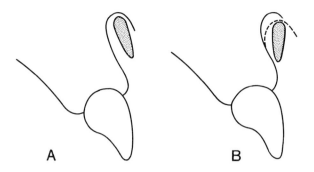

Figure 23-5. Fit of the upper labial pads. *A*, Correct fit. *B*, Incorrect fit. Notice that the upper labial pad is an inverted teardrop in sagittal view. The pad should lie three millimeters away from and parallel to the maxillary alveolus (after Fränkel[2]).

or reorient its growth in a vertical direction. To date, however, no clinical studies have documented a retardation of mandibular growth during treatment with the FR-3 appliance.

Wire Components

There are five wire components of the Fränkel FR-3 appliance, some of which are similar to those found in the FR-2 appliance. The upper labial pads are connected to the vestibular shields by a support wire that usually is formed by a series of three adjacent wires (Figs. 23-1 and 23-2). A lower labial wire that rests against the labial surface of the lower incisors connects the lower aspects of the vestibular shield. On the lingual surface, an upper lingual wire (Fig. 23-6) originates in the vestibular shields, traverses the interocclusal space, and rests against the cingula of the maxillary incisors. In contrast to the FR-2 appliance, the upper lingual wire does not lie between the canine and first deciduous molar (or first premolar), but rather lies in the interocclusal space between the maxillary and mandibular dental arches (Fig. 23-7).

The palatal wire (Fig. 23-6) originates in the vestibular shields and traverses the palate. In contrast to the FR-2 in which the palatal wire lies between the second deciduous molar and the first permanent molar, the

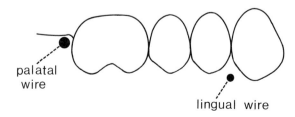

Figure 23-7. Position of the palatal and lingual wires of the FR-3 appliance (from McNamara and Huge[8]).

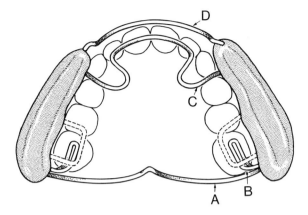

Figure 23-6. Schematic illustration of the FR-3 appliance in maxillary occlusal view. *A*, Palatal wire. *B*, Upper occlusal rest originating from the distal aspect of the maxillary first molar. *C*, Upper lingual wire. *D*, Lower labial support wire (from McNamara and Huge[8]).

palatal wire crosses the palate behind the last molar present (Fig. 23-7). Thus, the maxillary dentition is not restricted in its forward movement by the wires of the appliance.

Particular attention should be paid to the use of the occlusal rests in this appliance. All FR-3 appliances have lower occlusal rests that originate in the vestibular shield, make a gentle right angle bend along the central groove of the lower first molar, and then extend again back into the vestibular shield posteriorly (Fig. 23-8). The purpose of this type of occlusal rest is to prevent the eruption of the lower first molar, as has been advocated by Harvold[5] in the treatment of Class III malocclusion. Eirew[6] recommends that the mandibular occlusal rest be constructed to cover all erupted, or even partially erupted, mandibular molars.

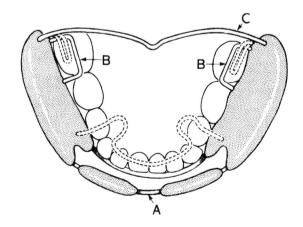

Figure 23-8. Schematic illustration of the FR-3 appliance in mandibular occlusal view. *A*, Support wire for the upper labial pads. *B*, Occlusal rest on the mandibular first molar. *C*, Palatal wire (from McNamara and Huge[8]).

It should be noted that the maxillary occlusal rests (Fig. 23-6) are necessary only in patients with anterior crossbite. These wires should be placed so that only the minimum necessary vertical opening is achieved, avoiding any positive vertical overlap of the maxillary and lower incisors. As soon as the anterior crossbite has been corrected, the upper occlusal rests should be removed from the appliance to close the bite, thus assuring positive horizontal and vertical overlap of the anterior teeth.

The upper occlusal rest originates in the posterior aspect of the vestibular shield, traverses the central groove of the maxillary first molars, and then recurves back on itself (Fig. 23-6). The upper occlusal rest is designed in this manner so as not to restrict the forward movement of the maxilla during functional appliance therapy.

TREATMENT EFFECTS

Both skeletal and dentoalveolar treatment effects have been reported following use of the FR-3 appliance (Fig. 23-9). These treatment effects include a more forward movement of maxillary skeletal and dental landmarks[1] as well as a backward rotation or repositioning of the mandible combined with an increase in lower anterior facial height.[7-9] Occlusal changes also have been noted, including proclination of the maxillary incisors and a lingual tipping of the lower incisors. Loh and Kerr[7] state that the best candidate for this type of treatment is the patient who initially has a deep overbite.

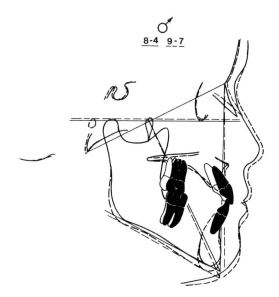

Figure 23-9. Typical treatment effects produced by the FR-3 appliance after 15 months of treatment. Serial superimposition of the tracings is on the basion-nasion line at the pterygomaxillary fissure (from McNamara and Huge[8]).

CLINICAL MANAGEMENT

As with any appliance that is primarily tissue-borne, successful FR-3 treatment depends upon the fit and comfort of the appliance. The following protocol is recommended for the proper fabrication and clinical management of the appliance.

Impression Technique

It is imperative that a proper impression technique be used in the fabrication of the FR-3 appliance. An accurate reproduction of the dentition and the associated soft tissue is essential for appliance fabrication. The extension of the buccal vestibule must be defined clearly, and the upper limits of the anterior maxillary region should be discernible.

Several different types of impression trays have been advocated for the construction of this type of appliance. Most clinicians today use a standard aluminum tray for impression taking. Customized trays such as those made from material such as "Form-a-Tray™" also can be used. A close fitting tray should be selected. Extensions of wax, compound, or custom tray material should be provided in the maxillary anterior region to obtain an accurate impression in this area. Care must be taken to avoid impingement of the tray on the soft-tissue structures of the maxilla and mandible.

It is extremely important that the impressions not be over- or underextended. The use of overextended trays, including Extendo-trays™ and Styrofoam trays, usually is contraindicated because of the vertical and lateral distortion of the soft tissue produced by these types of trays.

During impression procedure, the patient is seated in an upright position. A minimal to moderate amount of impression material should be used to prevent the lateral distortion of the soft tissue.

Construction Bite

A horseshoe-shaped wafer of medium-hard wax is used to orient the upper and lower dental arches in all three planes of space. A blue Projet™ bite fork, the use of which is described in Chapter 15, can be included to support the wax. It is important that this bite registration be accurate. Arbitrary adjustments in working model orientation during appliance fabrication can lead to an appliance that does not fit properly. The bite registration is made with the patient's mandible in the most comfortably retruded position. The wax bite is important, especially in patients who have a discrepancy between centric occlusion and centric relation (*e.g.*, pseudo-Class III individuals).

Approximately two millimeters of interocclusal space must be provided in the molar region for the construction of the lower and, when needed, upper occlusal rests. Excessive vertical opening should be avoided. In patients with an anterior openbite, only one millimeter of vertical bite opening in posterior regions is necessary.

Preparation of Work Models

After the impressions have been obtained, they are poured in either hard plaster or stone with a base of sufficient size to allow for adequate trimming (Fig. 23-10). It is important that an adequate base be present to allow for carving, particularly in the maxillary anterior region. The models are trimmed with a wax bite in place; the backs of the models should be trimmed flush with each other.

After removal of excess flash and bubbles, the models are carved by hand with a rotary instrument and a laboratory knife to help define the borders of the eventual vestibular shields. In most instances, it is not necessary to carve the mandibular work model, particularly if the border of the mandibular sulcus has been defined by the impression. It usually is necessary, however, to carve the maxillary vestibular region in the area of the tuberosity to allow for better definition of the superior extent of the vestibular shield (Fig. 23-10). It sometimes is advisable to define the areas of muscle attachment that appear adjacent to the maxillary first premolar.

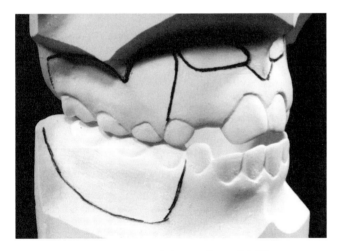

Figure 23-10. Preparation of the work model. The casts are poured in stone and trimmed similar to study models, with adequate bases for trimming. The maxillary model is carved to provide adequate extensions of the vestibular shields and upper labial pads. Typically, trimming of the mandibular model is not required. The future positions of the FR-3 components are marked on the model in pencil.

Usually it will be necessary to define the location of the upper labial pads. It is recommended that the maxillary labial vestibule be extended several millimeters (or more) above the outline achieved by the impression (Fig. 23-10). An acrylic bur in a slow speed handpiece and a sharp laboratory knife can be used to define the contours in this region.

When the preparation of the work model is completed, the wax bite is reinserted, and the posterior surfaces of the work models are checked to ascertain that the backs of the models are flush.

Prescription Sheet

The routine prescription for an FR-3 appliance is relatively simple, as there is little variation in appliance design. Any deviation from the standard three millimeters of wax relief in the maxillary region should be noted, and in contrast to the FR-2 prescription, notching of the teeth is not required.

Appliance Fabrication

In general, in-office fabrication of the FR-3 appliance is not recommended, due to the precise technical nature of appliance construction. A systematic protocol is outlined in McNamara and Huge[8] for the fabrication of this appliance; thus, the method of fabrication will not be described in detail in this chapter. In general, 3 mm of wax relief is applied not only to the maxillary buccal area but also to the maxillary labial area, the future site of the upper labial pads. Only a small amount of wax relief is applied to the mandibular alveolar area, due to the necessity for a close fitting appliance. The wire framework then is applied, and the acrylic parts of the appliance are formed from cold-cure acrylic with a "salt-and-pepper" method. Six views of the completed FR-3 appliance are shown in Fig. 23-11.

Delivery of the Appliance

At the delivery appointment, the clinician places the appliance in the patient's mouth to check for initial fit. Because there is no forward repositioning of the mandible, little adjustment usually is needed at the time of delivery. The upper labial pads should lie well above the maxillary incisors (Fig. 23-12). The appliance may cause the upper lip to appear somewhat full because of the position of the upper labial pads (Fig. 23-13). The clinician should tell the patient and parents that this fullness should disappear within a few weeks or months of full-time appliance wear. In patients with severe maxillary

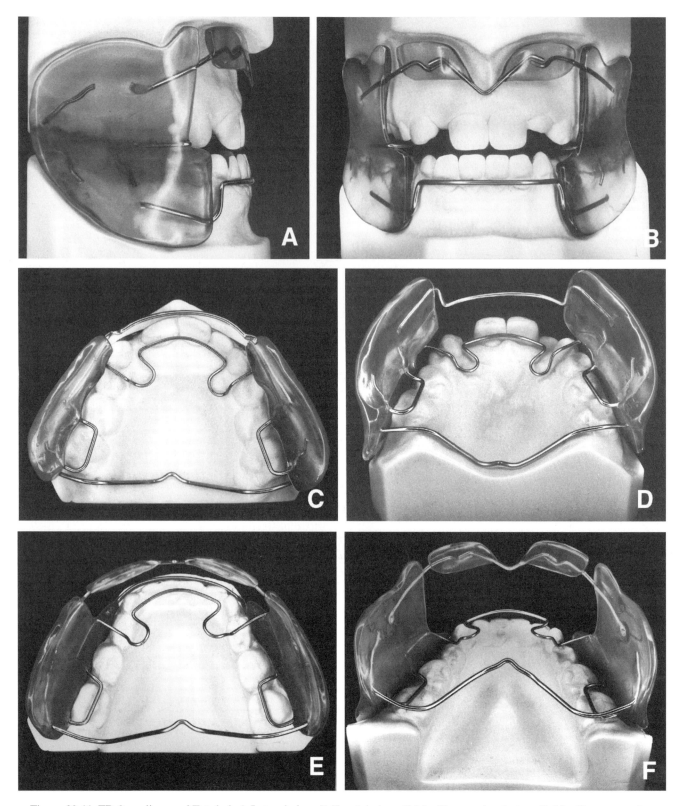

Figure 23-11. FR-3 appliance of Fränkel. *A*, Lateral view. *B*, Frontal view. *C*, Maxillary occlusal view. *D*, Maxillary posterior oblique view. *E*, Mandibular occlusal view. *F*, Posterior mandibular view (from McNamara and Huge[8]).

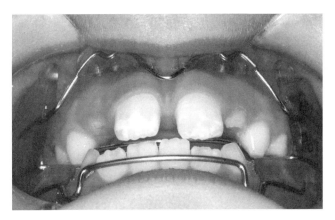

Figure 23-12. Intraoral view of the fit of the vestibular shields and the upper labial pads. The pads should lie above the clinical crowns of the maxillary incisors and anterior to the maxillary alveolus. A 3 mm space should exist between the posterior aspect of the pads and the maxillary mucosa. The lower vestibular shields fit closely to the mandibular alveolar mucosa.

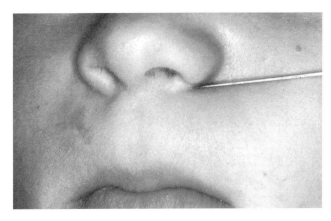

Figure 23-13. Fit of the upper labial pads. After initial appliance insertion, the tissue above the upper lip often is distended, due to the anterior displacement of the upper lip by the upper labial pad. The upper lip will assume a more normal appearance within a few weeks or months after appliance wear.

skeletal retrusion, the appearance of the patient actually may improve after the appliance is inserted.

Home Care Instructions

The patient should be told that this appliance is a full-time appliance. It eventually will be worn at all times except during eating, dental hygiene, playing contact sports, language lessons, or playing musical instruments that are held against the mouth. The patient is instructed to read aloud for one-half hour per day until normal speech can be accomplished when wearing the appliance. As there is no lingual shield, speech usually is not interrupted significantly.

During the break-in period, the patient is instructed to wear the appliance on an increasing basis. It usually is recommended that the appliance be worn for a few hours per day for the first few weeks; then the patient gradually increases wear until the appliance is worn on a full-time basis. As there is little change in mandibular position produced by the appliance, the occurrence of sore spots and other clinical problems are infrequent if the initial fit of the appliance is satisfactory.

After the initial break-in period, during which time the patient may be seen every two to six weeks, routine check-up appointments usually occur at six to ten week intervals. The purposes of the routine check-up appointments are to evaluate appliance fit and to motivate the patient. The duration of treatment with the FR-3 appliance, when worn as a primary treatment appliance, typically is 12–24 months of full-time wear followed by nighttime wear of the appliance until the transition to the permanent dentition is complete.

Appliance Activation

After the appliance has been worn on a full-time basis for three to five months, the distance between the upper labial pads and the underlying alveolus will decrease. Activation of the appliance becomes necessary. A crosscut fissure bur and a low-speed dental handpiece are used to free the ends of the support wires to the upper labial pads (Fig. 23-14A). Acrylic is removed around the ends of this wire to allow anterior advancement of the wire and the maxillary labial pads (Fig. 23-14B). The lingual surface of the upper labial pads should remain about three millimeters away from the underlying alveolus throughout treatment.

After the new position of the upper labial pad has been checked clinically for patient comfort, the holes in the vestibular shield are filled with acrylic to secure the support wire. In patients with severe maxillary skeletal retrusion, a second advancement of the maxillary labial pads may be necessary.

THE FR-3 AS A RETAINER

Although the original intent in design of the FR-3 was as an active treatment appliance, this device also can be used effectively as a retainer following orthopedic facial mask therapy.[10] Petit advocates the use of heavy orthopedic forces generated by the facial mask to achieve initial correction of the malocclusion. He suggests that an FR-3 appliance can be used as an active retention device to retain the maxillary anteroposterior correction and to retrain the associated musculature.

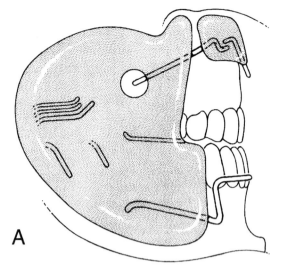 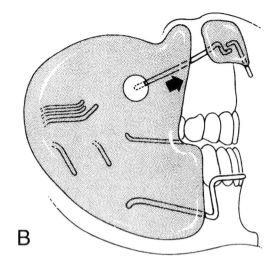

Figure 23-14. Activation of the FR-3 appliance. *A*, A crosscut fissure bur is used to remove the acrylic from around the ends of the upper labial support wire. *B*, A Weingart plier is used to grasp the upper labial support wire and move it anteriorly, so that once again there is a three-millimeter distance between the lingual surface of the upper labial pad and the underlying alveolus.

After treatment with the facial mask has been completed, the bonded acrylic splint expander is removed. The appropriate impressions are made for the FR-3 appliance, as described earlier in this chapter. The appliance can be worn as a nighttime retainer until the end of the transition of the dentition. Lingual arches and transpalatal arches can be used to maintain the space gained in the dental arches through the transition from the deciduous to permanent dentition.

Eirew and co-workers[11] also have stated that the FR-3 is an excellent retraining device and an aid to musculature re-education following surgical correction of Class III malocclusion.

CONCLUDING REMARKS

The FR-3 appliance of Fränkel effectively treats a wide variety of developing Class III malocclusions. As with the facial mask, the FR-3 appliance is much more effective in the early treatment of Class III problems than in the treatment of patients identified in the late mixed or permanent dentition.

The FR-3 provides an alternative to bonded RME/facial mask therapy in that both protocols can achieve the correction of a Class III malocclusion. Whereas FR-3 treatment may take longer to attain a satisfactory resolution of a malocclusion, it is much less invasive to the day-to-day activities of the young patient because it is worn intraorally. In addition, this type of function regulator treatment has a direct effect on the activity of the perioral musculature and the associated soft tissue, factors that otherwise may lead to the perpetuation of the Class III malocclusion over the long-term.

REFERENCES CITED

1. Fränkel R. Maxillary retrusion in Class III and treatment with the function corrector III. Trans Eur Orthod Soc 1970:46:249–259.
2. Fränkel R. Technik und Handhabung der Funktionsregler. Berlin: VEB Verlag Volk and Gesundheit, 1976.
3. Fränkel R, Fränkel C. Orofacial orthopedics with the function regulator. Munich: S Karger, 1989.
4. Fränkel R. Biomechanical aspects of the form/function relationship in craniofacial morphogenesis: a clinician's approach. In: McNamara JA Jr, Ribbens KA, Howe RP, eds Clinical alteration of the growing face. Ann Arbor: Monograph 14, Craniofacial Growth Series, Center for Human Growth and Development, The University of Michigan, 1983.
5. Harvold EP. The activator in interceptive orthodontics. St Louis: CV Mosby, 1974.
6. Eirew HL. Personal communication, 1984.
7. Loh MK, Kerr WJ. The function regulator III: effects and indications for use. Br J Orthod 1985;12:153–157.
8. McNamara JA Jr., Huge SA. The functional regulator (FR-3) of Fränkel. Am J Orthod 1985;88:409–424.
9. Yang KH. Fränkel appliance type III: Correct fabrication and case report of skeletal Class III malocclusion. J Clin Ped Dent 1996;20:281–292.
10. Petit HP. Adaptation following accelerated facial mask therapy. In: McNamara JA, Jr, Ribbens KA, Howe RP, eds. Clinical alterations of the growing face. Ann Arbor: Monograph 14, Craniofacial Growth Series, Center for Human Growth and Development, The University of Michigan, 1983.
11. Eirew HL, McDowell F, Phillips JG. The function regulator of Frankel: Clinical management. Br J Orthod 1976;3: 67–70.

Chapter 24

IMPACTED TEETH: ORTHODONTIC AND SURGICAL CONSIDERATIONS

By Vincent G. Kokich and David P. Mathews

Most permanent teeth erupt into occlusion. In some individuals, however, the permanent teeth may fail to erupt and become impacted within the alveolus. When this lack of eruption occurs, two alternative treatment plans are possible. The impacted tooth could be extracted; the removal of the tooth, however, might require the placement of an implant or fixed prosthesis to replace the missing tooth. The other alternative is to uncover the tooth surgically and move it into the dental arch orthodontically. The timing of orthodontic treatment, type of surgical procedure to uncover the impacted tooth, orthodontic mechanics necessary, and potential problems with treatment vary, depending on which tooth has become impacted.

This chapter will discuss the orthodontic and surgical management of impacted teeth. In order to elucidate the differences in treatment techniques, this chapter will be subdivided based on the specific tooth or teeth that commonly are impacted. In each subsection, the etiology, method of uncovering, timing of uncovering, preoperative and postoperative mechanics, and potential problems will be discussed.

SURGICAL TECHNIQUES

Four techniques can be employed to uncover impacted teeth. Subtle variations of each technique also are available for use in uncovering complex impactions. The type of impacted tooth and its location within the alveolus will dictate selecting the appropriate technique to uncover an impacted tooth.

Gingivectomy

A simple excision of gingiva can be accomplished with a sharp blade. This technique is indicated when there is a wide zone of attached gingiva, bone removal is not needed, and one-half to two-thirds of the crown can be exposed, leaving at least a 3 mm gingival collar. Unfortunately, there are only a few instances where this technique can be used. The most common area where this technique may be employed is over the labially impacted maxillary canine and/or central incisor.

Apically Positioned Flap

A split thickness flap is reflected from the area adjacent to the impacted tooth. Appropriate bone removal is accomplished, and the flap is sutured apically, exposing about two-thirds of the crown. This technique most often is employed on "simple" labially impacted teeth.

Flap/Closed Eruption Technique

A crestal incision is made and buccal and/or lingual flaps are reflected. Appropriate bone removal is accomplished, and a bracket or chain is attached to the impacted tooth. The flaps are returned to their original location for complete closure. The chain passes under the flap, exits at the mid-crestal incision area, and is attached to the archwire. This technique is best used with high labially impacted teeth and teeth that are impacted in the mid-alveolar area. With appropriate orthodontic mechanics, the tooth can be erupted, mimicking its natural eruptive path through the mid-crestal area.

Pre-Orthodontic Uncovering Technique

This technique is used on "simple" palatally impacted canines. A full thickness palatal flap is reflected from the premolar to the midline, and appropriate bone removal is accomplished. The flap is repositioned, and the area over the impacted canine is scalloped so the tooth remains uncovered. The canine will erupt on its own, and this eruption will facilitate final orthodontic positioning. This technique is used before placement of orthodontic appliances or during the initial stage of orthodontic treatment.

MAXILLARY CENTRAL INCISOR

Etiology

The most commonly impacted tooth is the maxillary canine,[1] followed by the maxillary central incisor. The usual cause of impaction of the maxillary central incisor is the presence of a supernumerary tooth or mesiodens.[2] If the supernumerary tooth is discovered early and extracted, the central incisor may erupt spontaneously. If the root of the impacted incisor forms completely and the mesiodens has not been removed, however, then the central incisor may not erupt spontaneously.

When the central incisor is impacted, it usually is located in the middle of the alveolus faciolingually. In most situations, the tooth is oriented vertically, with the incisal edge directed toward the dental arch. In some patients, however, the tooth bud of the central incisor becomes rotated and diverted, and the impacted tooth may be oriented in a horizontal direction parallel to the occlusal plane. Obviously, these complex impactions are much more difficult to treat.

Preoperative Orthodontics

Usually an impacted central incisor is recognized during the mixed dentition. At that time, all maxillary and mandibular central and lateral incisors are erupted, except for the impacted central incisor. The first step is to extract any supernumerary teeth as a separate procedure. In some patients, the impacted central incisor may erupt. If not, orthodontic treatment must be initiated to erupt the tooth. Brackets should be placed on the remaining central incisor and the two maxillary lateral incisors. This bracket placement typically provides sufficient anchorage to erupt the impacted tooth. If the contralateral central and adjacent lateral incisors have tipped toward one another, the space is opened with a coiled spring. Bands are cemented to the maxillary permanent first molars to help provide anchorage during the course of orthodontic treatment. After sufficient space has been established, a rectangular stabilizing archwire is placed in the maxillary brackets. A loop may be placed in the archwire to temporarily anchor the attachment that will be placed on the impacted central incisor during the uncovering procedure. At this point, the patient is referred to the surgeon to uncover the impacted central incisor.

Surgery

Impacted central incisors can be classified either as "simple," where the tip of the impacted tooth is near the adjacent cemento-enamel junctions (CEJ) (Fig. 24-1A), or "complex," where the impacted tooth is positioned high in the vestibule (Fig. 24-1B). Central incisors usually are impacted labially.

Simple

The simple labially impacted tooth can be uncovered with either the apically positioned flap or the flap/closed eruption technique. In the example shown in Fig. 24-2, the closed eruption technique is used. A crestal incision is made and joined with vertical incisions, and a pedicle flap is reflected from the edentulous ridge. Approximately two-thirds of the crown is exposed with appropriate bone removal by means of curettes and surgical round burs. The area is isolated with hemostatic agents such as Surgicel™ or Hemodent™. The tooth is etched and a bonding agent is placed. At this point, either a small button can be placed on the labial of the tooth with a gold chain or wire ligated to the button, or a gold chain can be bonded directly to the labial aspect of the tooth. The pedicle flap is returned to its original position and sutured. The chain is covered by the flap and exits at the mid-crestal incision. The chain can be ligated to the bracket on the adjacent tooth, and the orthodontist may begin erupting the tooth within one to two weeks.

Complex

If the tooth is impacted high in the vestibule on the labial aspect, then the closed eruption technique is the treatment of choice. In the example shown in Figure 24-3, the tooth is impacted high in the vestibule near the base of the nasal spine; it also is positioned horizontally. The use of an apically positioned flap in this situation is

MANAGEMENT OF IMPACTIONS

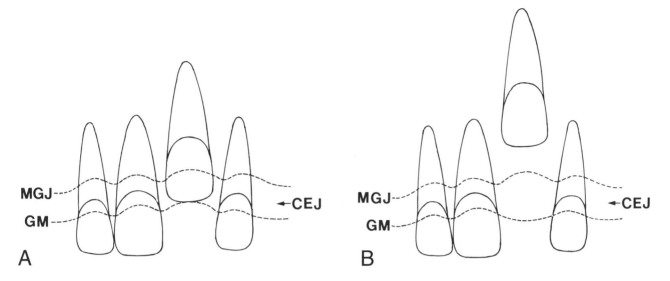

Figure 24-1. Diagrams indicating different positions for impacted maxillary central incisors. *A,* If the incisal edge of the maxillary central incisor is positioned coronal (incisal) to the mucogingival junction, an apically positioned flap, flap/closed eruption technique, or a gingivectomy procedure can be used to uncover the impacted central incisor crown. If the patient has insufficient attached gingiva, an apically positioned flap is chosen. If sufficient gingiva is present, a gingivectomy uncovering may be appropriate. *B,* If the incisal edge is positioned apical to the CEJ, a flap/closed eruption technique should be employed. With the latter technique, the tooth may be erupted through the crest of the ridge, and sufficient gingiva will be present over the labial of the central incisor.

injudicious. First, appropriate bone removal is accomplished. In this situation, the lingual aspect of the tooth is the only visible area. A bracket is bonded to the tooth, a wire or chain is attached, and the flap is returned to its original position. With appropriate orthodontic mechanics, this tooth can follow its normal eruptive pattern through the crest of the edentulous ridge, leaving adequate attached gingiva and a gingival margin that is esthetically harmonious with the adjacent central incisor.

In a third example (Fig. 24-4), an apically positioned flap was performed on this high labial impaction. This case points out the difficulty of using this technique to apically position tissue on a high labially impacted tooth. The tooth has been moved into its proper location, but as can be seen, the gingival margin is more apical than the adjacent central incisor. This example illustrates one reason why the flap/closed eruption technique is used to uncover most labially impacted teeth, except for the ectopic labially impacted tooth.

Postoperative Orthodontics

During the postoperative orthodontic treatment phase, the key to success is the eruption of the maxillary central incisor into the center of the alveolar ridge. In order to accomplish this maneuver, the orthodontic force must originate from the center of the edentulous alveolar ridge. If the clinician directs the force labially toward the archwire, the impacted tooth may erupt into the oral cavity in a more apical position. This movement may cause apical positioning of the gingival margin over the erupted central incisor, creating a difference in the crown lengths between the impacted and non-impacted central incisors and compromising the esthetic appearance of the teeth. In order to erupt the tooth into the center of the ridge, a Ballista loop (Fig. 24-5) is helpful. This loop can be activated, and its force is directed from the center of the ridge in a vertical direction. The use of this type of loop will help pull the tooth into its normal path of eruption and not toward the labial. After the tooth has erupted, a bracket is bonded to the labial surface, and the crown and root of the tooth are positioned properly.

MAXILLARY CANINE— LABIAL IMPACTION

Etiology

Labial impaction of the maxillary canine over the maxillary lateral incisor (Fig. 24-6) occurs occasionally. This type of impaction is due to one of two causes. Either the canine moves ectopically over the labial surface of the maxillary lateral incisor root and fails to erupt, or

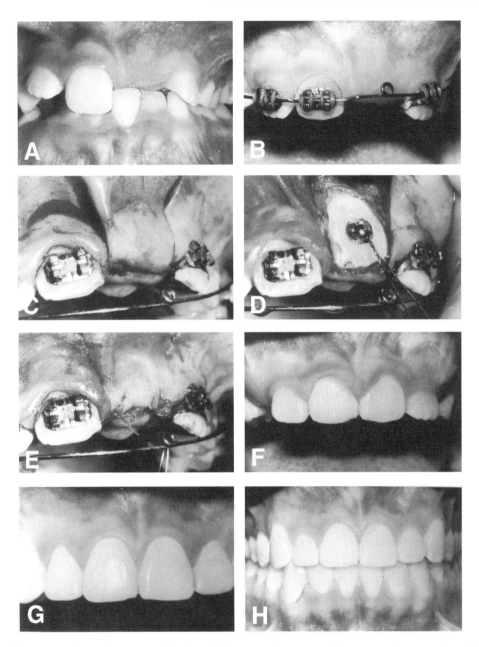

Figure 24-2. A labially impacted maxillary central incisor. *A*, The maxillary central incisor was impacted and had not erupted at age 10. *B*, Orthodontic treatment was initiated to create sufficient space between the maxillary right central and left lateral incisors. *C*, A pedicle flap was reflected from the crest of the ridge. *D*, A button was bonded onto the tooth, and a piece of ligature wire was attached. *E*, The flap was repositioned and sutured, and elastomeric chains were used to erupt the tooth. *F*, At the completion of this phase of orthodontic treatment, the gingival margins of both central incisors were identical, in that the left central was erupted through the crest of the ridge. *G*, At the end of the second phase of orthodontic treatment, the gingival margins of the two central incisors remained identical. *H*, Three years after orthodontic treatment, the positions of the central incisors and the gingival margins were at the same level.

the maxillary dental midline may shift toward the canine, causing it to be impacted labially. In some instances, the canine will erupt spontaneously and then can be moved orthodontically into the dental arch. In other patients, however, the tooth will not erupt and must be uncovered surgically and subsequently erupted into position orthodontically.

Preoperative Orthodontics

When the maxillary canine is labial to the maxillary lateral incisor, the root of the lateral incisor is oriented toward the palate. If brackets are placed on all maxillary teeth, including the lateral incisor, the root of the lateral may be forced toward the labial. If the canine crown is

MANAGEMENT OF IMPACTIONS

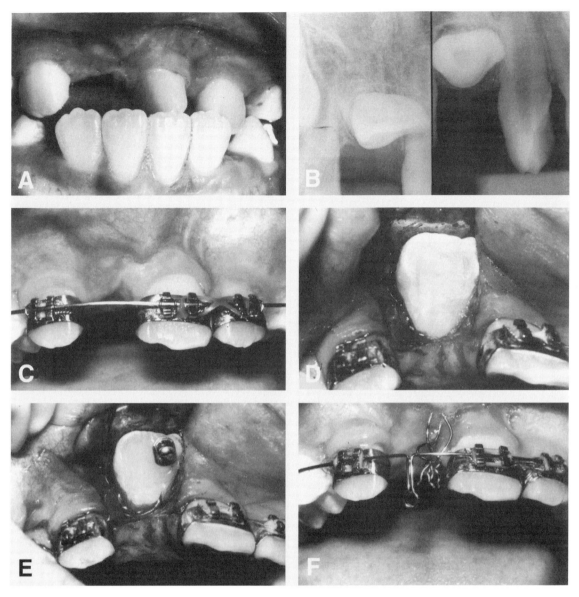

Figure 24-3. Horizontally impacted maxillary central incisor. *A*, The maxillary right central incisor was unerupted, and the maxillary left central incisor was rotated and in lingual crossbite. *B*, Pretreatment radiographs indicate the horizontal impaction of the maxillary right central incisor. *C*, Initially, brackets were placed on the teeth, and the teeth were aligned. *D*, A pedicle flap was reflected, and the tooth was uncovered. *E*, A button was bonded to the lingual surface of the central incisor, and the flap was repositioned in its original location. *F*, A Ballista loop was used to deliver an eruptive force to the impacted central incisor.

occupying this space, root resorption could occur on the labial surface of the lateral incisor. Therefore, in this situation, it is best not to bracket the maxillary lateral incisor initially. Bands and brackets are placed on the remaining teeth in the maxillary arch, and a coil spring usually is needed to move the first premolar and central incisor apart. The archwire bypasses the lateral incisor and does not attach to the lateral until after the canine has been uncovered and moved distally. After the remaining maxillary teeth have been positioned properly, the patient should be referred to the surgeon to uncover the maxillary canine.

Surgery

If the labially impacted tooth is located lateral to the edentulous area, *i.e.*, an ectopic labial impaction (Fig. 24-6*DE*), an apically positioned flap is the appropriate technique. It is rare that there is enough attached gingiva to allow use of the gingivectomy technique and still obtain an adequate collar of attached tissue. Use of the closed eruption technique would not be appropriate, because it would not allow the orthodontist to select the appropriate mechanics to move the tooth over the lateral incisor and into the edentulous area.

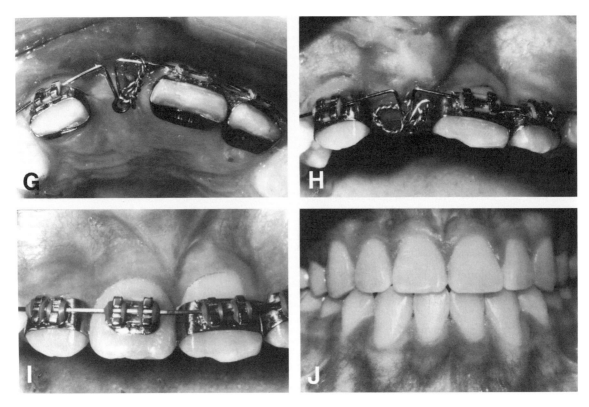

Figure 24-3 (continued). *G* and *H*, Other views of the activated Ballista loop. *I*, After the tooth had been erupted, a bracket was placed on the tooth, and it was aligned in its proper axial inclination. *J*, After orthodontic treatment, the gingival margins of the maxillary central incisors were nearly at the same level. In addition, the same amount of gingiva was present over both central incisors.

Ideally, to use the apically positioned flap on this type of impaction, there should be a minimum of 4 to 6 mm of gingiva on the adjacent central and lateral incisor. In this instance (Fig. 24-6), the donor tissue for the pedicle flap can be reflected from the central and lateral incisor by way of a split-thickness pedicle flap. Bone is removed from the crown of the impacted tooth, exposing approximately two-thirds of the enamel. The flap is ligated with resorbable gut suture to the periosteum, exposing approximately two-thirds of the tooth. It is important when using this technique to leave a 2 to 3 mm gingival collar around the incisor donor site (Fig. 24-6D). In addition, at least a 2 mm width of gingiva should be incorporated with the pedicle flap. This technique must be planned and employed carefully. The impacted tooth often is lying over the root of the incisor, and a significant bony dehiscence may be present.

If there is not adequate gingiva over the incisor donor site, then the edentulous area will need to be used.[3] Introduction of an incision into the edentulous area complicates the flap design, because of the distance from the edentulous ridge crest to the impacted tooth. The incisions must be planned very carefully to allow adequate exposure of the impacted tooth and to leave adequate gingiva over the central and lateral incisors.

Postoperative Orthodontics

After the labially impacted maxillary canine has been uncovered, the tooth must be moved into the dental arch. If sufficient space exists for the tooth, and the canine is positioned immediately above the edentulous space, a flexible nickel-titanium wire may be used to facilitate tooth eruption. If the canine is positioned mesially and has erupted labial to the lateral incisor, an elastomeric chain should be attached from the maxillary canine to the premolars and maxillary first molar on that side (Fig. 24-6F). It is helpful to attach the chain as far distally as possible to enhance anchorage. In some patients, it may be beneficial to place a maxillary Nance holding arch or a transpalatal arch to increase the amount of molar anchorage. Gradually, the maxillary canine is moved distally (Fig. 24-6G). It is important not to place a bracket on the lateral incisor during this movement in order to avoid root resorption of the lateral incisor. After the canine has been moved far enough distally, the lateral incisor can be bracketed, and space can be created for the canine by pushing the lateral incisor toward the mesial. After that movement has been accomplished, the maxillary canine may be erupted vertically into its position in the dental arch. At

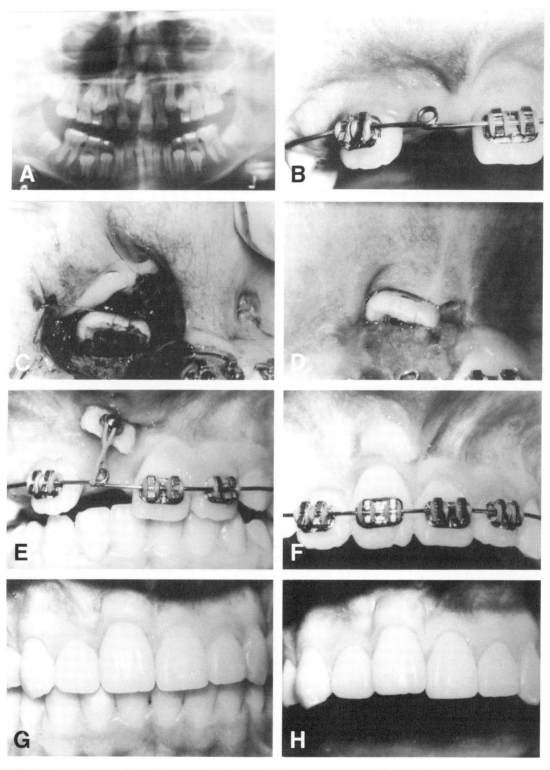

Figure 24-4. Horizontally impacted maxillary central incisor. *A*, The pretreatment radiograph shows the position of the impacted maxillary right central incisor. *B*, Brackets were placed on the adjacent teeth, and sufficient space was created for the right central incisor. *C*, An apically positioned flap was elevated. *D*, The flap was positioned near the CEJ of the impacted central incisor. *E*, An elastomeric chain was used to erupt the right central incisor, and brackets eventually were placed to position the crown and root of the formerly impacted tooth (*F*). *G*, After the completion of orthodontic treatment, the gingival margin of the right central incisor was more apical than the left central incisor. In addition, the gingiva is thicker over the formerly impacted tooth. *H*, Five years after treatment, the maxillary right central incisor had reintruded. This rebound probably was due to the pull of the mucosa, in that the apically positioned gingival flap had healed to the mucosa, well above the mucogingival junction of the adjacent teeth.

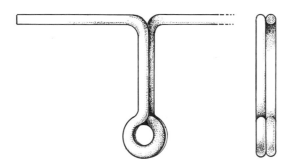

Figure 24-5. Diagrammatic representation of the Ballista loop, which is formed from .018" stainless steel wire.

that point, a rectangular archwire is helpful to complete the correction of tooth positioning and root angulation. During orthodontic finishing, the clinician also must move the root of the maxillary lateral incisor toward the labial to improve the axial inclination of the crown.

MAXILLARY CANINE— INTRA-ALVEOLAR IMPACTION

Etiology

Intra-alveolar impaction of the maxillary canine (Fig. 24-7) is more common than labial impaction; however, neither is more common than palatal impaction of the maxillary canine.[4] Intra-alveolar maxillary canine impactions usually are due to the presence of a supernumerary tooth in the path of eruption of the maxillary canine. Even when the supernumerary tooth is removed, the canine may fail to erupt. The tooth may be located within the center of the alveolar ridge, but the root forms completely, and the tooth becomes stalled and impacted in the alveolus.

Preoperative Orthodontics

The orthodontist should wait until all permanent teeth have erupted before beginning treatment. At that time, bands and brackets should be placed on all of the maxillary teeth. The dental arch should be aligned, and space must be created for the maxillary canine. After the proper amount of space has been apportioned, a rectangular archwire is placed in the maxillary arch, and the patient is referred to the surgeon to uncover the impacted tooth.

Surgery

When the tip of the labially impacted tooth is coronal to the adjacent CEJs, and there is a wide zone of attached gingiva, it may be possible to use the gingivectomy technique[5] (Fig. 24-7). In this patient, a simple gingivectomy was possible; two-thirds of the crown of the tooth was exposed, and no bone removal was necessary. There still is adequate remaining attached tissue. A dressing can be placed over the enamel to prevent tissue overgrowth. In one week, the dressing may be removed, and the patient is instructed to keep the exposed crown clean with a toothbrush or cotton swab, using a chlorhexidine rinse on the swab to prevent gingival proliferation. In three to four weeks, the tissue will be healed sufficiently to allow the orthodontist to place a bracket and begin tooth movement. If this technique is undertaken properly, there should be adequate attached gingiva and no recession, when the orthodontic treatment is completed (Fig. 24-7D).

If the tip of the labially impacted canine is near the adjacent CEJs, or slightly apical, then the apically positioned flap or closed eruption technique can be used. In this location, it would be impossible to perform an excisional gingivectomy and leave adequate attached gingiva. In the example shown in Figure 24-8, a split-thickness pedicle flap is reflected from the crest of the edentulous area, preserving as much gingiva as possible. The incisions are extended vertically into the vestibule, and the split-thickness flap is reflected (Fig. 24-8C). Occasionally a thin shell of bone covers the enamel, and this covering can be removed with a curette or surgical round bur. Two-thirds of the crown is exposed, and the connective tissue follicle is curetted from the periphery of the exposed portion of the crown. The flap is sutured to the periosteum with resorbable suture, exposing approximately two-thirds of the enamel. A small dressing can be placed over the enamel. If the patient employs good home care including the use of a chlorhexidine rinse, tissue overgrowth rarely is a problem. The orthodontist can place a bracket and initiate orthodontic therapy in four to six weeks after the uncovering procedure (Fig. 24-8E). If the tooth is impacted high in the vestibule or within the alveolus, then the closed eruption technique is the treatment of choice (Fig. 24-8D).

Before any surgery is initiated, it is important to determine the location of the impacted tooth. In the case of a labial impaction, locating the tooth often can be accomplished by palpation. If the tooth is positioned in the middle of the alveolus or palatally, however, it will be necessary to determine its location by taking two radiographs at different angles. The Buccal Object Rule[6] is helpful in determining the location of these impacted teeth. When two different radiographs are made of a pair of objects, the image of the buccal object moves, relative to the image of the lingual object, in the same direction that the X-ray beam is directed (see Figure 24-9B). In this instance (Fig. 24-9), the tooth was impacted

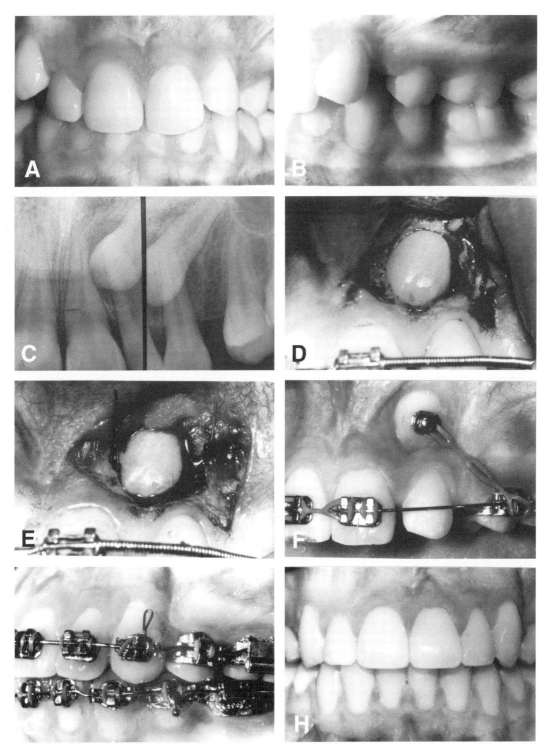

Figure 24-6. A 13-year-old patient with a maxillary left canine that is impacted mesial and labial to the left lateral incisor. *A* and *B*, Pretreatment intraoral photographs show that the maxillary left lateral incisor was proclined labially. The canine was impacted mesial to the root of the lateral incisor. Four premolars had been extracted previously, and the spaces were closed. *C*, Periapical radiographs indicate the location of the labially impacted canine. *D*, The adjacent incisors had adequate gingiva as a donor site for a split-thickness pedicle flap. Care was taken to leave a gingival collar over the central and lateral incisors. *E*, The flap was positioned apically and sutured to the periosteum, exposing two-thirds of the anatomic crown. *F*, An orthodontic attachment was placed on the canine, and the posterior teeth were used as anchorage to retract the canine distally. The lateral incisor was not bracketed to avoid moving the root of the lateral incisor into the crown of the canine and potential root resorption. *G*, After the canine was moved far enough distally, the lateral incisor was bracketed, and the proper occlusion and axial inclination of the teeth were established. *H*, At the end of orthodontic treatment, the maxillary left canine was well-positioned with sufficient attached gingiva. In addition, the gingival margin was only slightly higher than the contralateral canine that had erupted normally.

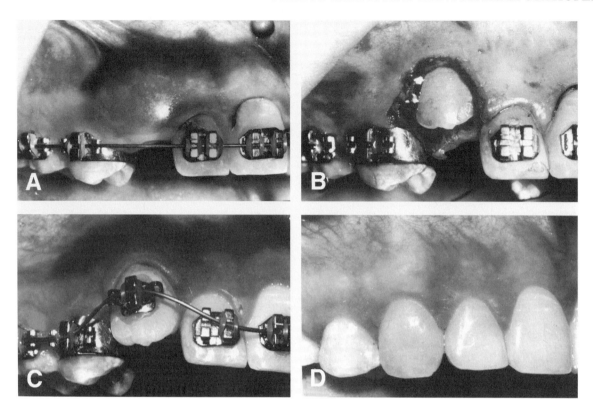

Figure 24-7. Intra-alveolar impacted maxillary canine. *A*, Initially, space was opened orthodontically to accommodate the canine into the dental arch. The gingiva had been stained with Schiller's solution. This solution temporarily stains the mucosa a dark brown, clearly delineating the mucogingival junction. The canine could be palpated, and a wide zone of attached gingiva was present. *B*, A gingivectomy was possible because of the wide zone of gingiva and location of the tooth. About two-thirds of the crown was exposed. *C*, An orthodontic bracket was placed, and a flexible wire was used to erupt the canine. *D*, Finished intraoral views show an adequate zone of attached gingiva over the erupted canine.

in the mid-alveolar area.[7-10] The flap/closed eruption technique is the treatment of choice in this situation. A crestal incision can be made, and vertical incisions can help release the flap on the labial aspect. Sulcular incisions can be made on the palatal aspect of adjacent teeth for better reflection. Curettes and surgical round burs are used to find the tip of the impacted tooth. Bone must be removed from the incisal aspect of the tooth to allow placement of a bracket and/or chain. The amount of bone removed must be sufficient to allow the widest part of the crown to pass through the bone unobstructed. The flaps are returned to their original location for complete closure with resorbable suture. The chain passes under the flap and exits at the mid-crestal incision area, where it is attached to the archwire or adjacent bracket. The orthodontist can activate force within one week. If proper mechanics are implimented, the tooth will erupt, as it would have naturally.

Postoperative Orthodontics

If the crown of the canine has been uncovered completely by means of excising the gingiva or apically positioning a flap, an orthodontic attachment may be bonded to the labial surface of the tooth. It is advantageous to place an orthodontic bracket. In some situations, however, a smaller attachment may be required if an insufficient area of enamel is available. After the bracket has been positioned, the objective of the orthodontic eruption process is to avoid distortion of the maxillary occlusal plane. In addition, the tooth must be erupted gradually to avoid potential recession of the gingiva. Flexible nickel titanium wires are advantageous for the eruption process. These wires will not distort permanently and will permit gradual eruption of the impacted tooth.

If the crown of the tooth is apical to the mucogingival junction, and a closed eruption procedure has been performed, a wire or chain will be extending through the gingiva at the crest of the alveolar ridge. The wire or chain will be connected to an attachment that has been bonded to the tooth. In this situation, the orthodontic objective is to erupt the tooth through the crest of the alveolar ridge. This movement will duplicate the normal eruption process. A Ballista spring or loop may be used to direct the eruption toward the crest of the ridge. This

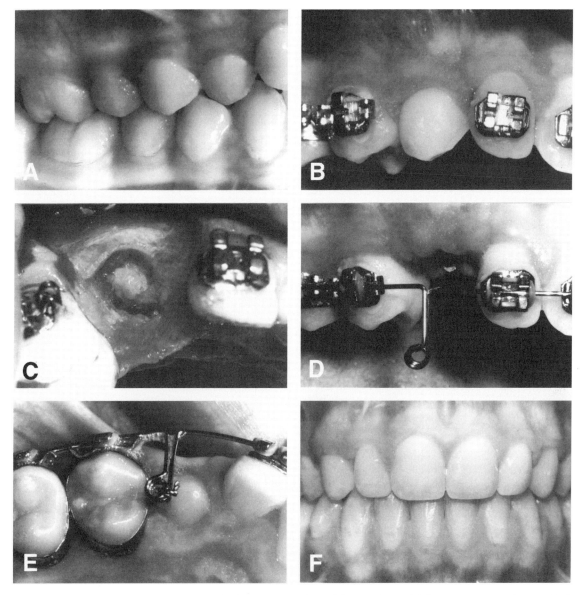

Figure 24-8. An adolescent patient with bilateral labially impacted maxillary canines. *A*, The pretreatment intraoral photograph shows that the maxillary primary canines still are present. *B*, Orthodontic treatment was initiated to make sufficient space for the permanent canines. *C*, A pedicle flap was reflected on the labial along with a small palatal flap to expose the tip of the canine. Sufficient bone was removed so that the crown was visible, and an attachment was placed on the crown. *D*, The flaps were reapproximated and sutured. This flap/closed eruption technique created sufficient gingiva labial to the tooth. *E*, A Ballista spring was used to erupt the tooth into position. *F*, At the end of orthodontic treatment, both canines were positioned properly, and the gingival margins were nearly identical with one another. Sufficient attached gingiva was present over the labial surfaces of the canines.

type of eruption system is easy to adjust as the tooth begins to erupt and move into the arch. As that process occurs, segments of the wire or chain are removed until the crown of the tooth protrudes through the gingiva. A bracket may be placed on the tooth, and the final positioning completed. After eruption of a labially impacted tooth, the root and crown of the tooth may require changes in axial inclination to position the tooth properly. This movement usually is accomplished best with a rectangular wire.

MAXILLARY CANINE— SIMPLE PALATAL IMPACTION

Etiology

The cause of palatal impaction of the canine is unknown. For some reason during tooth development, the direction of eruption of the canine becomes diverted toward the palate. Once this redirection of eruption oc-

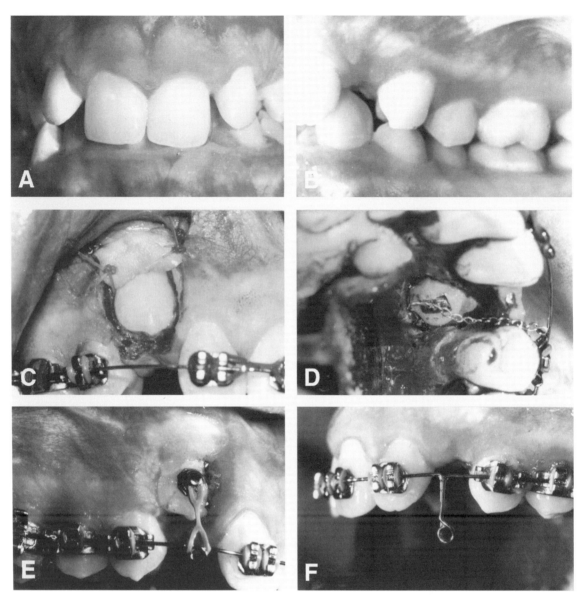

Figure 24-9. A patient with bilaterally impacted maxillary canines. *A*, and *B*, The pretreatment intraoral photographs show that the patient had a Class II malocclusion with deep anterior overbite. The maxillary right canine was impacted labially, and the left canine was impacted within the alveolus and slightly toward the palate. Two different types of uncovering procedure were used for this patient. *C*, Because the cusp tip of the right canine was positioned coronally relative to the mucogingival junction, and there was inadequate gingiva to perform gingivectomy, an apically positioned flap procedure was used to uncover the right canine. *D*, Because the left canine was impacted within the alveolus, a flap/closed eruption procedure was used. *E*, An elastomeric chain was used to erupt the right canine. *F*, A Ballista loop was used to erupt the left impacted canine.

curs, although the tooth may erupt, it usually will be positioned in crossbite.

Palatal impactions can be divided into two categories depending on the severity of the impaction. A *simple* palatal impaction is defined as a tooth that is diverted toward the palate, not deeply imbedded within the alveolus, and with the canine cusp tip located near the cemento-enamel junctions of the adjacent teeth (Fig. 24-10). A *complex* palatal impaction describes a canine that usually is oriented horizontally relative to the occlusal plane, with the canine cusp tip located near the middle to apical portions of the adjacent teeth (Fig. 24-11). The strategy for erupting these teeth and treating them orthodontically is different.

Preoperative Orthodontics

The timing of uncovering palatally impacted canines depends on the position of the tooth. If the impacted canine is not located high in the palate, but rather is positioned

MANAGEMENT OF IMPACTIONS

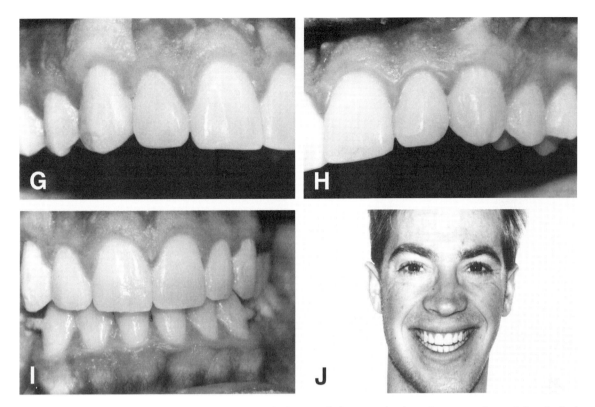

Figure 24-9 (Continued) *G-J*. After orthodontic treatment, the intraoral photographs show the comparison of the gingival margins and amount of gingiva around both canines. The maxillary right canine has more gingiva, because an apically positioned flap procedure was used; however, the left canine also has sufficient gingiva. The front intraoral photograph after treatment (*I*) shows the difference in the level of the gingival margins of the left and right canines. With the apically positioned flap, the gingival margin generally ends up more apical than the flap/closed eruption side. If the patient has a high lip line (*J*), then the discrepancy between the gingival margins of the right and left canines could be an esthetic compromise. In this patient, the difference in the levels of the gingival margins was not a problem.

near the alveolar ridge (*simple*), it may be advantageous to uncover the tooth prior to beginning orthodontic appliance placement. If the orientation of the crown and root are similar to the adjacent teeth, and the canine has been uncovered early, it usually will erupt partially into the palate. This pattern of eruption is advantageous, because the tooth can be moved laterally without dragging the crown through the palatal gingiva. If the canine is impacted near the roof of the palate (*complex*), early uncovering of the tooth may not be advisable. In this instance, the soft tissue probably will migrate over the crown, requiring a second surgical procedure.

In some patients, the primary canine still is present. It generally is advantageous to remove the primary canine when the permanent canine is uncovered. In that way, only one surgical procedure will be necessary.

During the preoperative orthodontic phase of treatment, sufficient space must be created for the permanent canine. Most maxillary canines are about 7.5 to 8.0 mm in width. Of course, the clinician can use the contralateral canine as a guide. If both canines are impacted, a radiographic assessment of the width of the tooth must be made. If the radiograph is distorted, the width of the permanent canine can be estimated from the relative size of the erupted first premolar. Permanent canines generally are about 1.0 to 1.5 mm wider than the first premolars. After sufficient interproximal space has been established, the patient is ready for surgical uncovering of the impacted canine.

Surgery

Two different techniques can be employed to uncover the palatally impacted tooth. Most palatal impactions are like those in Figure 24-10. These are *simple* impactions and are positioned palatal to the central and lateral incisors and not too deeply embedded within the alveolus. The *complex* situation shown in Figure 24-11 is positioned more horizontally and more deeply impacted within the alveolus, sometimes near the apices of the central and lateral incisor or even apical to them.

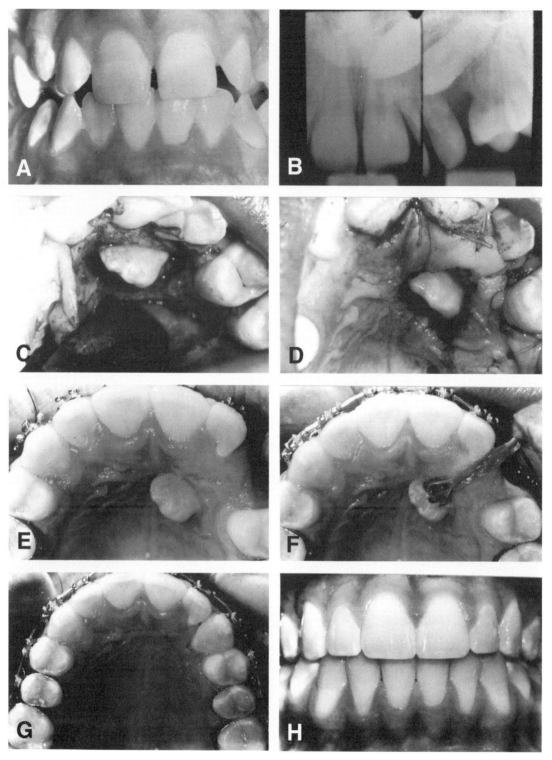

Figure 24-10. A patient with a palatally impacted maxillary left canine. *A*, The intraoral photograph shows that the patient had interdental spacing in the maxillary arch. *B*, The periapical radiographs confirmed that the maxillary canine was impacted palatally. In order to allow the canine to erupt during the initial stages of orthodontic treatment, the tooth was uncovered before placement of orthodontic brackets. *C*, A palatal flap was elevated in order to locate the impacted canine. The follicle was removed, and all of the bone was removed from around the crown. *D*, The flap was reapproximated, and a window was cut in the flap to allow the canine to protrude into the oral cavity. *E*, One year after uncovering, orthodontic treatment had begun, and space was created for the canine. By that time, the tooth had erupted farther into the oral cavity. *F*, The tooth then could be moved laterally into proper position. The independent eruption of the tooth facilitates movement of the tooth laterally. *G*, After movement into the dental arch, a bracket was placed and the root was positioned appropriately. *H*, After orthodontic treatment, the position of the canine on the left side matches the non-impacted canine on the right side.

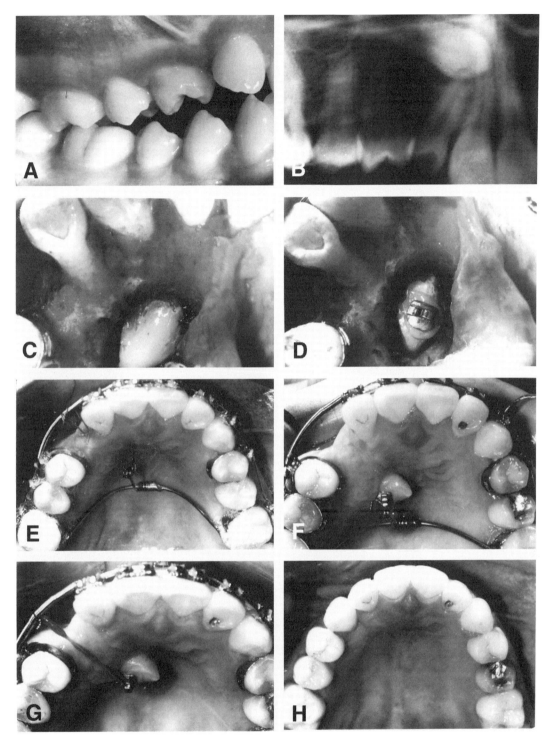

Figure 24-11. An adolescent patient with a complex palatally and horizontally impacted maxillary right canine. *A*, The impacted canine crown was located near the apices of the maxillary central incisors. *B*, Because the canine did not erupt, the maxillary first premolar and lateral incisor drifted toward one another, closing the space for the canine. Initially, orthodontic mechanics were used to open space for the impacted canine. *C*, A palatal flap was elevated to expose the crown of the canine. It was impacted next to the roots of the central and lateral incisors. All of the bone was removed over the crown. *D*, A cleat was bonded to the crown of the canine. The palatal flap was repositioned, and a window of tissue was removed over the eyelet. A dressing was placed on the exposed crown. *E*, A lingual arch was constructed and soldered to the maxillary first molar bands. *F*, A spring was soldered to the mid-portion of the palatal arch. This spring permitted eruption and posterior movement of the crown of the impacted canine to avoid damaging roots of the central and lateral incisors. *G*, After the crown of the canine had been moved away from the central and lateral incisors and into the oral cavity, an elastomeric chain was attached to the archwire to gradually move the canine into the dental arch. *H*, After orthodontic treatment, the position of the canine was corrected, and the shape of the dental arch was maintained.

Preorthodontic Uncovering Technique

Simple palatal impactions (Fig. 24-10) can be treated by an early uncovering technique before placement of orthodontic appliances. When these teeth are uncovered early and left uncovered, they will erupt into a more favorable location that will facilitate orthodontic movement.

The technique requires flap reflection and complete bone removal from the coronal aspect of the tooth. If the primary canines are present, they are extracted at the time of the uncovering procedure. A full-thickness palatal flap is reflected from the premolar to the midline (Fig. 24-10C). A curette or surgical round bur is used to locate the impacted tooth by gently removing the encasing bone. The follicle is curetted from the periphery. Before flap closure, the area of the flap over the impacted tooth is scalloped, so that it leaves the tooth uncovered after the flap is sutured (Fig. 24-10D). A dressing is placed over the enamel of the tooth and contoured flush with the surface of the palatal flap. A stent (Biostar™ or Omnivac™; see Chapter 27 for the fabrication of invisible retainers) can be made to cover the palate and the dressing to ensure that it will stay in place. This stent also minimizes postoperative discomfort and postoperative bleeding.

The dressing is removed in 7 to 10 days, and the patient is instructed in swabbing the area with a chlorhexidine rinse. On teeth that are embedded more deeply, the area may require slight degranulating with a curette at this appointment and replacement of the dressing for another week. The margins around the impacted tooth will be epithelialized in four to six weeks. The tooth will begin to erupt on its own and can remain unbracketed until the appropriate time determined by the orthodontist.

MAXILLARY CANINE—COMPLEX PALATAL IMPACTION

In this type of patient (Fig. 24-11), a different technique is used. These teeth usually are impacted high within the alveolus. They will not erupt on their own if left uncovered, because the tissue will grow over the tooth. A full-thickness palatal flap is reflected from the molar through the midline (Fig. 24-11C). A modification of the flap can be used when the tooth is impacted very high in the roof of the palate.[11,12] Bone is removed from the crown of the impacted tooth, being very careful not to damage the roots of the central or lateral incisor, especially around the apices of these teeth. The area is isolated to achieve a dry field for bracketing. Surgical notes should be made of the tooth and its bone relationship, and a photograph should be taken.[12] Documenting the surgery photographically or digitally will help the orthodontist choose the appropriate mechanics to erupt the tooth. A bracket is bonded to the tooth; pulling on the bracket with a hemostat will test the bond strength as well as verify the mobility of the tooth. If the canine is ankylosed, it should be luxated and loosened in the alveolus. The flap is returned to its original position. Before suturing, the flap is palpated to locate the bracket. This area of the flap is fenestrated with a #15 blade, so the bracket protrudes through the "window" in the flap[12] (Fig. 24-11E). The palatal flap then is sutured to its original position using 4-0 gut suture with a continuous sling technique. A ligating wire or gold chain is attached from the bracket and runs outside the flap to the archwire. In one to two weeks, the orthodontist can initiate tooth movement. If the tooth is ankylosed, immediate force should be applied.

Postoperative Orthodontics

In the instance of a simple palatal impaction, the canine will have erupted partially into the palate after pre-orthodontic uncovering. In most cases, an attachment can be bonded to the crown of the tooth. If the tooth has erupted sufficiently, an elastomeric chain can be used to move the canine laterally into the dental arch gradually. During this time, a non-resilient rectangular stainless steel archwire should be used to avoid arch distortion.

If the canine is impacted near the roof of the mouth, it is difficult to move the tooth directly into the arch. In these situations, it is advantageous first to erupt the tooth into the oral cavity and then to attach it to the archwire. A transpalatal arch connected to the maxillary molars provides suitable anchorage for the eruption process. A flexible spring or loop may be attached to the transpalatal bar. This attachment is activated to provide a vertical direction of eruption.

After the tooth has erupted sufficiently, it may be attached to the maxillary archwire and moved laterally into the dental arch. An important aspect during this process is to maintain the original arch width. There are several options for moving the canine laterally. Elastomeric chain or elastic thread is easy to attach and provides adequate force to move the canine into position. The disadvantage of the chain and thread is that the force levels produced by these materials diminish gradually, requiring frequent changing of the elastic modules. As the tooth nears its proper position in the arch, a double archwire may be used to move the canine into position. A flexible auxiliary wire made of nickel titanium may be attached in addition to the rectangular

MANAGEMENT OF IMPACTIONS

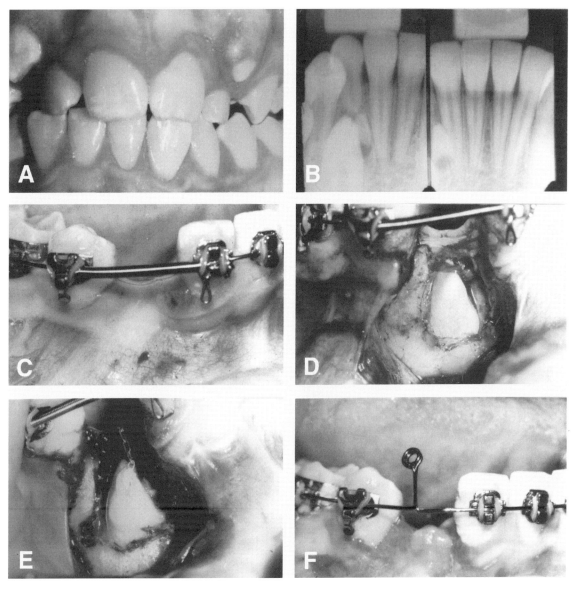

Figure 24-12. An adolescent patient with an impacted mandibular right canine. *A*, The pretreatment intraoral photograph shows that the patient had moderate arch length deficiencies with the maxillary canines erupting ectopically toward the labial. *B*, The pretreatment radiograph showed a supernumerary tooth that had impeded eruption of the mandibular right canine. The primary canine and supernumerary tooth were removed. *C*, Orthodontic treatment was initiated to open space for the permanent canine. *D*, A pedicle flap with a mid-crestal incision was reflected to uncover the impacted canine. The bone was removed from around the crown. *E*, A piece of gold chain was bonded to the cusp tip of the canine. *F*, A Ballista loop was used to deliver an eruptive vertical force to the impacted canine.

wire. The attachment of the auxiliary wire will ensure that the transpalatal width does not change as the tooth is brought into position.

After the canine has been moved into the arch, a radiograph should be taken. Final positioning of the root and crown requires placement of a rectangular wire. If the tooth has been moved from the palate, there usually is insufficient labial crown torque. The use of auxiliary torquing springs or rectangular archwires will accomplish the proper torque and angulation.

MANDIBULAR CANINE

Etiology

Impaction of the mandibular canine (Fig. 24-12) is uncommon. In some situations, the tooth bud of the mandibular canine will become rotated in the alveolus. As that happens, the canine root can develop in a horizontal direction. The canine then becomes impacted below the apices of the incisors. In these situations, it is

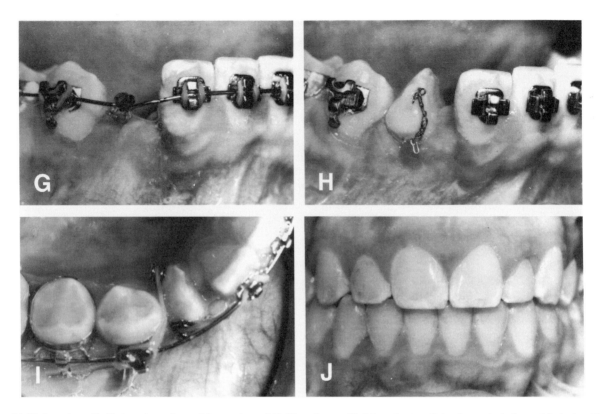

Figure 24-12 (continued) *G*, Another view of the activated Ballista loop. *H*, After the tooth had erupted, the gold chain still was visible at the cusp tip. The tooth was rotated. *I*, Stainless steel buttons and elastomeric chains were used to rotate the tooth into proper position. *J*, After orthodontic treatment, the mandibular right canine was positioned properly in the dental arch. The crown length and position of the gingival margin match the opposite unimpacted tooth. Use of a flap/closed eruption procedure allows tooth movement that closely matches natural tooth eruption.

very difficult to correct the impaction. In some of these patients, it is prudent to extract the canine to avoid damage to the roots of the incisors.

Occasionally, the mandibular canine will become impacted due to the presence of a supernumerary tooth. If the supernumerary is not removed early enough and the root of the canine forms completely, then the canine will lose its eruptive potential. In this situation, the tooth must be uncovered surgically and erupted orthodontically into position.

Preoperative Orthodontics

Initially, bands and brackets must be placed on all teeth, and space is opened for the mandibular canine. Usually 6.5 to 7 mm of space is adequate for most mandibular canines. After the space has been opened, a stabilizing rectangular wire is placed (Fig. 24-12*C*), and the patient is referred to the surgeon to uncover the tooth.

Surgery

When mandibular canines are impacted, they usually are in the intra-alveolar or labial position. It is very important that the surgeon has proper radiographs to determine the exact location of the tooth before surgery. Again, the Buccal Object Rule[6] can be used to locate the impacted tooth precisely.

The intra-alveolar impaction can be uncovered with the flap closed-eruption technique. To use this technique properly, it is imperative that orthodontic appliances have been placed on the teeth, and the patient is at the stage where the appropriate archwire size is present to help facilitate eruption of the tooth. The deciduous tooth and any supernumerary teeth should be extracted at the time of the uncovering. If the patient is too young to initiate orthodontic therapy, then these teeth should be removed at the appropriate times to help the impacted canine erupt on its own.

To uncover the intra-alveolar impaction, the flap closed-eruption technique is used. A crestal incision is made with conservative flap reflection (Fig. 24-12*DE*). Appropriate bone removal is accomplished and a bracket and/or chain, is bonded to the tooth. The flaps are returned to their original locations and sutured with resorbable suture. The orthodontist can initiate tooth movement in one week.

Postoperative Orthodontics

After the mandibular canine has been uncovered, a chain or wire will be extending through the gingival tissue into the oral cavity. The key in this situation is to erupt the tooth through the crest of the alveolar ridge. In order to accomplish this, it is advantageous to use a Ballista spring (Figs. 24-5 and 24-12F) to erupt the tooth in a vertical direction. This spring typically is made out of .018" round archwire. As the tooth erupts, the links of the chain can be removed until the crown has erupted sufficiently into the oral cavity. At that point, a bracket may be placed on the tooth.

Occasionally, the canine will erupt into a rotated position. Mechanics to derotate the tooth must be used before aligning the crown and root into the dental arch. During the finishing phase of orthodontic treatment, the root of the tooth must be positioned to match the axial inclination of the adjacent teeth.

MANDIBULAR SECOND PREMOLAR

Etiology

The most common mandibular impaction is the third molar, followed by the second premolar and the second molar. The second premolar impaction (Fig. 24-13) probably is due to idiopathic rotation of the tooth bud during development. If the tooth bud does not upright itself as the root develops, it eventually will become impacted horizontally. In this situation, surgical exposure of the tooth and orthodontic treatment will be necessary to properly position the tooth.

Preoperative Orthodontics

Prior to initiation of orthodontic therapy, the primary second molar should be removed to encourage eruption of the impacted second premolar. In some situations, the premolar may erupt spontaneously in response to the extraction of the primary tooth. If orthodontic treatment will be delayed, a mandibular space maintainer will hold the position of the first molar. If orthodontic treatment is necessary to erupt the second premolar, it generally is advisable to wait until all permanent teeth have erupted. It also is advantageous to wait until the root of the second premolar has formed completely. Often when second premolars are impacted, they also have delayed root formation.

During the preoperative orthodontic phase, it will be necessary to provide sufficient space for the second premolar. Usually the contralateral second premolar can be used as a guide for tooth size. If both second premolars are impacted, the size of the second premolars generally is about 0.5 to 1 mm larger than the first premolars. After sufficient space has been established, the patient is referred to the surgeon to uncover the second premolar.

Surgery

Second premolars usually can be located by palpation. They often are impacted on the lingual aspect of the mandibular corpus. If a tooth cannot be palpated, an occlusal radiograph or two differently angled periapical radiographs should be used to determine its exact location. When the tooth is impacted lingually, a full thickness lingual flap is reflected from the canine to the mesial of the second molar (Fig. 24-13D). Sometimes a vertical incision is needed when the impacted tooth is positioned near the apices of the adjacent teeth. Judicious bone removal is accomplished to create a hole wide enough for the widest dimension of the crown. The surgeon must proceed carefully when the tooth is displaced lingually, because it usually is located near the roots of the first molar (creating a bony dehiscence). A bracket and/or chain is placed and attached to the archwire (Fig. 24-13EF). The lingual flap is returned to its original location. Slight scalloping of the flap can be performed around the crown so it remains partially exposed. This *manipulation of the flap* will allow the orthodontist to use the necessary mechanics to erupt the tooth. If the impacted premolar is located within the alveolus, the closed eruption technique can be used.

Postoperative Orthodontics

Usually the crown of the impacted second premolar lies either within the alveolar housing or toward the lingual surface. If the tooth is positioned lingually, the crown will be visible after uncovering. In this situation, a bracket should be attached to the crown. Elastomeric chains or elastic thread may be used to move the tooth into position.

If the tooth is confined within the alveolar housing, a flap closed-eruption technique should be performed. The tooth will not be visible after the attachments have been placed. A wire or chain should extend through the gingiva at the crest of the alveolar ridge. In this situation, a Ballista spring may be used to erupt the tooth through the crest of the ridge. A radiograph should be made after the tooth is positioned in the dental arch. In some situations, the root of the second premolar is dilacerated. The angulation of the root should be assessed so the tooth may be positioned properly between the first premolar

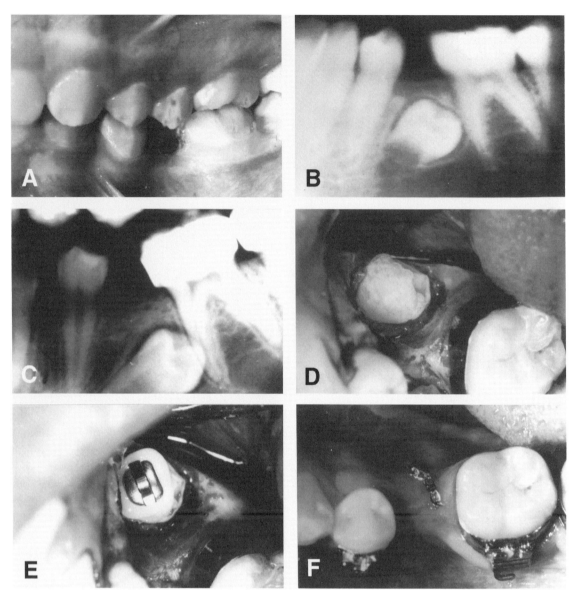

Figure 24-13. A patient with a horizontally impacted mandibular left second premolar. *A,* Pretreatment intraoral photograph. *B,* Although the maxillary and mandibular second molars had erupted, the pretreatment intraoral radiograph shows that the development of the mandibular left second premolar was delayed. The root had not developed. Orthodontic treatment was postponed for two years. *C,* After two years, the root of the second premolar had developed, but the tooth was impacted horizontally. *D,* Orthodontic appliances were placed on the teeth, and after sufficient space had been created, a lingual flap with vertical incisions was used to uncover the lingually and horizontally impacted mandibular second premolar. *E,* A cleat was bonded onto the crown of the premolar, and a gold chain was attached and extended out to the archwire. *F,* The flap was reapproximated and allowed to heal.

and first molar. A rectangular archwire often is needed to provide the proper torque and angulation.

MANDIBULAR FIRST MOLAR

Etiology

The etiology of mandibular first molar impaction (Fig. 24-14) is unknown. For some reason, the first molar fails to erupt. In some instances, this lack of eruption may be confused with ankylosis; however, many of these teeth probably are not ankylosed. The key in this situation is to diagnose the problem early. If the patient is seen in the early mixed dentition, it may be possible to uncover the tooth and erupt it into position. As time passes, however, the molar may need to be extracted if the tooth remains submerged to allow the second molar to drift mesially.

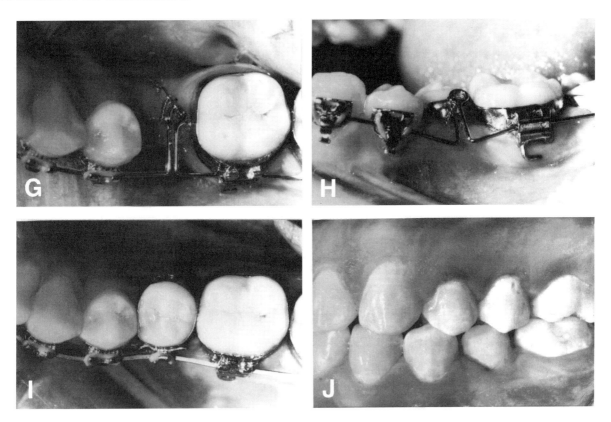

Figure 24-13 (Continued) *G* and *H*, A Ballista spring was used to erupt the canine and move it into position in the center of the alveolar ridge. *I*, Although the second premolar was rotated 180° in the alveolus, the decision was made to leave the premolar in its rotated position. The crown was positioned properly, and the occlusion was finished. *J*, After orthodontic treatment, the amount of gingiva labial to the formerly impacted premolar was adequate, as the tooth was erupted with a flap/closed eruption technique.

Preoperative Orthodontics

If the mandibular first molar is hopelessly impacted and is located significantly below the occlusal plane, extraction may be necessary. A mandibular lingual arch may help to avoid a change in the mandibular dental midline. Placing a lingual arch between the mandibular lateral incisor and first molar on the opposite side will maintain the dental midline. In that way, the posterior teeth may erupt more toward the mesial. When all teeth erupt, the second molar can be moved mesially and substituted for the first molar.

If the patient is seen at an early age, the impacted mandibular first molar may be uncovered and erupted. It is important, however, to have sufficient anchorage to erupt the impacted molar. During the preoperative orthodontic phase, a stabilizing appliance should be placed in the opposite arch, using the maxillary first molar as an anchor tooth to erupt the impacted mandibular first molar. A palatal expander or a transpalatal arch is helpful to obtain cross-arch anchorage. The ideal way to erupt the tooth would be with elastic or rubber band forces to the teeth in the opposite arch. Once the expander or stabilizing appliance has been cemented, the patient should be referred to the surgeon to uncover the impacted mandibular first molar.

Surgery

Fortunately, mandibular first molars rarely are impacted, and they can be very difficult to uncover adequately. It is a challenge to uncover the tooth completely and not damage adjacent teeth or tooth buds. A common error in uncovering teeth that are embedded in the mid-alveolar region is to not remove enough bone so that the greatest width of the tooth can be erupted through the opening. Due to the "bell" shape of posterior teeth, the widest dimension usually is found in the mid-coronal region (Fig. 24-14*E*).

These teeth usually are in the mid-alveolar region; however, appropriate radiographs need to be taken to verify the exact position of the tooth before uncovering. The closed-eruption technique is used, but more extensive flap reflection will be needed due to the severe apical position of the tooth (Fig. 24-14*D*). Vertical incisions can be used on the buccal aspect to facilitate access. Great care must be taken to avoid damage to the adjacent roots, tooth buds, and the mental nerve.

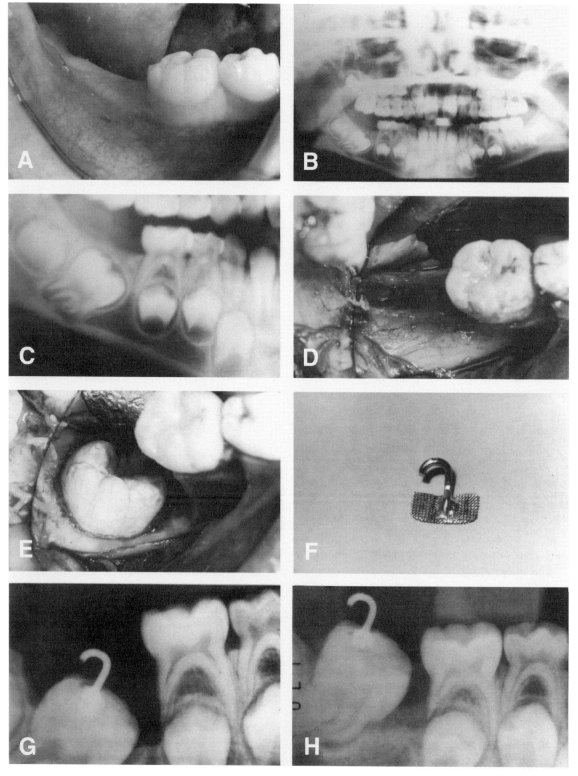

Figure 24-14. A young patient with an impacted mandibular right first molar. *A*, Pretreatment intraoral photograph. *B* and *C*, The pretreatment panoramic radiograph indicated that the mandibular right first molar was impacted and angulated mesially. The tooth was well below the level of the eruption of the contralateral first molar and maxillary first molars. The treatment plan involved uncovering the tooth, bonding an attachment, and using an elastic force from the maxillary arch to erupt the impacted molar. *D*, A flap was elevated over the ridge, distal to the mandibular right primary second molar. *E*, The bone over the first molar crown was removed. *F*, A piece of wire mesh was soldered to a segment of archwire shaped in the form of a hook, and this attachment was bonded to the buccal surface of the first molar (*G*). *H*, A palatal expander was placed in the maxilla, and a rubber band was used to erupt the first molar.

MANAGEMENT OF IMPACTIONS

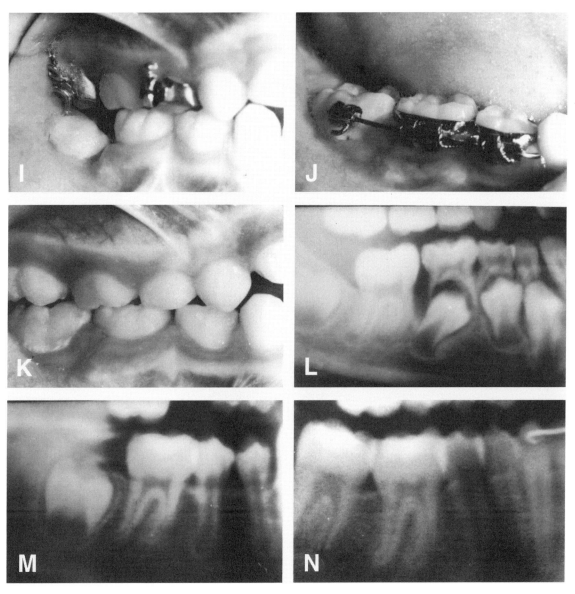

Figure 24-14 (continued). *I* and *J*, After the first molar had erupted, the bonded attachment was removed and a bracket was placed on the tooth. Segmental orthodontic techniques were used to complete the uprighting process. *K*, After bracket removal, the mandibular first molar was positioned in proper occlusion with the maxillary arch. *L*, The panoramic radiograph showed that the mandibular right second premolar had angulated somewhat mesially during the eruption of the first molar. *M* and *N*, After 12 months, the second premolar had erupted. The first molar also was erupting. The tooth appeared to be developing normally 1.5 years after the orthodontic treatment had been completed.

The tooth is isolated, and a bracket is bonded to the tooth. A chain is ligated to the bracket, exits through the crestal incision, and is attached to the archwire. The flaps are returned to their original location and sutured. Tooth movement can be initiated within a week.

Postoperative Orthodontics

After the surgical procedure, the patient will have an attachment protruding through the gingival tissue. Again, it is important to erupt the tooth through the crest of the ridge. In this way, the patient will have sufficient attached gingiva after it has erupted. Usually a hook (Fig. 24-14*F*) will be protruding through the gingiva. A rubber band can be worn from this hook to the palatal expander and the first molar in the opposite arch. When the patient chews and functions, the rubber bands will stretch, and the tooth will erupt. If the tooth does not move, the surgeon may not have removed enough bone around the crown of the tooth. After the tooth has erupted sufficiently, using an elastic force, a bracket may be placed on the crown of the first molar (Fig. 24-14*GH*). The adjacent posterior primary molars in that segment can be banded or bracketed and used as anchors to upright the permanent first molar. This technique of erupting the impacted mandibular first molar is efficient and avoids distortion of the occlusal plane in the opposing arch.

MANDIBULAR SECOND MOLAR

Etiology

Impaction of the mandibular second molars (Fig. 24-15) occurs in less than one percent of the population.[13-15] When it occurs, however, second molar impaction is a difficult problem to correct. Some second molar impactions occur spontaneously and may be related to the position of the third molar. The reason for the impaction may be due to differential development of the mesial and distal roots of the second molar. If the distal root develops first, the crown of the second molar may tip toward the mesial. Second molar impaction also may occur iatrogenically. Such an impaction may be the result of attempting to increase arch length in the mandibular arch. During this process, the mandibular first molar may tip distally and impact the second molar. In either situation, it often is necessary to uncover the tooth and position it orthodontically.

Preoperative Orthodontics

Prior to orthodontic treatment, the mandibular third molar should be evaluated. If the third molars will interfere with the eruption or distal movement of the second molars, they may need to be extracted. Another consideration may be possible. If the second molars are hopelessly impacted horizontally, and the third molars are in a reasonably good position, it may be prudent to extract the second molars. This is not a guaranteed solution, because in some situations, the third molars also may become impacted horizontally.

It is necessary to place orthodontic appliances on all remaining mandibular teeth to provide sufficient anchorage to move the second molars into their proper position. Once the mandibular teeth have been aligned and stabilized, the patient should be referred for uncovering of the second molar.

Surgery

Mandibular second molars usually are impacted in the mid-alveolar region. When they are "locked" under the first molar, they will need to be uncovered and left uncovered so that the orthodontist can apply appropriate mechanics to erupt the tooth. In the example shown in Figure 24-14, the flap closed-eruption technique cannot be used due to the mesial angulation. A modification of the technique is needed for proper exposure and orthodontic access.

A gingivectomy rarely is adequate to uncover enough of the buccal surface of these teeth. This inadequacy is due to the narrow width of the attached gingiva in this area and the mesial angulation of the tooth in the vestibule. Therefore, a conservative lingual flap and a buccal pedicle flap are reflected for access (Fig. 24-15D). Enough bone is removed to expose two-thirds of the crown. The lingual flap is positioned apically to uncover the lingual/coronal aspect of the molar. The buccal pedicle flap is positioned apically exposing two-thirds of the crown (Fig. 24-15E). A dressing then is placed on the buccal surface to keep the tissue in place and avoid hypertrophy of adjacent tissue. Within a week the tooth can be bracketed, and tooth movement can be initiated.

Postoperative Orthodontics

If the second molar is tipped severely to the mesial, it may be impossible to place a bracket on the buccal surface of the tooth. In those situations, a bracket or other attachment may be bonded to the occlusal or distal surface of the second molar. A spring from the first molar also can be used to push the second molar distally.

If the tooth is tipped moderately, a bracket may be placed on the buccal surface. A flexible nickel titanium wire is useful in engaging the bracket. These wires are very effective at producing gradual movement to upright the second molar. Again, it is important to assess the proximity of the third molars to determine if they will interfere with the movement of the second molars. After initial uprighting of the second molar, a rectangular wire usually is necessary to produce the proper axial inclination of the root.

POTENTIAL PROBLEMS

Lack of Movement

After uncovering an impacted tooth, orthodontic mechanics to erupt the tooth may be started within a few weeks. Occasionally the impacted tooth may seem immobile and resist orthodontic force. This situation occurs more commonly with palatal rather than intra-alveolar impactions. Usually this problem is temporary. Persistent orthodontic force in the proper direction usually will move the impacted tooth. In some patients,

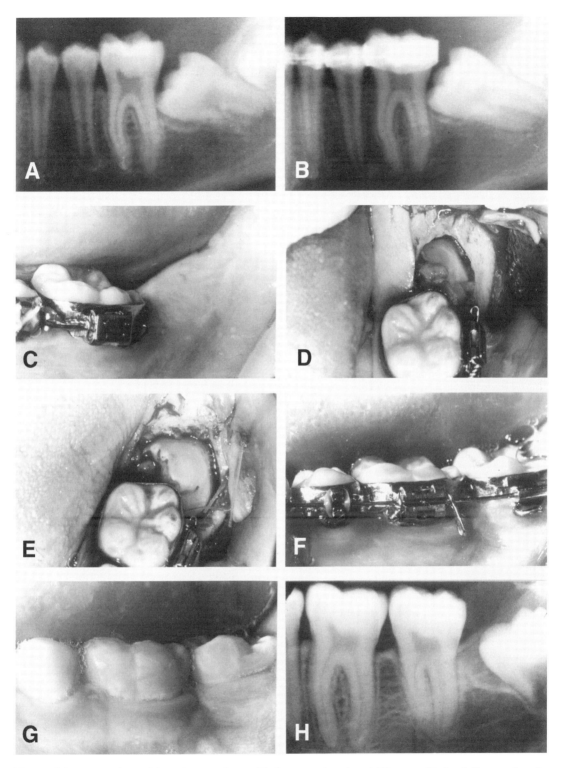

Figure 24-15. An adolescent patient with an impacted mandibular second molar. *A*, The mandibular left second molar was angulated mesially and impacted distal to the first molar. *B*, Orthodontic appliances were placed on all teeth, and initial alignment of the dental arches was achieved. The position of the impacted second molar did not improve. *C*, This preoperative intraoral photograph shows that the amount of gingiva distal to the first molar was not sufficient to permit a gingivectomy to expose the tooth. *D*, Therefore, a buccal pedicle flap and a lingual flap were elevated from the crest of the ridge to expose the second molar, which was covered by bone. *E*, The bone covering the buccal and occlusal portions of the second molar crown was removed. The buccal and lingual flaps were apically positioned to expose the second molar. *F*, After sufficient healing, the second molar was gradually erupted into position. *G*, The amount of attached gingiva buccal to the mandibular second molar has been increased with the apically positioned flap technique. *H*, The roots of the second molar have been positioned properly. The impacted third molar did not impede tooth movement and can be extracted later.

however, the impacted tooth will continue to resist movement. This problem has three possible causes. First, during the uncovering procedure, bone may have been left around the crown of the impacted tooth. As an orthodontic force is applied, there is no biologic mechanism for the enamel of the crown to resorb the surrounding bone. The tooth becomes wedge in the alveolus. It is important for the surgeon to remove sufficient bone to permit clearance of the crown of the impacted tooth as it erupts.

A second possible cause of lack of tooth movement is the use of inappropriate orthodontic mechanics. An impacted tooth may resist lateral movement because of its angulation within the alveolus. The solution for this problem is to erupt the tooth into the oral cavity initially. Extrusive mechanics do not require bone resorption. If the tooth can be erupted initially into the oral cavity, then it can be moved into position more easily.

The third possible cause of immobility is ankylosis. Although it is rare, ankylosis of an impacted tooth may occur. When the tooth is uncovered, it is important for the surgeon to test the mobility of the tooth. If the impacted tooth is mobile, it probably will erupt if the direction of force is correct. If not, the tooth may be ankylosed and should be luxated or loosened within its alveolar housing. Some ankylosed teeth will still not move and will require extraction.

During orthodontic finishing, it is important to position the root of an impacted tooth properly to avoid potential relapse. As a palatally impacted canine is moved laterally toward the alveolar crest, the root often tips toward the palate. If the root remains in this position after appliance removal, the crown will tend to migrate back toward the palate and into crossbite. Therefore, during orthodontic finishing, it is important to tip the root of the canine labially. This movement is performed with rectangular archwires or torquing springs. This process must be performed gradually, however. If the canine root is moved labially too rapidly, a dehiscence may occur at the labial crestal margin. If the tissue is thin over this defect, the gingival tissue may recede exposing the cementum of the root. In these situations, it may be necessary to refer the patient for gingival grafting to prevent recession.

In some situations, it may be more prudent to extract an impacted tooth rather than to attempt erupting it into the dental arch. Although this situation is rare, it may occur in patients with palatally impacted canines and horizontally impacted mandibular canines and second molars. If the maxillary canine is impacted horizontally and is high in the palate, and the patient has significant crowding of the maxillary teeth, it may be more judicious to extract an impacted canine instead of a first premolar. In this situation, the first premolar should be non-restored, non-carious, have good root form, and be in proper position to justify this unique extraction decision.

In the mandibular arch, a horizontally impacted mandibular second molar may be difficult to erupt. If the patient has third molars that are in reasonable relationship, it may be more judicious to extract the mandibular second molars. This extraction, however, does not ensure that the third molars will erupt into their proper position. Occasionally, the third molars also will be tipped to the mesial and require orthodontic uprighting.

Occasionally, the palatally impacted canine will be wedged against the root of the maxillary central or lateral incisor. In some of these patients, this close proximity of the impacted crown will cause resorption of the roots of the incisors. In this situation, it is important to develop orthodontic mechanics to move the crown of the impacted tooth away from the roots of the incisors. Usually, after proper positioning of the impacted tooth and completion of the orthodontic treatment, the root resorption will cease. If the root of the affected incisor has not shortened significantly, it may remain functional indefinitely.

A common question is whether or not to extract the third molars during the uncovering of the impacted second molars. If sufficient space exists for the third molars to erupt, they can be extracted at the time of uncovering; however, there are some possible disadvantages. The amount of trauma and postoperative discomfort will be greater and may delay bracketing of the second molars. Second, it may complicate flap management if both teeth are difficult impactions. The second molar will require considerable apical positioning of the flap, whereas the third molar site will require primary closure. These two adjacent flaps are not compatible. The primary goal is to uncover the second molar adequately. It may be more prudent to remove the third molars after completion of the orthodontic treatment.

Surgical Complications

Improper technique is the most common problem when impacted teeth are uncovered surgically. Inadequate surgery can complicate or even make orthodontic movement impossible. Inadequate flap reflection or operating through a "pigeon hole" can lead to damage to the crown or adjacent roots, inadequate or excessive bone removal, and poor isolation, causing a weakly bonded bracket.[11] Improper technique also can lead to loss of attached gingiva and damage to the attachment apparatus.[3,5,9] It also can lead to unesthetic gingival sequelae, seen most commonly when a gingivectomy is attempted in an improper situation.

The apically positioned flap has been the most common technique for uncovering labial impactions. Although this technique is appropriate for some labially impacted teeth (transposed labial impactions), the flap closed-eruption technique is the procedure of choice for most labial impactions and mid-alveolar impactions. When the apically positioned flap is not employed properly, the following problems may be encountered:

1. This technique produces a greater risk of recession and uneven gingival margins compared with the non-impacted contralateral tooth.[16,18-19]
2. Impactions located near the nasal spine are impossible to leave uncovered.[7-9]
3. When this technique is used for very high or laterally displaced impactions, accessory frena can be created in the vertical incision area, and orthodontic relapse has been observed in some patients.

The flap closed-eruption technique usually produces the best gingival esthetics.[17-19]

Two potential problems can arise with the flap closed-eruption technique if it is employed improperly. First, debonding of the bracket or chain can occur if proper isolation and bonding techniques are not used. Second, if improper orthodontic mechanics are used, a mucogingival problem can result. If the tooth erupts through mucosa or too near the mucogingival junction, it may have inadequate attached gingiva. This problem can be eliminated by properly using the Ballista spring to erupt the tooth through the mid-crestal area. When used properly, this technique mimics the normal eruptive pattern, eliminates potential recession, and leaves an adequate zone of attached gingiva.

The preorthodontic uncovering technique for palatally impacted canines has proved to be an excellent technique. Compared with other approaches, it requires considerably less time for the orthodontist to move the tooth into its proper location. It is also less traumatic to the teeth used for anchorage to erupt the tooth. There are also fewer instances of damage to the roots of adjacent teeth.

The problems with the preorthodontic uncovering technique center around postsurgical sequelae. The postoperative healing period is slower and more uncomfortable. Some teeth require deep, broad, scalloping of the palatal flap, and this type of surgical procedure can lead to bleeding problems during surgery and the postoperative period. Teeth in the "gray area" (i.e., higher in the roof of the palate and more deeply embedded) are more difficult to keep uncovered during the first few weeks. Sometimes they require degranulation of the tissue margins and replacement of the dressing until the tissue epithelializes. Most importantly, if bone is not properly removed from the crown of the tooth, the tooth will not erupt.

Some teeth are so deeply impacted that even if they can be uncovered, there is no possible orthodontic means to erupt them. There are times when it is preferable to extract the tooth than to create unnecessary surgical and orthodontic trauma. These situations usually can be diagnosed with proper records and consultation with the orthodontist.

It is the surgeon's responsibility to make detailed notes about the nature of the impacted tooth and its position and to take appropriate photographs. This information will assist the orthodontist in his/her efforts to erupt the tooth and will greatly facilitate the treatment.

REFERENCES CITED

1. Bass T. Observation on the misplaced upper canine tooth. Dent Practitioner 1967;18:25–33.
2. Witsenberg B, Boering G. Eruption of impacted permanent upper incisors after removal of supernumerary teeth. Int J Oral Surg 1981;10:423–431.
3. Vanarsdall RL, Jr, Corn H. Soft-tissue management of labially positioned unerupted teeth. Am J Orthod 1977;72: 53–64.
4. Johnston WD. Treatment of palatally impacted canine teeth. Am J Orthod 1969;56:589–596.
5. Boyd RL. Clinical assessment of injuries in orthodontic movement of impacted teeth. II. Surgical recommendations. Am J Orthod 1984;86:407–418.
6. Richards A. The buccal object rule. Dent Radiogr Photog 1980;55:37–56.
7. Fournier A, Turcotte JY, Bernard C. Orthodontic considerations in the treatment of maxillary impacted canines. Am J Orthod 1982;81:236–239.
8. Hunter S. Treatment of the unerupted maxillary canine. Br Dent J 1983;154:294–296.
9. Wong-Lee TK, Wong FC. Maintaining an ideal tooth-gingiva relationship when exposing and aligning an impacted tooth. Br J Orthod 1985;12:189–192.
10. Magnusson H. Saving impacted teeth. J Clin Orthod 1990; 24:246–249.
11. Abrams H, Gossett S, Morgan W. A modified flap design in exposing the palatally impacted canine. J Dent Child 1988;55:285–287.
12. Smukler H, Castellucci G, Goldman H. Surgical management of palatally impacted cuspids. Compend Cont Educ Dent 1987;8:10–17.
13. Montelius G. Impacted teeth. A comparative study of Chinese and Caucasian dentitions. J Dent Res 1932;12: 931–938.

14. Johnsen D. Prevalence of delayed emergence of permanent teeth as a result of local factors. J Am Dent Assoc 1977;94:100–106.
15. Grover P, Lorton L. The incidence of unerupted permanent teeth and related clinical cases. Oral Surg 1985;59:420–424.
16. Ranalli D, Buzzato J, Braun T, Jones R, Smith P. Long-term interdisciplinary management of multiple mesiodens and delayed eruption: Report of case. J Dent Child 1988;55:376–380.
17. Cangialosi TJ, Meistrell ME, Jr. A cephalometric evaluation of hard- and soft-tissue changes during the third stage of Begg treatment. Am J Orthod 1982;81:124–129.
18. Vermette ME, Kokich VG, Kennedy DB. Uncovering labially impacted teeth: Apically positioned flap and closed-eruption techniques. Angle Orthod 1995;65:23–32.
19. Kokich VG, Mathews DP. Surgical and orthodontic management of impacted teeth. Dent Clin N Am 1993;37:181–204.

Chapter 25

MANAGING ORTHODONTIC-RESTORATIVE TREATMENT FOR THE ADOLESCENT PATIENT

By Vincent G. Kokich

Most adolescent orthodontic patients have complete dentitions with few restorations, healthy periodontium, and lack of wear or trauma to their teeth. Therefore, orthodontists seldom need to interact with restorative dentists prior to or during orthodontic treatment. Some teenage orthodontic patients, however, have dental problems that require orthodontic-restorative interaction in order to produce an ideal functional and esthetic result.

Malformed maxillary lateral incisors, congenitally missing maxillary lateral incisors and mandibular second premolars, and major or minor trauma to the anterior teeth resulting in partial or complete fracture of permanent anterior teeth may require combined orthodontic, restorative, surgical, and periodontal intervention. As a result, orthodontists must know how to interact with other members of the dental team in the management of these types of problems. This chapter will use many examples to illustrate the key steps in managing the adolescent patient who requires orthodontic and restorative treatment.

MALFORMED MAXILLARY INCISORS

The most common malformed tooth is the maxillary lateral incisor. It often is referred to as "pegged" or a "peg lateral." These malformed laterals generally have two different shapes. Some are cone-shaped (Fig. 25-1). Others resemble the shape of a normal lateral incisor (Fig. 25-2), but are significantly narrower, thinner, and shorter. If a lateral incisor is only slightly narrower than normal, and the problem is bilateral, the orthodontist may decide not to provide space to restore the tooth during orthodontic treatment. If the width discrepancy is only slight, the influence on the anterior occlusion, and the impact on esthetics may be indistinguishable. If the malformation is unilateral, however, or if the width discrepancy is significant, esthetics and occlusion could be affected adversely if the malformed tooth or teeth are ignored.[1-5]

Before the advent of composite bonding, restorative treatment of malformed maxillary lateral incisors was much more challenging and required a full crown to enlarge the size of the malformed tooth. If the dentist attempts to place a full crown, an adolescent patient with a large pulp may be at substantial risk for irreversible damage.

Bonding has permitted much more conservative restoration without extensive preparation of the lateral incisor. Either composite or porcelain veneer restorations, or complete composite or porcelain crowns may be bonded to the enamel with minimal tooth reduction. The orthodontist, however, must position the malformed tooth in the proper position in order to facilitate ideal restoration.

If the malformed lateral incisor merely is narrower, thinner, and shorter than the contralateral incisor, the final restoration probably will be a composite or porcelain veneer. In this situation, the orthodontist must position the tooth precisely prior to restoration. If sufficient space exists, a composite restoration may be placed before orthodontic treatment (Fig. 25-1). In most situations, however, there is insufficient space to restore the malformed lateral incisors (Fig. 25-2). Therefore, orthodontic treatment often is necessary to create space to build-up malformed lateral incisors.

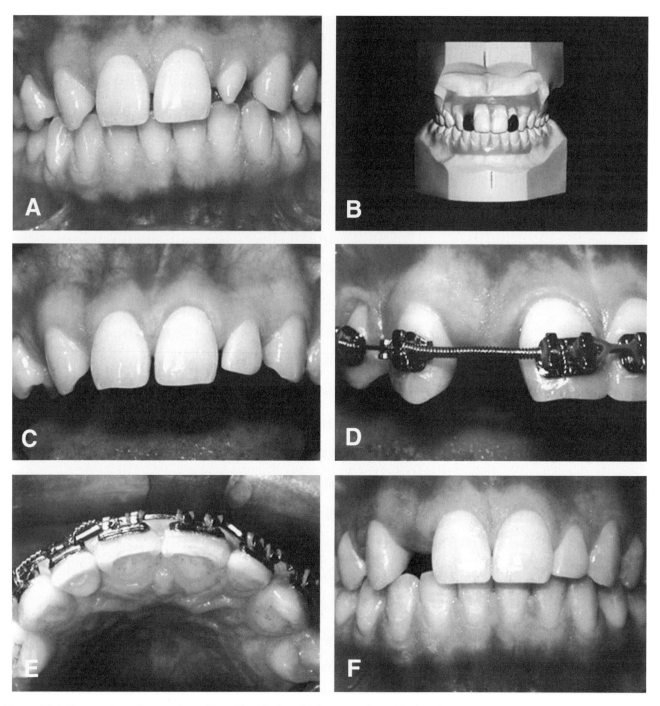

Figure 25-1. Restoration of a peg-shaped maxillary incisor. If the contralateral incisor is missing and sufficient space exists to restore the peg-shaped tooth (*A*), the restoration should be completed before orthodontic bracketing. The correct size of the lateral incisor restoration is determined by constructing a diagnostic wax set-up (*B*). The restorative dentist uses the diagnostic set-up as a guide (*C*). Then during the orthodontic treatment, the orthodontist creates the same amount of space for the contralateral missing lateral (*D,E,F*). Relying on the diagnostic set-up will insure that the size of the laterals will be symmetrically identical and the teeth will occlude properly. A pontic tied to the archwire is shown in Figure 25-1*E*.

Creating a Space for a Restoration

The orthodontic mechanics to open space mesial and distal to the lateral incisor are relatively simple. Compressed coil springs are placed between the central incisor, lateral incisor, and canine to push the central and canine away from the lateral incisor (Fig. 25-2*C*). Space will be generated in a few weeks. As space is created, four questions must be answered. First, how much space is required to restore the lateral incisor? If the patient is congenitally missing the opposite lateral incisor, a diagnostic wax-up should be constructed. This set-up will de-

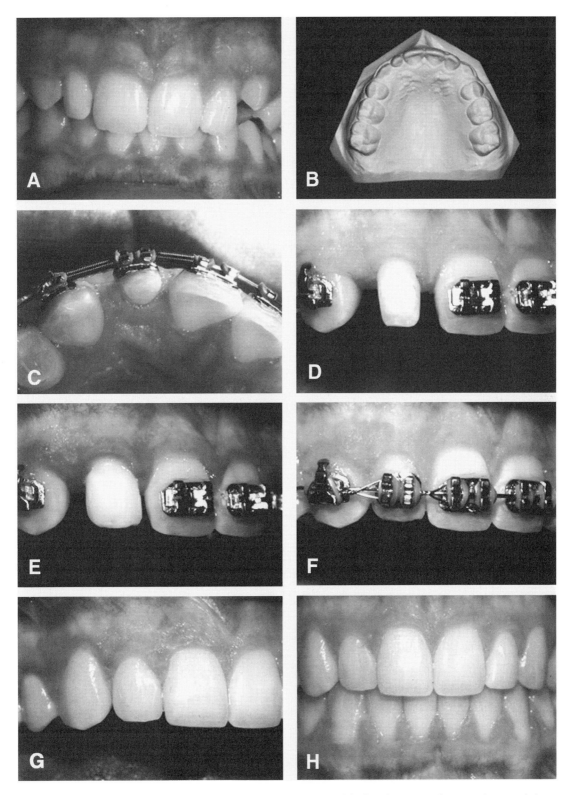

Figure 25-2. Restoration of a narrow maxillary lateral incisor. If one lateral incisor has normal proportions, and the contralateral tooth is narrow (*A,B*), the narrower tooth should be restored to proper dimension during the orthodontic treatment. Compressed coil springs (*C*) are used to create space for the restoration. The narrow lateral is positioned nearer to the central than the canine (*D*), so the form of the restoration can be flat on the mesial and overcontoured on the distal (*E*). This shape mimics the natural lateral incisor and allows creation of a more natural papilla between the central and lateral incisor (*F,G*). The gingival margin of the narrow lateral incisor is aligned with the gingival margin of the contralateral lateral incisor, so the eventual crown length, as well as the width, will be identical to the natural lateral incisor (*H*).

termine the correct size for the restoration of the peg-shaped lateral incisor. If the patient has an existing lateral incisor of normal width on the opposite side, it is appropriate to create the same amount of space. Occasionally, it is advantageous to create extra space temporarily. This additional space will allow the restorative dentist to contour and polish the interproximal surfaces of the temporary composite restoration, so it matches the width of the opposite lateral. Any residual space may be closed after the restoration has been placed.

When creating space orthodontically, a second question arises. Where should the maxillary lateral incisor be positioned mesiodistally relative to the central incisor and canine? If the lateral incisor is positioned too close to the canine, the mesial surface of the lateral must be overcontoured to achieve the appropriate crown width; the result could be unesthetic. The emergence profile or contour of the mesial surfaces of lateral and central incisors is relatively flat. The distal surfaces of central and lateral incisors are more contoured or convex. Therefore, the peg-shaped lateral incisor should be positioned nearer the central incisor[2] than the canine during orthodontic treatment.

Where should a lateral incisor be positioned buccolingually: toward the labial, in the center of the ridge, or toward the lingual? The answer to this question depends on the type of permanent restoration that eventually will be constructed for the tooth. In most instances during orthodontic treatment, a temporary composite build-up is placed on a peg-shaped lateral incisor. Eventually, this tooth may be restored with either a porcelain veneer or a porcelain crown. If the eventual restoration will be a porcelain crown, the lateral incisor should be positioned in the center of the ridge buccolingually, leaving 0.50 to 0.75 mm of overjet. Positioning the tooth in this manner will avoid additional tooth preparation of the lingual of the lateral and permit space for gold and/or porcelain in the final restoration. If the final restoration will be a porcelain veneer, however, then the peg-shaped lateral should be positioned lingually to contact the mandibular incisors in centric occlusion.[2] Sufficient space will be available on the labial to construct both the temporary composite build-up and the eventual porcelain veneer.

Finally, where should the lateral incisor be positioned incisogingivally? This relationship is determined by the relative positions of the gingival margins. Most peg-shaped lateral incisors not only are narrower mesiodistally and buccolingually; they also are shorter than normal lateral incisors incisogingivally. If the incisal edge is aligned with the opposite lateral incisor, the crown could be too short. Therefore, the gingival margins of the peg-shaped lateral should be aligned with the contralateral lateral incisor.[2] The restorative dentist will restore proper length, width, and thickness of the tooth, when the temporary composite build-up and final restoration are constructed.

Gingival Surgery Prior To Restoration

In some adolescent patients, the clinical crown length of the malformed lateral incisor may appear unusually short (Fig. 25-3A). This situation could affect the ability of the restorative dentist to build-up the tooth, and the restoration may not represent the true anatomical crown length accurately. If the malformed lateral incisor is short, the orthodontist should take a periapical radiograph of the tooth to determine the actual position of the cementoenamel junction (Fig. 25-3B). Many of these situations require gingival surgery[6] to lengthen the malformed incisor crown (Fig. 25-3C) prior to restoration (Fig. 25-3D).

In most instances, the surgery will involve simple excisional removal of gingiva. The orthodontist may confirm the need for crown lengthening by probing the sulcus around the lateral incisor to determine if the sulcular depth is greater than one millimeter on the labial surface. In some situations, if the alveolar bone level is near the cementoenamel junction and the zone of gingiva is narrow, the surgery could be more involved and require an apically positioned flap and bone removal to achieve the proper crown length. Creating proper crown length facilitates the construction of the provisional restoration and enhances placement of orthodontic brackets on the peg-shaped tooth (Fig. 25-3DEF).

MULTIPLE MALFORMED INCISORS

Occasionally, both central and lateral incisors may be malformed and narrower than normal (Fig. 25-4). This abnormal morphology will create a substantial anterior tooth-size discrepancy and a compromised esthetic result if the teeth are not restored to a larger size at some time either before or during the orthodontic treatment. If centrals and laterals are malformed bilaterally, there are no guides for the correct size of these teeth. This situation is complicated further if the patient has a significant posterior malocclusion (Fig. 25-4AB). In these patients, it is mandatory that the orthodontist create a diagnostic wax set-up (Fig. 25-4F) prior to restoration to simulate the correct size of the centrals and laterals in order to provide not only the correct anterior and posterior occlusal relationship (Fig. 25-4EG), but also to provide the correct esthetic balance between the widths of the central and lateral incisors (Fig. 25-4HIJ).

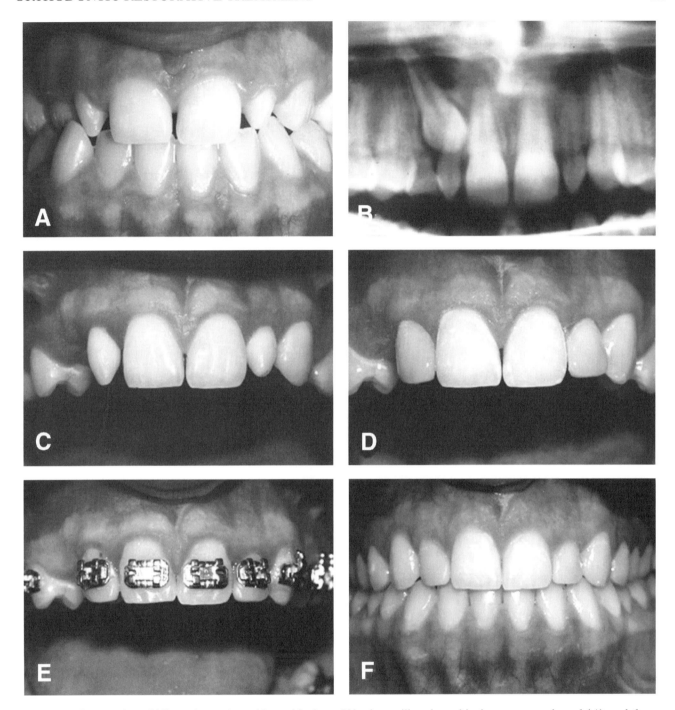

Figure 25-3. Restoration of bilateral peg-shaped lateral incisors. If both maxillary lateral incisors are peg-shaped (*A*), and the canine is impacted in the palate (*B*), a diagnostic wax set-up constructed to determine the appropriate size of lateral incisor restorations may be inaccurate. In addition, the peg-shaped laterals may not be erupted completely, making restoration difficult. In these situations, gingival surgery to lengthen the clinical crowns (*C*) is beneficial. The size of the lateral incisor restoration is estimated from the width of the central incisor, and should be about two-thirds the width of the central (*D*). By restoring the lateral incisors in this way, orthodontic bracketing (*E*) is much easier, the esthetic result is improved, and the occlusion fits properly (*F*).

CONGENITALLY MISSING MANDIBULAR SECOND PREMOLARS

Often adolescent patients are congenitally missing mandibular second premolars. The options for replacing these teeth depend on several factors. First of all, the clinician must decide if the patient has an arch length deficiency. If so, and the patient's profile will not be adversely affected, extraction of maxillary premolars and mandibular primary second molars along with complete space closure may be the best alternative to eliminate

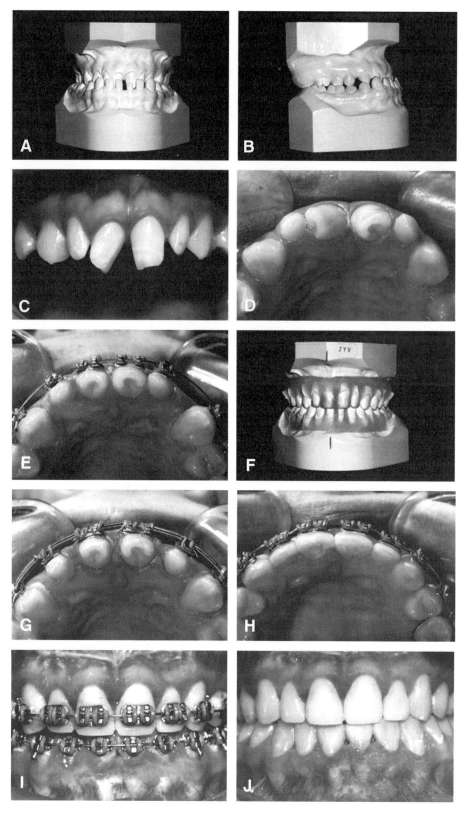

Figure 25-4. Restoration of multiple malformed maxillary incisors. Occasionally, both the maxillary central and lateral incisors are narrow. If the patient has a skeletal malrelationship (*A,B*), it may be difficult to estimate the correct width for restoration of the malformed incisors (*C,D*). In these situations, creating the correct spacing during orthodontic treatment (*E*), is determined by constructing a diagnostic wax set-up that simulates the result of both the orthodontics and orthognathic surgery (*F*). The set-up is used by the orthodontist to open interproximal spaces (*G*) and by the restorative dentist to restore the malformed incisors to their proper width during orthodontics (*H*). If the set-up is accurate, the orthognathic surgery will produce the correct anterior and posterior occlusion (*I*) as well as the appropriate esthetic relationship of the maxillary incisors (*J*).

the need for restorations. Alternatively, if the arch length deficiency is not severe, or if the patient has a satisfactory profile, extraction of teeth and space closure may be disadvantageous. In these situations, the space from the congenitally missing premolars must be maintained and restored with either a bridge or an implant.

Retaining Primary Molars

If an implant is planned for the congenitally missing mandibular second premolar, the space and bone support must be monitored and maintained. It is ideal to allow the mandibular primary molar to remain in position as long as possible in order to maintain the bone support. The primary molar, however, may be too wide (mesiodistally) to occlude properly with the opposing dentition (Fig. 25-5*AB*). In this situation, it may be advantageous to reduce the width of the primary molar so it approximates the width of a second premolar (Fig. 25-5*CD*).[7]

The reduction can be performed efficiently with a fissure bur. It is important for the clinician first to determine the width of the primary molar at the cervical region. By examining a bitewing radiograph, the clinician can estimate the width of the primary molar. Then that distance is transferred to the occlusal table of the primary molar, and a thin fissure bur should be used to reduce its width. Usually local anesthetic is not necessary, because this type of procedure typically is performed around age 14 to 15 years, when the pulp chamber of the primary molar has constricted significantly.

After the width of the molar has been reduced, it is advantageous to cover the exposed dentin on the mesial and distal surfaces by means of a light-cured composite (Fig. 25-5*E*). Then the composite restoration may be trimmed to simulate the shape and size of a mandibular premolar. In this way, the primary molar may be bracketed (Fig. 25-5*FG*) and remain in position to maintain the alveolar bone prior to implant placement (Fig. 25-5*H*).

Timing Primary Tooth Extraction

If the primary molar has remained in position for several years, and the patient chooses to have the implant placed, then the primary tooth must be extracted prior to implant placement. The implant should be placed about two months after the primary tooth extraction to allow for soft tissue healing over the extraction socket, but avoid narrowing of the edentulous ridge (Fig. 25-6).

Extracting Ankylosed Primary Molars

Occasionally, the mandibular primary second molar will become ankylosed (Fig. 25-7) and fused to the alveolus. In these situations, leaving the primary molar may result in a significant bone defect in the edentulous ridge. If an implant is planned in the edentulous site, the vertical defect may make implant placement difficult.

The decision to extract an ankylosed primary molar depends on the patient's age and gender.[7] If the second premolar is congenitally missing, and the primary molar is ankylosed and submerging at ages 7 through 12 in either males or females, the ankylosed tooth should be extracted. At these ages in both genders, the patient has considerable facial growth remaining. As the mandibular ramus grows, the posterior teeth will erupt, except in the ankylosed site. This condition eventually will cause a vertical alveolar defect.

If the ankylosed tooth is extracted, however, research[8] has shown that the alveolar ridge will move occlusally with the adjacent teeth as they continue to erupt (Fig. 25-8). The stretching of the periosteum over the ridge provides the osteoblastic activity to continue alveolar ridge growth.

If the patient is a male aged 12 to 15, the ankylosed and submerging primary molar also should be extracted, as males may have significant mandibular ramus growth until the late teenage years. In contrast, females generally complete facial growth earlier, and an ankylosed primary second molar may not be submerging after 13 years of age in females, thus not creating a vertical alveolar defect.[7] In general, it always is advantageous to maintain the mandibular primary second molar, but reduce its mesiodistal dimension, in order to preserve the width of the alveolus for the future implant. The primary second molar should only be extracted if it is submerging.

Determining The Age For Implant Placement

The age for implant placement in adolescent males and females is totally dependent on the completion of facial growth.[7] As the mandibular ramus continues to grow, the posterior teeth erupt. If an implant is placed too early, before growth is completed, it will mimic an ankylosed tooth and become submerged in the alveolus. This situation could lead to a periodontal defect between the implant and adjacent teeth, if the submersion is severe enough.

The most precise method for determining if facial or

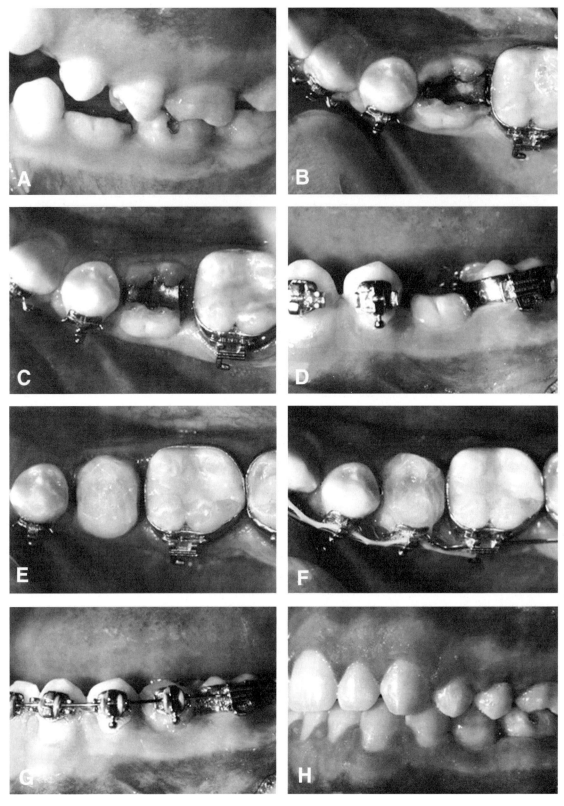

Figure 25-5. Reshaping and restoring primary mandibular second molars. If the mandibular second premolar is congenitally absent, it is advantageous to retain the primary second molar in order to preserve the width of the alveolar ridge for eventual implant placement. The deciduous molar is too wide mesiodistally, however, and often is submerged relative to the adjacent permanent first molar (A,B). In these situations it is helpful to reduce the width of the primary molar (C) to produce the correct posterior occlusion. To facilitate orthodontic bracketing of the primary molar, it is necessary to restore it temporarily with composite (D,E). Then the spaces can be closed (F,G), and the resulting occlusion will improved (H). The primary molar not only retains the correct amount of space for the eventual implant, but prevents overeruption of teeth in the opposing arch, until the implant is placed.

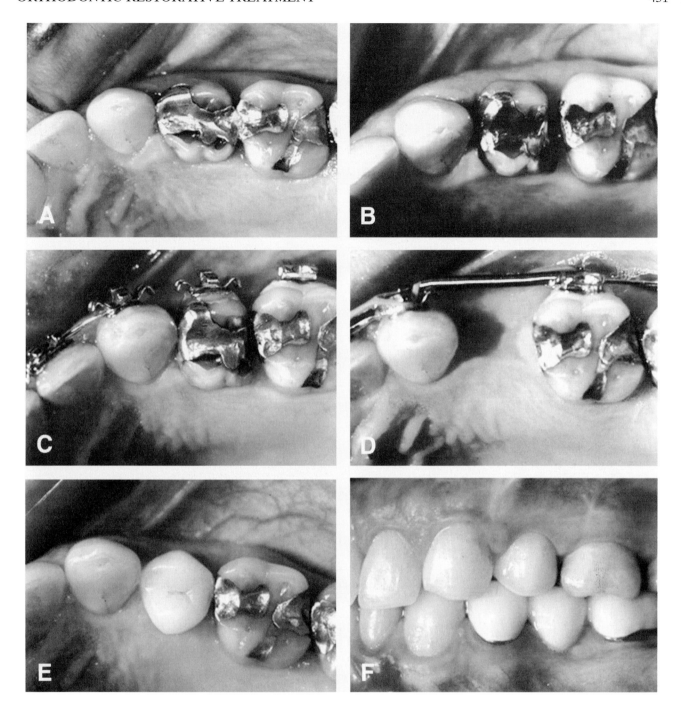

Figure 25-6. Timing the extraction of primary molars before implant placement. Eventually retained primary molars will be extracted to facilitate placement of implants. If primary teeth are extracted too early, however, the alveolar ridge will narrow significantly, possibly complicating later implant placement. In this patient, both maxillary premolars were congenitally missing, and the primary second molars had been retained (A). The width of the primary tooth was reduced (B), and the excess space was consolidated orthodontically to produce the correct width for a premolar implant crown (C). The primary tooth was extracted six weeks prior to implant placement to preserve the width of the alveolar ridge (D). By retaining the primary molar, the final maxillary premolar crown has the appropriate esthetic dimension, and the posterior occlusion fits properly (E,F).

ramal growth is completed is to superimpose sequential cephalometric radiographs. If growth is continuing, the distance between nasion and menton will continue to increase, indicating that it is too early to place the implant. The implant should not be placed until the there is no change in facial vertical dimension taken on two headfilms one year apart. As a general rule, implants should not be placed in boys until after 21 years of age and in females until after 17 years of age. The final decision regarding the timing of implant placement, however, should be made on the basis of longitudinal radiographic (cephalometric) data from the individual patient.

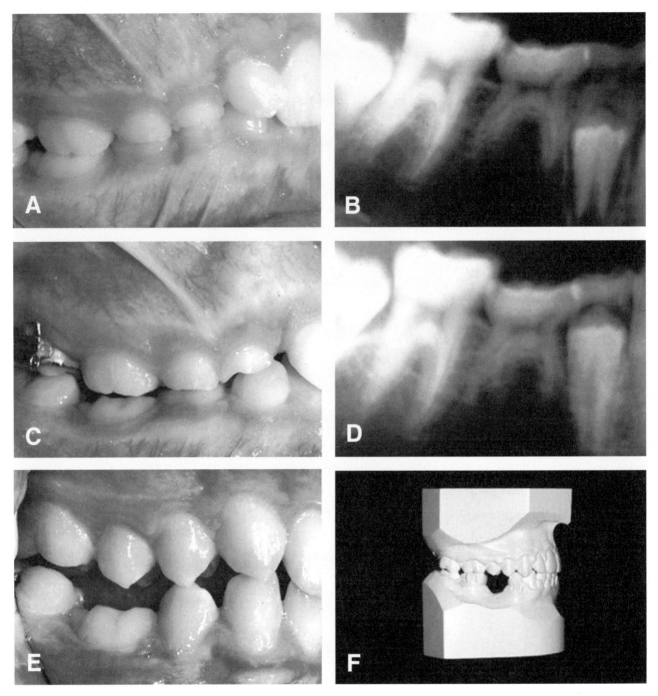

Figure 25-7. Timing the extraction of primary second molars to facilitate implant placement. If mandibular second premolars are congenitally missing, an ankylosed primary molar must be extracted at the appropriate time to avoid alveolar ridge deformation. This patient was initially examined at 9 years of age (*A,B*), and was treated with a headgear and maxillary incisor brackets for one year. At age 10 years (*C,D*), the mandibular primary molar was submerged, the alveolar crestal bone level was angled obliquely between the permanent and primary molars, but the ankylosed tooth was left in place. At 14 years of age (*E*), a second phase of orthodontic treatment was begun. The primary molar was not removed, however, until after orthodontic therapy had been completed at 16 years of age (*F*). As a result, the alveolar ridge has a severe vertical defect that makes implant placement extremely challenging and likely requiring a bone graft.

ORTHODONTIC-RESTORATIVE TREATMENT

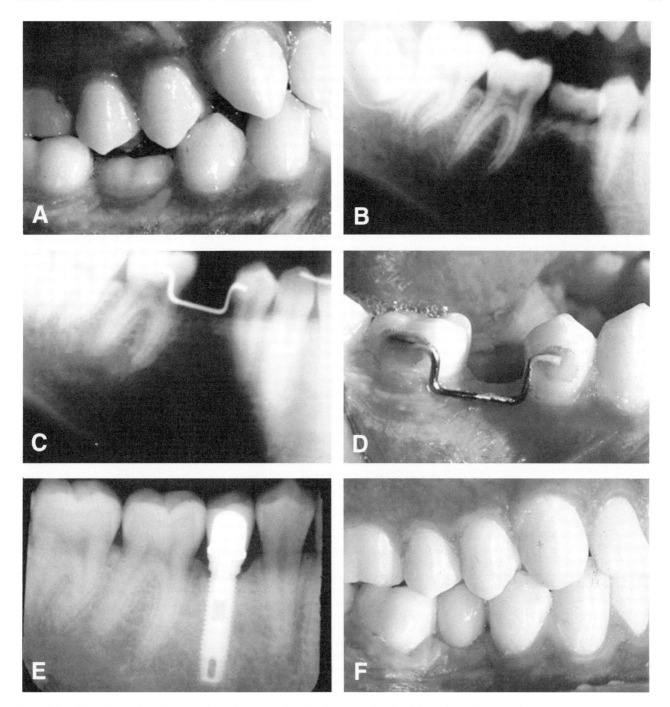

Figure 25-8. The effect of early extraction of an ankylosed primary molar. In this patient, the mandibular right second premolar was congenitally absent, and the primary molar was retained, ankylosed, and submerging (A,B). In order to avoid ridge deformation, the primary molar was extracted prior to orthodontic treatment. After the completion of orthodontics, the radiograph (C) shows that the edentulous alveolar ridge moved coronally as the adjacent premolar and molar erupted (D). This produced the appropriate vertical position of the alveolar ridge to facilitate implant placement (E) and restoration (F).

Other Restorative Options

The other option for replacing a congenitally missing mandibular second premolar is preserving the space and placing a conventional full-coverage bridge or a resin-bonded bridge. Neither of these options, however, is desirable in young patients. First of all, most adolescent patients do not have caries in the first premolar or first molar. Therefore, it is destructive to prepare these teeth for full crowns simply to replace a missing second premolar. Resin-bonded bridges generally do not have a high success rate in the posterior region, especially in the mandibular arch.[9,10] Posterior resin-bonded bridges require frequent re-bonding.

Orthodontic Development Of The Implant Site

If an ankylosed primary molar is not extracted early enough, and a vertical ridge defect is produced, another option is to move the mandibular first premolar into the second premolar position[7] and to place the implant in the first premolar position (Fig. 25-9). Previous studies have shown that it is possible, within limits, to move a tooth into a narrower edentulous ridge[11,12] in order to create an implant site. The bone that is created behind the moving tooth typically will be the width of the root of the tooth that was moved. This type of orthodontic movement, termed "orthodontic implant site development," may eliminate the need for a bone graft in the edentulous site.

CONGENITALLY MISSING MAXILLARY LATERAL INCISORS

Indications For Canine Substitution

Many orthodontic patients are congenitally missing their maxillary lateral incisors. If this problem occurs, there are two general options for treatment. One option involves opening space for a pontic or implant; the other option involves substitution of maxillary canines for lateral incisors and closure of the maxillary edentulous spaces (Fig. 25-10).

Three criteria should be evaluated before choosing the latter treatment option. First of all, the patient's occlusion or malocclusion must be appropriate. The ideal situation for canine substitution is a patient with a Class II molar relationship, minimal crowding of the mandibular teeth, and an acceptable facial profile. Substitution of the permanent canines for the lateral incisors will eliminate the need for any major restorations.

The second criterion for selecting canine substitution is the anterior tooth-size relationship. When canines are substituted for lateral incisors, maxillary anterior tooth-size excess is created. The widths of the maxillary six anterior teeth often must be reduced in size to create the correct overbite and overjet relationships. A diagnostic wax set-up is necessary to determine if canine substitution is a reasonable treatment plan for congenitally missing lateral incisors.

The third criterion is the length, shape, and color of the maxillary canine crowns. If canines are substituted for lateral incisors, their gingival margins must be positioned more incisally relative to the central incisors, because the crown lengths of lateral incisors typically are shorter than central incisors. Therefore, the canines must be erupted, and their cusps must be equilibrated to create the illusion that they are lateral incisors (Fig. 25-10). If the shape of the canine cusp is unusually long and pointed, it could be impossible to reduce the cusp enough to simulate the incisal edge of a lateral incisor.

One of the most difficult aspects of canine shape to overcome is the labial contour. Some maxillary canines have relatively flat labial surfaces. This type of contour more closely resembles the labial contour of a lateral incisor. Some maxillary canines, however, have convex or rounded labial surfaces. It is challenging to make these teeth look like laterals because of the rounded labial contour. Restoration of the labial surface with a porcelain or composite veneer will create a much more acceptable esthetic result.

Esthetic Crown Lengthening

A common esthetic problem with maxillary canine substitution is the gingival discrepancy between the canine and first premolar (Fig. 25-11). If a canine is substituted for a lateral incisor, the premolar is located in the maxillary canine position. In this situation, the premolar may appear too short compared to the canine. Crown lengthening of the premolar by gingival surgery may create a better relationship between the gingival levels of the maxillary anterior teeth and also enhance anterior esthetics.

Positioning Teeth For Resin-Bonded Bridges

A second option for congenitally missing lateral incisors is a maxillary resin-bonded or Maryland bridge. These restorations typically are easy to construct if the orthodontist positions the central incisor and canine in their proper relationships (Fig. 25-12). First, the angulation of the central incisors should be more upright and vertically oriented.[2] In this position, the occlusal force transmitted through the crown of the central incisor produces a shear force at the restoration-tooth interface.

A second important aspect of tooth position for the resin-bonded bridge is the amount of overbite. Typically, the amount of overbite in any orthodontic patient should be determined by evaluating protrusive function of the mandible. The amount of overbite is sufficient when the posterior teeth disclude as the mandible is protruded in an end-to-end incisor relationship. In a patient with an anterior resin-bonded bridge, however,

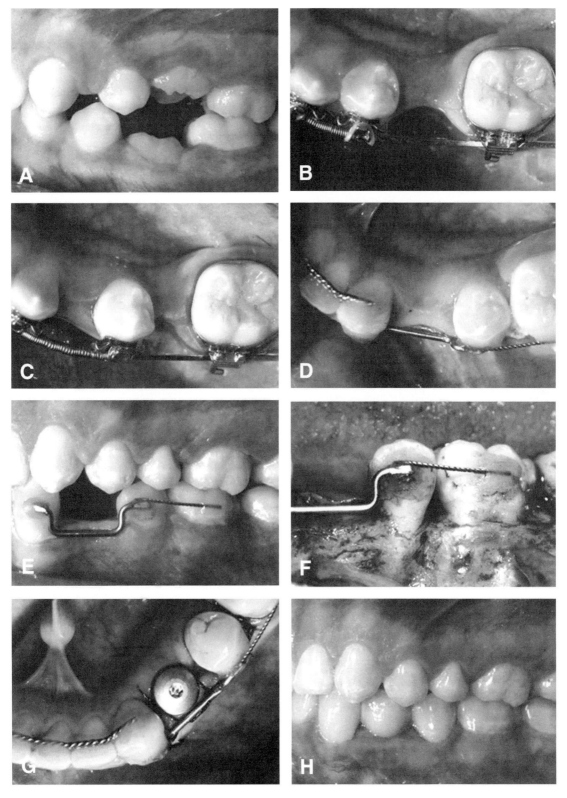

Figure 25-9. Orthodontic implant site development. In this patient, the mandibular left primary second premolar was congenitally absent, and the mandibular left primary second molar was ankylosed and submerged (*A*). After extraction of the primary second molar, the alveolar ridge resorbed significantly (*B*), jeopardizing implant placement. In order to create the appropriate width of bone for an implant and avoid bone grafting, the first premolar was pushed distally (*C*) into the second premolar position (*D,E*). When the surgery was performed to place the implant, the bone distal to the first premolar did not show any dehiscence (*F*). By moving the first premolar distally, the implant site was created mesial to the first premolar, and permitted placement (*G*) and restoration (*H*) of the implant without bone grafting.

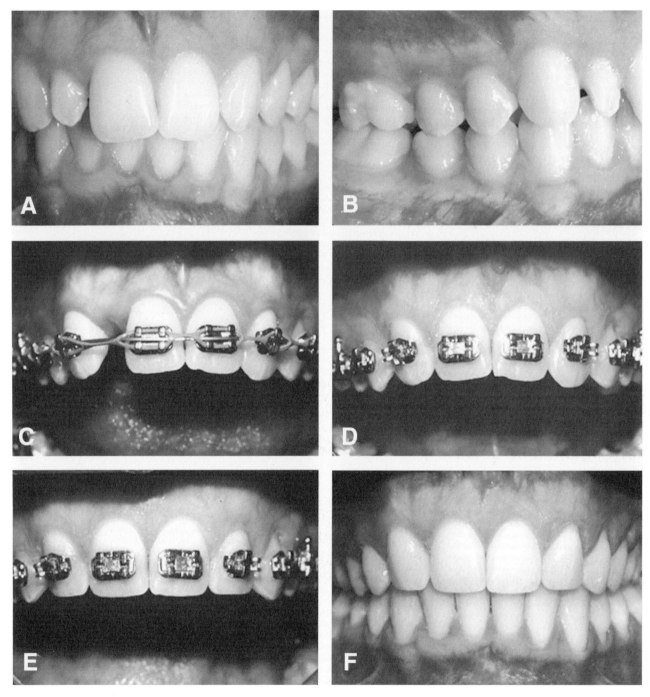

Figure 25-10. Canine substitution. Occasionally, canine substitution may be the best option for treating a patient with a congenitally missing maxillary lateral incisor. Certain criteria should be evaluated, however, before choosing this option. In this patient, the maxillary left lateral incisor was congenitally absent, and the right lateral was peg-shaped (*A*). The molar relationship was Angle Class II (*B*), and the patient had a good facial profile. In addition the size, shape, and color of the maxillary canines were acceptable. Therefore, the right lateral was extracted (*C*), and the space was closed (*D*). The maxillary canines were extruded (*D*), and the cusps were equilibrated (*E*) to simulate the length and shape of lateral incisors. The final orthodontic result (*F*) shows a reasonably good proportion of size between the canine and central, and the shape tends to simulate a lateral incisor. This plan, if appropriate, is advantageous, because it obviates the need for an implant or bridge.

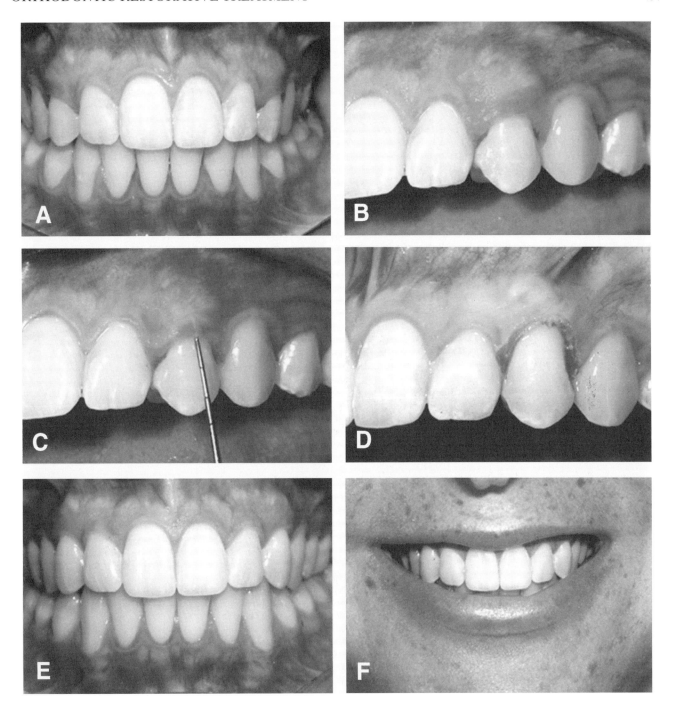

Figure 25-11. Improving gingival levels with canine substitution. If the premolars are placed in the canine position after orthodontic therapy, their esthetic appearance is compromised, because they are shorter than the typical canine crown (A,B). If the labial sulcular depth of the premolar is greater than one millimeter (C), however, the excess gingiva can be removed surgically (D). This relatively simple procedure will add length to the premolar crown, improve the esthetic balance of the anterior gingival margins, and help create the illusion that the premolar is a canine.

the amount of overbite is even more critical. If the overjet is zero with the maxillary and mandibular incisors are in contact, then minimal space is present for the bonded metal connector of the resin-bonded bridge. Therefore, in a patient with a resin-bonded bridge, the clinician should create minimal overbite,[2] with just enough overlap to provide disclusion of the posterior teeth in protrusive function (Fig. 25-12).

Positioning Teeth For Conventional Bridges

Although resin-bonded bridges appear esthetic, they are highly technique sensitive. If not constructed properly, this type of fixed restorations has a short clinical life. Even under ideal conditions, the average life of a resin-bonded anterior bridge replacing a missing maxil-

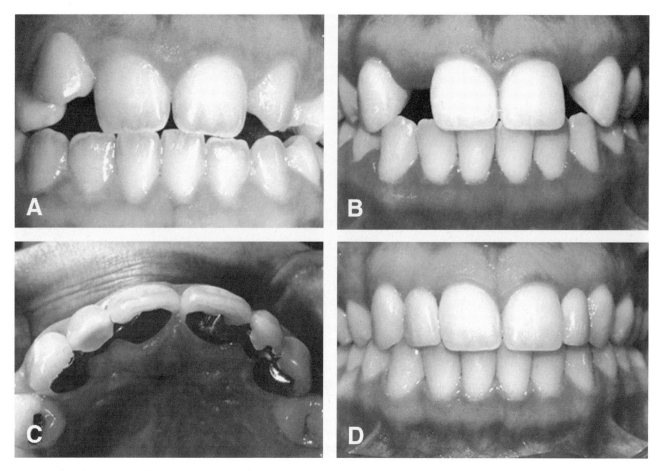

Figure 25-12. Resin-bonded bridges to replace missing maxillary lateral incisors. In this patient, the maxillary lateral incisors were congenitally absent (*A*). Analysis of profile and occlusion showed that opening space (*B*) for resin-bonded bridges (*C,D*) was the best solution. In these situations, the overbite of the central incisors must be minimal, and should only be enough to produce posterior disclusion in anterior protrusive occlusion. In addition, the central incisor and canine abutments should be positioned more upright so the forces of occlusion will produce a shear force on the metal connectors resulting in fewer failures of the bridge due to debonding.

lary lateral incisor is less than ten years.[9,10] Another option for restoring an edentulous space in the maxillary anterior region in an adolescent or young adult is a conventional fixed bridge. These generally are used, however, only if the adjacent teeth require crowns, have had significant trauma, or have had root canal therapy. If extensive restorations are planned for the adjacent teeth, it is reasonable to consider a conventional bridge in the anterior region in an adolescent patient.

The abutments for a conventional bridge must be positioned appropriately, so the crown preparations of the two abutments will have parallel walls to permit seating of the soldered bridge. If the patient's central incisors or canines are proclined relative to one another (Fig. 25-13), the abutments could require extensive reduction to achieve parallel preparations. This relationship could reduce the retention of the preparation, and in some instances require root canal therapy of the abutment teeth. As a general rule, the axial inclinations of the abutment crowns should be perpendicular to the occlusal plane. This orientation will result in the least amount of tooth reduction and the greatest amount of retention of the preparations.

Timing Of Lateral Incisor Implant Placement

A third option for replacing a missing maxillary lateral incisor is an implant. If this option is chosen, several factors must be considered. First of all, the age of the patient is vitally important. If an implant is placed before a patient has completed facial growth, then the adjacent teeth will continue to erupt as the maxilla and mandible continue to grow. A recent study[13] has shown that facial growth continues on average until about 17 years of age in females and about 21 years of age in males. There are males and females who complete facial growth before

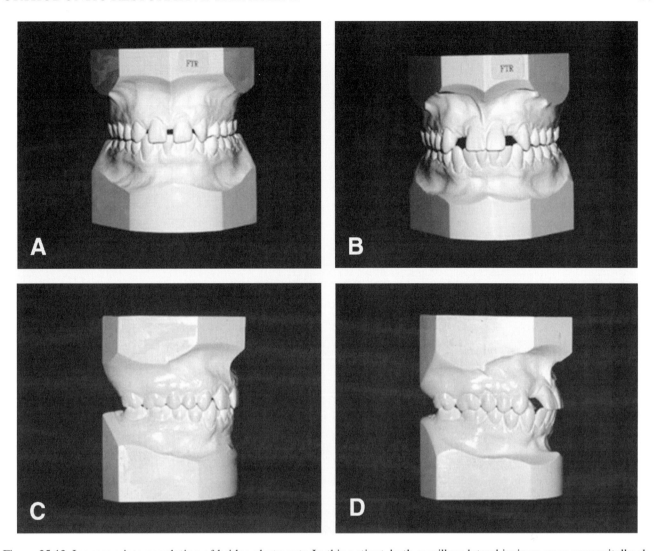

Figure 25-13. Inappropriate angulation of bridge abutments. In this patient, both maxillary lateral incisors were congenitally absent (A). The patient had a Class I occlusion (C), an acceptable facial profile, and minimal mandibular arch length deficiency. Therefore, space was opened for two anterior conventional bridges with pontics for the lateral incisors (B,D). Unfortunately, the teeth were proclined significantly to create pontic space. As a result, the central and canine crowns are not parallel, and therefore crown preparations will not draw without severely over-reducing the teeth. The orthodontist must be aware of abutment crown angulation during preparation for conventional bridges and make certain that the crowns are parallel with one another to facilitate bridge construction.

and after these average ages, so the orthodontist must help the surgeon to determine whether or not facial growth has ceased.

The best means for assessing the completion of facial growth is to superimpose sequential lateral cephalometric head radiographs.[7,13] By registering the superimposition on the base of the skull (sella, greater wings of the sphenoid, and cribriform plate), the clinician may determine if the distance between nasion and menton has increased between successive films. The radiographs should be taken least six months to one year apart. If no change has occurred in the nasion menton distance in one year, then facial growth is complete, and the implant may be placed.

Creating Space For A Lateral Incisor Implant

A second factor that the orthodontist must be aware of is the amount of mesiodistal space that is created for the lateral incisor implant.[7] First of all, if a normal-sized contralateral incisor is present, the space for the missing lateral incisor crown should match the width of the natural lateral incisor. In general this space should be at least 5.5 mm wide. If the contralateral lateral incisor is malformed or peg-shaped and is smaller than 5.5 mm, then the crown should be built-up to a width that is 67–75% the width of the central incisor. The width of most central incisors ranges from 8 to 10 mm wide.

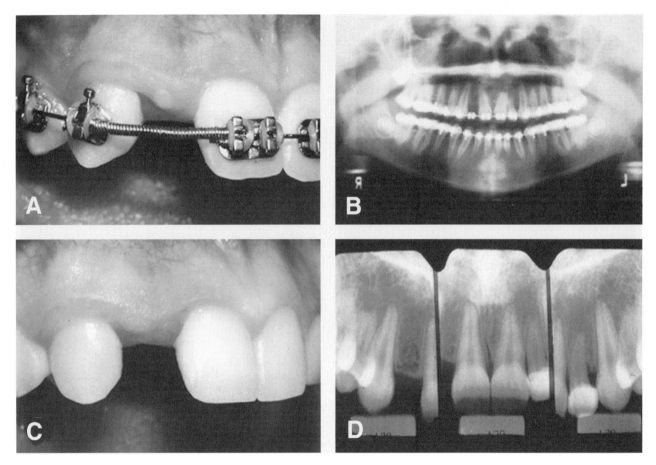

Figure 25-14. Root angulation for anterior implants. This patient is missing the maxillary right lateral incisor, and space is being opened for an implant (*A*). As the crowns move apart (*A*), the root apices move closer together (*B*). During orthodontic finishing, the roots must be moved apart to create sufficient space for the eventual crown (*C*) and implant (*D*).

Therefore, the width of the lateral incisor implant crown should range from about 5.5 to 7.0 mm.

The width of the edentulous space should allow at least 1 mm between the implant and the adjacent teeth. If the distance between implant and tooth is less than 1 mm, the interproximal bone could be jeopardized, and the space for the papilla between the implant crown and the adjacent teeth will be constricted and could appear much shorter than the contralateral papillae.[7] This situation will make the implant crown more obvious and appear less esthetic.

The space between the roots of the adjacent central incisor and canine must be sufficient to permit placement of the implant (Fig. 25-14). As space is created between a central incisor and canine by pushing the crowns apart, the roots tend to move toward one another. This root proximity must be corrected prior to implant placement. This type of tooth movement is accomplished by progressively bending the archwires to move the apices of the roots in opposite directions.

Implant Site Development

The labiolingual dimension of the alveolar ridge must be wide enough to place the implant in its proper position. If insufficient ridge width exists, a bone graft may be necessary before or during implant placement (Fig. 25-15). The type of bone may be either autogenous or freeze-dried cadaver bone. Both types of graft material will become remodeled and form an adequate osseous housing for the implant.[14-18]

A bone graft can be avoided if the central incisor and canine erupt adjacent to one another (Fig. 25-16). As the space is opened orthodontically for the future implant, bone is laid down along fiber tracks of the periodontal membrane.[7] The labiolingual width of the alveolar ridge formed in this manner generally is stable over time. Therefore, if implant placement is delayed until an adolescent has completed facial growth, the ridge will not become narrower.

ORTHODONTIC-RESTORATIVE TREATMENT

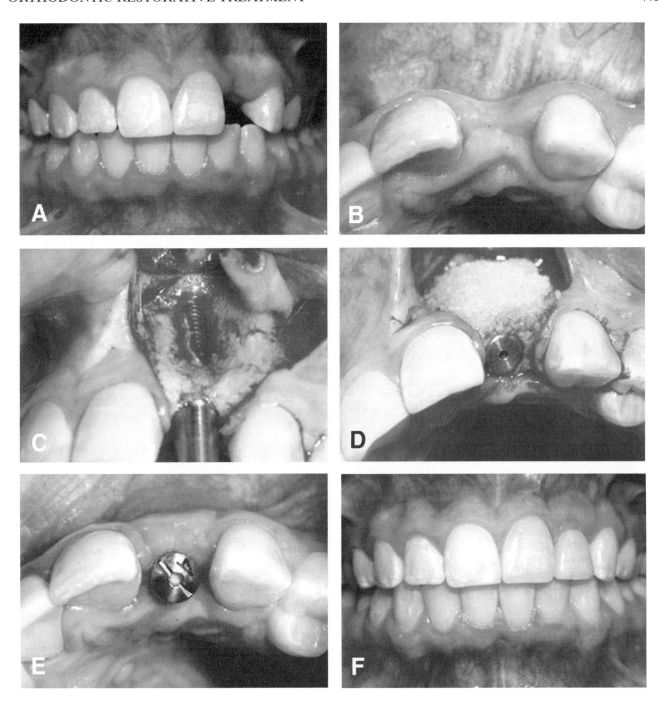

Figure 25-15. Bone grafting to create an implant site. Orthodontic treatment had been completed on this patient, and her maxillary left lateral incisor was avulsed in a sports accident (*A*). Her alveolar ridge narrowed significantly (*B*), before the implant could be placed. A significant fenestration was produced (*C*) during the implant placement, so a freeze-dried, decalcified bone graft was placed to re-enforce the implant (*D*). The bone graft created a wider labiolingual dimension to the ridge (*E*), and produced a more esthetic final restoration (*F*).

Retaining The Implant Space

The edentulous space for the implant should be maintained during and after orthodontic therapy. A plastic tooth with a bracket may be placed in the edentulous space during orthodontic therapy to maintain the space for the future implant (Fig. 25-17). The plastic tooth should be contoured so it does not impinge on the gingiva near the adjacent teeth.[7] It also must be contoured to maintain the health of the future papilla between the implant and the adjacent dentition.

After orthodontic treatment, a retainer with a prosthetic tooth in the implant site should used to maintain the implant space (Fig. 25-17). The tooth should be se-

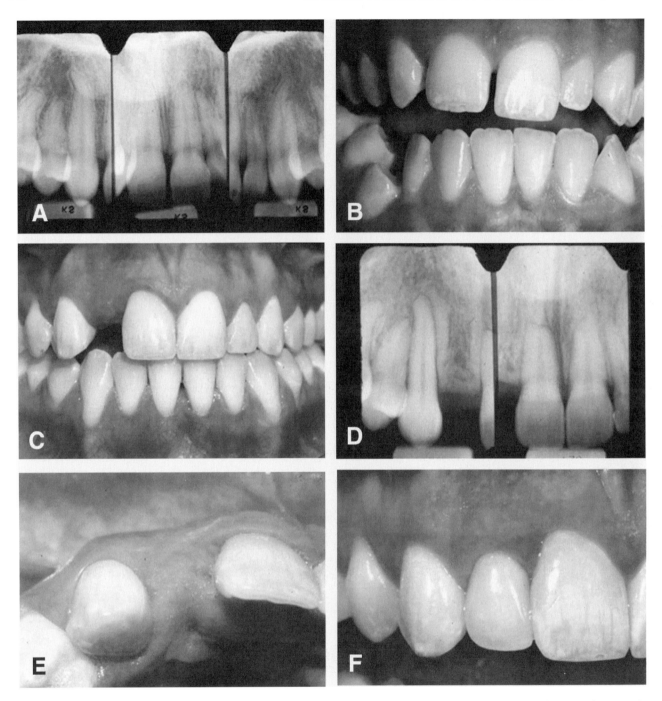

Figure 25-16. Orthodontic implant site development. This patient has an ideal situation for developing an implant site to replace her congenitally absent maxillary right lateral incisor (*A*). The central and canine have erupted adjacent to one another (*B*). As space was opened for the implant (*C*), bone was laid down between the roots, as they were moved apart (*D,E*). This produces an excellent ridge for the surgeon to place the implant, eliminates the need for a bone graft, thereby reduces the surgical trauma to the implant site, and results in better papillae adjacent to the implant crown.

cured to the retainer with a wire embedded into the acrylic and the tooth.[7] This wire will reinforce the retainer and prevent accidental fracture of the tooth from the retainer if the acrylic in this area is reduced when the implant is uncovered. If the implant placement will be delayed for several years, while the clinician is waiting for growth to be completed, a temporary resin-bonded bridge may be used instead of a removable retainer.

Need For Gingivectomy Before Implant Placement

Another aspect of implant placement that is more important in adolescents than in adults is the level of the gingival margin at the conclusion of the orthodontic therapy (Fig. 25-18). In most implant systems, the head of the implant must be placed 4 millimeters from the fu-

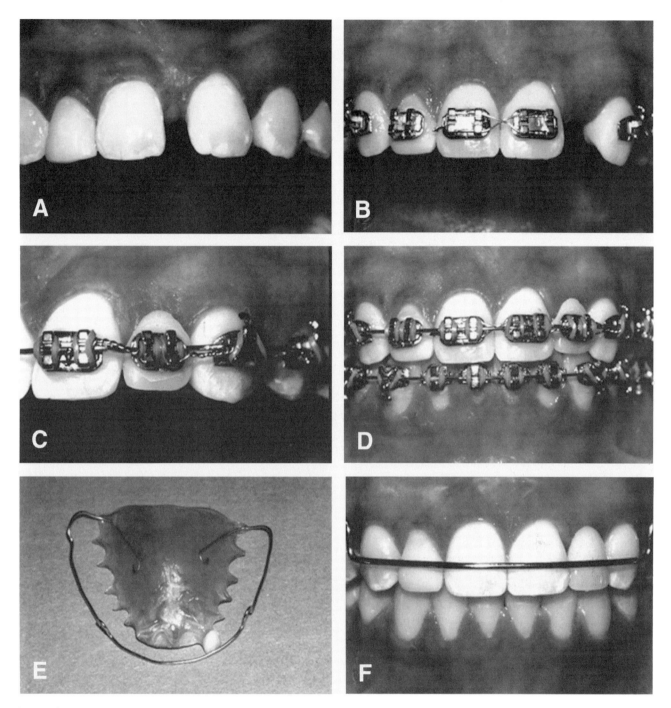

Figure 25-17. Retaining the implant site during and after orthodontics. This patient is congenitally missing her maxillary left lateral incisor (A). Space was opened for an implant (B). In order to maintain the space during orthodontic finishing and provide an esthetic replacement for the patient, a plastic pontic was constructed and placed in the edentulous site (C). The gingival embrasures on the pontic were opened to avoid damaging the ridge in the future implant site. In addition, the occlusion was adjusted (D) so the pontic tooth did not occlude with the opposing arch. After orthodontics, an acrylic circumferential retainer with a prosthetic tooth (E) is used to hold the space for an eventual implant. The plastic retainer tooth was also shaped at the gingival to avoid impinging on the tissue in the implant site (F).

ture gingival margin of the implant crown. In some late-adolescent patients, however, the level of the labial gingival margin may not have achieved its adult position. In most adolescents, the alveolar bone may be positioned at the level of the cementoenamel junction of the adjacent teeth. In contrast, the crest of the bone generally is about 2 mm apical to the CEJ in most adults. Therefore, it is critical to know the exact position of the labial gingival margin prior to implant placement. Because the head of the implant must be 4 mm from the

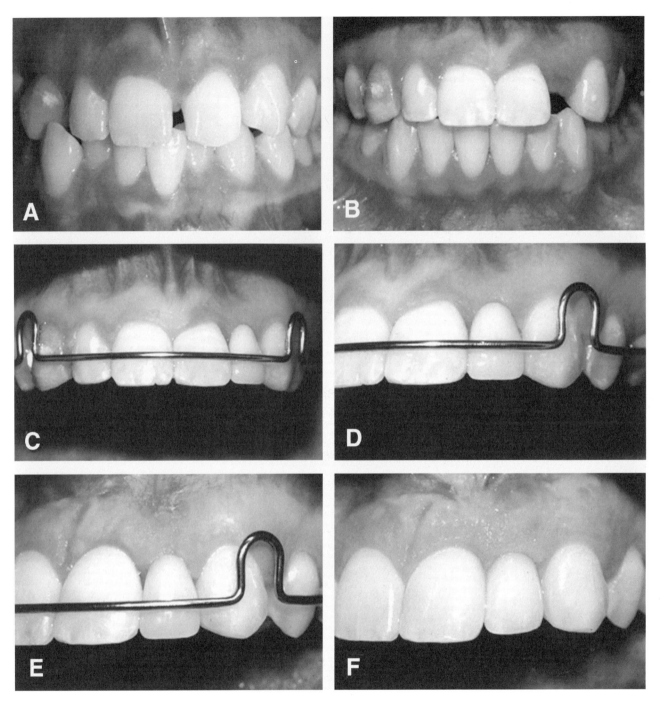

Figure 25-18. Gingival surgery prior to implant placement. This patient was congenitally missing her maxillary left lateral incisor (A), and space was opened for an implant (B). Although the length of the plastic pontic matches the crown length of the contralateral lateral incisor (C), the central incisor appears shorter than the pontic tooth (D). Because the head of the implant must be placed 4 mm from the ultimate gingival margin of the lateral incisor, and because the adjacent central should appear longer than the lateral, gingival surgery was required prior to implant placement to lengthen the central incisor crown (E). By sequencing the gingival surgery prior to implant placement, the final restoration on the implant (F) has the correct gingival margin relationship with the adjacent central incisor and canine.

eventual gingival margin, some adolescent patients require gingival surgery (Fig. 25-18), with or without bone removal before implant placement, so that the implant can be positioned in its proper vertical relationship relative to its expected gingival margin.[7]

Implants have become an important part of restorative dentistry for patients who are congenitally missing teeth as well as for those patients in whom teeth were extracted due to extensive caries, trauma, or periodontal disease. If all members of the team participate correctly, the results can be outstanding. On the other hand, if the team of surgeon, orthodontist, and restorative dentist do

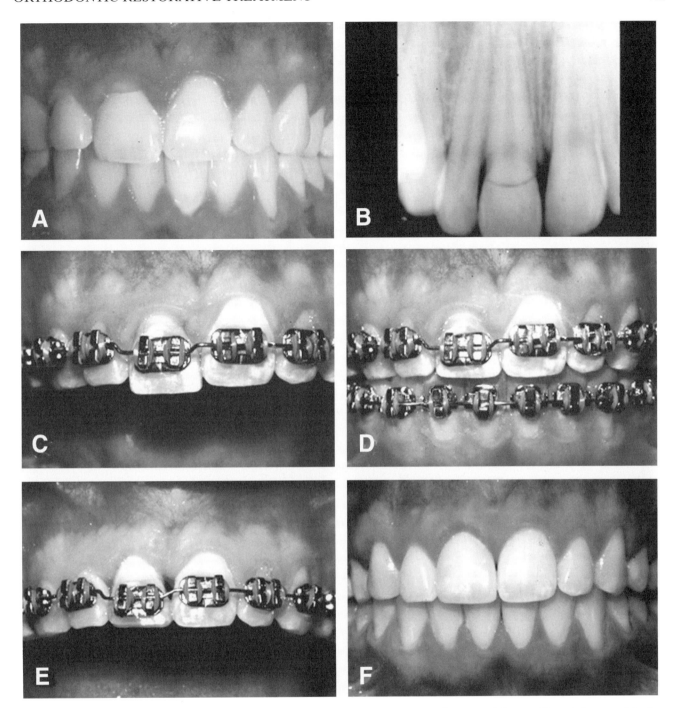

Figure 25-19. Forced eruption of a fractured tooth. This young patient had a severe fracture of the maxillary right central incisor (A) that extended apically to the level of the alveolar crest on the lingual (B). In order to restore the tooth adequately and avoid impinging on the periodontium, the fractured root was extruded four millimeters (C). As the tooth erupted, the gingival margin followed the tooth (D). Gingival surgery was required to lengthen the crown of the central incisor (E), so the final restoration had sufficient ferrule for resistance and retention, and the appropriate gingival margin relationship with the adjacent central incisor (F).

not coordinate their efforts properly, the results potentially could be disastrous.

TRAUMATIC FRACTURE OF TEETH

Occasionally, children and adolescents will fall and accidentally injure their anterior teeth. If the injuries are minor and result in small fractures of enamel, these irregularities can be restored with light-cured composite or porcelain veneers, and in some instances camouflaged through enamel reshaping. In some situations, however, the fracture may extend beneath the level of the gingival margin and terminate at the level of the alveolar ridge (Fig. 25-19). In these situations, restoration of the fractured crown is impossible, because the tooth preparation would extend to the level of the bone. This overextension could result in an invasion of the biologic width of the tooth and cause persistent inflammation of the marginal gingiva.

In these situations, it may be beneficial to erupt the fractured root out of the bone and move the fracture margin coronally, so that it can be restored without creating gingival inflammation.[19] In some situations, if the fracture is too severe, it may be better to extract the tooth and replace it with an implant or bridge. The orthodontist and restorative dentist should evaluate six criteria to determine if the tooth should be forcibly erupted or extracted.[19]

Criteria For Selecting Forced Eruption

Root Length. The first criterion is root length. Is the root long enough, so that a one-to-one crown-root ratio will be preserved after the root has been erupted? In order to determine the answer to this question, the clinician must know how far to erupt the root. If a tooth fracture extends to the level of the bone, it must be erupted four millimeters.

The first two and one-half millimeters will move the fracture margin far enough away from the bone to prevent a biologic width problem. The other one and one-half millimeters will provide the proper amount of ferrule (*i.e.,* coping) for adequate resistance form of the crown preparation. Therefore, if the root is fractured to the bone level and must be erupted four millimeters, the clinician must evaluate a periapical radiograph (Fig. 25-19) and subtract four millimeters from the end of the fractured tooth root. Then the length of the residual root should be compared with the length of the eventual crown on this tooth. The root to crown ratio should be about one to one. If the root to crown ratio is less than this amount, too little root may remain in the bone for stability. In the latter situation, it may be more prudent to extract the root and place a bridge or implant.

Root Form. Root form is the second criterion that determines whether forced eruption is feasible. The shape of the root should be broad and non-tapering rather than thin and tapered. A thin, tapered root will provide a narrower cervical region after the tooth has been erupted four millimeters; the shape of the cervical region could compromise the esthetic appearance of the final restoration.

The internal root form also is important. If the root canal is wide, the distance between the external root surface and root canal filling will be narrow. In these situations, the walls of the crown preparation will be thin, which could result in early fracture of the restored root. The root canal should not be more than a third of the overall width of the root. In this way, the root still could provide adequate strength for the final restoration.

Level of Fracture. A third criterion that determines whether a fractured root should be erupted is the level of the fracture. If the entire crown is fractured 2 to 3 mm apical to the level of the alveolar bone, it is difficult if not impossible to attach to the root in order to erupt it.

Relative Importance. The fourth criterion is the relative importance of the tooth. If the patient were 70 years of age, and both adjacent teeth had prosthetic crowns, then it could be more prudent to simply construct a bridge attaching to the crowned teeth. If the patient were 15 years of age, however, and the adjacent teeth were unrestored, then forced eruption would be much more conservative and appropriate.

Esthetics. The fifth criterion to evaluate prior to beginning forced eruption of a fractured root is esthetics. If the patient has a high lip line and shows 2 to 3 mm of gingival when smiling, then any type of restoration in this area will be more obvious. In this situation, keeping the patient's own tooth would be much more esthetic than any type of implant or prosthetic replacement.

Prognosis. The sixth and final criterion to determine whether or not a tooth should be erupted is the endo/perio prognosis. If the tooth has a significant periodontal defect, it may not be possible to salvage the root. In addition, if the tooth root has a vertical fracture, then it is hopeless and must be extracted.

Mechanics For Forced Eruption

If all of these factors are favorable, then forced eruption of the fractured root is indicated. The orthodontic mechanics necessary to erupt the tooth can vary from elastic traction to orthodontic banding and bracketing.[19] If a large portion of the tooth still is present, then orthodontic bracketing will be necessary. If the entire crown has fractured leaving only the root, then elastic traction from a bonded bar may be possible.

The tooth root may be erupted rapidly or slowly. If the movement is performed rapidly, the alveolar bone will be left behind temporarily, and a circumferential fiberotomy may be performed to prevent bone from following the erupted root. On the other hand, if the root is erupted slowly, the bone will follow the tooth. In this situation, the erupted root will require crown lengthening, and an apically positioned flap to expose the correct amount of tooth to create the proper ferrule (coping), resistance form, and retention for the final restoration.

Stabilization After Extrusion

After the tooth root has been erupted, it must be stabilized to prevent it from intruding back into the alveolus. The reason for re-intrusion is the orientation of the principal fibers of the periodontium. During forced eruption, the periodontal fibers become oriented obliquely and are stretched as the tooth root moves coronally. These fibers eventually will reorient themselves after about six months. Before this time, the tooth root can re-intrude significantly. Therefore, if this type of treatment is performed, an adequate period of stabilization is necessary to avoid significant relapse and re-intrusion of the root.

Need For Gingival Surgery

As the root erupts, the gingiva will move coronally with the tooth. As a result, the clinical crown length will become shorter after extrusion. In addition, the gingival margin may be positioned more incisally than adjacent teeth. In these situations, gingival surgery is necessary to create ideal gingival margin heights. The type of surgery varies depending on whether or not bone removal will be necessary. If bone has followed the root during eruption, the surgeon will elevate a flap and remove the appropriate amount of bone to match the bone height of the adjacent teeth. If the bone level is flat between adjacent teeth, a simple excisional gingivectomy will correct the gingival margin discrepancy.

After gingival surgery, an open gingival embrasure may exist between the erupted root and adjacent teeth (Fig. 25-19). This space occurs because the narrower root portion of the erupted tooth has been moved into the oral cavity. This space may be closed in two different ways. One method involves overcontouring of the replacement restoration. The other method involves reshaping of the crown of the tooth, and movement of the root to close the space. This latter method often helps to improve the overall shape of the final crown on the restored tooth.

UNEVEN GINGIVAL MARGINS

Background

Ideally, the gingival margins of the maxillary central incisors should be at the same level. The gingival margins of the lateral incisors should be positioned slightly coronal to the centrals, and the gingival margins over the canines should be at the same level as the central incisors.[20] In some adolescents, however, the gingival margins are uneven (Figs. 25-20 and 25-21). If the patient has a high lip line during smiling, this discrepancy in gingival margin heights can produce an unesthetic smile in spite of well-aligned teeth. In order to correct this discrepancy, the clinician must determine if the gingival margin discrepancy is due to abnormal wear and compensatory eruption of the teeth, or abnormal gingival margin location requiring gingival surgery.

Orthodontic Intrusion Of Short/Abraded Teeth

In order to diagnose this problem adequately, the clinician first must evaluate the labial sulcular depth of the maxillary incisors. If the sulcular depths uniformly are one millimeter, then the discrepancy in gingival margins may be due to uneven wear or trauma of the incisal edges of the anterior teeth (Fig. 25-20). Although most adolescents do not have significant attrition of their incisal edges, it does occur occasionally. In these situations, the clinician must decide if the amount of gingival discrepancy will be noticeable. If so, bracketing and alignment of these teeth must be accomplished in a way that improves the esthetics and restorability of the abraded teeth.[21-24] In these instances, the gingival margins are used as a guide in tooth positioning, not the incisal edges. As the gingival margins are aligned, the discrepancy in the incisal edges becomes more apparent. These incisal discrepancies are restored with composite restorations temporarily and then are restored permanently with porcelain veneer restorations when the adolescent patient reaches adulthood.

If the gingival margin discrepancies are corrected by leveling the gingival margins orthodontically, these tooth positions should be maintained for at least six months to avoid relapse. As teeth are intruded, the orientation of the periodontal fibers changes and becomes more oblique. It typically takes at least six months for these fibers to re-orient themselves in the horizontal position and stabilize the tooth position.

Surgery To Level Gingival Margins

If the discrepancy in gingival margin position is due to differences in the sulcular depths over the maxillary incisors, then the correct method for dealing with these discrepancies is with gingival surgery (Fig. 25-21). If the level of the alveolar bone is positioned 1–2 mm apical to the cementoenamel junction, and the patient has sufficient attached gingiva, then the surgical procedure should be a simple excisional gingivectomy. If the bone

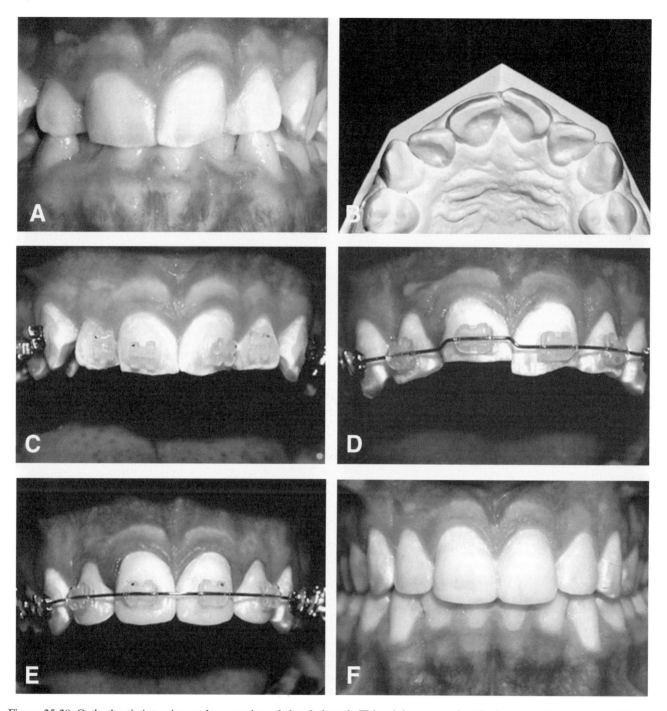

Figure 25-20. Orthodontic intrusion and restoration of abraded teeth. This adolescent patient had a protrusive bruxing habit that resulted in extensive wear of the maxillary central and lateral incisors (A,B). In order to provide the restorative dentist with sufficient space to add length to the central incisors, the brackets were positioned initially near the incisal edges of the centrals and laterals (C). As the teeth aligned, the incisors were intruded (D), using the gingival margins of the canines and central incisors as a guide. When the gingival margins were positioned correctly, the incisal edges were restored (E), and the brackets were replaced to complete the orthodontics. The final result shows crown lengths (F) that are proportional with the widths of the anterior teeth.

level is located at the CEJ, however, or if the patient has insufficient attached gingiva, then an apically positioned flap is the correct procedure. In either situation, the change in the position of the gingival margins can be a tremendous improvement in the esthetic appearance of the patient's smile.[25–30]

OPEN GINGIVAL EMBRASURES

Occasionally, at the end of orthodontic therapy, an adolescent patient may have an open gingival embrasure between the maxillary central incisors (Figs. 25-22 and 25-23). This space usually is due to one of three causes:

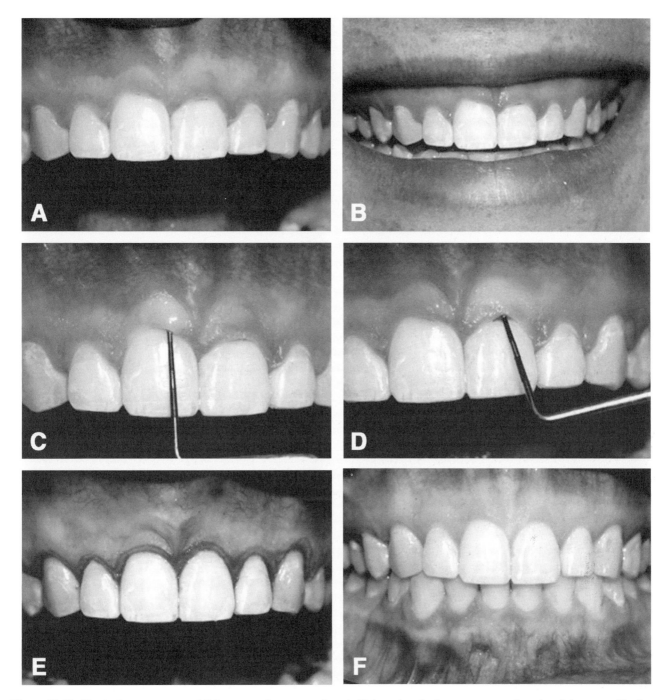

Figure 25-21. Gingival surgery to establish appropriate crown length. This patient had uneven crown lengths of the central incisors (*A*), and this unesthetic relationship was apparent when she smiled (*B*). In order to determine the correct solution for this discrepancy, the sulci of the two central incisors were measured (*C,D*) with a periodontal probe. Because the sulcus of the left central was deeper than the right, gingival surgery (*E*) could be used to establish the correct gingival levels between the centrals, laterals and canines (*F*).

tooth shape, root angulation, or periodontal bone loss. As most adolescent patients do not have significant periodontal problems, open gingival embrasures in teenagers are due to tooth shape or root angulation.

The interproximal contact between the maxillary central incisors consists of two parts. One portion is the tooth contact, and the other portion is the papilla. The ratio of papilla to contact is one to one. In other words, half the space is occupied by papilla and half is formed by the tooth contact. If the patient has an open embrasure, the first aspect that the clinician should evaluate is whether the problem is due to the papilla or the tooth contact. If the papilla is the problem, then the cause is usually a lack of bone support due to an underlying periodontal prob-

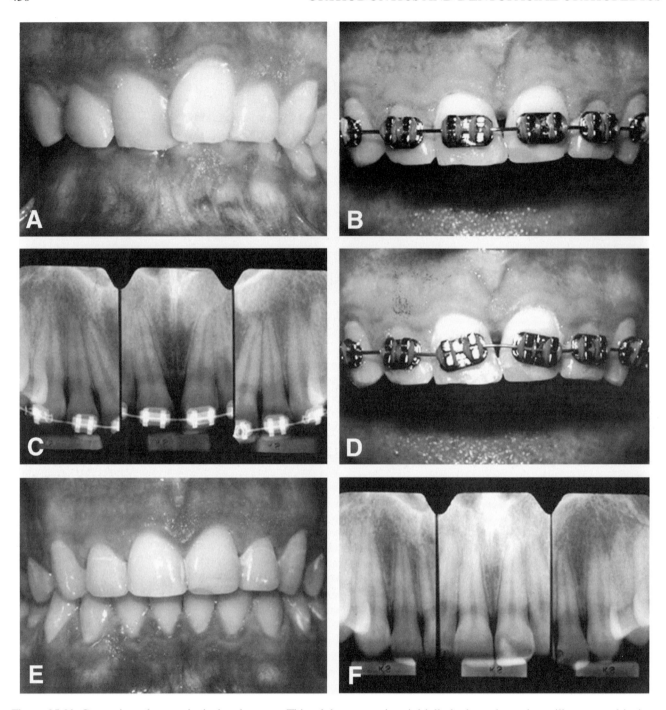

Figure 25-22. Correction of open gingival embrasures. This adolescent patient initially had overlapped maxillary central incisors (*A*), and after initial orthodontic alignment of the teeth, an open gingival embrasure appeared between the centrals (*B*). A radiograph showed that the open embrasure was caused by divergence of the central incisor roots (*C*). In order to correct this problem, the central incisor brackets were repositioned (*D*), and the roots were moved together. This required restoration of the incisal edges after orthodontics (*E*), since these teeth had worn unevenly prior to orthodontic therapy. As the roots were paralleled (*F*), the tooth contact moved gingivally, and the papilla moved incisally, resulting in the elimination of the open gingival embrasure.

lem. Most adolescents, however, do not have periodontal bone loss between the maxillary central incisors.

Correcting Root Angulation

Therefore, most open embrasures between the central incisors are due to problems with tooth contact.[6] The first step is to evaluate a periapical radiograph of the central incisors. If the root angulation is divergent (Fig. 25-22), then the brackets should be repositioned so the root position can be corrected. In these situations, the incisal edges may be uneven and require restoration with either composite or porcelain restorations. If the periapical radiograph shows that the roots are in their

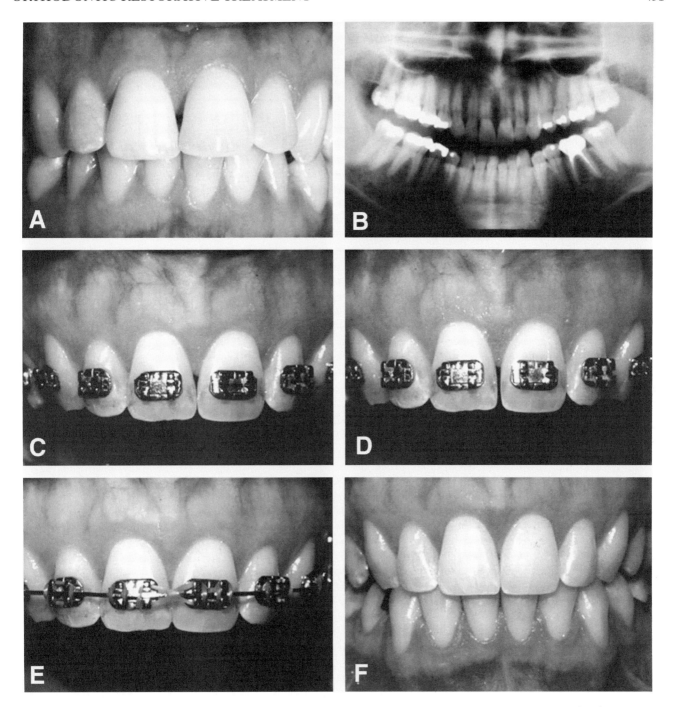

Figure 25-23. Correction of open gingival embrasures. This patient initially had triangular-shaped central incisors (*A,B*), which produced an open gingival embrasure after orthodontic alignment (*C*). As the roots of the central incisors were parallel with one another, the appropriate solution for the open gingival embrasure was to recontour the mesial surfaces of the central incisors (*D*). As the diastema was closed (*E*), the tooth contact moved gingivally, and the papilla moved incisally, resulting in the elimination of the open gingival embrasure (*F*).

correct relationship, then the open gingival embrasure is due to triangular tooth shape.

Reshaping/Restoring Teeth

If the shape of the tooth is the problem, two solutions are possible. One possibility is to restore the open gingival embrasure. The other option is to reshape the tooth (Fig. 25-23) by flattening the incisal contact and closing the space.[6] This reshaping will result in lengthening of the contact until it meets the papilla. In addition, if the embrasure space is large, closing the space will squeeze the papilla between the central incisors. This compression will help to create a one to one relationship between the contact and papilla and restore uniformity to the heights between the midline and adjacent papillae.

CONCLUDING REMARKS

This chapter has focused on the interrelationship between the orthodontist, periodontist, and restorative dentist in the management of adolescent patients with restorative problems. It is important for the orthodontist to think like a restorative dentist during the planning of treatment for adolescent patients. It is no longer adequate to simply align the incisal edges of teeth and expect to obtain an ideal result. Many adolescent patients can benefit from a coordinated approach of orthodontic tooth positioning and adjunctive restorative dentistry to overcome common restorative and esthetic dilemmas.

It also is important for the orthodontist to educate their restorative colleagues about those types of restorative problems that could benefit from pre-restorative tooth positioning prior to final restoration. Teamwork is truly an important concept.

REFERENCES CITED

1. Kokich VG. Anterior dental esthetics: An orthodontic perspective: Mediolateral relationships. J Esthet Dent 1993;5:200–207.
2. Kokich VG, Spear F. Guidelines for managing the orthodontic-restorative patient. Semin Orthod 1997;3:3–20.
3. Lombardi AR. The principles of visual perception and their clinical application to denture esthetics. J Prosth Dent 1973;29:358–382.
4. Ricketts RM. The biologic significance of the divine proportion and Fibonacci series. Am J Orthod 1982;81:351–70.
5. Chiche G, Pinault A. Replacement of deficient crowns. In: Pinault A, Chiche G, eds. Esthetics of fixed prosthodontics. Chicago: Quintessence, 1994:53–73.
6. Kokich VG. Esthetics: The orthodontic-periodontic-restorative connection. Semin Orthod. 2:21–30, 1996.
7. Spear F, Mathews D, Kokich VG. Interdisciplinary management of single-tooth implants. Semin Orthod 1997;3:45–72.
8. Ostler MS, Kokich VG. Alveolar ridge changes in patients congenitally missing mandibular second premolars. J Prosthet Dent 1994;71:144–149.
9. Creugers N. Seven year survival study of resin-bonded bridges. J Dent Res 1992;71:1822–1825.
10. Boyer D. Analysis of debond rates of resin-bonded bridges. J Dent Res 1993;72:1244–1248.
11. Stepovich ML. A cephalometric positional study of the hyoid bone. Am J Orthod 1965;51:882–900.
12. Hom BM, Turley PK. The effects of space closure of the mandibular first molar area in adults. Am J Orthod 1984;85:457–469.
13. Fudalej P. Determining the cessation of facial growth to facilitate placement of single-tooth implants, Seattle: Unpublished Master's thesis, Department of Orthodontics, The University of Washington, 1998.
14. Nyman S, Lang N, Buser D, Brägger U. Bone regeneration adjacent to titanium dental implants using guided tissue regeneration: A report of two cases. Int J Oral Maxillofac Implants 1990;5:9–14.
15. Becker W, Becker B, Handlesman M, Celletti R, Ochsenbein C, Hardwick R, Langer. Bone formation at dehisced dental implant sites treated with implant augmentation material: A pilot study in dogs. Int J Periodont Rest Dent 1990;10:93–101.
16. Jovanovich S, Nevins M. Bone formation utilizing titanium-reinforced barrier membranes. J Periodont Rest Dent 1995;15:57–69.
17. Buser D, Dula K, Belser U, Hirt HP, Berthold H. Localized ridge augmentation using guided bone regeneration. I. Surgical procedure in the maxilla. J Periodont Rest Dent 1993;13:29–45.
18. Adell R, Lekholm U, Grondahl K, Branemark PI, Lindstrom J, Jacobson M. Reconstruction of severely resorbed edentulous maxillae using osseointegrated fixtures in immediate autogenous bone grafts. Int J Oral Maxillofac Implants 1990;5:233–246.
19. Kokich VG. Enhancing restorative, esthetic and periodontal results with orthodontic therapy. In: Schluger S, Youdelis R, Page R, Johnson R, eds. Periodontal diseases. Phil-adelphia: Lea & Febiger, 1990.
20. Rufenacht C. Structural esthetic rules. In: Rufenacht C, ed. Fundamental of esthetics. Chicago: Quintessence, 1990:67–135.
21. Kokich VG, Nappen DL, Shapiro PA. Gingival contour and clinical crown length: their effect on the esthetic appearance of maxillary anterior teeth. Am J Orthod 1984;86:89–94.
22. Kokich VG. Anterior dental esthetics: An orthodontic perspective I. Crown length. J Esthet Dent 1993;5:19–23.
23. Chiche G, Kokich VG, Caudill R. Diagnosis and treatment planning of esthetic problems. In: Pinault A, Chiche G, eds. Esthetics in fixed prosthodontics. Chicago: Quintessence, 1994.
24. Kokich VG. Esthetics and vertical tooth position: The orthodontic possibilities. Compend Cont Ed Dent 1997; 18:1225–1231.
25. Orban B. Indications, technique and postoperative management of gingivectomy in the treatment of periodontal disease. J Periodontol 1941;12:88–91.
26. Goldman H. The development of physiologic gingival contour by gingivoplasty. Oral Surg 1950;3:879–888.
27. Ramfjord SJ. Gingivectomy—its place in periodontal therapy. J Periodontol 1952;23:30–35.
28. Prichard J. Gingivectomy, gingivoplasty, and osseous surgery. J Periodontol 1961;32:257–262.
29. Gargiulo A, Wenz F, Orban B. Dimensions and relation at the dentogingival junction in humans. J Periodontol 1961;32:261–267.
30. Maynard J, Wilson R. Physiologic dimension of the periodontium fundamental to successful restorative dentistry. J Periodontol 1979;50:170–174.

Chapter 26
FINISHING AND RETENTION

With Patrick J. Nolan and Kristine S. West

Earlier chapters have discussed routine orthodontic and orthopedic treatment procedures, including band and bracket placement and archwire sequencing. It is assumed, regardless of the technique used and whether teeth have been extracted, that the orthodontic treatment eventually will reach a satisfactory state in which only minor (but important) adjustments in the occlusion are necessary.

Finishing and retention are two continuous phases of orthodontic treatment, with some retention procedures being initiated before the completion of active orthodontic treatment with fixed appliances. We seek to detail the occlusion according to the standards established by the *American Board of Orthodontics*.[1] Thus, although both simple and complex treatment protocols are described within this chapter, we favor the option of using one or more of the complex protocols that allow for optimizing the overall functional and esthetic result.

EVALUATION OF THE TREATED DENTITION

Before the removal of the fixed appliances, the clinician should evaluate the occlusion thoroughly to determine if further adjustments in tooth position are necessary. Such an evaluation can be performed chairside, or better, a set of progress models (termed "debond evaluation" models) can be obtained. In addition, a panoramic radiographic examination of root angulation is suggested before appliance removal, usually after the final finishing archwire is placed (*i.e.*, 4–6 months before the anticipated end of active treatment).

A number of criteria have been used to evaluate the treated occlusion, and deviations from such guidelines may indicate that further changes in tooth position are necessary.

Keys to Optimal Occlusion

In 1972, Andrews[2] published "The six keys to normal occlusion," an article based on his evaluation of 120 sets of study models obtained from individuals who had ideal occlusions and no history of orthodontic treatment. In a later publication,[3] Andrews explained his concepts further and termed his observations the "The six keys to optimal occlusion." These criteria represent guidelines for evaluating the treated occlusion.

1. *Interarch Relationships*. The mesiobuccal cusp of the maxillary first molar occludes in the groove between the mesial and middle buccal cusps of the mandibular first molar, and the distal marginal ridge of the maxillary first molar occludes with the mesial marginal ridge of the mandibular second molar (Fig. 26-1). The buccal cusps of the maxillary premolars have a cusp-embrasure relationship with the mandibular premolars. The cusp tip of the maxillary canine is slightly mesial to the embrasure between the mandibular canine and first premolar. The lingual cusps of the maxillary premolars have a cusp-fossa relationship with the mandibular premolars.

2. *Crown Angulation* represents the mesiodistal relationship of the clinical crown. For all teeth, the gingival portion of the long axis of each crown is distal to the occlusal portion of the long axis of each crown.
3. *Crown Inclination* represents the faciolingual relationship of the clinical crown. The maxillary central incisors are inclined so that the gingival portions of the crowns of the teeth are lingual to the incisal surfaces. The gingival portions of all the other crowns are inclined labially or buccally, although the mandibular incisor roots are inclined lingually. In the maxillary arch from canine to molar, all crowns are lingually inclined, with the molars slightly more lingually inclined than the premolars and canines. In the mandibular posterior segment, all the crowns are lingually inclined, progressively increasing in inclination from canine through the molars.
4. *Rotations*. All teeth should be free of undesirable rotations.
5. *Tight Contacts*. Teeth should be in contact in the interproximal region, with no spaces present.
6. *Curve of Spee*. The curve of Spee should range from a flat plane to a slight arc in the second molar region.

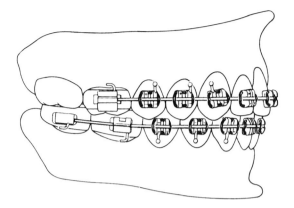

Figure 26-1. Diagrammatic representation of treated occlusion before debonding. Elastomeric chain also may be used at this stage.

Other Occlusal Keys

Okeson[4] and Roth,[5,6] among others, have suggested that patients be treated to a "mutually protective occlusion." When moving from centric occlusion in either a protrusive or lateral direction, the contact of the anterior teeth should serve to disclude the posterior teeth very gently, but immediately, in all movements away from full closure. In centric, the posterior teeth should have equal and even contact of the central cusps, with the forces being directed as nearly as possible down their long axes. The anterior teeth should not be in contact in centric, but rather they should have .005" of clearance. Other clinicians[10] prefer to finish an occlusion with very light contact between the maxillary and mandibular anterior teeth. Roth[5,6] states that the anterior teeth protect the posterior teeth from lateral stress during movement, and the posterior teeth protect the anterior teeth from lateral stress during closure.

The general concepts of Andrews,[2,3] Okeson,[4] and Roth[5,6] regarding the fit of the occlusion are consistent with our views, and thus these concepts are used as guidelines when evaluating a patient nearing the completion of orthodontic treatment. Of course, the position of the dentition must be compatible with the skeletal and soft tissue elements of the patient's face, as is discussed in Chapters 2 and 28.

American Board of Orthodontics Criteria

Another set of criteria was developed in 1998 by the directors of *The American Board of Orthodontics* (ABO) for objectively evaluating the dental casts and panoramic radiographs presented by candidates during the Phase III portion of the ABO examination.[1] Because the ABO standards represent a method of determining excellence in treatment above the so-called standard of care (*i.e.*, "Board quality" result rather than a "clinically acceptable" result), the criteria are described and discussed below.

1. *Alignment*. Attention is paid to the incisal edges and lingual surfaces of the maxillary anterior teeth and the incisal edges and labioincisal surfaces of the mandibular anterior teeth. The mesiodistal central grooves of the maxillary premolars and molars are used to assess the adequacy of alignment, as are the buccal cusps of the mandibular premolars and molars. The most common errors noted by the directors were the orientations of the lateral incisors and second molars in both arches.[1]
2. *Marginal Ridges*. Marginal ridges of adjacent teeth should be at the same level or within 0.5 mm of the same level. Radiographically, the cementoenamel junctions should be at the same relative height, resulting in a flat bone level between adjacent teeth. The most common mistakes in marginal ridge alignment occurred between the first and second molars in both arches.
3. *Buccolingual Inclination*. The buccolingual inclination of the maxillary and mandibular posterior teeth is assessed by using a flat surface that is extended between the occlusal surfaces of the right and left posterior teeth. There should not be a significant dif-

FINISHING AND RETENTION

ference between the heights of the buccal and lingual cusps of the maxillary and mandibular premolars and molars, with all cusps within 1 mm of the straight edge. Significant problems have been observed by the ABO directors in the buccolingual inclination of the maxillary and mandibular second molars.

4. *Occlusal Relationship.* In concordance with the occlusal scheme of Angle,[7] the mesiobuccal cusp of the maxillary first molar must coincide within 1 mm of the buccal groove of the mandibular first molar. In addition, the buccal cusps of the maxillary molars, premolars, and canines must align within 1 mm of the interproximal embrasures of the mandibular posterior teeth.

5. *Occlusal Contacts.* Maximum intercuspation should be established between the buccal cusps of the mandibular posterior teeth and the lingual cusps of the maxillary posterior teeth. Each functional cusp should be in contact with the opposing arch. The most common problem has been inadequate contact between maxillary and mandibular second molars.

6. *Overjet.* Overjet is used to assess the relative relationship of the posterior teeth and the sagittal relationship of the anterior teeth. Posteriorly, the mandibular buccal cusps and the maxillary lingual cusps are used to determine proper position within the fossa of the opposing arch. Anteriorly, the mandibular incisal edges should lightly contact the lingual surfaces of the maxillary anterior teeth. The most common mistakes in overjet have been observed in the incisor and second molar regions.

7. *Interproximal Contacts.* The study models are evaluated from an occlusal perspective. All spaces within the dental arches should be closed. Open spaces not only are unesthetic, but also may lead to food impaction. In general, spacing has not been a problem in past ABO cases.

8. *Root Angulation.* Generally, the roots of the maxillary and mandibular teeth should be parallel to each other and perpendicular to the occlusal plane, as viewed in the panoramic radiograph. If roots are properly angulated, sufficient bone will be present between adjacent roots, an important consideration in periodontal health. The most common errors are in the angulation of the roots of the maxillary lateral incisors, canines, and second premolars and mandibular first premolars.

The above eight criteria can be used to determine whether "American Board quality" results are being produced in the treatment of a given patient. This grading system for the first time provides objective criteria against which the occlusion of a patient nearing the end of treatment can be evaluated. The past experiences of the directors of the ABO in evaluating treatment results indicate the importance of banding or bonding second molars and paying specific attention to such matters as incisal alignment, premolar and molar rotation, marginal ridge heights of adjacent teeth, and flattening of the curve of Wilson during treatment. All of these issues have been addressed in previous chapters. During the finishing phase of treatment, the occlusion should be examined, either clinically or by way of "debond evaluation" models, according to the criteria established by *The American Board of Orthodontics.*[1]

SIMPLE PROTOCOL FOR FINISHING AND RETENTION

Worldwide, the most frequently used (but not necessarily the most effective) finishing and retention protocol of an orthodontic patient involves detailing of the occlusion with fixed appliances, followed by their removal and the delivery of a wire and acrylic retainer.

Most clinicians use a heavy rectangular archwire as a finishing archwire before debonding. First, second, and third order bends are placed in the archwires as needed to provide detailing of the occlusion. A final archwire with multiple bends at the end of treatment may be proof of excellent wire bending skills, but unfortunately also is evidence of poor bracket placement at the beginning of fixed appliance treatment. The number and extent of first, second, and third order bends necessary for the fine detailing of an occlusion are, in part, due to the nature of initial bracket and band placement.

In Chapter 9, we described a method of bracket positioning that, when combined with the use of a transpalatal arch, eliminates most undesirable rotations, particularly in the maxillary premolar and molar regions. If these rotations are not eliminated during fixed appliance treatment, the finishing process is made more difficult.

Triangular elastics (Fig. 26-2) also can be used to settle the occlusion in the buccal segments, often used in association with lighter wires in one or both arches. Seating of the canines as well as anterior vertical space closure often are left until the final stages of finishing.

After a satisfactory occlusion has been achieved, the patient is debonded and debanded, with the excess bonding material and cement removed from the dental arches. A fluoride treatment may be administered after appliance removal.

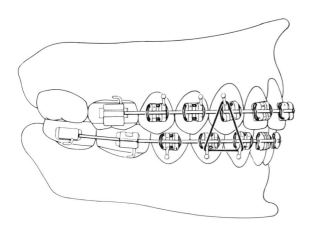

Figure 26-2. Triangular elastics that extend from the maxillary canine to the mandibular canine and first premolar. A light archwire (e.g., .0175" coaxial) may be inserted in one or both arches to facilitate settling of the occlusion.

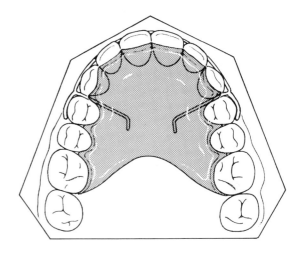

Figure 26-3. Occlusal view of maxillary Hawley retainer. Clasps extend posteriorly from the labial wire to the first premolars. Optional ball clasps and circumferential clasps can be used posteriorly to increase retention.

Removable Retainers

Several types of orthodontic retainers are used during the retention period. All wire retainers have the advantage of being reasonably durable, although wire fatigue, solder joint failure, and breakage occur occasionally. These types of retainers provide a variable amount of settling of the posterior occlusion, depending on the amount and nature of the clasping and the trimming of the acrylic.

The most significant drawback to wire and acrylic retainers in general is the inability to maintain precise incisor alignment. Often, although the labial wire contacts the incisors, some rebound toward the original incisor position occurs, particularly in the maxillary lateral incisor region. The return of mandibular incisor rotations and overlap also can be troublesome.

Full-time retainer wear is recommended for the first year, after which wear decreases to nighttime only. The retainers are removed for eating and oral hygiene procedures.

Hawley Retainer

The most widely used type of removable retainer is the Hawley retainer. The maxillary Hawley appliance has full palatal coverage contoured at the posterior margin to avoid the patient's gag reflex (Fig. 26-3). The upper labial wire crosses from the palate facially between the maxillary first premolar and the maxillary canine. A vertical loop is formed that reaches 2–3 mm above the gingival margin. A parallel vertical leg then extends inferiorly to the middle of the canine, at which point the wire crosses the labial surface of the maxillary incisors at about their midpoint (Fig. 26-4). The wire continues to the other side of the arch in a similar fashion and recurves through the interproximal area to the palate.

The Hawley retainer can be used with or without posterior clasping. Posterior clasps are not needed if wire extensions are soldered to the upper labial wire distal to the posterior leg of the vertical loop. These wires lie above the height contour of the first premolar and provide sufficient retention of the appliance. Acrylic can be removed judiciously from the posterior surface of the retainer to allow for setting of the buccal segments as well as for band space closure. In addition, sufficient acrylic must be present along the lingual surface of the anterior teeth to prevent rotation during the retention period.

If clasps are used posteriorly, a number of options exist. Either arrow clasps or ball clasps can be placed between the maxillary second premolars and maxillary first molars, or Adams clasps[8] can be placed on the first molars. A circumferential clasp also can be used, espe-

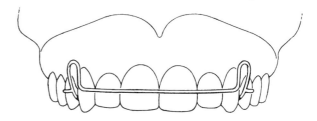

Figure 26-4. Frontal view of maxillary Hawley retainer. Note clasps on maxillary first premolars.

FINISHING AND RETENTION

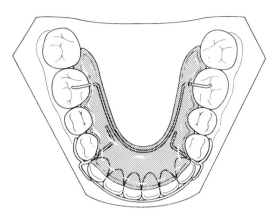

Figure 26-5. Occlusal view of mandibular Hawley retainer. Note occlusal rests on the mandibular first molars.

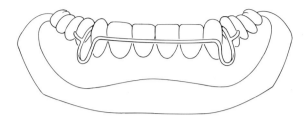

Figure 26-6. Frontal view of mandibular Hawley retainer, including clasps to the premolars.

cially in instances in which teeth have been extracted, and there is a concern about the maintenance of extraction space closure.

As is standard with most retainers that are composed of acrylic, the "salt and pepper" method of acrylic application can be used during the fabrication process. Alternatively, Biocryl™ can be applied to the occlusal surface of the work model, by way of a thermal pressure machine (Biostar™, Great Lakes Orthodontics, Tonawanda NY). If needed, an anterior bite plate can be incorporated into the maxillary Hawley in patients who had a deep bite at the beginning of treatment.

The mandibular Hawley retainer (Figs. 26-5 and 26-6) has the same basic design as the maxillary Hawley. The labial wire crosses through the interproximal space between the mandibular first premolar and the mandibular canine, forms a vertical loop inferiorly, and then crosses the lower incisors at their midpoint incisogingivally (Fig. 26-6).

One design variation is the placement of occlusal rests on the mandibular first molars (Fig. 26-5). These rests are formed from one continuous piece of wire that passes along the lingual aspect of the alveolus, providing added support to the appliance. Segmenting the wire frequently creates a weak point in the acrylic, resulting in acrylic fracture during the retention phase of treatment.[9] As with the maxillary Hawley appliance, an extension that incorporates the first premolar can be added to the distal aspect of the vertical loop.

Circumferential Retainer

An alternative retainer design, used particularly in the maxillary arch, is the circumferential retainer (Figs. 26-7 and 26-8). The circumferential retainer is ideal in closing interproximal spaces that may be present following removal of bands from the posterior teeth. This type of retainer also is helpful in keeping extraction spaces closed, as the labial bow does not cross over the arch in the extraction regions.

The circumferential wire, formed from .030" stainless steel, originates from the palate and passes immediately behind the most distally positioned molar. The wire courses anteriorly until the region of the maxillary canine, at which point a vertical loop that is similar to the Hawley loop is placed in the wire (Fig. 26-8). The wire

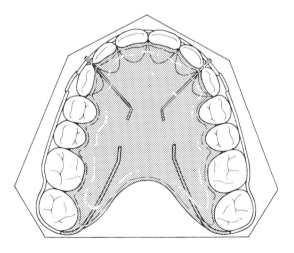

Figure 26-7. Occlusal view of maxillary circumferential retainer. The support wires lie either distal to the lateral incisors or they can cross the arch more posteriorly.

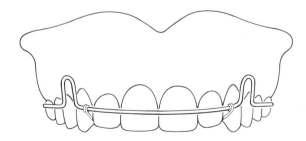

Figure 26-8. Frontal view of circumferential retainer. Note support wires extending interproximally distal to the lateral incisors and wrapping around the anterior wire.

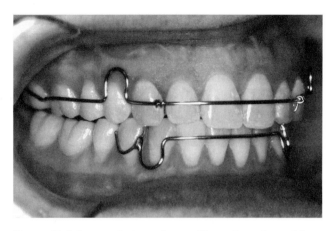

Figure 26-9. Intraoral view of a maxillary circumferential retainer and a mandibular Hawley retainer. The support wire of the circumferential retainer lies between the maxillary lateral incisors and canines. Most acrylic and wire retainers may open the bite slightly, as is shown here.

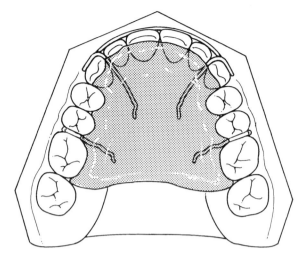

Figure 26-10. Occlusal view of Ricketts retainer. Arrow or ball ended clasps are placed anterior to the first molars.

then contacts the anterior teeth at their midpoint incisogingivally. The wire is stabilized anteriorly with two support wires (.020" stainless steel) that extend from the palatal area and cross interproximally between the maxillary lateral incisors and the maxillary canines (Figs. 26-7 and 26-8). Alternatively, these support wires can be placed distal to the canines or between the premolars[10] (Fig. 26-9), according to the preference of the clinician.

The acrylic is added to the work model in a manner similar to that previously described for the Hawley retainer. Again, care is taken to ensure that the posterior aspect of the palatal acrylic is contoured to prevent initiating the patient's gag reflex (Fig. 26-7).

Ricketts Retainer

A variation in retainer design is the Ricketts retainer, named after its developer Robert M. Ricketts. The Ricketts retainer is similar to a Hawley retainer except that the labial wire originates from the palatal surface and crosses interproximally between the maxillary lateral incisors and maxillary canines (Fig. 26-10). The labial wire then curves distally around the canine, returning mesially, at which point a Hawley-type adjustment loop is placed (Fig. 26-11). This type of retainer is useful in patients treated with extractions, as the labial wire does not cross through the embrasure between the maxillary canine and maxillary premolar.

Van der Linden Retainer

Another type of retainer that has gained popularity in Europe is the van der Linden retainer (Figs. 26-12 and 26-13), developed by Frans van der Linden of the Netherlands.[11] This retainer is similar to a Hawley retainer, with the major modification occurring in the labial bow at the canines. The labial wire, made from .028" stainless steel, crosses the midportion of the incisors and then extends posteriorly to cover the canines. At this point, the wire forms a loop that contacts the canines, and then the wire crosses through the embrasure distal to the maxillary lateral incisors. The recurrent parts of the labial wire function as clasps, coursing into the undercuts at the cervical region of the canines. The incisors are held firmly in position by the lingual acrylic.

The developer of this retainer[11] recommends that the anterior teeth should contact the palate in centric occlusion, whereas the premolars and molars should occlude without interference. The three-quarter clasp that curves distally around the last molar can be used to move a buccally erupted second molar palatally and distally. The palatal acrylic adjacent to the maxillary second molar should be removed, but not the acrylic adjacent to the first molar. In those patients with a good occlusion of

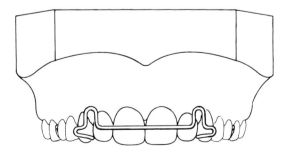

Figure 26-11. Frontal view of Ricketts retainer. The labial wire passes interproximally distal to the lateral incisors.

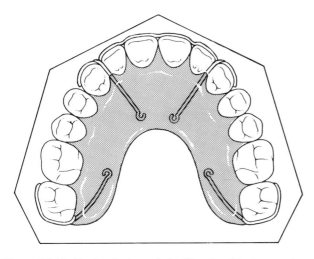

Figure 26-12. Occlusal view of the Van der Linden retainer. The anterior crossover wires pass distal to the lateral incisors. Circumferential clasps are present on the distal molars.

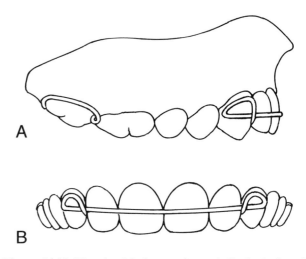

Figure 26-13. Van der Linden retainer. *A*, Sagittal view. *B*, Frontal view.

the second molars and a solid occlusion of the other posterior teeth, Van der Linden[12] recommends removing the acrylic medial to the first molars and premolars to allow for further settling of these teeth.

The retainer offers full control over the anterior teeth as the clasp function on the canines keeps the plate and the labial bow in place. In addition, the closed loops do not deform and provide a rigidity that is lacking in open loops. Furthermore, the position of the canines is well controlled.

The Van der Linden retainer is not designed to move teeth; however, small changes needed after bracket removal can be accomplished by the appliances. By scraping away plaster on the labial surfaces and by placing a corresponding number of tinfoil layers on the palatal surfaces, an instant correction can be realized when the retainer is inserted. The wide periodontal spaces at the end of active treatment offer this possibility. The instant correction does not reduce the rigidity of the fixation of the adjusted and the other teeth involved.

COMPLEX FINISHING AND RETENTION PROTOCOLS

Depending on the severity of the initial malocclusion and the quality of the orthodontic result achieved through fixed appliance therapy, additional treatment protocols may be indicated during the final stages of treatment. The implementation of some of these protocols may allow for earlier fixed appliance removal than if all detailing of the occlusion is accomplished with fixed appliances.

Some of the protocols are implemented in the majority of patients in our practice, including enamoplasty and interproximal reduction, vertical elastics or serpentine wires, positioners, and invisible retainers. Fixed lingual retainers and supracrestal fiberotomy procedures are used infrequently, but are indicated in some patients.

Evaluation for Permanent Mandibular Incisor Retention

If the original malocclusion was characterized in part by significant irregularities in mandibular incisor position, a fixed lower lingual retainer may be desirable for long-term retention. It may be preferable to place a bonded lingual retainer *before* appliance removal to insure that the position of the mandibular incisors is as ideal as possible. We use this type of fixed retention sparingly, however, because of the need for continued supervision of the patient during the post-treatment period. Typically, we choose to place patients on "inactive retention" status (*i.e.*, patients do not have a scheduled retention appointment) after one year, and a bonded lingual retainer usually requires supervision by the orthodontist or family dentist as long as it remains bonded.

There are a number of retainers that have been advocated for stabilizing the position of the mandibular incisors, including the bonded lingual wire of Zachrisson[13–15] (Fig. 26-14), which typically involves a dead-soft braided wire attached to the lower canines. This type of retainer maintains the intercanine distance while allowing some settling of the occlusion.

A more rigid type of bonded lingual retainer is that designed by Krause,[16] which features bonded metallic lingual pads on the cingula of each incisor and canine connected by a wire soldered to each pad (Fig. 26-15).

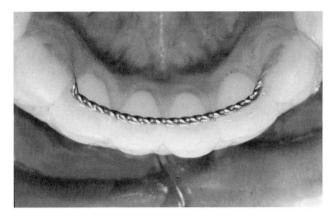

Figure 26-14. Occlusal view of bonded lingual retainer of Zachrisson.[13] (Photo courtesy of Bjorn Zachrisson.)

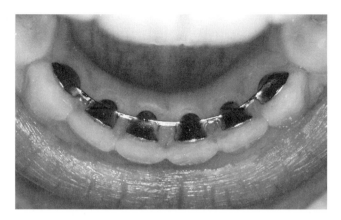

Figure 26-15. Occlusal view of bonded lingual retainer of Krause.[16] This type of retainer can be used in either arch.

As with the Zachrisson retainer, the original Krause retainer can be placed in either arch. This type of retainer is particularly useful in adult patients in whom the overjet is not reduced completely. The position of the maxillary dentition can be stabilized with a fixed lingual retainer.

One of the difficulties with the original Krause retainer, however, is difficulty in retainer removal. Often the bonded bases must be ground off the teeth with a diamond stone, because of problems with grasping the retainer with appropriate bond removing pliers. Thus, we recommend the so-called "Krause-Lite" retainer (Specialty Appliances, Norcross GA), an acrylic and wire version of the Krause retainer with pads that are bonded to the cingula of the six mandibular anterior teeth (Fig. 26-16). Using acrylic instead of metal pads facilitates efficient removal of this bonded appliance as well as ease in repairing a single loose pad.

A bonded lingual retainer such as a Krause-Lite is indicated after the lower incisors have been aligned properly and are oriented satisfactorily relative to the maxillary incisors. An impression is taken with the fixed appliances in place, and the subsequent work model is sent to the laboratory. The technician places a small amount of acrylic on each tooth and incorporates a .0195" round or .016 × .022" rectangular braided stainless steel wire. A two-part transfer tray is fabricated (Fig. 26-17) with an outer part made of 1mm thick Biocryl™ (harder acrylic) and the inner part of 2 mm thick Bioplast™ (softer acrylic). When removed, the carrier tray contains the Krause-Lite retainer.

At the time of appliance delivery, the teeth are prepared for bonding. The lingual surfaces of the mandibular anterior teeth are etched, rinsed, and dried. After placing the appropriate sealant, either a light-cured ad-

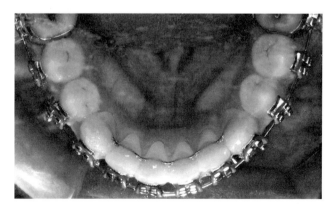

Figure 26-16. Occlusal view of Krause-Lite retainer that consists of a braided wire and acrylic pads that are bonded to the lingual surfaces of the mandibular six anterior teeth. The fixed appliances were removed after this photo was taken.

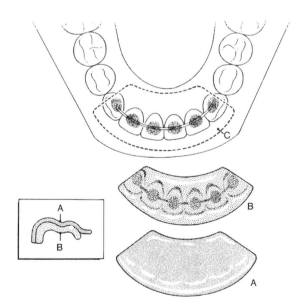

Figure 26-17. Transfer tray used to place Krause-Lite retainer. A, Outer hard part of transfer tray. B, Softer inner lining of transfer tray. C, Future placement of transfer tray.

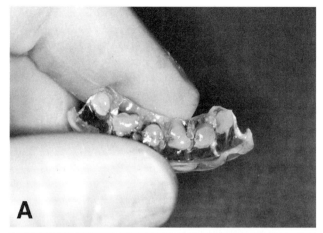

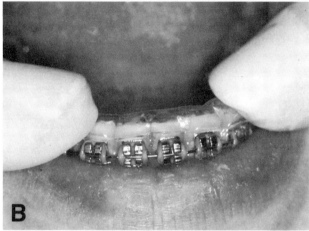

Figure 26-18. *A*, Krause-Lite retainer in a transfer tray after a minimal amount of light-cure adhesive has been placed on each acrylic pad. *B*, A single transfer tray is used to position the retainer on the mandibular teeth. The adhesive then is hardened by way of a high intensity curing light (not shown).

hesive (*e.g.*, Light-bond™, Reliance Orthodontic Products, Itasca IL) or a mixed acrylic (*e.g.*, Excel™, Reliance Orthodontics) can be used to fix the bonded retainer to the mandibular anterior teeth (Fig. 26-18). The use of a light-cured acrylic is advantageous, as the carrier tray is transparent and lends itself to incisor transillumination. Proper light curing of the acrylic also can be accomplished while fixed appliances are in place. The Krause-Lite retainer bonded intraorally is shown in Figure 26-16.

A bonded lingual retainer can be used in the maxillary arch to stabilize incisor position and to maintain closures of previously existing diastemas.[16] Care must be taken, however, to ensure that there is no interference between the maxillary bonded retainer and the mandibular incisors. If interference exists, the bonded retainer may be dislodged. Bonded lingual retainers should be checked routinely (*e.g.*, every 6-12 months) for leakage or decay. If a problem is identified, the retainer should be removed immediately.

Supracrestal Fiberotomy

In patients whose original malocclusion was characterized by significant anterior crowding or rotation of teeth (*e.g.*, Class II division 2 malocclusion with flared and rotated lateral incisors), gingival surgery may be indicated. The procedure of choice is the circumferential supracrestal fiberotomy (CSF), as advocated by Edwards.[17-19] The research of Reitan,[20] among others, has shown that the supracrestal tissues (free gingival and transseptal fibers) remain stretched for months or years after tooth movement. The remodeling period for the transseptal fibers contrasts with other fibers of the periodontal ligament that remodel within 2–3 months after orthodontic rotation of teeth.[20,21]

We recommend that the CSF procedure ideally be carried out 1–4 months before appliance removal, after the anterior teeth are aligned properly. This procedure can be performed by the orthodontist or can be referred to the general dentist, the periodontist, or the oral and maxillofacial surgeon. A narrow, tapered scalpel blade is placed into the gingival sulcus, severing the epithelial attachment surrounding the involved teeth (Fig. 26-19). According to Edwards,[19] the blade also transects the transseptal fibers interdentally by entering the periodontal ligament space (Fig. 26-20). Edwards states that surgical dressings are not required and that clinical healing usually is completed in 7–10 days. CSF procedures are contraindicated in patients who have active periodontal disease, gingival recession, lack of attached gingiva, and/or poor oral hygiene.[18,19]

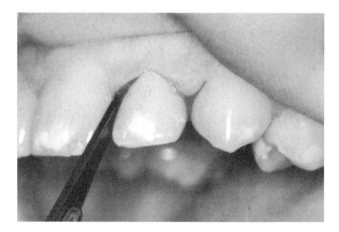

Figure 26-19. Intraoral view of circumferential supracrestal fiberotomy, which severs the transseptal fibers. (Photo courtesy of John G. Edwards.)

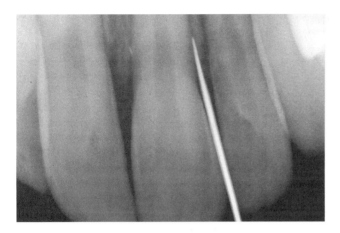

Figure 26-20. Periapical radiograph of scalpel position when performing a CSF procedure (Photo courtesy of John G. Edwards).

Gingivectomy

Another periodontal procedure that has found increased use in our practice is the gingivectomy,[22-25] the removal of excess gingival tissue that sometimes occurs in orthodontic patients during treatment, particularly in patients with poor oral hygiene. Other patients, particularly female patients, experience gingival changes associated with altered hormonal levels during puberty or pregnancy.

Hypertrophied or hyperplastic tissue leads to many problems, the first of which is unfavorable esthetics. Gingival tissue may become inflamed or fibrous, leading to an unsightly appearance when the patient smiles (Figs. 26-21A). The surgical removal of excess tissue dramatically improves the appearance of the smile within a week or two (Figs. 26-21B). This immediate improvement in esthetics often is a prime reason why a patient and his or her family may choose to have this surgical procedure performed. Typically, this type of esthetic gingivectomy is carried out by a periodontist.

Of even greater concern, however, is the possibility of decalcification and decay in areas of the enamel covered by the hypertrophied tissue. The enamel becomes highly susceptible to plaque and debris build-up, both under and adjacent to the enlarged gingiva, and decalcification or decay may result. The patient also has an increased risk for periodontal disease. Further, conservative gingivectomy may serve in a manner similar to the CSF procedure in improving the long-term stability of teeth that have been rotated orthodontically.[26]

One of the dilemmas facing the orthodontist is the timing of the gingivectomy procedure. Should the procedure be performed while the fixed appliances are in place, or should the patient be reevaluated for this procedure several months following the removal of the fixed appliances? In instances of severe gingival hypertrophy or hyperplasia that result in pronounced esthetic problems and that appear to be causing enamel decalcification or periodontal disease, gingivectomy during treatment is recommended. In those patients who have experienced mild to moderate gingival enlargement but no significant damage to the associated hard or soft tissue, the decision may be deferred until after the fixed appliances are removed. Often simply removing the fixed appliances allows an improvement in oral hygiene, and the tissue shrinks without further intervention. Further, the use of a tooth positioner (to be described in detail below) encourages the recontouring of enlarged gingival tissue through the intermittent application pf pressure to the tissue.

Regardless of the timing during or after active treatment, each patient should be evaluated not only for the straightness of his or her teeth, but also for the quality and quantity of the associated gingival tissue. Fiberotomy and gingivectomy procedures should be performed when indicated.

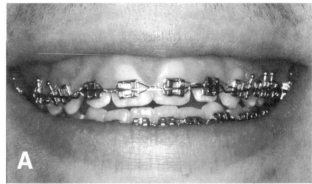

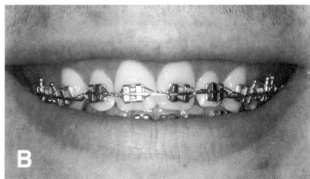

Figure 26-21. Esthetic gingivectomy. *A*, Smiling view of patient prior to periodontal surgery. Note the excess gingival tissue, particularly in the maxillary lateral incisor regions. *B*, smiling view of same patient two weeks following surgery.

Enamoplasty

One of the most overlooked procedures that should be used routinely in comprehensive orthodontic therapy is enamoplasty, a mechanical reshaping of teeth with a rotary instrument.[27] As Kokich stated during the 2000 Moyers Symposium,[28] we should be striving to attain "a beautiful alignment of beautiful teeth." Thus, the orthodontist, in tandem with the restorative dentist or prosthodontist, should pay close attention to the morphology and color of the individual teeth to be straightened, making whatever changes are necessary before, during, and after treatment.

Ideally, tooth recontouring should be an ongoing process, beginning before bracket placement. It makes little sense clinically to place brackets before obvious abnormalities in tooth morphology are eliminated. Unusual patterns of wear should be adjusted and mamelons removed whenever necessary. The patient is told that his or her anterior teeth will benefit from a "manicure,"[29] and minor changes in tooth contour are achieved easily and painlessly without anesthesia by way of a diamond stone in either a high-speed or low-speed handpiece.

The patient also should be evaluated for enamoplasty throughout the period of active treatment, especially as rotated and tipped teeth become aligned. In virtually every patient, all changes in tooth shape should be completed before impressions for a positioner are made.

Interproximal Reduction

Interproximal reduction[30-33] (Figs. 26-22 to 26-24) is a version of enamoplasty that involves reducing the mesiodistal width of teeth, either to resolve intraarch problems such as crowding or interarch relationships such as Bolton discrepancies[34,35] and residual Class II or Class III relationships.

Interproximal reduction classically has been used to resolve minor problems in mandibular incisor crowding during retention. For example, it is common to note a slight shifting in the position of the mandibular incisors following treatment (Fig. 26-22A), a phenomenon that occurs in the majority of the population regardless of whether orthodontic treatment has been performed.[36,37] A diamond disk in a slow speed handpiece can be used to gain a modest amount of arch space, while flattening the contact points interproximally (Fig. 26-22B).

The occlusion also should be evaluated for residual Bolton discrepancies[34] that become evident during the fine detailing of the occlusion. Typically, these imbalances between the aggregate tooth sizes of the maxillary and mandibular dentitions become obvious in subtle ways. The following case example illustrates this point. A patient is nearing the end of treatment, and a Class I molar and canine relationship has been attained; however, excessive overjet remains (Fig. 26-23), indicating a "Bolton discrepancy". This situation is handled easily through interproximal reduction distal to the maxillary lateral incisors.

We have found it convenient to perform interproximal reduction on the left side while holding the handpiece in the right hand (Fig. 26-24AB). On the opposite side, the handpiece is held in the opposite hand (Fig. 26-24CD). Most clinicians can learn to become ambidextrous when performing this procedure within a short period.

Another example of the need for interproximal reduction near the end of treatment is shown in Figure 26-25. In this clinical situation, the patient has achieved a Class I interdigitation on the left side and a Class I molar and premolar relationship on the right side; however, the right canine still is slightly toward Class II.

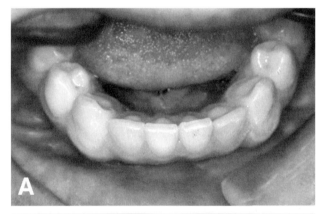

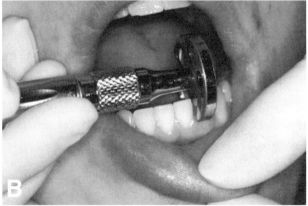

Figure 26-22. Interproximal reduction used to correct minor mandibular incisor crowding. A, The mandibular lateral incisor is slightly labial. B, a diamond disk in a low speed handpiece used to flatten the contacts interproximally, gaining additional space for the alignment of the mandibular anterior teeth.

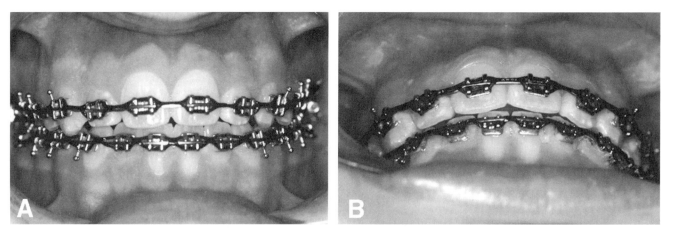

Figure 26-23. Intraoral views of patient nearing the end of treatment with a normal posterior occlusion and excessive overjet, indicating an interarch tooth-size ("Bolton") discrepancy. A, Frontal view. B, Inferior oblique view.

Logically, interproximal reduction should be performed distal to the maxillary right canine to facilitate retraction of the maxillary canine and incisors. Minimal overjet, however, is present anteriorly. The solution to this problem is straightforward. Interproximal reduction is performed on the distal aspect of the maxillary right canine and between the six lower anterior teeth. The interarch tooth size imbalance is eliminated, and the occlusion can be detailed appropriately as the space is closed.

An additional example is the discoordination between the arches (usually the maxillary arch appears

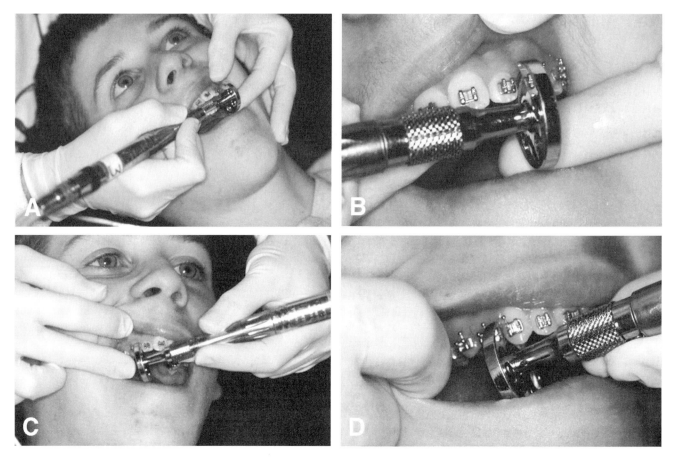

Figure 26-24. Technique of interproximal reduction. *AB*, stripping the distal surface of the maxillary left lateral incisor with the handpiece held in the right hand. *CD*, stripping the distal surface of the maxillary right lateral incisor with the opposite hand.

FINISHING AND RETENTION

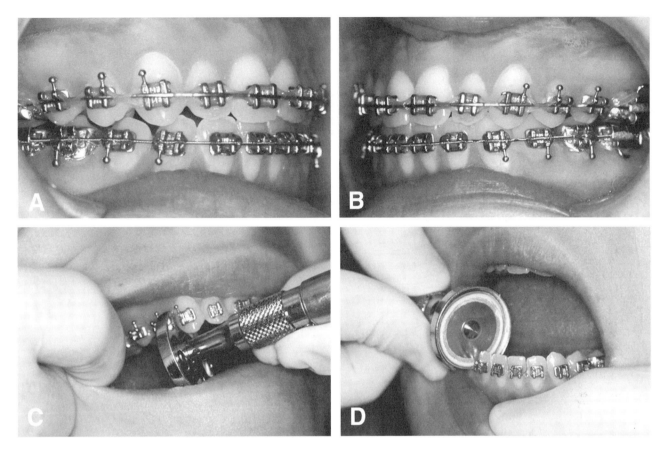

Figure 26-25. Problems in finishing. *A*, Slight Class II tendency in the right canine region, although the right premolars and molars are Class I. *B*, Normal left side occlusion with minimal overjet. *C*, Stripping the distal of the maxillary right canine. *D*, Stripping the mandibular incisors.

slightly wider than the mandibular arch) that occurs near the end of treatment. Often this problem can be eliminated by judicious interproximal reduction in the maxillary canine and first premolar regions. Triangular elastics (Fig. 26-2) are used to seat the canines, as can so-called Buffalo elastics, which are described in the next section.

Transpalatal ("Buffalo") Elastics

Another technique for coordination of the arches at the end of treatment involves the use of what we have termed "Buffalo" elastics (Fig. 26-26). These transpalatal elastics are used to constrict the maxillary arch by producing a transpalatal force in the maxilla.[38] The elastics, which typically are 3/8", 8-ounce in size and strength ("Buffalo" elastics, Ormco Corp., Orange CA), extend across the palate and attach to ball hooks or Kobayashi hooks on the maxillary first premolar bands (Figs. 26-27 and 26-28). These elastics typically are not worn full-time, but rather only at night because of interruption of speech patterns, although some patients have worn Buffalo elastics on a fulltime basis with little difficulty. These elastics can constrict the maxillary dental arch within a few months, if worn conscientiously at night by the patient.

This type of elastic also can be useful in orthognathic surgery patients, particularly those with Class III malocclusion, who require maxillary constriction as part of their presurgical orthodontic preparation. Buffalo elastics can be worn fulltime for 2–4 months, producing 3 or more millimeters of reduction in the distance between the maxillary premolars (Fig. 26-29).

Impressions for Immediate Positioner

We routinely (~80% of patients) deliver a tooth positioner following debonding/debanding. The tooth positioner is used to close band space and to detail (settle) the occlusion. The positioner also can be used effectively as a retainer in openbite patients, and it is useful in shrinking and recontouring hyperplastic gingival tissue.

One month before appliance removal, both archwires are removed. First, the clinician evaluates the patient for enamel recontouring, performing this procedure if indicated. Maxillary and mandibular alginate impres-

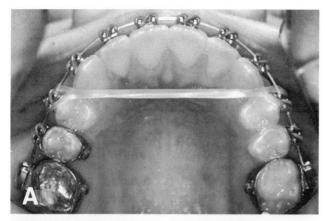

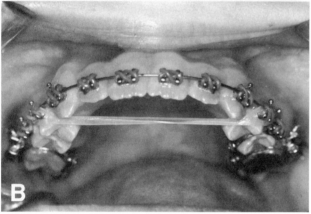

Figure 26-26. Buffalo elastics. This intraarch elastic typically is worn across the palate between the maxillary first premolars in order to narrow the maxillary dental arch. *A*, Occlusal view. *B*, Oblique frontal view.

sions are made over the fixed appliances. These models are used to fabricate a positioner that will be delivered at the time of appliance removal. At the same appointment, a lateral headfilm is taken, and a hinge-axis tracing is made that is sent to the laboratory as part of the positioner set-up.

At the laboratory, each tooth in the maxillary and mandibular work model is freed, carved, and reset in wax to an ideal occlusion (Fig. 26-30). The bite then is opened sufficiently to allow for the construction of the positioner.

The positioner (Fig. 26-31) can be made from a number of clear elastomeric materials including silicone, vinyl, and urethane. The positioner is formed so that it covers the facial and lingual surfaces of the teeth. The material itself is flexible so that the teeth can be guided into an ideal relationship.

Detailing the Occlusion

One week before appliance removal, the occlusion is evaluated and a decision is made regarding the need for

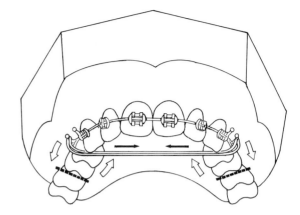

Figure 26-27. Schematic representation of the placement of the transpalatal elastics on the ball hooks of the maxillary first premolars. The elastics can be worn either at night or fulltime, depending on the magnitude of the desired reduction in palatal width.

further vertical closure of the dentition. If the occlusion is near ideal, serpentine wires are placed. If additional vertical closure is required, the patient wears what are termed "spaghetti elastics." The first procedure requires minimal patient cooperation, whereas the second requires maximal cooperation.

Serpentine Wires

One week before appliance removal, the maxillary and mandibular archwires are removed, as are all bands and the TPA, if present. The teeth are ligated together in a serpentine fashion from second premolar to second premolar (Fig. 26-32) with standard ligature wire.[39] The use of ligature wire allows the occlusion to settle without creating any interdental spacing. The patient is instructed to chew gum as much as possible during the

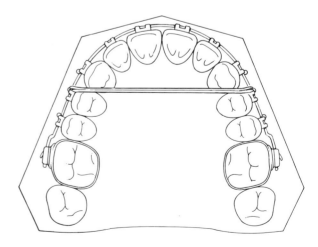

Figure 26-28. Occlusal view of the placement of Buffalo elastics between the maxillary first molars. This type of elastic can be placed on the maxillary second premolars as well.

FINISHING AND RETENTION

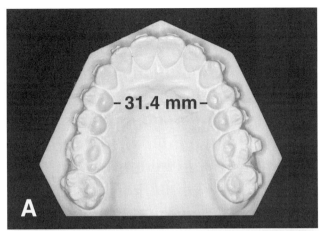

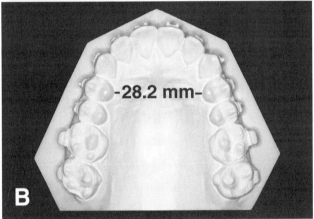

Figure 26-29. Maxillary progress models of a Class III patient being prepared for orthognathic surgery. She required maxillary width reduction as part of her pretreatment orthodontic treatment. She wore transpalatal elastics continuously for three months, producing a 3.2 mm decrease in the width between the maxillary first premolars. *A*, Before elastics. *B*, After wearing transpalatal elastics for three months.

following week. This method of fine detailing is ideal if there are only minimal discrepancies remaining in tooth position or if patient cooperation has not been optimal during treatment.

Vertical ("Spaghetti") Elastics

One week before appliance removal, the maxillary and mandibular archwires are removed, and the interproximal contacts between the maxillary six anterior teeth are stripped (if needed). A .016" stainless steel wire is secured in place in the mandibular arch with light steel ligatures.[40] No archwire is placed in the maxillary brackets. Then, using 3/16", 2 or 3 1/2 ounce elastics (Quail or Otter elastics, Ormco Corp., Orange CA), a series of triangular elastics are placed between the two dental arches (Fig. 26-33). The three arms of the triangular elastic include the distal bracket wing of one maxillary tooth, the mesial bracket wing of the tooth posterior to

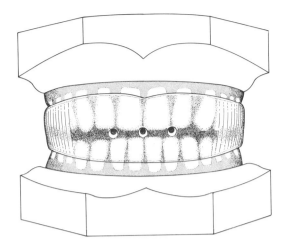

Figure 26-30. Frontal view of positioner set-up with positioner in place. Note serrations on lateral aspect of positioner for ease of placement. Air holes also are evident in the anterior region.

it and the entire bracket of the mandibular tooth closest to the two maxillary teeth (Fig. 26-34*A*).

The only exception to the placement of the triangular elastics is in the region of the central incisors (Fig. 26-34*B*). Two triangular elastics are placed in the midline, each encompassing the mesial tie wings of both central incisors, one elastic extending to the mandibular right central incisor, and one elastic extending to the mandibular left central incisor.

The patient is instructed to wear the spaghetti elastics on almost a full-time basis for the week before appliance removal. The proper wearing of the elastic facilitates a rapid settling of the occlusion. If there is a tendency toward an anterior openbite remaining at this stage, judicious interproximal stripping is recommended as well, a protocol that also facilitates the management of any remaining "Bolton discrepancies."[34] The patient

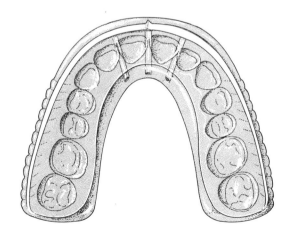

Figure 26-31. Maxillary occlusal view of positioner. Note lateral serrations and air holes anteriorly.

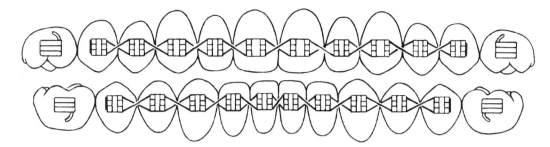

Figure 26-32. Serpentine wires. All archwires and bands are removed. Then .008″ ligature wire is extended in a serpentine configuration from second premolar to second premolar in both arches. The patient is instructed to clench and chew gum as much as possible until the debonding appointment.

is instructed to avoid wide opening movements with the elastics in place to minimize discomfort. The elastics are removed during meals and when oral hygiene procedures are being performed.

Spaghetti elastics in general are very useful in those patients in whom there is difficulty closing the bite, whether anteriorly or posteriorly. This type of elastic is contraindicated in malocclusions that originally were characterized by a deep bite (*e.g.*, Class II, division 2 malocclusion). In these situations, the use of serpentine wires is indicated.

Delivery of Immediate Positioner

At the time of appliance removal, the remaining archwire(s) is (are) removed as are the bands, cement, bonds and the bonding agent. After the appropriate hygienic procedures have been performed, the patient is given the positioner (Fig. 26-35).

It is our intention to have the patient wear the positioner as much as possible for a relatively limited time. Thus, the patient is told to wear the positioner full-time for the first 24 hours (except during meals), as much as possible for the next five days, and then four hours per day plus nighttime for two to six weeks. The patient also is told that if patient cooperation is not sufficient, or even if patient cooperation is sufficient but the occlusal result is not acceptable, fixed appliances may be replaced. This possibility proves to be a formidable factor in encouraging patient motivation.

Post-treatment Evaluation

Ideally, two or three weeks after appliance removal (certainly within the first six-eight weeks), the patient is seen for a follow-up visit. The occlusion is checked to verify that the positioner is being worn properly and that the occlusal result is satisfactory. Before obtaining post-treatment records, however, the patient once again should be evaluated for an enamoplasty and even for further interproximal reduction.

Routine post-treatment records are obtained at this appointment. These records include a lateral cephalogram, study models, and photographs. As mentioned earlier, we strongly recommend that the post-treatment panoramic film be taken several months *before* removal of appliances to check root angulation and for pathology. If the panoramic film was not taken before appliance removal, it also is obtained at this appointment. A panoramic film also should be obtained if further substantial root paralleling has been undertaken since the earlier (pre-debond) film was taken. The need for adequate documentation of the post-treatment status of the patient has become more important in recent years, es-

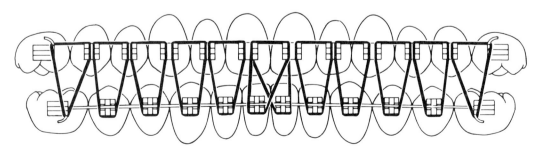

Figure 26-33. Schematic diagram of vertical ("spaghetti") elastics. The mandibular arch wire is ligated in place with steel ligatures (not shown).

FINISHING AND RETENTION

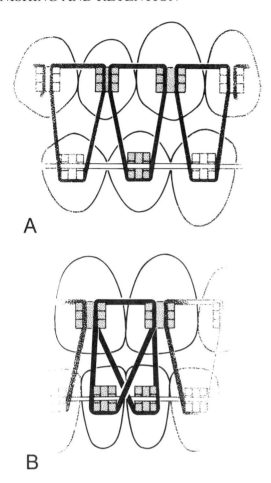

Figure 26-34. Placement of triangular ("Spaghetti") elastics. *A*, Typical configuration. An elastic extends from the distal wing of the more anterior maxillary bracket to the mesial wing of the more posterior bracket to both wings of the mandibular bracket. *B*, Configuration in the central incisor region. The elastics extend from the mesial wings of the maxillary central incisor brackets to both wings of one of the mandibular central incisor brackets.

pecially due to the litigious environment in which the orthodontist now practices.

If positioner wear has been satisfactory and the occlusal results are acceptable, upper and lower impressions are taken for the fabrication of invisible retainers (Fig. 26-36). These retainers typically are made from 1-mm thick splint Biocryl™ that has been trimmed 1–2 mm from the gingival margin. These retainers are worn fulltime for at least one year and then indefinitely at night.

The use of this type of retainer also allows for the correction of subtle deviations from ABO standards[1] noted in the occlusion of a patient after appliance removal. As discussed in detail in the next chapter, one tooth per quadrant can be reset to optimize the occlusion. In certain situations, impressions are taken every six to eight weeks, and new invisible retainers are fabricated until

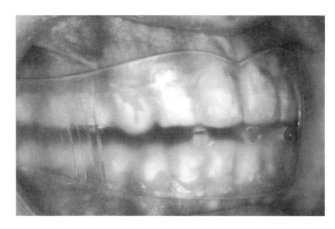

Figure 26-35. Intraoral view of positioner at the time of appliance delivery.

ideal tooth position is achieved. Usually, however, only one or two sets of retainers are necessary to obtain a satisfactory occlusion if proper finishing techniques have been employed.

Long-term Retention

Long-term retention usually is achieved by having the patient wear retainers on a full-time basis for at least one year, then at night for an indefinite period. Nighttime retainer wear is the only way of maintaining the achieved orthodontic result over the long-term. It is well known that craniofacial growth continues long after the teenage years,[41,42] so continued retainer wear must be stressed, even after the patient has been placed on inactive status in the orthodontic practice.

In most instances, patients simply continue to wear invisible retainers on a nighttime basis. Alternatively, a removable Hawley retainer, circumferential retainer, or

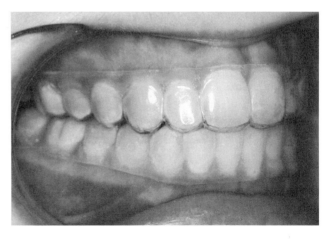

Figure 26-36. Intraoral view of patient wearing maxillary and mandibular invisible retainers. The retainers are trimmed so that the acrylic covers 1-2 mm of the gingival margin.

bonded lingual retainer can be used, depending on the particular needs of the patient (*e.g.*, poor patient compliance, need for posterior settling, interproximal space closure).

Retention Protocol

In recent years, retention protocols have been refined substantially to streamline our practice. Following the delivery of retainers, typically invisible retainers, the patient is recalled in four months. The integrity of the retainers is determined, and the occlusion is checked. If there is any tendency toward crowding in the lower anterior region, judicious interproximal reduction is performed, particularly at the distal surface of the lower lateral incisors (Fig 26-22). In some instances, another set of invisibles is indicated to fine detail the occlusion, and impressions are obtained at this time for new retainers.

The patient is seen six months later, now about one year after appliance removal and is evaluated for "inactive retention" status. At this appointment, the patient is formally evaluated in a number of areas and a written form is completed (Fig. 26-37). During this exit examination, the patient again is evaluated for enamoplasty and interproximal reduction, any needed changes in tooth morphology are made, and appropriate notes are made on the form.

If not evaluated previously, the status of the third molars is determined, either by writing a prescription to the oral and maxillofacial surgeon for their removal or by deferring the decision until later. If the patient is to be placed on inactive status and the decision regarding the third molars is deferred, a letter is written to the family dentist, asking her or him to assume responsibility for the third molar decision. A digital or duplicate copy of the most recent panoramic radiograph is included with the letter.

At this appointment, the status of the temporomandibular joints and associated musculature is determined first by asking the patient if s/he has any complaints about his/her jaw function. Most do not, and this observation is recorded on the form (Fig 26-37). Maximal interincisal opening is measured with a flexible ruler (Fig. 26-38) or a Therabite™ range of motion scale (Therabite Corp., New Town Square PA). As described in detail in Chapter 2, the typical maximal incisal opening ranges from 40–60 mm. The opening in millimeters is recorded on the form.

If the patient reports symptoms of temporomandibular disorders, appropriate treatment should be taken, including the fabrication of a flat plane splint that is worn at night. Such patients typically are not placed on inactive retention status, but rather are monitored on an intermittent basis. The primary responsibility for the management of the temporomandibular disorder typically remains with the family practitioner, although the orthodontist may choose to manage the patient's care or refer the patient to a practitioner focusing on the diagnosis and treatment of temporomandibular disorders.

After the form has been completed, the form is signed by the orthodontist and, after reading the document, the patient (or his or her parent, if necessary) also signs the form. The form also states that from this point forward, there will be a charge for retention visits and replacement retainers.

Correction of Lower Incisor Irregularity

A common observation during the post-treatment period, regardless of whether or not permanent teeth have been extracted, is the occurrence of mandibular incisor irregularity.[36,43–46] Two types of retainers can be used to correct mandibular incisor crowding, combined with the use of interproximal reduction.

Invisible Retainers

The simplest type of retainer to fabricate is the invisible retainer (Fig. 26-36), which is described in detail in the next chapter. One tooth per quadrant can be reset and the invisible retainer fabricated with the teeth in reset positions. The invisible retainer then acts like a minipositioner, facilitating rapid tooth realignment. If a tooth must be moved substantially, then sequential invisible retainers may be necessary.

Spring Retainer

A more durable type of retainer that can facilitate the simultaneous movement of the mandibular incisors is the spring retainer, developed by Barrer.[47] The original design of this retainer has been modified in a manner similar to a Hawley retainer (Fig. 26-39).

After an impression is made and a work model is poured, the four mandibular incisors (or whatever teeth need to be reset) are removed from the model, trimmed, and then reset in wax (Fig. 26-40). The anterior and posterior parts of the retainer are united only by the distal extension of the anterior wire framework. The labial surface of the anterior wire also is covered with acrylic (Fig. 26-40) to aid in the alignment of the mandibular anterior teeth. Posteriorly, occlusal rests begin on the lingual groove of the mandibular first molar, cross anteriorly along the lingual contour of the mandibular alveolus, and then end in the lingual groove of the opposite molar. This type of retainer can be used not only to move teeth, but

INACTIVE RETENTION STATUS

You have completed orthodontic treatment in our office some time ago. You report no major concerns about your teeth and face, and therefore active orthodontic supervision is no longer necessary.

We are placing you on inactive status. This simply means that you are no longer in need of routine supervision in our office. We will be happy to see you at any time, however, if you notice any problems developing.

Virtually all patients are given retainers at the end of active orthodontic treatment. We encourage our patients to wear retainers on a full time basis for at least one year and then on a nighttime basis after that time. We encourage you to continue wearing your retainers at least on a part-time basis at night to maintain the bite that was achieved through orthodontic treatment.

The mouth is no different than other parts of the body, in that the bones and teeth gradually shift with time. For example, the lower front teeth often develop mild crowding as a person gets older, whether or not he or she has undergone orthodontic treatment. Thus, we recommend the long-term wearing of retainers.

We will be happy to see you at any time if you have any orthodontic concerns. As mentioned in your financial agreement, there is a charge for these retention visits. Please contact us if we can be of further service to you.

_____   _____
Patient/Parent Signature   Date

_____   _____
Orthodontist Signature   Date

Clinical Notes:

Enamoplasty: _____

Interproximal reduction: _____

Third molar status: _____

TMD complaints: _____ Max Interincisal opening: _____mm

Other concerns: _____

Figure 26-37. Inactive retention form. This form is completed and signed by the orthodontist and read and signed by the patient or parent at this visit.

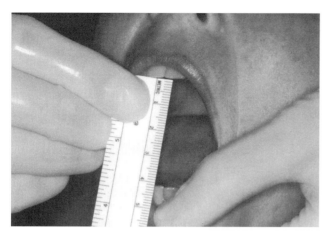

Figure 26-38. Maximum incisal opening. This measurement is made by way of a flexible ruler (shown here) or a Therabite™ disposable ruler (see Chapter 2).

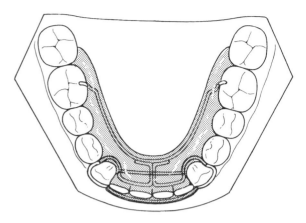

Figure 26-39. Modified spring retainer of Barrer. Note the separation between the posterior and anterior parts of the acrylic.

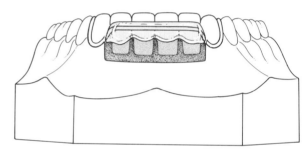

Figure 26-40. Frontal view of mandibular spring retainer. The mandibular incisors have been reset in wax. An acrylic cap covers the anterior wire on the labial surface.

also to stabilize severely rotated teeth after they have been aligned during orthodontic treatment.

CONCLUDING REMARKS

This chapter has dealt with the final months of fixed appliance therapy and the subsequent post-treatment period. One of the most important aspects of this chapter was the presentation of criteria that can be used for the evaluation of the occlusion of a patient as s/he approaches the end of treatment. The six keys to optimal occlusion of Andrews[2,3] and the concept of a mutually protected occlusion[4–6] are well-known guidelines of occlusal evaluation, and should be incorporated into the patient's overall treatment plan. Further, the 1998 guidelines of the *American Board of Orthodontics*[1] provide specific criteria for determining the adequacy of the fine detailing of the occlusion. Obviously, it is much better if these criteria are used in evaluation of an occlusion before the appliances are removed, through direct clinical inspection or better through a close examination of so-called "debond evaluation" models, obtained 1–3 months before anticipated appliance removal.

In this chapter, two general treatment protocols are outlined, one relatively simple and one more complex. The first protocol involves fixed appliance therapy and the use of wire and acrylic retainers for detailing and stabilizing of the dentition. This protocol is relatively inexpensive to implement as it requires the fabrication of only one set of maxillary and mandibular removable retainers. Patient compliance is minimal, but only limited tooth movement is possible after the fixed appliances are removed.

The second protocol is much more detailed and involves significant patient cooperation, especially if vertical ("spaghetti") elastics and a positioner are used. These finishing mechanics, however, allow for the earlier removal of the fixed appliances than if all tooth positioning had to be accomplished through detailed adjustments of the archwires.

Another advantage of using the positioner at the end of treatment is in the closure of band spaces that may remain between the posterior teeth after appliance removal. Further, the positioner has a positive effect on gingival health, especially in instances of gingival hypertrophy during treatment. The use of a positioner, on the other hand, usually is contraindicated in patients who have preexisting signs and/or symptoms of temporomandibular disorders.

This chapter also describes a number of removable retainers, including invisible retainers and wire and acrylic retainers. Invisible retainers are extremely well received by patients and are our retainer of choice. The ability to control tooth position is greater with invisible retainers than with wire and acrylic type retainers (except perhaps for the spring retainer); however, invisible retainers have the drawback of excessive wear of the retainers in some patients with parafunctional habits, sometimes resulting in the need to replace these retainers once or twice each year. In these individuals, a retainer such as the Hawley or circumferential retainer may be preferred.

This chapter provides information on a number of other treatment protocols that can be used in conjunction with fixed appliance treatment to finely detail the occlusion, both immediately before the removal of appliances as well as during the early parts of the retention period. The specific choice of which of the many protocols outlined in this chapter are to be used on a given patient, of course, depends on the quality of the occlusion near the end of active orthodontic therapy.

REFERENCES CITED

1. Casko JS, Vaden JL, Kokich VG, Damone J, Cangialosi TJ, Riolo ML, Owens SE, Bills ED. Objective grading system for dental casts and panoramic radiographs. Am J Orthod Dentofac Orthop 1998;114:589–599.
2. Andrews LF. The six keys to normal occlusion. Am J Orthod 1972;62:296–309.
3. Andrews LF. Straightwire: The concept and appliance. San Diego: LA Wells, 1989.
4. Okeson JP. Management of temporomandibular disorders. St Louis: Mosby Year Book, 1993.
5. Roth RH. Functional occlusion for the orthodontist. J Clin Orthod 1981;15:32–40, 44–51.
6. Roth RH. Treatment mechanics for the straight wire appliance. In: Graber TM, Swain BF, eds. Orthodontics: Current principles and techniques. St Louis: CV Mosby, 1985.
7. Angle EH. Classification of malocclusion. Dent Cosmos 1899;41:248–264.
8. Adams CP. The design and construction of removable orthodontic appliances. Bristol: John Wright and Sons, 1970.
9. Berger EV. Personal communication, 1992.
10. Winshall AI. Personal communication, 1987.
11. Van der Linden FPGM. Doelmatige retentie. Practische Orthodontie 1997;1:1–16.
12. Van der Linden FPGM. Personal communication, 2000.
13. Zachrisson BU. Clinical experience with direct-bonded orthodontic retainers. Am J Orthod 1977;71:440–448.
14. Dahl EH, Zachrisson BU. Long-term experience with direct-bonded lingual retainers. J Clin Orthod 1991;25:619–630.
15. Zachrisson BJ. Third-generation mandibular bonded lingual 3-3 retainer. J Clin Orthod 1995;29:39–48.
16. Krause FW. Bonded maxillary custom lingual retainer. J Clin Orthod 1984;18:734–737.
17. Edwards JG. A study of the periodontium during orthodontic rotation of teeth. Am J Orthod 1968;54:441–461.
18. Edwards JG. A surgical procedure to eliminate rotational relapse. Am J Orthod 1970;57:35–46.
19. Edwards JG. A long-term prospective evaluation of the circumferential supracrestal fiberotomy in alleviating orthodontic relapse. Am J Orthod Dentofac Orthop 1988;93:380–387.
20. Reitan K. Tissue rearrangement during retention of orthodontically rotated teeth. Angle Orthod 1959;29:105–122.
21. Beertsen W. Remodeling of collagen fibers in the periodontal ligament and the supra-alveolar region. Angle Orthod 1979;49:218–224.
22. Orban B. Indications, technique and postoperative management of gingivectomy in the treatment of periodontal disease. J Periodontol 1941;12:88–91.
23. Ramfjord S. Gingivectomy - its place in periodontal therapy. J Periodontol 1952;23:30–35.
24. Prichard J. Gingivectomy, gingivoplasty, and osseous surgery. J Periodontol 1961;32:257–262.
25. Monefeldt I, Zachrisson B. Adjustment of clinical crown height by gingivectomy following orthodontic space closure. Angle Orthod 1977;47:256–264.
26. Boese LR. Increased stability of orthodontically rotated teeth following gingivectomy in *Macaca nemestrina*. Am J Orthod 1969;56:273–290.
27. Zachrisson BU, Mjor IA. Remodeling of teeth by grinding. Am J Orthod 1975;68:545–553.
28. McNamara JA, Jr, Kelly KA (eds). Frontiers of dental and facial esthetics. Ann Arbor: Monograph 37, Craniofacial Growth Series, Center for Human Growth and Development, The University of Michigan, 2001.
29. Mayes JH. Personal communication, 1998.
30. Hudson A. A study of the effects of mesiodistal reduction of mandibular anterior teeth. Am J Orthod 1956;42:615–624.
31. Peck H, Peck S. An index for assessing tooth shape deviations as applied to the mandibular incisors. Am J Orthod 1972;61:384–401.
32. Tuverson DL. Anterior interocclusal relations. Part I. Am J Orthod 1980;78:361–370.
33. Tuverson DL. Anterior interocclusal relations. Part II. Am J Orthod 1980;78:371–393.
34. Bolton WA. Disharmony in tooth size and its relation to the analysis and treatment of malocclusion. Angle Orthod 1958;28:113–130.
35. Bolton WA. The clinical application of a tooth-size analysis. Am J Orthod 1962;48:504–529.
36. Little RM. Stability and relapse of dental arch alignment. Br J Orthod 1990;17:235–241.
37. Carter GA, McNamara JA, Jr. Longitudinal dental arch changes in adults. Am J Orthod Dentofac Orthop 1998;114:88–99.
38. Mayers CA. Personal communication, 1997.
39. Schaal DM. Personal communication, 1976.
40. Savage RA, Schaal DM. Personal communication, 1985.
41. Behrents RG. Growth in the aging craniofacial skeleton. Ann Arbor: Monograph 17, Craniofacial Growth Series, Center for Human Growth and Development, The University of Michigan, 1985.
42. West KS, McNamara JA, Jr. Changes in the craniofacial complex from adolescence to adulthood: A cephalometric study. Am J Orthod Dentofac Orthoped 1999;115:521–532.
43. Little RM, Wallen TR, Riedel RA. Stability and relapse of mandibular anterior alignment-first premolar extraction cases treated by traditional edgewise orthodontics. Am J Orthod 1981;80:349–365.
44. Little RM, Riedel RA, Årtun J. An evaluation of changes

in mandibular anterior alignment from 10 to 20 years postretention. Am J Orthod Dentofac Orthop 1988;93:423–428.
45. Little RM, Riedel RA, Engst ED. Serial extraction of first premolars—postretention evaluation of stability and relapse. Angle Orthod 1990;60:255–262.
46. McReynolds DC, Little RM. Mandibular second premolar extraction—postretention evaluation of stability and relapse. Angle Orthod 1991;61:133–144.
47. Barrer HG. Protecting the integrity of mandibular incisor position through keystoning procedure and spring retainer appliance. J Clin Orthod 1975;9:486–494.

Chapter 27

INVISIBLE RETAINERS AND ALIGNERS

The most versatile of all retainers used in our practice is the invisible retainer (Fig. 27-1), often termed "invisibles." This type of thin acrylic retainer was developed originally by Henry Nahoum in the late 1950s, and an article on this subject (unknown to us until very recently) was published in the *New York State Dental Journal* in 1964.[1]

The invisible retainer, as we use them, was developed by Robert Ponitz of Ann Arbor, Michigan.[2] Typically this retainer is formed from a sheet of thin Biocryl™ or other similar material that is heated and forced by suction[1,2] or pressure[3] on to a work model of the dentition.

This type of retainer has many uses in routine orthodontic practice, not only as a finishing and retention appliance, but also as an active treatment adjunct. The development of the Invisalign® System of aligners for comprehensive movement, a logical outgrowth of this technology, will be discussed later in this chapter.

FUNCTIONS OF INVISIBLE RETAINERS

The invisible retainer can be used for three purposes: minor tooth movement, long-term retention, and as a transitional retainer.

Minor Tooth Movement

Invisible retainers can produce minor tooth movements effectively, whether used immediately after debonding, after positioner wear is concluded, or in instances of minor relapse during the retention period. When used after the end of active fixed appliance treatment, even though the vast majority of dental irregularities have been eliminated, small inter-arch and intra-arch discrepancies often remain in the treated occlusion. Fine detailing of the occlusion can be accomplished by resetting up to one tooth per quadrant in the work model prior to invisible retainer fabrication.

Small adjustments in tooth position (*e.g.,* tipping, rotation, intrusion) can be achieved most easily for incisors and premolars, due to the morphology of these teeth. For example, a slightly rotated lower incisor can be reset into an ideal relationship before fabricating the appliance. The elasticity of the acrylic used in the fabrication of the invisible retainer can help force the rotated tooth into a new, aligned position.

Conical shaped teeth (*e.g.,* some canines) are more difficult to reposition with an invisible retainer. Although simple tipping movements are accomplished easily as is minor tooth intrusion, the correction of rotations is more difficult. Extrusive movements are difficult to produce in all teeth, except if significant undercuts are present.

Only very minor changes in the position of the molars should be attempted with conventional invisible retainers. Occasionally, a remaining band space can be closed by repositioning the molar more anteriorly; however, gross changes in the position of the molar usually are not possible, because the invisible retainer simply will not fit on the patient's dental arch with the molar in its new position. In addition, it should be noted that adjacent teeth (*e.g.,* both maxillary central incisors) typically cannot be repositioned simultaneously with a conven-

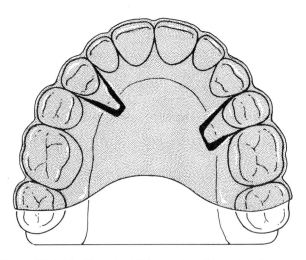

Figure 27-1. Maxillary invisible retainer. Note that the posterior extension is contoured to prevent evoking the patient's gag reflex. Alternatively, the invisible can be trimmed so that all or part of the palate is left uncovered.

tional invisible retainer, because the retainer will not snap into place at the time of delivery.

Usually a set of invisible retainers is worn for one or two months before a new set of retainers is made. The number of sets of retainers necessary, is, of course, dependent on the quality of the orthodontic result at the time of debonding. If multiple teeth have to be reset in a quadrant, multiple sets of invisibles will be necessary.

Long-term Retention

The second function of the invisible retainer is to stabilize the dentition in its current position. Invisible retainers are used as a long-term retention appliance after minor tooth movements have been achieved. These acrylic retainers usually will last for six to twelve months or longer, depending on the parafunctional activities of the patient. Some patients use these retainers indefinitely, whereas the invisible retainers of others (especially heavy bruxers) show a high degree of wear and/or breakage. In the latter case, wire and acrylic retainers (*e.g.,* Hawley retainer, circumferential retainer) can be used effectively.

Many clinicians are concerned about using any retainer that provides occlusal coverage. It has been our experience that, in general, the occlusal coverage provided by the invisible retainer does not appear to pose many clinical problems. The patient usually "self-equilibrates" the maxillary and mandibular appliances within a few days, and symptoms of temporomandibular joint disorders are rare. As with any removable appliance, patients are instructed to discontinue invisible retainer wear if any problems with their temporomandibular joints are encountered. Also, if a patient has chronically poor oral hygiene, decalcification under the retainer may occur. Patients should be instructed to brush their teeth prior to the insertion of invisible retainers.

One of the major advantages of the invisible retainer is that it provides a positive positioning of the teeth, thus aiding in the prevention of relapse. This is particularly true with the position of the incisors, specifically the mandibular incisors and the maxillary lateral incisors. Using many types of conventional wire retainers, minor changes in tooth position often are observed; this is not the case when invisible retainers are worn as directed. In addition, if the invisible retainers are not worn for some time, resuming retainer wear on a fulltime basis should eliminate minor undesirable changes in tooth position.

Invisible retainers can be used for minor space closure or perhaps, better stated, for space reallocation. For example, a small diastema between the maxillary central incisors may be closed by repositioning one of the central incisors. The angulation of one of the incisors may be altered, or alternatively the space may be relocated to another part of the dental arch. After several invisible retainers have been fabricated, bonding material may be placed at the distal of the lateral incisors to ensure that the midline diastema does not reopen.

If a patient has significant interproximal spacing at the end of treatment, the use of invisible retainers is contraindicated, as no space closure is possible with traditional invisible retainers. Prior finishing with a positioner is advisable. If a positioner is not used, a retainer such as a circumferential retainer is recommended.

Transitional Appliance

As mentioned elsewhere in this book, the invisible retainer also can be used as a transitional appliance between phases of orthodontic treatment. If, for example, incisor intrusion and protrusion have been accomplished successfully prior to the fabrication of a functional appliance, the invisible retainer is used as a transitional retainer until fulltime functional appliance wear has been achieved.

Generally, the transitional retainer should be used without the resetting of any teeth. Even though minor irregularities may remain, changing the position of certain teeth while a functional appliance is being fabricated may lead to problems with the fit of the functional appliance. This is particularly true if an acrylic splint Herbst appliance is used, because of the precise reproduction of the anatomy of the teeth in this type of appliance.

INVISIBLE RETAINERS AND ALIGNERS

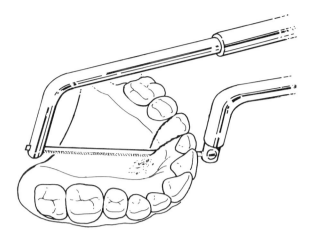

Figure 27-2. A laboratory saw is used to remove the canine from the model. Note the tapered cuts.

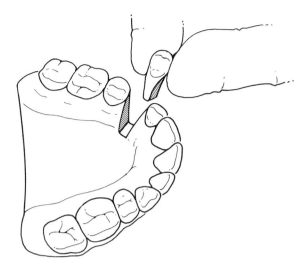

Figure 27-3. Finger pressure or a laboratory knife is used to break the remaining plaster, freeing the tooth. The cut in the stone is trimmed so that the tooth can be repositioned, allowing enough space for wax.

Another common use of the conventional invisible retainer as a transitional appliance is in the adolescent patient who is to receive a dental implant after active craniofacial growth has ceased. In this situation, a pontic may be incorporated into the invisible, or alternatively, an invisible retainer can be fabricated over a flipper to which a pontic is attached. The pontic holds the space that was established for the implant during orthodontic treatment. The invisible retainer with the pontic is worn until implant replacement of the missing tooth has been completed.

FABRICATION OF INVISIBLE RETAINERS

The steps in invisible retainer fabrication have been described previously by McNamara and co-workers[3] in the *Journal of Clinical Orthodontics*. This article is updated below. In this summary, the possibilities of making minor changes in tooth position with invisible retainers will be stressed.

Preparation of the Work Models

Upper and lower alginate impressions are made with standard aluminum trays, and a wax bite registration is obtained in centric occlusion to articulate the models, if the correct occlusion is not obvious. The impressions are poured in plaster and trimmed as standard work models with minimal base (Fig. 27-2). Before articulating the maxillary and mandibular work models, excess plaster and any bubbles on the articulating surfaces of the teeth should be removed carefully with a laboratory kinfe or waxing instrument.

The orthodontist then checks the hand articulated models for resets by placing the models together in centric occlusion. The teeth to be reset are indicated on the laboratory slip, with specific instructions as to the direction of movement or the percentage of rotation, if necessary.

Minor Tooth Repositioning on Work Models

One of the limitations of using a conventional invisible retainer as a tooth-moving device, in contrast to the series of aligners to be discussed later, is that in order to insure appliance fit, usually only one tooth per quadrant can be reset in each retainer. In the four premolar extraction case used as an example (Fig. 27-2), it is necessary to reposition the maxillary right canine. Interdental cuts that approximate the long axis of the tooth are made on the maxillary work model with a laboratory saw. Gentle finger pressure is used to fracture the remaining plaster and free the tooth from the model (Fig. 27-3).

A laboratory knife is used to trim the area of the model in which the tooth is to be repositioned. Stone also must be removed from the sides of the "extracted" tooth (Fig. 27-4) to allow repositioning of this tooth in a more ideal position. Medium-hard pink wax is melted and placed into the area where the tooth has been removed (Fig. 27-5), and the tooth is repositioned temporarily in the wax (Fig. 27-6).

In this example the lower premolar also needs repositioning; it is removed from the mandibular work

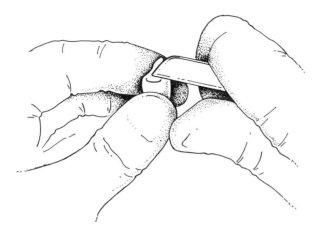

Figure 27-4. Tooth trimmed with laboratory knife.

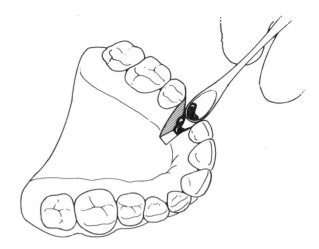

Figure 27-5. Melted wax placed in tooth space.

model in a similar manner. The dental casts are occluded, and the final changes in tooth position are achieved. The wax contours are smoothed, and the models are ready for retainer fabrication (Fig. 27-7) If interproximal undercuts are present, particularly in adult patients, they should be eliminated with wax. Similarly, any missing teeth that are not being replaced with a pontic should be waxed out as well.

Application of Acrylic

The invisible retainers are formed from 1 mm thick acrylic by means of a Biostar™ positive pressure thermal forming machine (Great Lakes Orthodontic Products, Tonawanda, NY). Splint Biocryl™ is used for maxillary retainers because of its transparancy. Invisacryl C™, also available through Great Lakes Orthodontics, is used for the fabrication of mandibular retainers because of its durability.

The work model is placed into the large (125 mm) model holder of the Biostar™, with the occlusal plane horizontal. Lead pellets are placed around the model to a point 1 mm below the desired margin of the appliance. The holding frame is placed on the pressure chamber, with the gasket and the four holding pins facing upward. A piece of 1 mm acrylic is placed inside the four pins of the holding frame, and acrylic is secured in position by placing the clamping frame over the holding frame. The handle of the clamping frame is turned to the left and secured with light pressure to lock it in place.

The heating element is moved into position over the pressure chamber and left in place for 25-30 seconds for splint Biocryl™ and 80 seconds for Invisacryl C™ to soften the acrylic. The heating element is removed, the pressure chamber is rotated over the model holder, and the pressure chamber handle is engaged. Air pressure, rather than partial vacuum pressure as originally advocated by Ponitz,[1] is used to push the softened Biocryl™ onto the work model at about five atmospheres of pressure.

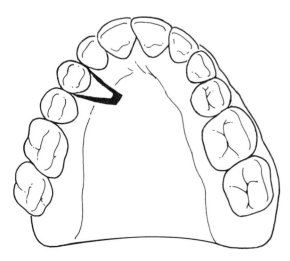

Figure 27-6. Tooth secured in preliminary corrected position.

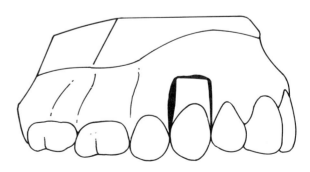

Figure 27-7. After the occlusion has been checked and the tooth is properly positioned, the wax is smoothed to a final contour.

INVISIBLE RETAINERS AND ALIGNERS

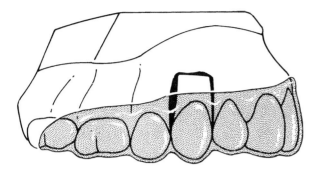

Figure 27-8. Finished trim of the maxillary invisible retainer. Care should be taken not to encroach on the gingival margin.

Trimming of Acrylic

After two minutes, the pressure chamber handle is unlocked and the pressure chamber is rotated out of position. The clamping frame is removed and the acrylic with the embedded work model is taken off the Biostar™. The work model is removed from the acrylic with a laboratory knife, destroying the model. Excess acrylic is trimmed with a sturdy pair of scissors, and the general contour of the invisible retainer is established with a carborundum disk. The invisible is soaked in warm (not hot) water to eliminate the wax.

A pair of scissors is used for the final trimming and finishing of the appliance. No further polishing or trimming usually is necessary, although a light sanding, pumicing, or polishing of the edges of the appliance may be required in some instances.

It is extremely important always to cover at least part of the last molar in each arch (including third molars) to prevent extrusion of these teeth with full-time appliance wear. The invisible retainer usually is trimmed to include full palatal coverage (Fig. 27-1), although all or part of the palate can be removed, if necessary. The facial surface is trimmed to follow the approximate contour of the gingival margin (Fig. 27-8).

The mandibular invisible retainer is trimmed in a horseshoe shape, again covering part of the last molar (Fig. 27-9). The facial and lingual surfaces are trimmed to approximate the gingival margins (Fig. 27-10). Invisible retainers require virtually no adjustment at the time of delivery, except for trimming with scissors in areas of soft tissue impingement. Often invisible retainers can be mailed to the patient with instructions to trim the acrylic at any point at which irritation occurs.

If teeth have been reset in the invisible retainer, the patient should be told that the appliance will take a few hours to a few days to seat completely. If too much tooth movement has been carried out on the work model or more than one tooth per quadrant has been reset substantially, the appliance will not fit and will have to be remade.

If a pontic is to be incorporated into an invisible retainer, the size and the appropriate shade are determined at chairside. After the correct pontic is obtained, it is trimmed to fit the available space on the work model, and then it is positioned on the cast with me-dium hard pink wax. The invisible retainer is fabricated as usual. As a final step, the pontic is glued to the invisible with an adhesive (*e.g.,* MDS Adhesive™, Great Lakes Orthodontic Products, Tonawanda NY), letting the adhesive dry thoroughly before delivery.

NEW TECHNOLOGY: The Invisalign® System

One of several new treatment approaches presented in this text is the methodology developed by Align Technology (Santa Clara CA). The Invisalign® System is a technologically advanced esthetic approach to treating

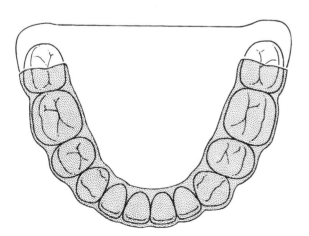

Figure 27-9. Finished contour of mandibular invisible retainer. Note that at least part of the last tooth is incorporated into the retainer bilaterally.

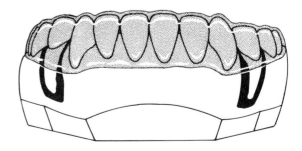

Figure 27-10. Final contour of the mandibular retainer. Typically the gingival margin is not scalloped, but rather forms gentle curves.

malocclusion. This approach brings the concept of the invisible retainer into the 21st century by linking these relatively simple and easy to fabricate retainers (Figs. 27-11 and 27-12) with three-dimensional graphic imaging and CAD/CAM technology.

The Invisalign® System was introduced commercially in June 1999. At this writing, over half of all U.S. and Canadian orthodontists have been certified to use the Invisalign® System.[4] During the certification process, the orthodontist becomes familiar with case selection criteria, receives training in poly-vinyl siloxane impression taking, and learns communication skills via the company's treatment planning forms and website.[5]

Methodology

The basic concept of using one or more removable semi-flexible appliances to move teeth is not new, as suggested by the use of tooth positioners[6] as well as various overlay types of appliances such as invisible retainers.[1-3,7,8] The amount of tooth movement possible with a traditional invisible retainer, however, is limited. As mentioned earlier, it has been our experience that routinely only one tooth per quadrant can be moved effectively and that moving molars with traditional invisible retainers is very difficult. Because of the 3D graphical imaging and precise computer manipulation of "virtual" models, more precise tooth movements involving a greater number of teeth are possible with the Invisalign® System. This includes tooth movement in the molar region.

A variety of tooth movement options are available, at the discretion of the clinician. For example, dental expansion can be accomplished in several ways. In the first method, all the teeth move at the same time; expansion occurs as teeth move to eliminate the crowding. With the second method, the first premolars through second molars expand first. When space appears distal to the canines, the canines move distally, creating space anteriorly. This latter space can be used to alleviate crowding in the incisor region.

According to current case selection criteria, a candidate for the Invisalign® System should have fully erupted permanent teeth, for whom growth has minimal or no effect on treatment (*i.e.*, late adolescents and adults).[9] Currently, Align Technology does not include continued craniofacial growth of the patient as a factor within its software.

Occlusal problems that are amenable to Invisalign® orthodontic appliance treatment include mild spacing (1–3 mm), moderate spacing (4–6 mm), mild crowding (1–3), moderate crowding (4–6), narrow arches that are dental in origin (4-6 mm), as well as patients who have relapsed following conventional orthodontic treatment.[9] Such treatment decreases the time that the the patient is in fixed appliances.

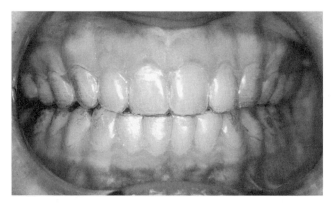

Figure 27-11. Frontal view of the maxillary and mandibular aligners of the Invisalign® System.

Align Technology reports that orthodontic movements which can be produced effectively with aligners include space closure, tooth movement following interproximal reduction (*i.e.*, stripping), dental (not skeletal/sutural) expansion, flaring, and distalization. In addition, space closure following the extraction of a lower incisor can be produced successfully. The Invisalign® System also can be used in conjunction with fixed appliances (*e.g.*, following an initial phase of treatment with fixed appliances to correct severe tooth rotations and malalignments prior to aligner fabrication).

Clinical studies are underway to evaluate the treatment of more complex orthodontic problems, including premolar extraction treatment, severe deep bite, anteroposterior corrections greater than 2 mm, and uprighting of severely tipped teeth.[5,11] At present, such treatments do not fall within the criteria for case acceptance by Align Technology, but may be acceptable in the future. Orthodontic problems not expected to become appropriate for the Invisalign® System include skeletal expansion, patients with significant temporomandibular joint pathology, severe anterior or posterior open bites, and tooth impaction/forced eruption problems.[10]

Invisalign® Components

The Invisalign® System has a number of components, some familiar to the average orthodontist and some not. The appliances used in the treatment, termed "aligners" (Figs. 27-11 and 27-12), are comparable to the invisible retainers described earlier in this chapter. The aligners are made from a thin (.030″) proprietary medical-grade plastic material that is a mixture of plastics comparable to polycarbonate. This material also is similar to the 1 mm thick splint Biocryl™ described earlier.

INVISIBLE RETAINERS AND ALIGNERS

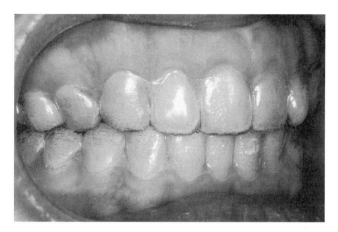

Figure 27-12. Right lateral view of maxillary and mandibular aligners. The aligners are scalloped to reflect the gingival contours.

The aligners are trimmed at the level of the gingival margin, so that both aligners are of horseshoe shape (Figs. 12-13 and 27-14). Each aligner is worn for a two-week period prior to being replaced by the next aligner in the series. Each aligner covers a patient's teeth fully and is nearly invisible when in place. Aligners typically are worn in pairs, one for each arch. Single arch treatment can be undertaken as well.

The second component of the Invisalign® System is the patented software, the technology that enables the design and manufacture of the aligners. The software includes Treat 2.x© software, which is an in-house manufacturing program that generates a simulated treatment outcome and then a series of intermediate stages of movement from the initial malocclusion to the final treatment result. All manipulations of the occlusion are

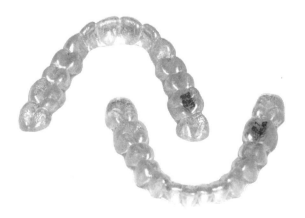

Figure 27-13. Finished contour of maxillary and mandibular aligners. A patient identifier and the series number in the sequence are incorporated into the aligners in the first molar region.

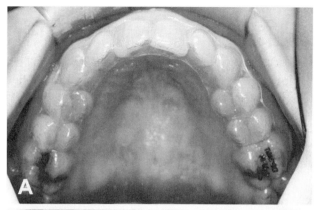

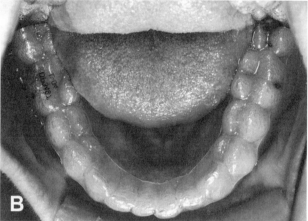

Figure 27-14. Intraoral views of the maxillary and mandibular aligners in a patient with mild crowding.

performed in accordance with the instructions of the orthodontist, as written in the treatment planning form.

The company interacts with the orthodontist by way of ClinCheck®, an Internet-based treatment planning tool that relies on 3D-graphical and manipulation techniques. ClinCheck® allows the orthodontist to view a computerized simulation of the entire course of treatment with a level of accuracy and from angles that are not possible using traditional diagnostic methods. Each patient sent into Align Technology, has a "ClinCheck®" file associated with it that is downloaded from the website (www.invisalign.com).

Sequence of Treatment

A course of treatment using the Invisalign® system involves the following steps.

After performing a clinical examination and gathering the necessary diagnostic records, the orthodontist establishes a diagnosis for the patient's malocclusion and determines whether the patient is a candidate for the Invisalign® System. If appropriate, the orthodontist obtains polyvinyl siloxane (PVS) impressions of the patient's teeth, as well as a bite registration (see below for a detailed description of the impressing-taking technique), and sends them to Align Technology. Polyvinyl siloxane is the impression material of choice because it yields highly accurate impressions that remain stable for as long as three weeks and allows for multiple pours.[9]

The orthodontist submits copies of the lateral cephalogram, the panoramic radiograph (or full-mouth radiographs), and intraoral and extraoral photography. The photographic and radiographic records can be submitted either in hard copy form or over the Internet. In addition, the orthodontist prepares an Invisalign® treatment-planning form (*i.e.* prescription) to specify the goals of treatment and to suggest the specific path of tooth movements required to achieve the desired corrections. Any limitations or compromises should be described as well. This form can be filled out by hand and mailed to the company, or it can be sent electronically via the Align Technology website.

After the company receives the impressions, bite registration, patient records, and the prescription provided by the orthodontist, two sets of dental casts are derived from the PVS impression. The first set of models (termed "scan models") is used to prepare a three-dimensional computer graphic image of the patient's teeth and associated soft tissues. The second set of models is used for validation of the orthodontist's diagnosis and treatment plan by Align Technology clinical staff. The PVS impressions then are archived for purposes of model duplication or replacement.

The technologies involved in the manufacturing of the Invisalign® System are evolving rapidly. At this writing, the scan models (which are poured in die stone rather than in laboratory plaster) are used to produce the three-dimensional computer models that later will be manipulated for simulated tooth movement and ultimately used as the basis for the production of a series of aligners.

The creation of a three-dimensional graphical image of the dental casts is a multi-step process. After the scanning model has been poured and trimmed, the upper and lower models are oriented to each other, first by means of a registration bite typically made from wax or polyvinyl siloxane (*e.g.*, Blue Mousse™), the latter being the preferred material due to its higher accuracy. PVS material has also been successful in that it is less susceptible to heat and cold changes during transport and does not break. Currently, however, most types of wax bites are acceptable for the Invisalign® process.

The patient's bite is taken and registered in centric occlusion. Patients with discrepancies between centric occlusion and centric relation should be told by the treating orthodontist that the aligners are not intended to resolve such discrepancies; other treatment may be required to address this issue.

Custom-made imaging software then is used to create a digital three-dimensional model of the arch (*i.e.*, the virtual study model) through a proprietary scanning technique. Align's Treat 2.x© software is used to prepare the graphical images for manipulation. Virtual tools in the form of planar and curved cutters that are part of the Treat 2.x® software are used to isolate each tooth within the arch. This procedure in virtual reality is similar to the initial preparation of a tooth positioner in a traditional commercial orthodontic laboratory, a process in which each tooth is removed from the stone or plaster model and prepared for reassembly in final form.

The difference with the digital image, however, is that the reassembly of the teeth in the arch creates an exact replica of the original arch without any deviation in dimensional accuracy. At this point, the trained computer technician manipulates the virtual images, much in the same way that a laboratory technician creates a positioner set-up from an original set of work models. Based on the instructions from the orthodontist, the final occlusion is established virtually by way of the proprietary software, and the "forecast" model representing the final treated occlusion is created, once again in virtual reality.

The next step in the process is to determine the number of intermediate stages (and thus the number of aligners) between the original malocclusion and the final treatment result. The two factors governing the number of treatment stages required are the path of tooth movement and the velocity at which the teeth are to be moved. The maximum velocity of tooth movement currently is 0.20-0.25 mm per tooth per stage. The particular magnitude of the movement is dependent on the nature of the tooth repositioning (*e.g.*, distalization versus simple flaring or space closure). The path of correction will depend on which teeth impede each tooth from moving to its final position. In other words, the movement of a tooth may be delayed until adjacent teeth are moved out of the way.

Obviously, the greater the distance that the teeth need to be moved or rotated and the more complicated the movement path, the greater the number of aligners needed to treat the patient. The number of aligners varies from ten or less for relatively simple problems to fifty aligners or more in complicated malocclusions. Distalization cases, midline discrepancies, and expansion cases typically require more stages than less complicated movements.

Figures 27-15 and 27-16 illustrate a representative sequence in virtual reality of malocclusion correction for a patient requiring 31 sets of aligners. In addition to the forecast model, the entire sequence of tooth movement is established. The gradual changes in tooth alignment can be observed in the six stages shown. Aligners usually are changed every two weeks; treatment for this patient should take 15-16 months to complete. Thus, in addition to the forecast model, the entire sequence of tooth movement is established before the actual treatment begins.

After the forecast model and treatment sequence have been generated, this information is sent over the Internet to the orthodontist, who reviews the forecast model and sequence by way of the ClinCheck® software program. The orthodontist can view the initial malocclusion, the intermediate stages of treatment, and the final forecast model from multiple perspectives, including some views that are not readily obtainable by conventional methods. The orthodontist then approves the treatment plan, or alternatively, may request modifications in the position of specific teeth.

Following the orthodontist's approval of the treatment plan, Align Technology uses the sequence of graphical images combined with computer-aided design and manufacturing (CAD/CAM) in producing the aligners. Specifically, stereolithography (i.e., polymerization of liquid resin with laser technology) is used to make a physical three-dimensional model for each stage out of resin. An aligner is made from each of these physical models. At present, the fabrication of the aligners is performed by hand, a process similar the fabrication of invisible retainers described earlier in this chapter. It is the intention of Align Technology to automate the fabrication process and the trimming of the aligners in the future.

In about half of treatment protocols, it is necessary to add one or more "attachments" to the teeth (Fig. 27-15). Currently, these attachments, which are simply buttons of restorative composite (e.g., Herculite™, Kerr, Orange CA) or light-cure bonding material, are used in instances of significant tooth rotation or for any absolute dental intrusion (i.e., attachments are placed on teeth adjacent to segments being intruded[5]). The attachments provide undercuts that facilitate tooth movement. In some instances, attachments may be used for the retention of the aligners in patients with short clinical crowns. In addition, this methodology has been shown to improve the movement of individual teeth by placing attachments on the teeth adjacent to an extraction site.

The attachments are formed on the teeth using a plastic template (similar to an aligner, but thinner), where each attachment well has been generated in virtual space and will follow the movement of the tooth exactly until the final stage of treatment.

Another issue of significance in many patients with minor to moderate crowding undergoing Invisalign® orthodontic appliance treatment is interproximal reduction (IPR). Because of the nature of the virtual graphical images, Align Technology recommends that as much interproximal reduction (stripping) as possible is carried out prior to time that the polyvinyl siloxane impressions are obtained. By performing reproximation prior to the impression-taking procedure, the precise amount of reduction in tooth width is established before treatment is initiated. Thus, there is no confusion regarding how much stripping actually is required. Miller[5] advises that if significant interproximal reduction is performed before the PVS impressions, the patient should be given an aligner or invisible retainer to wear at night until the treatment begins.

If interproximal reduction is part of the patient's treatment plan, we recommend that as much stripping as possible is carried out following the the completion of initial diagnostic record taking, preferably during the same appointment. Often agressive IPR leads to localized gingival bleeding which may compromise the PVS impressions if they are obtained during the same appointment. Thus, stripping ideally should be performed at an appointment separate from the PVS impression appointment.

Reducing the mesiodistal width of the teeth prior to the impression, however, sometimes is not possible without severely compromising the anatomy of certain teeth. In such instances, interproximal reduction may be performed during the course of treatment, instead of before treatment. A reproximation form is sent by Align Technology in these situations, indicating the amount of interproximal reduction required and the stages at which the teeth should be stripped. Significant stripping performed during treatment can result in the necessity of retaking the PVS impressions and remaking the aligners not yet used, obviously incurring added expense and extending the length of treatment. Also, unwanted side effects, such as tooth intrusion can occur when the clinician does not perform interproximal reduction as advised.[5]

Impression Technique

Perhaps the biggest paradigm shift concerning the patient management aspect of the Invisalign® System is the impression-taking technique. Alginate impressions

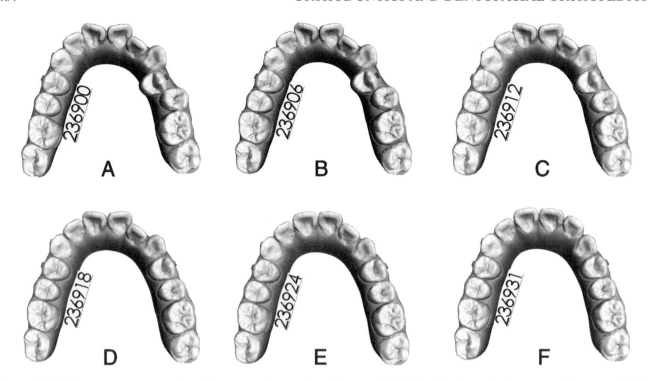

Figure 27-15. Treatment sequence of maxillary correction produced by way of the Treat 2 software. The sequence begans at *A*, the initial malocclusion and progresses to *F*, the forecast result. This treatment sequence has 31 stages. The first four numbers next to each image is the patient identification number, The last two numbers indicate the stage of treatment. Attachments can be seen on the facial surfaces of the canines and first premolars. (Images courtesy of Ross J. Miller)

that traditionally have been used by the profession have proven to be inadequate for this procedure. At the time of this writing, Align Technology recommends the use of polyvinyl siloxane (ESPE America, Norristown PA) for generating the model used during the scanning procedure. Polyvinyl siloxane takes far longer to set than does alginate, and the patient should be informed ahead of time about the length of the impression-taking procedure. We also recommend that the patient be draped (*e.g.*, protective drape from a hair salon) in order to protect the clothing of the patient from damage.

The recommended protocol is a two-step technique. The first step involves making the equivalent of a loose-fitting custom tray from a heavy body impression material. The second step is the actual impression itself, made from a light body material that produces a highly accurate negative reproduction of the hard and soft tissue anatomy of the dental arch.

A perforated rim lock metal tray is selected that approximates the size of the patient's dental arch. The tray must be long enough to capture all the teeth in the arch, including second molars and any erupted third molars. In addition, a three-inch square section of Saran Wrap™ plastic film also is cut and set aside for future use.

Prior to beginning the impression procedure, it also is very important to block out the undercuts of any bridge pontics with wax. Removing PVS trays can be difficult, due to the amount of suction generated. Old crowns with underlying decay and temporary crowns can be pulled off with this material. In order to avoid these problems, the clinician should make sure that any questionable restorations are fixed prior to taking the impressions.

Once the impression material is mixed, the clinician has about two minutes of working time. The tray should be loaded with ESPE Dimension® Penta H tray material, keeping the tip of the dispenser immersed in the material to avoid introducing air bubbles. At the same time, the dental assistant should make sure that the patient's mouth remains isolated and dry.

After the heavy body material has been inserted into the tray, the three-inch square of Saran Wrap™ is placed over the tray and gently smoothed across the impression material. Keeping the Saran Wrap™ in place, the impression is seated fully in the patient's mouth, starting with the posterior region. The tray should be moved slightly from front to back and side to side as the tray is seated to place. Fully seating the heavy body material is crucial, because it is this material that provides the hydraulic pressure necessary to capture the anatomical detail with the light body material. The tray should

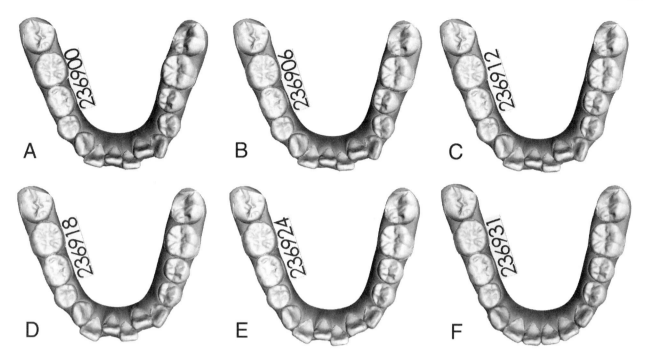

Figure 27-16. Treatment sequence of mandibular correction of the same patient shown in Figure 27-15. The sequence begins at *A*, the initial malocclusion and progresses to *F*, the forecast result. This treatment sequence has 31 stages. The first four numbers next to each image is the patient identification number, The last two numbers indicate the stage of treatment. (Images courtesy of Ross J. Miller.)

not be removed from the mouth until the 3½ minute setting time has elapsed, even though the material may appear to have set.

An alternative approach to this technique (which we recommend) is to use the patient's study models for the first step of the procedure. The purpose of the first impression is to create a tray that fits closely to the patient's dental arch; the study model can serve adequately in this regard. The obvious advantage is that the first impression can be obtained without the patient being present, thus saving chair time, and it is easier for the patient.

As the study model is seated into the Saran Wrap™ lined heavy body material, the midline of the study model should be centered in the tray. The model should be seated fully and then moved front to back and side to side. The impression material should be pushed against the study model, as there are no cheeks or lips to do so.

After the impression material has hardened, the study model is removed carefully from the impression tray, guarding against fracturing any of the teeth on the cast. Any excess impression material, especially in the posterior region must be trimmed and removed; otherwise, the tray will not seat in the patient's mouth. The tray always should be placed in the patient's mouth for a preliminary try-in to check for comfort and for the ability to seat the tray fully, before attempting to take the impression with the light body material. If necessary, the heavy body material can be added to the tray to extend it distally.[5]

The next step in the impression-taking technique involves placing the light-body impression material inside the impression tray containing the heavy body material. The tip of a disposable impression syringe should be cut with scissors to the appropriate size of the opening. A disposable impression syringe should be back-filled with ESPE Dimension™ Garant L light-bodied material, with one-half of a cartridge used per arch. The timer is set for 5½ minutes, with two minutes of working time available. The Saran Wrap™ is removed, and any excess impression material is trimmed from the tray with a sharp instrument. The light-body impression material is loaded on top of the hardened heavy-bodied PVS with the impression gun. Additional light-bodied material is placed in the tray distal to the last molars, as it is difficult to do so in the mouth. Again, it is important not to introduce air bubbles into the material during the loading process.

After the patient's mouth has been suctioned and air-dried thoroughly and before the tray is inserted, the disposable impression syringe should be used to place additional light-bodied material around the gingival margin as well as on the buccal, lingual and occlusal sur-

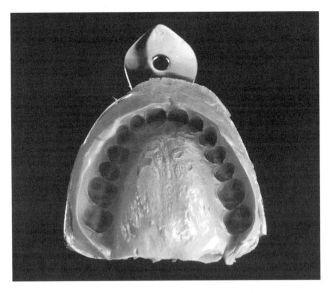

Figure 27-17. Impression made from polyvinyl siloxane. Virtually all of the visible impression is magenta in color, indicating that the light body impression material contacted the teeth and adjacent soft tissue. (Photo courtesy of Ross J. Miller.)

faces of the teeth. In addition, it is very important to place additional impression material by way of the syringe into undercuts of overlapping teeth in patients with moderate to severe crowding.[5]

The syringe tip should be kept in light contact with the teeth. The impression tray then should be reseated in the patient's mouth with light pressure, starting posteriorly and moving forward.

When the timer sounds, the impression tray is removed from the patient's mouth. To aid in tray removal, the clinician should grasp the tray with one hand, and place one finger of the other hand in the patient's vestibule. Having the patient open his or her mouth while rolling the finger in the vestibule will break the seal and facilitate tray removal. The tray is "popped" out of the mouth as the patient opens.

The quality of the impressions then should be evaluated. An accurate impression should show all the gingival margins and the anatomical occlusal surfaces, all in the magenta-colored light-bodied material (Fig. 27-17).

Aside from determining the proper diagnosis and treatment plan, perhaps the most critical step in the fabrication of aligners from the perspective of the orthodontist is obtaining accurate PVS impressions. Attention to detail is extremely important.

CONCLUDING REMARKS

Traditional invisible retainers have had a high level of patient acceptance because they are inconspicuous. The invisible retainer is simple to construct, easy to deliver, and inexpensive. In addition, when the invisible retainer is used as a finishing appliance, minor changes in tooth position also can be obtained. These appliances are not as durable as wire-acrylic retainers, but they provide control over tooth position when worn over the long term.

Combining invisible retainer wear with 3-D technology, as has been developed in the Invisalign® System, provides new opportunities to treat adult patients who otherwise would not consider conventional orthodontic treatment. It must be remembered, however, that the Invisalign® technology is new and evolving constantly. Based on our 30 years of experience routinely using invisible retainers, it is not a question of whether invisible retainers or aligners will move teeth (they will), but rather for which cases this technology is appropriate. It is very important to continue to expand clinical understanding of those cases appropriate for Invisalign® treatment through ongoing clinical studies in university and private practice settings.

REFERENCES CITED

1. Nahoum HI. The vacuum formed dental contour appliance. New York State Dent J 1964;9:385–390.
2. Ponitz RJ. Invisible retainers. Am J Orthod 1971;59:266–272.
3. McNamara JA, Jr, Kramer KL, Juenker JP. Invisible retainers. J Clin Orthod 1985;19:570–578.
4. Abolfathi A. Personal communication, 2000.
5. Miller RJ. Personal communication, 2000.
6. Kesling HD. The philosophy of the tooth positioning appliance. Am J Orthod 1945;31:297–304.
7. Sheridan JJ, LeDoux W, McMinn R. Essix retainers: fabrication and supervision for permanent retention. J Clin Orthod 1993;27:37–45.
8. Rinchuse DJ, Rinchuse DJ. Active tooth movement with Essix-based appliances. J Clin Orthod 997;31:109–112.
9. Boyd RL, Miller RJ, Vlaskalic V. The Invisalign System in adult orthodontics: Mild crowding and space closure cases. J Clin Orthod 2000;34:203–212.
10. Align Technology. Orthodontist workbook: Embark on a whole new movement in adult orthodontics. Santa Clara: Align Technology, 2000.
11. Boyd RL. Personal communication, 2000.

Chapter 28
CEPHALOMETRIC EVALUATION

In studying a case of malocclusion, give no thought to the methods of treatment or appliances until the case shall have been classified and all peculiarities and variations from the normal in type, occlusion, and facial lines have been thoroughly comprehended. Then the requirements and proper plan of treatment become apparent.

Edward H. Angle

This chapter describes a method of cephalometric evaluation that has been used by us in the diagnosis and treatment planning of patients undergoing orthodontic, orthopedic and orthognathic surgical treatments. Originally developed nearly 25 years ago, this cephalometric analysis has been used to describe the components of various types of malocclusions,[1-8] as well as studies of untreated adults with ideal facial and occlusal relationships.[9,10] In addition, this cephalometric approach can be incorporated into the analysis of treatment effects produced by various orthodontic and orthopedic appliance systems.[11-16] Studies of the effects of various pharyngeal soft-tissue surgical procedures, using this cephalometric analysis, also have been reported.[17,18]

DEVELOPMENT OF THE ANALYSIS

Since Broadbent's introduction of radiographic cephalometrics in 1931, a number of different lateral headfilm analyses have been devised. Those of Downs,[19-21] Steiner,[22-24] Tweed,[25,26] and Ricketts,[27-29] as well as the so-called "Wits" appraisal, originally developed by Jenkins[30] and later described by Johnston[31] and Jacobson,[32,33] probably have gained the widest acceptance. Other analyses such as those of Wylie,[34] Coben,[35] Sassouni,[36,37] Jarabak,[38] Bimler,[39] and Enlow and coworkers[40] perhaps are used less widely, but they are, nevertheless, well known.

The purpose of this chapter is to describe and update a method of cephalometric analysis that has evolved gradually during the last two and a half decades, while being used in the evaluation and treatment planning of orthodontic, orthopedic, and orthognathic surgery patients. This cephalometric analysis is but one of many diagnostic tools used to determine the type and focus of therapy for an individual patient.

The reader may question the necessity of presenting yet another cephalometric analysis. Cephalometrics must be put into the context of the wide variety of treatments now available in the 21st century. Most of the analyses mentioned earlier were conceived during the period from 1940 to 1970, when significant alterations in craniofacial structural relationships were thought impossible. Especially during the last three decades, however, clinical orthodontics has seen the advent of numerous orthognathic surgical procedures that allow three-dimensional repositioning of almost every bony structure in the facial region. Similarly, facial orthopedic therapies (*e.g.,* functional jaw orthopedics, facial mask treatment) have become part of everyday clinical practice. Both surgical and orthopedic procedures offer numerous possibilities in the treatment of skeletal discrepancies.

Therefore, we perceived a need for a method of cephalometric analysis that is sensitive not only to the position of the teeth within a given bone, but also to the relationship of the maxilla, mandible, and cranial base structures, one to another. In short, the method of analysis described in this chapter is an effort to relate teeth to teeth, teeth to jaws, each jaw to the other, and the jaws to the cranial base. This method of cephalometric analysis was published originally in 1984 in the *American Journal of Orthodontics.*[41] This revised chapter updates and supplements that article.

Cephalometrics is not an exact science. Even though headfilms can be measured with precision, the measurement error can vary greatly with any given landmark, as illustrated by the work of Baumrind and Frantz.[42] Thus, the method of analysis described in this chapter is presented more as a *language*. The clinician can use this language to communicate to other clinicians and, perhaps more importantly, to herself or himself the identification and description of a set of structural relationships that are critical to the diagnosis and treatment planning of a given patient. In addition, the basic principles of this analysis are communicated easily to laypersons (*e.g.*, patients, parents) and to other dental professionals who do not have a detailed knowledge of cephalometrics. One does not have to have an in-depth experience with cephalometric measurement to understand the general relationships being discussed here.

This analysis is derived in part from the principles of the cephalometric analyses of Ricketts[27-29] and of Harvold.[43,44] Other aspects of this analysis, such as the construction of the nasion perpendicular and the Point A vertical, are presumed to be original.

BASIS OF ANALYSIS

This method of cephalometric analysis is conventional in that it consists of a predetermined set of measurements applied to each cephalometric tracing. This approach is useful in the diagnosis and treatment planning of the individual patient, when the values derived from the tracing of the patient's initial headfilm are compared to established norms. Therefore, composite normative standards based on three cephalometric samples are presented in this chapter. These values have been tested empirically and redefined over the last 25 years and have been found useful in determining treatment protocols. An analysis of treated patients indicates that these protocols appear to have been appropriate.

The first sample provides normative data derived from lateral cephalograms of the children comprising the Bolton Standards,[45] subjects who were followed longitudinally from 4 to 18 years of age. These records were retraced and digitized by Behrents and McNamara[48] to include all the landmarks necessary for the present analysis.

The second normal data set (the Burlington Sample) is derived from a group of untreated children from the Burlington Orthodontic Research Centre who were followed longitudinally from 6 to 20 years of age.

The third group considered is an Ann Arbor sample of nearly 200 young adults who, in the opinion of the senior author and his co-workers,[9] have excellent facial configurations. As can be seen in Figure 28-1, there is a much wider variation in soft tissue profile than in the underlying skeletal relationships. These subjects had what was judged to be good skeletal balance with an orthognathic facial profile and would gain either minimal or no benefit from orthodontic treatment.

In addition to establishing an initial diagnosis of a patient, lateral headfilms can be used serially to monitor normal growth and to determine the effects of treatment. In this regard, we have found that the four-point superimposition developed by Ricketts[27,28] is useful. This protocol involves the systematic use of regional superimpositions, including mandibular, maxillary, and cranial base regions. Bony remodeling and translation as well as differential tooth movement can be evaluated using this technique. A detailed description of the analysis of serial films will be provided later in this chapter.

ANALYSIS OF A SINGLE FILM

The analysis of a single lateral cephalogram is presented in this section. An attempt will be made to differentiate between the skeletal and the dentoalveolar components of a malocclusion. For example, a well-balanced skeletal and dental relationship is represented diagrammatically in Figure 28-2. A Class II relationship characterized by maxillary skeletal prognathism is represented in Figure 28-3*A*. This latter type of occlusion can be treated effectively by extraoral traction in a young patient or by a Le Fort I osteotomy or, in certain instances, by an anterior maxillary ostectomy in an adult patient. Of course, some clinicians might choose to camouflage this skeletal discrepancy by extracting two maxillary premolars.

A similar dental condition, that is, an anterior position of the upper dentition, is represented diagrammatically in Figure 28-3*B* In this example, however, the incisor relationship is a reflection of dentoalveolar protrusion rather than maxillary skeletal protrusion. This type of malocclusion can be treated most easily by dental extraction. In certain instances, both skeletal and dental protrusion can contribute to the overall condition. Thus, it is extremely important to differentiate skeletal abnormalities from dentoalveolar abnormalities.

Relating the Maxilla to the Cranial Base

In the analysis to be presented in this section, the position of the maxilla relative to the cranial base is evalu-

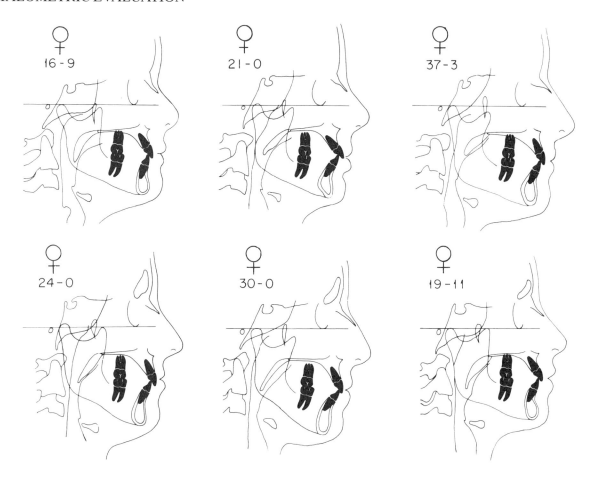

Figure 28-1. Six representative faces from the Ann Arbor sample of patients with well-balanced faces and good occlusions. There is greater variation in the soft tissue profile than in the underlying skeletal and dentoalveolar structures.

ated in two ways: The skeletal relationship of Point A to the nasion perpendicular and, more importantly, the patient's soft tissue profile as viewed clinically.

Soft Tissue Evaluation

The position of the maxilla can be evaluated best at the time of the clinical examination, but it also can be evaluated while analyzing the lateral cephalogram. In particular, the nasolabial angle and the cant of the upper lip should be examined both clinically and cephalometrically.

The nasolabial angle is formed by the intersection of a line tangent to the base of the nose with a line tangent to the upper lip (Fig. 28-4). Scheideman and co-workers[46] reported that the nasolabial angle was approximately 110° in their sample of so-called "dentofacial normals." In our Ann Arbor adult sample of individuals with a well-balanced soft tissue profile and of European ancestry, the average nasolabial angle was 102°±8° for both males and females.[10] An acute nasolabial angle may be a reflection of dentoalveolar protrusion, but it also can be a reflection of the orientation of the base of the nose.

The upper lip should be evaluated relative to the vertical orientation of the face. The upper lip should form about a 14° (13.7°±8.2° in the Ann Arbor sample) angle with the nasion perpendicular (Fig. 28-5A). In the companion sample of males (Fig. 28-5B), the upper lip was slightly less protrusive (8.4°±7.8°).[10] Regardless of whether the nasolabial angle or the cant of the upper lip is used for evaluation, the upper lip should have a slight forward cant. A vertical or retruded upper-lip orientation is a contraindication for any mechanics that would distalize the maxilla or the maxillary dentition.

It should be noted that the values for both the nasolabial angle and the cant of the upper lip vary greatly among various racial and ethnic groups. For example, Miyajima and co-workers[47] compared the European-American subjects from the previously mentioned Ann

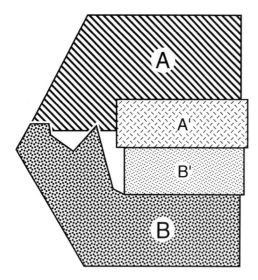

Figure 28-2. Idealized skeletal and dental components of the face. *A*, Maxillary skeletal position. *A'*, Maxillary dentoalveolar position. *B'*, Mandibular dentoalveolar position. *B*, Mandibular skeletal position.

Arbor sample with a group of untreated Japanese individuals, who were judged by a panel of Japanese orthodontists to have ideal occlusions and well-balanced faces. On average, the subjects in the Japanese sample were more protrusive dentally, with a more acute nasolabial angle and a greater tendency toward bilabial protrusion. These differences, evident even in groups of individuals with so-called "well-balanced faces," indicate that fundamental variations exist in the craniofacial morphology of Japanese and European Americans. The results of Miyajima and co-workers[47] support the premise that a single standard of facial esthetics is not appropriate for application to diverse racial and ethnic groups. In fact, European Americans in general have a straighter facial profile than do Asian Americans and African Americans, indicating the necessity of using standards that are racially and ethnically specific for the population group being studied.

Hard Tissue Evaluation

The anteroposterior orientation of the maxilla is determined first by constructing the nasion perpendicular.[41] This construction begins by defining the Frankfort horizontal (FH) plane or line (Fig. 28-6), using anatomical porion (the superior aspect of the *external* auditory meatus; Fig. 28-7) and orbitale (the inferior border of the orbit of the eye) as reference points. As Ricketts[27] has advocated for many years, anatomical porion, not machine porion, should be used to determine the Frankfort horizontal. Machine porion, the top of the ear rods of the cephalometric headholder, can be located as much as a centimeter away from the actual position of anatomical porion and can vary greatly between serial films. A similar radiolucency, the *internal auditory meatus*, is located posterior and superior to the external auditory meatus and must not be confused with the external auditory meatus. After porion and orbitale have been identified, the Frankfort horizontal is drawn, and a perpendicular line (the nasion perpendicular) is erected through nasion inferiorly (Fig. 28-6).

The first measurement to be made is the linear distance from Point A, the most posterior point on the anterior contour of the maxilla adjacent to the root apices of the maxillary incisors, to the nasion perpendicular.

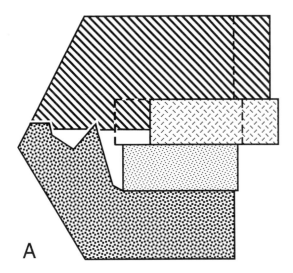 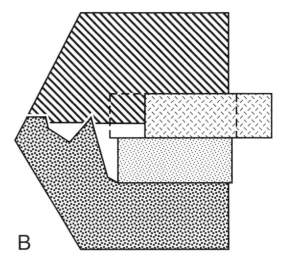

Figure 28-3. Skeletal and dentoalveolar components of the face. *A*, Maxillary skeletal protrusion. *B*, Maxillary dentoalveolar protrusion. Note that the teeth are in the same positions in both conditions although the position of the maxilla varies.

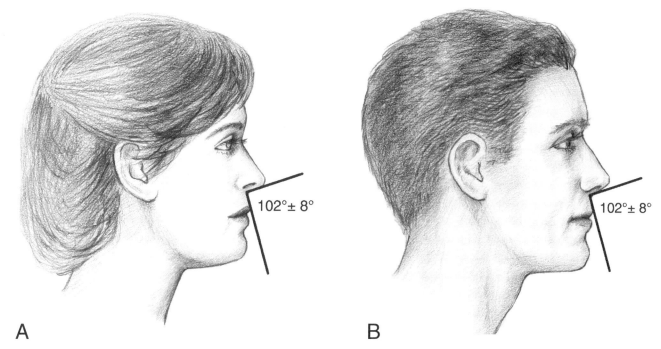

Figure 28-4. Nasolabial angle. This angle is constructed by drawing lines tangent to the base of the nose and to the contour of the upper lip. In the Ann Arbor Sample, this angle was 102°±8° in males and females. *A*, Female. *B*, Male.

An anterior position of Point A is a positive value, and a posterior position of Point A is a negative value. In the Ann Arbor sample of adults with well-balanced faces, Point A is in front of the nasion perpendicular by 0.4 mm in females and 1.1 mm in males (Table 28-1). Our composite norm for adults of both genders is Point A one mm anterior to the nasion perpendicular (Table 28-2).

Data derived from the subjects comprising the Bolton Standards[48] indicate that the SNA angle increases minimally with age (approximately 1° from ages six to eighteen). Because a 1° change in SNA is equiva-

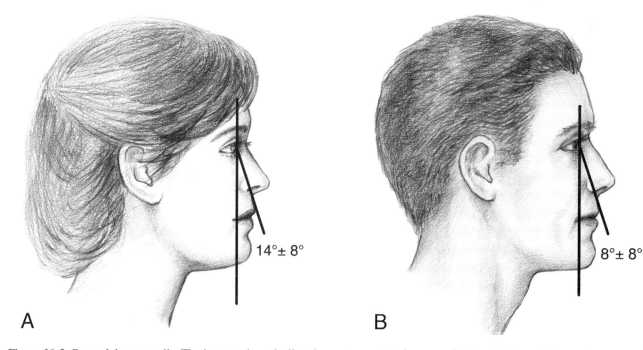

Figure 28-5. Cant of the upper lip. The intersection of a line drawn tangent to the upper lip should intersect the nasion perpendicular at about 14°±8° in adult females and 8°±8° in adult males with well-balanced faces. *A*, Female. *B*, Male.

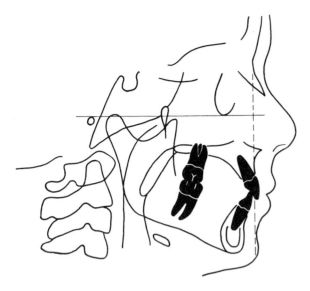

Figure 28-6. Construction of the Frankfort horizontal plane using anatomical porion and orbitale. The nasion perpendicular (dashed line) is constructed by dropping a line vertically inferior to nasion and perpendicular to the Frankfort horizontal.

lent to a 1 mm linear change in the position of Point A relative to nasion, one can extrapolate the position of Point A relative to the nasion perpendicular during the mixed dentition. Thus, a composite norm for the relationship of Point A to the nasion perpendicular is 0 mm in the mixed dentition individual (Fig. 28-8A), and 1 mm in the adult male and female (Fig. 28-8B).

Usually, separate evaluations of the hard and soft tissues lead to the same diagnostic conclusions. A patient with maxillary prognathism or maxillary dentoalveolar

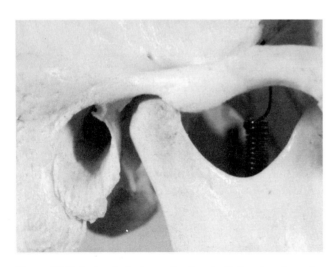

Figure 28-7. Lateral photograph of a skull showing the relationship of the mandibular condyle to the external auditory meatus (articular disk is absent). Note that the superior aspect of the external auditory meatus (porion) lies just inferior to the superior aspect of the mandibular condyle.

Table 28-1. Cephalometric Values of 111 untreated adults with well-balanced faces and good occlusions (Ann Arbor sample, 1984)

	Female (N=73)		Male (N=38)	
	Mean	SD	Mean	SD
Maxilla to Cranial Base				
Nasion Perp. to Point A (mm)	0.4	2.3	1.1	2.7
SNA Angle	82.4	3.0	83.9	3.2
Mandible to Maxilla				
Effective Mandibular length (mm) (Condylion to Gnathion)	120.2	5.3	132.3	6.8
Effective Maxillary length (mm) (Condylion to Point A)	91.0	4.3	99.8	6.0
Maxillomandibular Differential (mm)	29.2	3.3	32.5	4.0
Lower Anterior Facial Height (mm) (ANS to Menton)	66.7	4.1	74.6	5.0
Mandibular Plane Angle	22.7	4.3	21.3	3.9
Facial Axis Angle	0.2	3.2	0.5	3.5
Mandible to Cranial Base				
Pogonion to Nasion Perp. (mm)	−1.8	4.5	−0.3	3.8
Dentition				
Upper Incisor to Point A Vert. (mm)	5.4	1.7	5.3	2.0
Lower Incisor to A-Po line (mm)	2.7	1.7	2.3	2.1
Airway				
Upper Pharynx (mm)	17.4	3.4	17.4	4.3
Lower Pharynx (mm)	11.3	3.3	13.5	4.3

Table 28-2. Composite Norms

	Mixed Dentition	Change per year	Adult
Maxillary Skeletal			
Nasion Perp. to Point A (mm)	0	0.1	1
Maxillary Dental			
Upper incisor to Point A Vert. (mm)	4–6	no change	4–6
Mandibular Dental			
Mandibular incisor to A-Po) line (mm	1–3	no change	1–3
Mandibular Skeletal			
Pogonion to Naison Perp. (mm)	−8 to −6	0.5	−2 to +4
Vertical Measures			
Mandibular Plane Angle	25°	−1° every 3–4 years	22°
Facial Axis Angle	0° (90°)	no change	0° (90°)

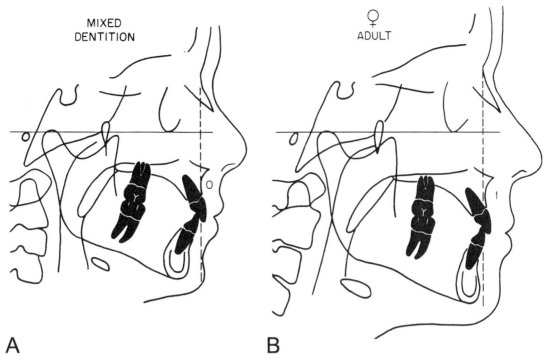

Figure 28-8. Relationship of the nasion perpendicular to the maxilla at Point A. *A*, Ideal mixed dentition. *B*, Ideal adult female (from McNamara[55]).

protrusion routinely displays a relatively acute nasolabial angle, whereas a patient with maxillary retrusion often displays an obtuse angle.

A discrepancy sometimes exists, however, between the clinical and cephalometric observations. For example, this discrepancy could be due to an excessive thinness or thickness of the overlying soft tissues. In these patients, it is advisable to use the soft tissue profile as the *primary* guide. Whenever a discrepancy exists between findings derived during a clinical examination and findings from a cephalometric evaluation regarding maxillary position, *the findings from the clinical examination should take precedence.* Treating a patient only to specific cephalometric norms must be avoided.

In this chapter, a number of clinical examples of maxillary skeletal position are presented to illustrate variations from normal. Figure 28-9 is a tracing of a patient with the clinical appearance of maxillary prognathism and a relatively acute nasolabial angle. In addition, the upper lip is proclined relative to the nasion perpendicular, and the maxilla at Point A lies 5 mm ahead of the nasion perpendicular. The patient also has an anterior open bite and a prolonged history of thumb sucking.

In the patient example shown in Figure 28-10, the values derived imply a retrusive maxilla and mandible. This type of patient often is characterized clinically as having a steep mandibular plane angle, a convex facial profile, an obtuse nasolabial angle, and a dorsal hump or con-

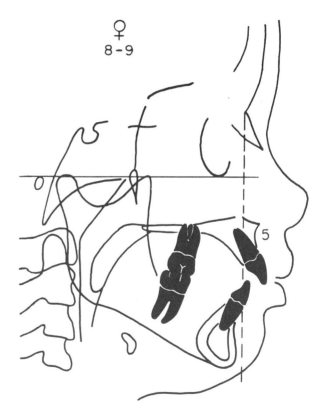

Figure 28-9. Maxillary skeletal protrusion, as indicated by the 5 mm distance from Point A to the nasion perpendicular (from McNamara[55]). This 8-year-old girl had a history of persistent thumb sucking, which may have contributed to the maxillary skeletal protrusion.

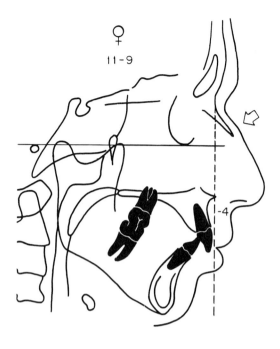

Figure 28-10. Maxillary skeletal retrusion. The arrow indicates a bump (dorsal hump) on the external contour of the nose. This patient has a steep mandibular plane angle and mandibular skeletal retrusion as well. The nasolabial angle is within normal limits (from McNamara[55]).

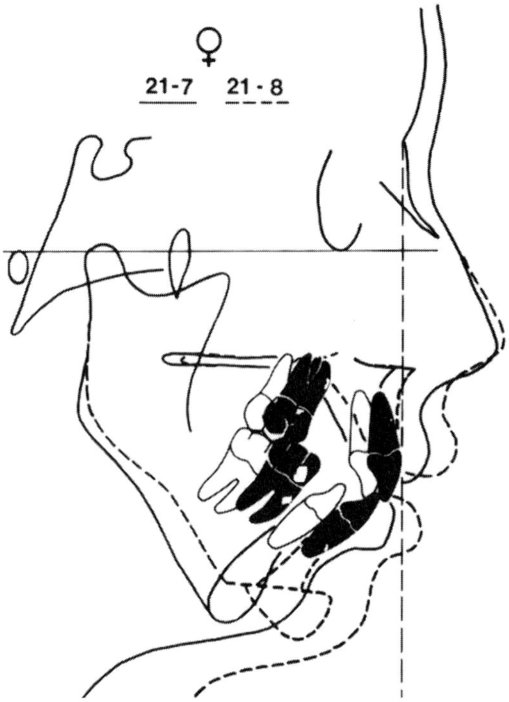

Figure 28-11. Change in nasal shape after orthognathic surgery. This severely retrognathic patient underwent maxillary and mandibular advancement with augmentation genioplasty. The nasal contour became straighter following surgery as the maxilla was advanced.

vex superior nasal ridge (see arrow). Clinically, the appearance of the patient's large nose is exaggerated by the retrusive position of both the upper and lower jaws. In spite of the retrusive position of the maxilla, however, the nasolabial angle of this individual is within normal limits.

Figure 28-11 depicts the pre- and post-surgical cephalometric tracings of a 21-year-old female who presented with a retrusive maxilla, severe mandibular skeletal retrusion, and a very receding chin point. A two-jaw surgical procedure combined with a genioplasty was used to advance the maxilla and mandible. Pogonion was repositioned 19 mm anteriorly; note the change not only in the maxilla but in the dorsal hump region as well. As the maxilla was advanced, the nasal tip moved forward.

A retrusive maxilla occurs more frequently than usually is recognized in Class II malocclusions. In a study of 277 untreated juvenile Class II subjects, McNamara[1] noted that individuals with maxillary retrusion outnumbered those with maxillary protrusion. This observation held true regardless of whether the SNA angle or the relationship of Point A to the nasion perpendicular was used to evaluate maxillary position.

The 13 year-old male shown in Figure 28-12 also has a retrusive maxilla, as well as a Class III molar relationship and an obtuse nasolabial angle. In addition, the upper lip is retroclined relative to nasion perpendicular. In this patient, the length of the mandible should be estimated following a "theoretical" correction of the position of Point A relative to the nasion perpendicular, as will be described later in this chapter.

The nasion perpendicular is not always a reliable line of orientation for determining the position of the maxilla. One such exception is the Class III patient in whom there is a short anterior cranial base (see Fig. 28-29 later in the text). In that instance, the posterior position of nasion, which can be evaluated clinically by examining the soft tissue profile, results in the construction of a misleading nasion perpendicular, thereby giving the appearance that the maxilla and mandible are positioned more anteriorly than normal.

Another problem using Point A can arise when there is lingual tipping of the crown of the maxillary incisor, as in Class II, division 2 malocclusions. In this instance, the position of Point A will be displaced labially by the anterior tipping of the root. If so, a 1–2 mm "theoretical" adjustment also can be made to reflect more accurately the position of the maxilla relative to the nasion perpendicular.

CEPHALOMETRIC EVALUATION

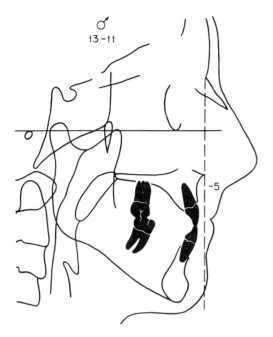

Figure 28-12. Class III patient with a retruded maxilla and an obtuse nasolabial angle (from McNamara[55])

In summary, no single cephalometric measure, such as SNA or Point A to nasion perpendicular, should be the sole determinant of treatment decisions regarding the position of the maxilla. The nasolabial angle, the angle of the upper lip relative to the nasion perpendicular, and the overall soft tissue profile are the most significant determinants of maxillary skeletal position.

Relating the Mandible to the Midface

Midfacial and Mandibular Lengths

The next step in the analysis characterizes the relationship of the mandible to the midface. The determination of midfacial and mandibular lengths can be accomplished using a modification of a method developed by Harvold.[43,44] First, the *effective length*, not the actual anatomical length of the midface, is determined by measuring the distance from condylion (the most posterosuperior point on the outline of the mandibular condyle; Fig. 28-13) to Point A. Then, the *effective length* of the mandible is determined by measuring the distance from condylion to anatomical gnathion (the most anteroinferior aspect of the mandibular symphysis). A linear relationship exists between the effective length of the midface and that of the mandible. Any given effective midfacial length corresponds to an effective mandibular length within a given range.

The reader may have concerns about using condylion as a point of reference, as this landmark often is difficult to find. Two replies must be made to this concern. First, every effort should be made (*e.g.,* soft tissue shield, intensifying screen) to improve the quality of the radiographs routinely taken by the clinician. Any metallic registration rings present on the ear rods must be removed as well. Second, condylion is used as a common landmark in the measurement of the lengths of both the midface and mandible. A slight error in the

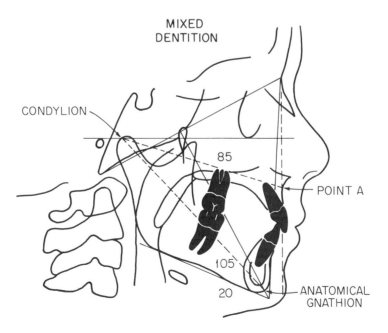

Figure 28-13. Effective midfacial and mandibular lengths. Effective midfacial length is constructed from Point A to condylion. Effective mandibular length is constructed from anatomical gnathion (on the contour of the symphysis) to condylion (from McNamara[55]).

Table 28-3. Skeletal values derived from the Bolton Standards (N=16) for each sex at each age. Standardized 8% enlargement. (mm)

	6 years		9 years		12 years		14 years		16 years		18 years	
	X̄	SD	X̄	SD	X̄	SD	X̄	SD	X̄	SD	X̄	SD
Female												
Mandibular Length (Co-Gn)	97.7	3.4	106.1	3.4	113.1	3.6	118.9	5.0	120.0	3.4	121.6	4.5
Maxillary Length (Co-Point A)	79.8	2.2	85.0	2.3	89.6	2.4	92.1	2.7	92.7	2.3	93.6	3.2
Maxillomandibular Differential	17.9	8.1	21.1	2.7	23.5	3.0	26.8	4.1	27.3	3.0	28.0	3.2
Lower Anterior Facial Height	57.9	3.7	60.0	2.9	62.6	4.5	65.6	4.9	66.1	4.3	67.2	4.7
Male												
Mandibular Length (Co-Gn)	99.3	3.6	107.7	3.8	114.4	4.3	120.6	4.3	126.8	4.7	131.0	4.6
Maxillary Length (Co-Point A)	81.7	3.4	87.7	4.1	92.1	4.1	95.2	3.2	98.9	4.4	100.9	3.9
Maxillomandibular Differential	17.5	2.2	20.0	2.6	22.3	3.1	25.4	3.5	27.9	3.3	30.1	3.9
Lower Anterior Facial Height	58.4	3.1	61.1	3.6	64.3	3.6	66.8	3.9	69.7	4.3	71.6	4.9

estimation of condylion will not affect the linear relationship between the sizes of the upper and lower jaws dramatically.

The relationship between the effective length of the midface and that of the mandible can be observed in the longitudinal studies of the Bolton Standards (Table 28-3) and of the Burlington Orthodontic Research Centre (Table 28-4). Composite norms (Table 28-5) have been extrapolated from the values derived from the Burlington and Bolton samples, as well as from the Ann Arbor Sample (Table 28-1). These norms represent the relationship between the effective midfacial length and the effective mandibular length and *are not directly related to the age or sex of the individual*. The impor-

Table 28-4. Values derived from the Burlington Orthodontic Research Centre. Standardized 8% enlargement (mm)

	6 years		9 years		12 years		14 years		16 years		18 years		20 years	
	X̄	SD	X̄	SD	X̄	SD	X̄	SD	X̄	SD	X̄	SD	X̄	SD
Female														
Mandibular length (Co-Gn)	94.1	3.3	103.3	5.3	110.2	6.4	114.9	7.1	117.7	4.5	118.9	4.7	116.8	7.3
Midfacial length (Co-Point A)	78.6	3.1	88.3	4.0	87.3	4.6	89.2	5.2	90.9	4.1	91.1	3.1	90.7	5.2
Maxillomandibular Differential	15.5	—	15.0	—	22.9	—	25.7	—	26.8	—	27.8	—	26.1	—
Lower Anterior Facial Height	57.2	3.4	61.2	3.9	63.4	4.7	66.2	5.1	66.6	4.7	68.5	4.7	66.7	5.7
Male														
Mandibular length (Co-Gn)	96.6	3.83	105.0	4.15	113.0	5.11	119.2	5.7	124.5	5.97	127.2	6.0	128.2	4.2
Midfacial length (Co-Point A)	80.5	2.4	84.9	2.5	90.3	3.6	93.9	4.6	96.6	4.4	96.6	4.7	98.8	4.3
Maxillomandibular Differential	16.1	—	20.1	—	22.7	—	25.3	—	27.9	—	30.6	—	29.4	—
Lower Anterior Facial Height	59.9	2.7	63.0	3.0	65.7	2.5	68.8	4.0	73.1	4.4	73.1	4.4	72.0	3.0

Table 28-5. Composite norms.

Midfacial Length (mm) (Co—Point A)	Mandibular Length (mm) (Co—Gn)	Lower Anterior Facial Height (mm) (ANS—Me)
80	97–100	57–58
81	99–102	57–58
82	101–104	58–59
83	103–106	58–59
84	104–107	59–60
85	105–108	60–62
86	107–110	60–62
87	109–112	61–63
88	111–114	61–63
89	112–115	62–64
90	113–116	63–64
91	115–118	63–64
92	117–120	64–65
93	119–122	65–66
94	120–124	66–67
95	122–125	67–69
96	124–127	67–69
97	126–129	68–70
98	128–131	68–70
99	129–132	69–71
100	130–133	70–74
101	132–135	71–75
102	134–137	72–76
103	136–139	73–77
104	137–140	74–78
105	138–141	75–79

tance of having the reader understand that last statement cannot be overemphasized.

The effective midfacial length is measured first. Once the position of Point A has been determined, the length of the midface of that patient is used to determine the expected mandibular length, regardless of the age or sex of the patient. In other words, the length of the mandible is not estimated from age and gender related norms, as has been advocated by Harvold.[43] Rather, the "ideal" length of the mandible is determined based on the length of the midface of the given patient, as is described below.

Once the effective length of the midface is measured, the range of comparable mandibular lengths can be determined. For example, if a mixed dentition subject with a balanced face has a midfacial length of 85 mm (Fig. 28-13), the range of normal values for the mandible is 105–108 mm (Table 28-5). If the effective midfacial length is subtracted from the effective mandibular length, the *maxillomandibular differential* can be determined. In this instance, the maxillomandibular differential is 20–23 mm (Fig. 28-13).

If the effective length of the maxilla in a medium-sized individual, such as an adult female, is 94 mm, the range of effective mandibular lengths is 120–124 mm (Fig. 28-14A; Table 28-5). In this example, the maxillomandibular differential is 26–30 mm. If the effective midfacial length of a large individual, such as an adult male, is 100 mm, the range of effective lengths of the mandible is 130–133 mm with a differential of 30–33 mm (Fig. 28-14B). It is important to reemphasize that the linear relationship of the components is the most important consideration, not the age or sex of the patient, as is illustrated in Figure 28-15. A midface of a given length (regardless of gender) corresponds to a given mandibular length (or range of mandibular lengths).

Examples of variation in the relationship between the midface and the maxilla will be demonstrated by analyzing the pretreatment cephalometric tracings of three patients. The first tracing (Fig. 28-16) shows a 22-year-old male who presented with a Class II, division 1 malocclusion. The effective length of his midface is 96 mm; thus the effective length of his mandible should be 124–127 mm (Table 28-5) with a maxillomandibular differential of 28–31 mm. In fact, however, his mandible is approximately 12 mm too short, with the discrepancy primarily in the size of the mandible. The midface is normally positioned (0 mm relative to the nasion perpendicular).

Figure 28-17 shows the cephalometric tracing of a 22-year-old female who has an effective midfacial length of 93 mm. The predicted effective length of the mandible for a maxilla of this size is 119–122 mm (Table 28-5). According to the relationship of Point A to the nasion perpendicular, the maxilla is normally positioned anteroposteriorly (0 mm) relative to the cranial base, as indicated by the anteroposterior position of the nasion perpendicular. Therefore, the mandible, at 129 mm, is approximately 10 mm too long.

Figure 28-18 shows the tracing of a 25-year-old male who has a Class III malocclusion characterized clinically by a retrusive maxilla (indicated by the measurement of −3 mm from Point A to the nasion perpendicular) and a prognathic mandible. The maxillomandibular differential is about 11 mm greater than the norms estimate. The jaw discrepancy is due to a combination of a retruded position of the upper jaw and a protruded position of the lower jaw. In this instance, a theoretical adjustment should be made in the effective length of the midface. For example, if the maxilla were moved forward (*e.g.,* surgically) to its normal relationship with the cranial base (1 mm ahead of the nasion perpendicular), the effective midfacial length then would be 95 mm, corresponding to a mandibular length of 122–125 mm. Even if the position of the midface were corrected, there still would be relative mandibular prognathism remaining.

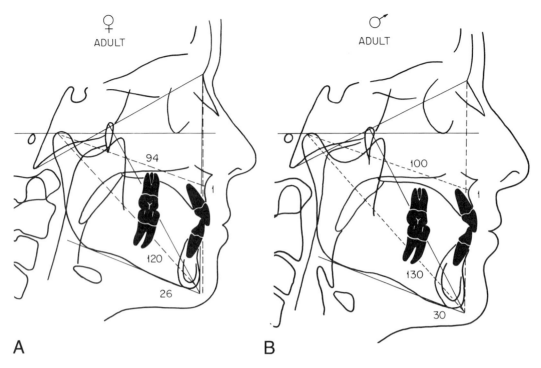

Figure 28-14. Effective midfacial and mandibular lengths in: *A*, Ideal female adult. *B*, Ideal male adult. The maxillomandibular differential is determined by subtracting effective length from effective mandibular length (from McNamara[55]).

Vertical Dimension

This far, we have considered changes in the horizontal dimensions of the face. Of course, it is evident, however, that the clinical appearance of the relationship between the upper and lower jaws is affected largely by lower anterior facial height (note: upper anterior facial height is not considered unless there is an obvious abnormality). An increase in lower anterior facial height can result in a downward and backward position of the chin (Fig. 28-19*A*), whereas a decrease in vertical dimension can lead to an autorotation of the chin in a forward and upward direction (Fig. 28-19*B*).

The vertical dimension of the lower face has a profound influence on the anteroposterior position of the chin. Patients who are congenitally missing most or all of their permanent teeth (Figure 28-20) or who have lost their teeth through decay or periodontal disease can illustrate the effect of increasing or decreasing lower anterior facial height (LAFH) on chin prominence. Increasing LAFH makes the chin less prominent; decreasing LAFH makes the chin more prominent and the mentolabial sulcus more defined.

In the analytical method presented here, lower anterior facial height is measured from anterior nasal spine to menton. This linear measurement increases with age and is correlated with the effective length of the midface (Tables 28-1, 28-4, 28-5). The lower anterior facial height for the ideal mixed dentition subject with an 85 mm effective midfacial length is 60–62 mm (Fig. 28-21). An effective midfacial length of 94 mm (Fig. 28-22*A*) corresponds to a lower anterior facial height of 66–67 mm in the medium-sized subject. In the large individual

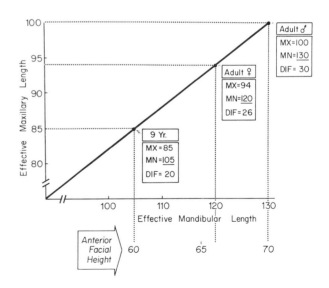

Figure 28-15. The relationship between effective midfacial length and effective mandibular length. This relationship generally is linear and is dependent on the size, rather than the age and sex, of the individual.

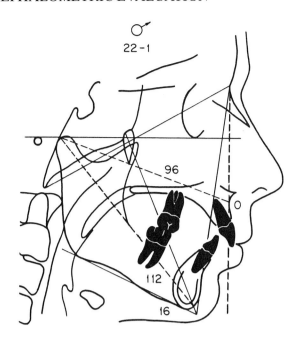

Figure 28-16. Cephalometric tracing of a 22-year-old male with a skeletal mandibular deficiency of 12 mm. The position of the maxilla is normal (from McNamara[55]).

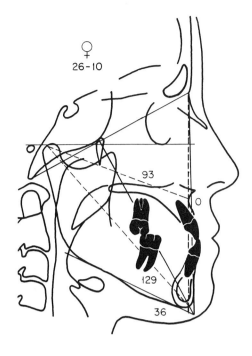

Figure 28-17. Cephalometric tracing of a 26-year-old female with skeletal mandibular excess of 10 mm (from McNamara[55]).

with an effective midfacial length of 100 mm, lower facial height is approximately 70–74 mm (Fig. 28-22B).

The relationship between lower anterior facial height and the horizontal position is relatively constant. For example, if the mandible is rotated downward and backward concomitant with a 15 mm increase in lower facial height (Fig. 28-23A), the chin point moves downward and backward from the nasion perpendicular (−13 mm) because of the rotation. If the anterior facial height is shortened by 15 mm (Fig. 28-23B), autorotation of the mandible will move the chin point forward by 15 mm. Thus, if lower facial height is increased, the mandible will appear to be more retrognathic; if lower facial height is decreased, the mandible will appear more prognathic. In a growing individual, an increase in lower anterior facial height will camouflage a similar increase in mandibular length, which may result in the appearance that the chin in is the same relationship anteroposteriorly to cranial base structures.

The relationship between the anteroposterior and vertical dimensions will be demonstrated further by considering three clinical examples. Figure 28-24 represents the cephalometric tracings of a 15-year-old female with a Class II, division 2 malocclusion. The effective length of the midface in this patient is 99 mm (this length should be adjusted by subtracting 2 mm because of the anterior position of the roots of the maxillary incisors). If the adjusted *effective length* of the midface then is 97 mm, the effective mandibular length is expected to be approximately 126–129 mm (Table 28-5). Even though the actual effective mandibular length is 5 or 6 mm short of the expected value, pogonion lies on the nasion perpendicular. The explanation for this ob-

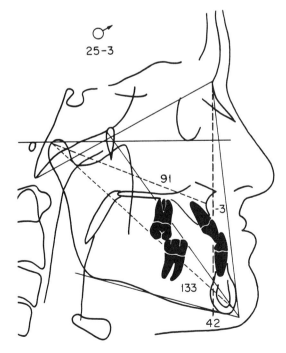

Figure 28-18. Cephalometric tracing of a 25-year-old male with a skeletal midfacial deficiency of 4 mm and a skeletal mandibular excess of 11 mm (from McNamara[55]).

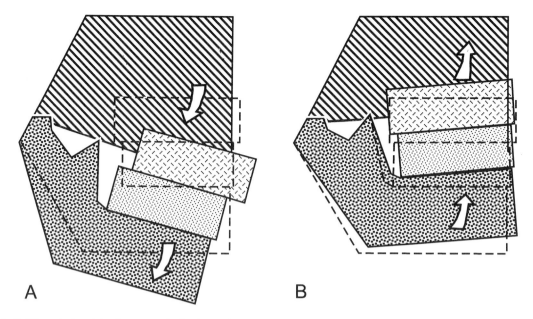

Figure 28-19. The relationships between the horizontal and vertical facial dimensions. *A*, Excessive anterior facial height is related to a downward and backward positioning of the mandible and vertical maxillary excess. *B*, Deficient lower anterior facial height is related to an overclosure of the mandible and vertical maxillary dentoalveolar deficiency.

servation is that the patient has a deficient lower anterior facial height of 9 or 10 mm that allows for autorotation of the mandible into a more forward position, thus masking the severity of the mandibular deficiency. If the lower anterior facial height will correct relative to the midfacial length, pogonion would be 6 or 7 mm posterior to the nasion perpendicular.

A patient with a severe skeletal discrepancy is seen in Figure 28-25. This eight-year-old male has a slightly retrusive maxilla, as indicated by the −2 mm measurement relative to the nasion perpendicular (normal values are 0–1 mm). Given the existing midfacial length of 91 mm, the mandible should be 115–118 mm in length (actual value is 101 mm). In addition, lower anterior fa-

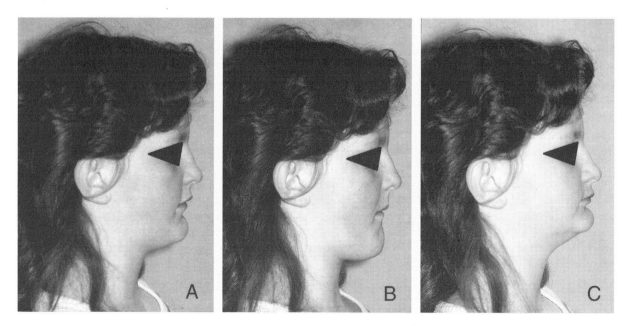

Figure 28-20. The effect of changing the vertical dimension on the anteroposterior position of the chin. This 16-year-old patient was congenitally missing most of her permanent teeth. Note the alteration in chin prominence with the approximation of *A*, "Normal" vertical dimension, *B*, Increased vertical dimension, *C*, Decreased vertical dimension.

CEPHALOMETRIC EVALUATION

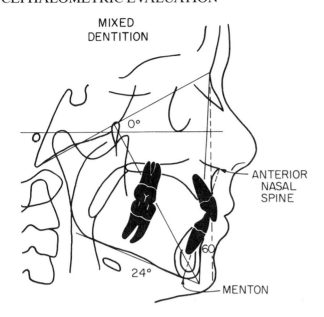

Figure 28-21. Determination of lower anterior facial height as measured from anterior nasal spine to menton (from McNamara[55]).

cial height for a patient with a 91 mm midfacial length should be 63–64 mm (the actual value is 69 mm). Thus, this patient has a severe skeletal discrepancy, in which pogonion is in a retrusive position, due not only to the deficiency in the anatomical length of the mandible, but also to the autorotation associated with an increase of 5 mm in lower anterior facial height.

The next example (Fig. 28-26) is a 25-year-old male with a chief complaint of dislike of the appearance of his face, particularly in the nose and chin area. His maxilla is slightly retruded relative to the nasion perpendicular, and he has an unfavorable nasolabial angle. The 93 mm effective midfacial length in this patient should correspond to an effective mandibular length of approximately 119 mm (Table 28-5); however, the actual value for this measurement is 128 mm. This measure indicates that the mandible is prognathic. Because his lower anterior facial height is 82 mm (more than 15 mm greater than expected), the net effect of the excessive mandibular length and the even greater excess in anterior facial height is the appearance of a long face with an apparent mandibular retrusion. Once again, however, lower anterior facial height is altering the appearance of the horizontal relationship of the maxilla and mandible. It is evident that one must assess lower anterior facial height before classifying a given malocclusion, due to the interrelationship of lower anterior facial height and the anteroposterior position of pogonion.

The relationship of anteroposterior and vertical measurements indicates the inadequacy of using horizontal measurements such as the ANB angle[22] as an indicator

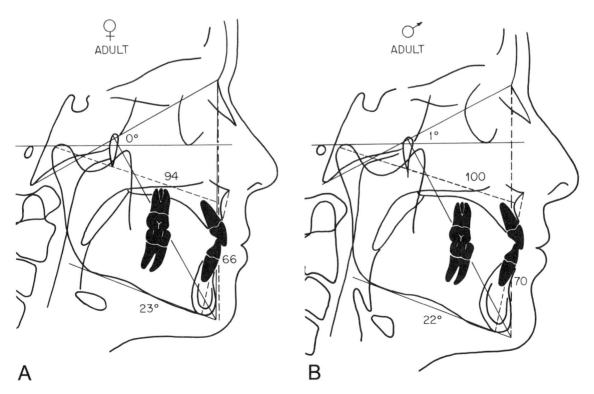

Figure 28-22. Lower anterior facial height as measured from anterior nasal spine to menton. *A*, Ideal adult female. *B*, Ideal adult male (from McNamara[55]).

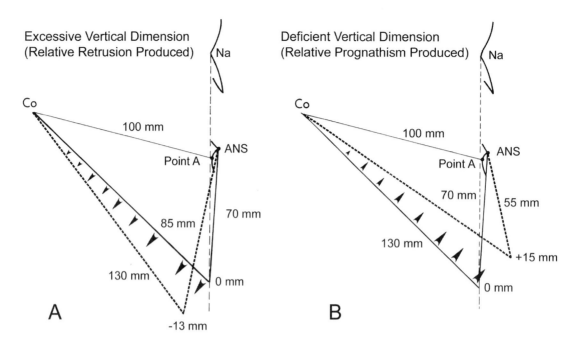

Figure 28-23. The relationship between lower anterior facial height and effective mandibular length. *A*, Using adult male proportions, an increase in lower anterior facial height of 15 mm results in an effective mandibular retrusion of 13 mm. *B*, A reduction in vertical dimension of 15 mm produces a relative mandibular protrusion of 15 mm (from McNamara[55]).

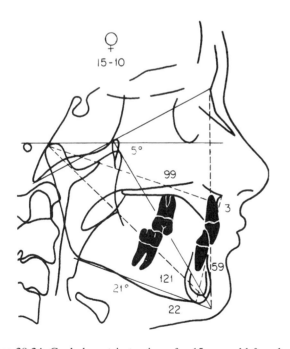

Figure 28-24. Cephalometric tracing of a 15-year-old female with a Class II, division 2 malocclusion. The labial position of the roots of the maxillary central incisors necessitates an adjustment in effective midfacial length from 99 to 97 mm. This indicates a relative mandibular deficiency of 8 mm that is masked by a forward rotation of the mandible. The patient has a 5° facial axis angle and a relatively low (21° mandibular plane angle (from McNamara[55]).

of skeletal change, particularly when evaluating the treatment effects produced by certain types of functional appliances. For example, the correction of many Class II malocclusions necessitates the correction of not only the anteroposterior discrepancy but also of excessive overbite. If it is necessary to open the bite 4 mm vertically in order to attain a normal incisal relationship, approximately 4 mm of increased mandibular length is necessary merely to keep the chin in the same position relative to cranial base structures. Thus, actual measurements of changes in midfacial, mandibular, and lower anterior facial dimensions are necessary if a proper understanding of the treatment effects produced by a specific type of therapy is to be achieved.

Two other cephalometric measurements are shown in Figures 28-21 and 28-22, the mandibular plane angle (the angle between the anatomical Frankfort plane and the mandibular plane constructed through gonion and menton) and the facial axis angle of Ricketts.[27,28] The latter measurement is determined by constructing a line from basion to nasion, a line that represents the cranial base. Then, a second line (the facial axis) is constructed from the posterosuperior aspects of the pterygomaxillary fissure (PTM point) to constructed gonion (the intersection of the facial plane and the mandibular plane). The angle measured is from basion to the pterygomaxillary fissure to gnathion. A 90° or perpendicular relationship of the basion-nasion and the facial axis is to

CEPHALOMETRIC EVALUATION

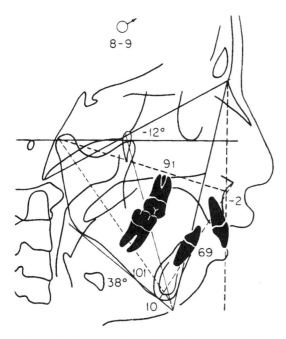

Figure 28-25. Cephalometric tracing of an 8-year-old male with a mild maxillary skeletal retrusion (-2 mm) and a deficiency in effective mandibular length of 16 mm. The patient appears more retrognathic because of the 5 mm excess in lower anterior facial height (from McNamara[55]).

be expected in a balanced face. When the facial axis angle deviates from 90° in its relationship to the cranial base, horizontal or vertical facial development can be assessed. Excessive vertical development is indicated by negative values (90° subtracted from the actual values, resulting in negative numbers). For example, the patients shown in Figures 28-25 and 28-26 demonstrate a vertical direction of growth with facial axis angles of −12° and −7° respectively. Deficient vertical development is indicated by positive values (90° subtracted from the actual angular measurement), as indicated, for example, in the patient shown in Figure 28–24 who has a horizontally directed facial axis angle of 5°.

Relating the Mandible to Midfacial and Upper Facial Structures

The relationship of the mandible to the cranial base is determined by measuring the distance from pogonion to the nasion perpendicular. For example, in a mixed dentition subject with a balanced face, pogonion lies posterior (−8 mm to −6 mm) to the nasion perpendicular (Fig. 28-27A; Table 28-2). In the individual with a medium-sized face (Fig. 28-27B), pogonion usually lies −4 mm to 0 mm relative to the nasion perpendicular (Tables 28-1 and 28-2). In the large individual, such as an adult male, the measurement of the chin position is usually from −2 mm to +4 mm relative to the nasion perpendicular (Fig. 28-27C; Tables 28-1 and 28-2). More variation in the anteroposterior position of the chin is observed in adult male subjects than in adult female subjects.

Figure 28-28 is an example of an adult patient with a retrusive maxilla (−7 mm), a retrusive mandible, a steep mandibular plane angle (45°), and a −30 mm distance from pogonion to the nasion perpendicular. A prognathic patient with pogonion positioned 16 mm ahead of the nasion perpendicular is shown in Figure 28-29.

Relating the Maxillary Incisor to the Maxilla

The precise determination of the position of the anterior teeth relative to the maxilla and mandible is of interest not only in the treatment planning of routine orthodontic patients, but perhaps more importantly in determining the pre-surgical or pre-orthopedic positioning of the upper and mandibular incisors. The anteroposterior and vertical determinants of upper and mandibular incisor position are described in detail below.

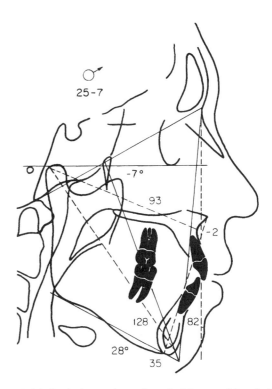

Figure 28-26. Cephalometric tracing of a 25-year-old male. The patient has a relative maxillary skeletal retrusion of −2 mm and a mandibular skeletal protrusion of 7 mm. The patient appears retrognathic, however, because of the 15 mm excess in lower anterior facial height (from McNamara[55]).

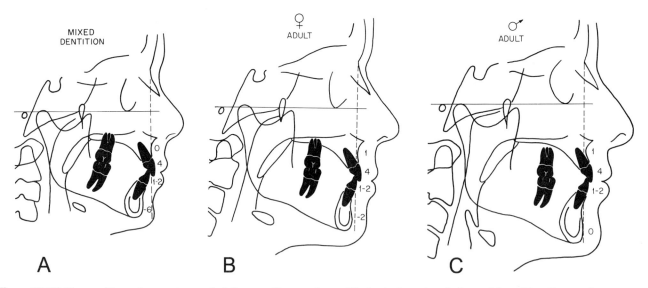

Figure 28-27. The position of pogonion and of the maxillary and mandibular incisors in a balanced face. The distance from pogonion to the nasion perpendicular is variable according to the age of the patient. Regardless of the patient's age, the maxillary incisors should be 4–6 mm ahead of a vertical line dropped perpendicular to Frankfort horizontal through Point A. The facial surface of the mandibular incisors should be 1–3 mm ahead of a line constructed through Point A and pogonion. *A*, Mixed dentition. *B*, Adult female. *C*, Adult male (from McNamara[55]).

Anteroposterior Position

In instances of malrelationships between the maxillary and mandibular skeletal structures, serious errors may result if the position of the upper incisor is determined by any measurement that uses the mandible as a point of reference. If the chin point is in a retrusive position relative to mid- and upper-facial structures, the orientation line will make the upper incisor appear as if it were in a more protrusive position than it actually is, relative to the maxilla. An example of this type of measurement is the Point A-pogonion line (Fig. 28-30) used in the Ricketts analysis.[27,28] The mandible can be used as a reference for maxillary incisor position only if the unchanged position of the mandible is acceptable as a treatment goal.

A similar statement can be made regarding any measure that uses cranial base structures for reference to determine the position of the upper incisor. For example, a measurement of the position of the upper incisor relative to a line drawn through nasion and Point A[22–24] is valid only if the maxilla is in a neutral position anteroposteriorly relative to the cranial base. A retrusive position of the maxilla relative to nasion will make the upper incisor appear more protrusive, whereas a protrusive position of the maxilla will make the upper incisor appear more retrusive.[4]

It is extremely important to be able to differentiate whether or not the dentition is in a neutral, protrusive or retrusive position relative to skeletal structures (Fig.

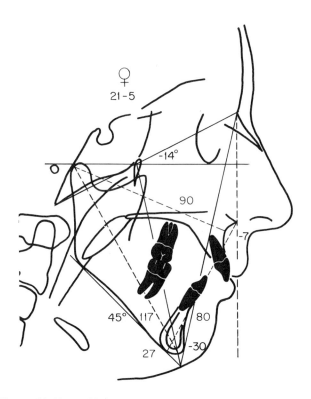

Figure 28-28. A 21-year-old female with maxillary skeletal retrusion, severe mandibular skeletal retrusion, and excessive lower anterior facial height. Clinically, the patient's nose is quite prominent, although the prominence is due in great part to the retrusion of the mid and lower face (from McNamara[55]).

CEPHALOMETRIC EVALUATION

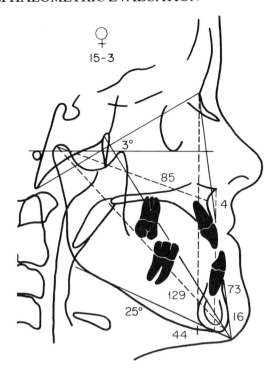

Figure 28-29. Cephalometric tracing of a 15-year-old female with mandibular prognathism. This tracing represents an example of a Class III patient who appears clinically to be deficient in the upper facial area, particularly at nasion. Therefore, the nasion perpendicular is positioned posteriorly and is subject to adjustment (from McNamara[55]).

28-31). In determining the position of the upper incisors, measures that relate the dental portion of the maxilla to the skeletal portion of the maxilla are used. A vertical line is drawn through Point A parallel to the nasion perpendicular (Fig. 28-32). The distance from this constructed *Point A vertical* to the facial surface of the upper incisor is measured. The ideal distance from Point A to the facial surface of the upper incisor horizontally is 4–6 mm (Tables 28-1 and 28-2). Figure 28-33 shows a patient who has protruded upper incisors and a normally positioned maxilla (1 mm ahead of the nasion perpendicular). Figure 28-34 shows a patient with maxillary skeletal protrusion and maxillary dentoalveolar protrusion. A patient with retruded upper incisors is illustrated in Figure 28-35.

Vertical Position

The vertical position of the maxillary incisor is best determined at the time of the clinical examination, although a headfilm taken with the lips at rest also may be useful. Typically, the incisal edge of the maxillary incisor should lie 2–3 mm below the upper lip at rest. In addition, the upper lip of the patient should be at the junction between the incisors and the associated gingiva when smiling.

Some adjustment may need to be made in interpreting the meaning of these measurements according to the functional state of the lip musculature and the axial inclination of the tooth before treatment. In some instances, particularly following either functional appliance therapy or orthognathic surgery, a hypotonic lip musculature may increase in activity, thus changing its functional state.

Relating the Mandibular Incisor to the Mandible

Relating the mandibular incisor to the mandible is analogous to relating the maxillary incisor to the maxilla. Both anteroposterior and vertical relationships of the mandibular incisor are considered.

Anteroposterior Position

The anteroposterior position of the mandibular incisor must be determined relative to the mandible. A clear differentiation must be made between, for example, a Class II malocclusion in which the mandibular dentition is well related to a retrusive mandible (Fig. 28-36A), and a mandibular dentition that is retruded relative to a normally positioned mandible (Fig. 28-36B). In the first diagrammatic representation, an increase in mandibular length during treatment would be the obvious goal, whereas in the latter, a forward movement of the mandi-

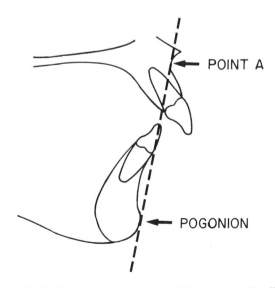

Figure 28-30. The construction of the Point A-pogonion line. The distance from the incisal edge to the A-Po line is measured. The maxillary incisors appear flared if the mandible is in a retruded position.

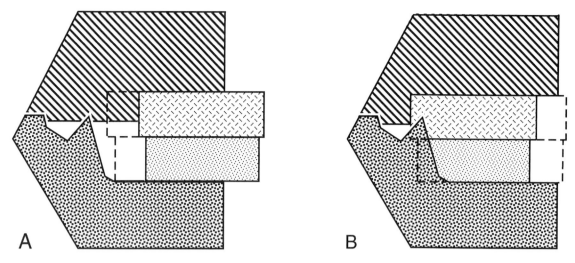

Figure 28-31. Schematic representations of A, Bialveolar protrusion. B, bialveolar retrusion.

bular dentition relative to the mandible would be the treatment goal of choice. In certain instances, both mandibular skeletal retrusion and mandibular dentoalveolar retrusion may exist in the same individual.

In our opinion, the estimation of the anteroposterior position of the mandibular incisor numerically is the weakest and most cumbersome part of this analysis. For practical purposes, a subjective evaluation of lower incisor position can be made by the clinician to determine whether the incisor is well positioned within the mandibular symphysis. The treating of mandibular incisor position to a precise angular relationship with the mandibular plane angle (*e.g.*, treating the lower incisor to a 90–95° angulation with the mandibular plane) is not recommended. The position of the lower incisor in part is related to the functional state of the associated soft tissue (particularly the relationship of the upper and lower lips as well as to the position of the maxilla).

If a precise measurement of the position of the lower incisor is desired, the anteroposterior position of the incisor can be determined using two measures. The first uses a traditional version of the Ricketts[27-29] measurement of the facial surface of the lower incisor to a line drawn through Point A and pogonion (Fig. 28-30). The facial surface of the lower incisor should lie 1–3 mm ahead of the A-pogonion line. In a well-balanced face, such as those comprising the Bolton Standards (Table 28-6), the facial surface of the mandibular incisor is approximately 1.5 mm anterior to the A-pogonion line. In the Ann Arbor sample (Table 28-1), the lower incisor is in a slightly more protrusive position (2.3–2.7 mm).

If a discrepancy exists in the anteroposterior or vertical positioning of the mandible or maxilla, modifications in this measurement procedure are necessary. For example, in instances of mandibular skeletal retrusion, it is necessary to evaluate the position of the mandibular incisor relative to the predicted repositioning of the mandible, regardless of whether repositioning is through surgical or functional intervention. A second tracing of the mandible and the incisor is made, and the tracing is positioned so that the mandible is in the desired orientation

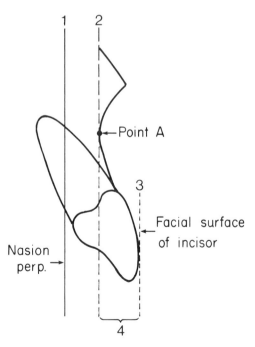

Figure 28-32. The method of determining the anteroposterior position of the maxillary incisor relative to Point A. This measurement should be 4–6 mm. 1) Nasion perpendicular. 2) Point A vertical constructed parallel to the nasion perpendicular through Point A. 3) Line drawn parallel to the nasion perpendicular through the most labial point on the maxillary incisor crown. 4) The anteroposterior distance from the maxillary incisor to Point A. (From McNamara[41].)

CEPHALOMETRIC EVALUATION

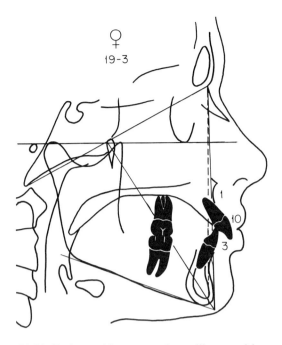

Figure 28-33. Patient with a normal maxillary position and protruded maxillary teeth. The maxillary incisors are 4-6 mm forward of their ideal position. The mandibular incisors are well related to the mandibular symphysis.

relative to the maxilla (Fig. 28-37A). A new line from Point A to pogonion is drawn. The incisor is expected to lie 1-3 mm anterior to the constructed A-Po line.

Another way in which mandibular incisor position can be determined relative to a constructed A-pogonion line is to estimate first the distance (*i.e.*, number of millimeters) that the mandible will be brought forward relative to the maxilla at the end of treatment. Then, a new Point A is constructed the same distance in the opposite direction (Fig. 28-37B). This method provides an approximate post-treatment A-pogonion line that then can be used to evaluate the predicted mandibular incisor position without making a template tracing.

Figure 28-34 shows a patient with maxillary and mandibular incisor protrusion. This is indicated by a 7 mm relationship of the maxillary incisor to the maxilla and a 7 mm relationship of the mandibular incisor to the A-pogonion line. In this instance, the mandible is in a normal orientation while the maxilla has some degree of skeletal protrusion evident (4 mm to the nasion perpendicular). Figure 28-35 is an example of a patient who has dentoalveolar retrusion in both arches.

Vertical Position

The vertical position of the mandibular incisor is evaluated based on existing lower anterior facial height. The pre-treatment overbite relationship is first evaluated by relating the mandibular incisor tip to the functional occlusal plane. If there is an excessive curve of Spee, a decision must be made as to whether the mandibular incisors should be intruded or the mandibular molars allowed to erupt. The determining factor is lower anterior facial height relative to the effective midfacial length (Table 28-5). If the existing lower anterior facial height is either excessive or normal, the mandibular incisors are *intruded*. If, on the other hand, lower anterior facial height is inadequate and the mandibular incisors are extruded, *further eruption* of the molars is desired.

Anterior repositioning of the mandible in a patient with a deep overbite (as occurs following a surgical advancement of the mandible or during functional appliance treatment) will require a significant increase in lower anterior facial height. This repositioning may be detrimental to patients with pre-treatment normal or excessive anterior vertical dimensions. If so, the mandibular incisors must be intruded prior to surgical or orthodontic intervention (see Fig. 28-25 for an example of such a patient).

A patient who presents with an inadequate lower anterior facial height and a deepbite may benefit from anterior and inferior repositioning of the mandible to an edge-to-edge incisor position, followed by posterior tooth eruption. Such eruption would close the transient open bite. Through the anteroposterior and vertical

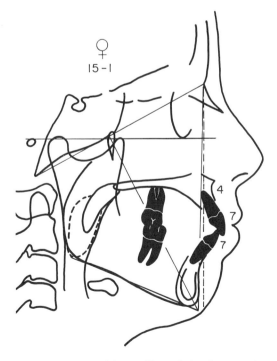

Figure 28-34. Patient with maxillary skeletal protrusion and bialveolar protrusion.

508 ORTHODONTICS AND DENTOFACIAL ORTHOPEDICS

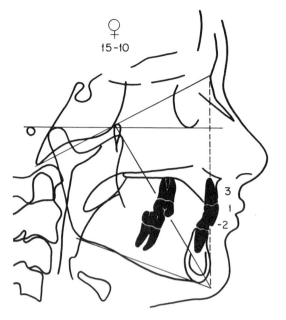

Figure 28-35. Patient with bialveolar retrusion.

control of the position of the mandibular incisor, repositioning of the osseous elements can be maximized.

In conclusion, the vertical position of the mandibular incisor should be one of the key factors considered in planning treatment strategies.

Airway Analysis

One of the most controversial areas in orthodontic diagnosis and treatment planning today is the relationship between upper airway obstruction and craniofacial growth.[17,49-52] Conflicting evidence exists as to this interrelationship. For the purpose of this analysis, two measurements are used to examine the *possibility* of airway impairment.

Upper Pharynx

Upper pharyngeal width (Fig. 26-38) is measured from a point on the posterior outline of the soft palate to the closest point on the posterior pharyngeal wall. This measurement typically is made from the anterior half of the soft palate outline because the area immediately adjacent to the posterior opening of the nose is critical in determining upper respiratory patency. It must be noted, however, that the headfilm outline of the nasopharynx is only a two-dimensional representation of a three-dimensional structure.

If a patient is swallowing when the radiograph is taken, the soft palate takes on the appearance of an inverted "V," as the tensor and levator veli palatini muscles pull the palate upward and backward during closure. This configuration of the soft palate observed in a given headfilm suggests only limited usefulness of the upper pharyngeal measurement.

Warren[53,54] has determined that 40 square millimeters of nasopharyngeal airway must be present in order for nasal breathing to occur without an oral component. Because the average nasopharynx is approximately 15–20 mm in width, a distance of 2 mm or less in the upper pharyngeal measurement may be used as an indicator

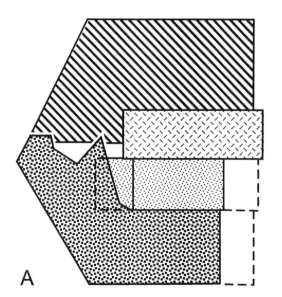
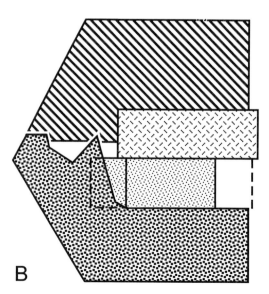

Figure 28-36. Schematic representation of mandibular incisor position. *A,* Retrusive mandible with normally positioned mandibular incisors. *B,* Normal mandible with retruded position of mandibular incisors. A patient with the latter type of morphology clinically would have a strong chin point. This condition is often related to hypertonic perioral musculature.

Table 28-6. Dental variables from the Bolton Standards N=16 for each sex at each age. Standardized 8% enlargement.

Variable (mm)	6 years		9 years		12 years		14 years		16 years		18 years	
	$\overline{X}$	SD	$\overline{X}$	SD	$\overline{X}$	SD	$\overline{X}$	SD	$\overline{X}$	SD	$\overline{X}$	SD
Female												
Maxillary Dental												
(Upper Incisor to Point A)	−2.1	1.4	2.9	0.9	3.3	1.0	4.2	1.5	4.0	1.3	4.2	1.3
Mandibular Dental												
(Lower Incisor to A-Po line)	0.02	1.4	0.9	1.1	1.3	0.7	1.4	1.6	1.1	1.6	1.2	1.4
Male												
Maxillary Dental												
(Upper Incisor to Point A)	0.8	1.4	3.1	1.3	3.8	1.3	3.8	1.4	4.1	2.1	3.7	1.3
Mandibular Dental												
(Lower Incisor to A-Po line)	0.5	1.3	1.1	1.5	1.4	1.6	1.4	1.8	1.3	2.3	0.4	1.8

of possible airway impairment. (This value is in contrast to 5 mm or less stated in the 1984 McNamara article[55] in the *American Journal of Orthodontics*.) A more accurate diagnosis can be made only by an otorhinolaryngologist during a clinical examination or more accurately by a measurement of oral and nasal airflow.

In the Ann Arbor Sample of adult individuals with well-balanced faces, the average upper airway measurement for adults of both sexes is 17.4 mm (Table 28-1). This measurement increases with age. Figure 28-38 shows a patient who demonstrates *possible* adenoid obstruction of the upper airway, as the upper pharyngeal width is only 2 mm. This observation was verified through clinical examination by an otolaryngologist. A typical upper pharyngeal measurement in a mixed-dentition patient is shown in Figure 28-39.

Lower Pharynx

Lower pharyngeal width is measured from the intersection of the posterior border of the tongue and the inferior border of the mandible to the closest point on the

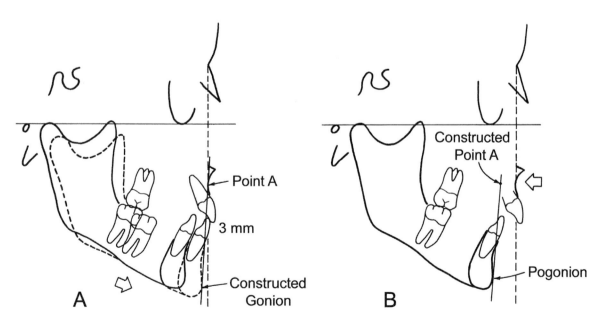

Figure 28-37. Determination of mandibular incisor position in patients with co-existing skeletal discrepancies. *A*, A tracing of the mandible and mandibular dentition is constructed. This tracing is moved so that the mandible is in the expected position relative to the maxilla and cranial base. An idealized A-Po line can be constructed and the position of the mandibular incisor evaluated. In this example, the mandibular incisor now lies 3 mm ahead of the idealized A-Po line. *B*, The amount of desired anterior movement of pogonion is measured. Point A then is moved in the opposite direction the same amount. The idealized A-Po line is constructed through the new Point A and the existing pogonion, and the position of the mandibular incisor is then measured (from McNamara[55]).

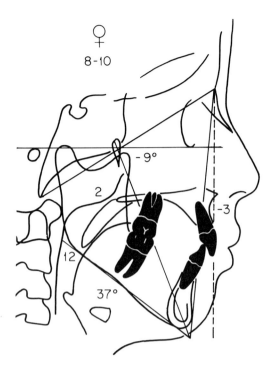

Figure 28-38. Indications of possible upper airway obstruction in a patient with an excessive adenoidal mass. The distance between the posterior aspect of the soft palate and the closest point on the posterior pharyngeal wall is 2 mm. The lower airway measurement is within normal limits (12 mm). Note that this patient has a steep mandibular plane angle and a negative facial axis angle (from McNamara[55]).

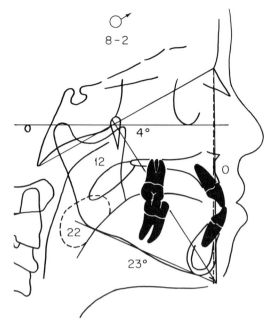

Figure 28-39. Patient with enlarged tonsils and a forward tongue position. The distance from the intersection of the posterior outline of the tongue and the lower border of the mandible and the closest point on the posterior pharyngeal wall is 22 mm. The upper airway measurement of 12 mm is within normal limits. This patient has a positive facial axis angle and a relatively normal mandibular plane angle (from McNamara[55]).

posterior pharyngeal wall. According to the data derived from the Ann Arbor Sample (Table 28-1), the average value for this measurement is 11–14 mm, and it does not change appreciably with age. In contrast to the upper pharynx, a smaller-than-average value for the lower pharynx is not remarkable. It is rare to see an obstruction of the lower pharyngeal area because of the position of the tongue against the pharynx. A lower pharyngeal width of greater than 18 mm, however, suggests a possible anterior positioning of the tongue, either because of habitual posture, or due to an enlargement of the tonsils.

Determination of tongue position is important in the diagnosis of certain clinical conditions, such as mandibular prognathism, dentoalveolar anterior crossbite, and bialveolar protrusion of the teeth. These clinical conditions can be associated with a forward tongue position and/or enlarged tonsils. A recent article by Trotman and colleagues[52] has shown an association between a forward tongue position due to enlarged tonsils and altered craniofacial morphology (see also Chapter 8 for a discussion of this issue).

Figure 28-38 shows a tracing of a patient with a normal lower pharyngeal measurement. Figure 28-39 shows a patient with excessive lower pharyngeal width and a forward position of the tongue.

Overview

The combined normative values for adult male and female patients are presented in Figure 28-40. These values present the senior author's conceptualization of cephalometric tracings of an ideal male and an ideal female face. The growing patient is considered next.

ANALYSIS OF SERIAL FILMS

In orthodontics, it is important not only to establish a diagnosis and treatment plan, but it is of equal importance to determine the effects of the prescribed treatment once performed. A treatment effect can be defined as the skeletal and dentoalveolar changes that are measured in serial headfilms after expected normal growth has been taken into consideration.

The following analytical steps are used to assess growth or treatment changes occurring between serial

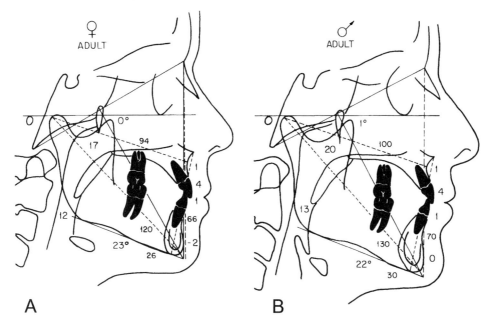

Figure 28-40. Composite values for the adult patient. A, Ideal female. B, Ideal male (from McNamara[55]).

headfilms. A tracing of a headfilm of an ideal mixed-dentition patient is presented in Figure 28-41A. The effective length of the midface is 85 mm, the effective length of the mandible is 105 mm, and the maxillomandibular differential is 20 mm. Lower anterior facial height is 60 mm, and the maxilla is in its expected relationship relative to the cranial base (0 mm to the nasion perpendicular). The maxillary incisor is in its expected position relative to the maxilla (4 mm to the Point A vertical) and the mandibular incisor is positioned ideally with respect to the mandible (1 mm to Point A-pogonion). The mandibular plane angle and the facial axis angle of Ricketts[27,28] also are shown.

Figure 28-41B presents a tracing of the same subject two years later. It is estimated that the effective length of the midface will increase approximately 1–2 mm per year, the effective length of the mandible will increase approximately 2–3 mm per year, and lower anterior facial height as measured from anterior nasal spine to menton will increase approximately 1 mm per year.

An analysis of the incremental values derived from the Bolton Standards (Table 28-7) indicates evidence of sexual dimorphism and age-related differences in growth increments. Midfacial and mandibular lengths increase steadily in girls until about age 14, at which time the rate of growth drops dramatically. In contrast, male subjects demonstrate growth increments to the oldest ages studied (18 years), with the highest rates of growth occurring between ages 12 and 16.

The relationship of the maxilla to the cranial base, of the maxillary incisor to the maxilla, and of the mandibular incisor to the mandible does not change during the two-year time period evaluated. The distance from pogonion to the nasion perpendicular usually decreases approximately 0.5–1 mm per year. The facial axis angle remains relatively unchanged, whereas the mandibular plane angle decreases slightly.

Superimposition Technique

In the analysis of serial films, care must be taken to ensure that identification of landmarks in serial films from the same subject or patient is consistent. Thus, the four-point superimposition method of Ricketts[27,28] is used not only to analyze growth changes, but also to check for errors in landmark identification.

Cranial base superimposition

The first superimposition (Fig. 28-42) is along the basion-nasion line at the posterosuperior aspect of the pterygomaxillary fissure. This superimposition shows the downward and forward movement of the facial structures during a two-year period. The chin moved downward and forward, as did the maxillary and mandibular teeth. A relatively parallel progression of the profile in a downward and forward direction also is observed.

Mandibular superimposition

Superimposition of the mandible, using internal structures, such as the outline of the inferior alveolar canal

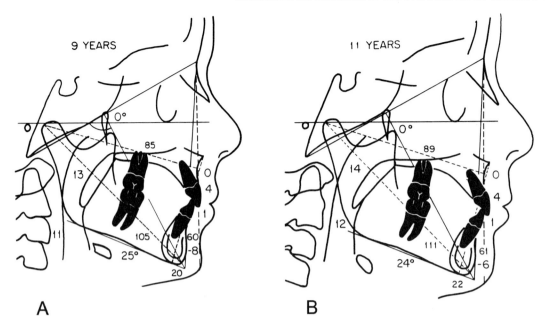

Figure 28-41. Composite values for the growing individual. *A*, Cephalometric tracing of an ideal mixed dentition patient. *B*, Cephalometric tracing of the same patient two years later (from McNamara[55]).

and the lingual surface of the symphysis (Fig. 28-43), demonstrates the amount of eruption and the horizontal movement of the teeth. The amount and direction of condylar growth and the degree of localized remodeling also can be measured.

Maxillary superimposition

Superimposition of the maxilla on internal structures (Fig. 28-44) shows the movement of the maxillary dentition and the amount of localized remodeling that occurred in various regions of the maxilla.

Maxillary displacement

Superimposition along the basion-nasion line at nasion (Fig. 28-45) allows evaluation of the position of the maxillary complex relative to the upper face. As mentioned earlier, nasion and Point A move forward at approximately the same rate during growth. With this type of superimposition, downward movement is observed in the growing person, but there is little forward or backward movement.

The effect of treatment on the maxilla also can be measured when this last method of superimposition is used. Point A may be moved forward with the use of an orthopedic appliance, such as a facial mask combined with a rapid palatal expansion appliance.[56] Conversely, if an orthopedic headgear were used to move the maxilla posteriorly, Point A would appear to be displaced posteriorly in the second tracing.

DISCUSSION

As mentioned earlier, although some cephalometric landmarks can be located with a high degree of reproducibility, cephalometrics itself is an inexact science. The information gathered from the analysis is highly dependent upon the landmarks and measures chosen. Thus, the information gathered from any conventional cephalometric analysis is limited by the analysis itself.

An attempt has been made to tailor this analysis to the current needs of the orthodontist, taking into consideration the wide variety of treatment techniques available today. This method depends primarily upon linear measurements rather than angles, so that treatment planning (particularly treatment planning for the

Table 28-7. Mandibular and maxillary lengths (Bolton Sample) (mm)

	Age in Years					
	6	9	12	14	16	18
Male						
Mand. Length	96.9	105.5	112.1	118.2	124.5	128.7
Max. Length	79.8	86.1	90.2	93.4	97.1	99.1
Differential	17.1	19.4	21.9	24.8	27.4	29.6
Female						
Mand. Length	95.2	103.7	110.1	116.4	117.6	119.1
Max. Length	77.8	83.0	87.9	90.3	90.8	91.7
Differential	17.4	20.7	22.2	26.1	26.8	27.4

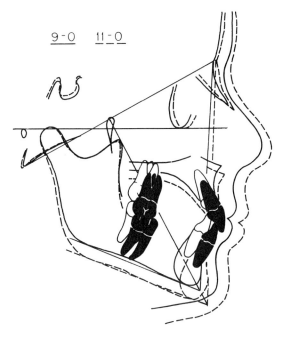

Figure 28-42. The analysis of serial films. The overall changes in facial growth are indicated by superimposing subsequent tracings along the basion-nasion line at the intersection of the pterygomaxillary fissure (from McNamara[55]).

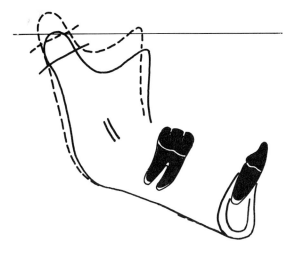

Figure 28-43. Changes in the mandible and the mandibular dentition can be displayed by superimposing serial tracings on internal structures of the mandible (from McNamara[55]).

orthognathic surgery patient) is made easier. The percentage of cephalometric enlargement must be known if normative data are to be used correctly.

This method of analysis is more sensitive to vertical changes than is an analysis that relies on the ANB angle, such as that of Steiner.[22–24] As mentioned earlier, the use of the ANB angle can be misleading, as it tends to be insensitive to the vertical component of jaw discrepancies. Similarly, changes in growth pattern, which include both horizontal and vertical adaptations, may be missed completely if only a change in the ANB angle is measured.

This analytical procedure also provides guidelines relative to normally occurring growth increments. Therefore, the norms derived from the Bolton Standards, the Burlington Sample, the Ann Arbor Sample, and the composite norms presented can be used to evaluate treatment results. These values have been derived and tested for nearly twenty-five years and appear to be clinically useful in most instances.

Finally, the principles of this analysis are easily explained to non-specialists and to laypersons such as patients and parents. Many times, a simple version of the analysis is used in patient consultation, with only the Frankfort horizontal and the nasion perpendicular drawn on the film. Anteroposterior relationships of the

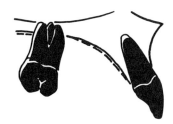

Figure 28-44. Changes in the maxilla and the maxillary dentition can be examined by superimposing serial tracings on internal structures of the maxilla (from McNamara[55]).

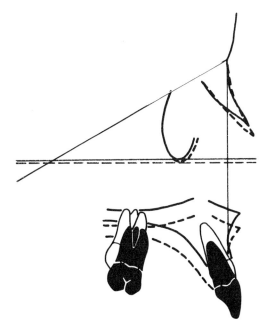

Figure 28-45. The measurement of anteroposterior maxillary displacement can be determined by superimposing serial tracings along the basion-nasion line with superimposition at nasion. During normal growth, nasion and Point A move forward at about the same rate (from McNamara[55]).

maxilla and mandible to the cranial base are described easily by way of this simple construction.

This analysis has proved to be useful in a variety of clinical situations; however, not all possible measurements are included in this analysis. Therefore, variations and additions to the analysis may be made according to the clinical situation. The analysis described provides the clinician with a specific language that assists in the diagnosis, treatment planning, and treatment evaluation of clinical patients.

STEP-BY-STEP PROCEDURE

The previous presentation of this analysis has been conceptual rather than practical. The actual performance of the analysis is carried out in an order based on the actual process of tracing the cephalogram. The following is a description of the systematic procedures involved in completing the static and dynamic parts of the analysis.

Analysis of a Single Film

This part of the procedure is used in diagnosis and treatment planning. The use of the Ricketts template (Dome Orthodontics, Thousand Oaks CA) is recommended when performing the analysis by hand. Definitions of landmarks used are found in Table 28-8. The tracing and measurement of a single headfilm should be carried out in the following sequence.

1. Draw the outline of the soft tissue profile from soft tissue glabella (forehead) to the base of the throat.
2. Identify anatomical porion (the most superior aspect of the external auditory meatus) and orbitale (the most inferior point on the bony orbit).
3. Draw the Frankfort horizontal.
4. Define the bony nasal structures including nasion, the junction of the frontal bone, and the nasal bone.
5. Construct the nasion perpendicular, a line extending vertically downward from nasion perpendicular to the Frankfort horizontal.
6. Define the superior and inferior outlines of the maxilla.
7. Define the outline of the mandible, including the symphysis, the gonial region, the condyle, and the coronoid process.
8. Define the position of the maxillary and mandibular teeth. The most anteriorly positioned incisor should be used, whereas the outline of the molars should be bisected if double images are present. Particular attention should be paid to the mesial and occlusal outlines of the posterior teeth.
9. Measure the following distances:
    a. Point A to the nasion perpendicular (ideal is 0.1 mm)
    b. Point A vertical to the facial surface of the maxillary incisor (ideal is 4-6 mm)
    c. Facial surface of the mandibular incisor to the Point A-pogonion line (ideal is 1–3 mm)
    d. Pogonion to the nasion perpendicular (ideal: small, −8 to −6 mm; medium, −4 to 0 mm; large, −2 to 4 mm)
10. Identify the pterygomaxillary fissure and basion.
11. Construct:
    a. The basion-nasion line
    b. The facial plane (nasion-pogonion)
    c. The mandibular plane (gonion-menton)
12. Construct the facial axis by connecting the most posterosuperior aspect of the pterygomaxillary fissure (PTM point) with constructed gnathion, the intersection of the facial and mandibular planes.
13. Measure the facial axis angle (basion-PTM-gnathion) and subtract this value from 90°. A value of 0° is normal for this measure. A negative number indicates a vertical direction of facial development; a positive number indicates a horizontal direction of facial development.
14. Measure the angle between the mandibular plane and the Frankfort horizontal plane.
15. Identify condylion (the most posterosuperior point on the condylar outline).
16. Measure the effective midfacial length from condylion to Point A and the effective mandibular length from condylion to anatomical gnathion. All normative values include an eight percent enlargement factor.
17. Subtract the effective midfacial length from the effective mandibular length, determining the maxillomandibular differential (ideal: small, 20 mm; medium, 25–27 mm; large, 30–33 mm).
18. Identify anterior nasal spine and menton. Measure the distance between these two landmarks (ideal: small, 60–62 mm; medium, 65–67 mm; large, 70–73 mm).
19. Define the posterior pharyngeal wall, the soft palate, and the posterior border of the tongue.
20. Bisect the distance from posterior nasal spine to the tip of the soft palate. Measure the closest distance from the anterior half of the soft palate to the posterior pharyngeal wall (measurements of 3 mm or less are of interest).

CEPHALOMETRIC EVALUATION

21. Identify the intersection point between the posterior outline of the tongue and the inferior border of the mandible (near the gonial angle).
22. Measure the distance from this intersection point to the posterior pharyngeal wall. Average values are 10–12 mm; any value over 15–16 mm is of interest. Larger than normal values usually are accompanied by an enlarged tonsil that typically can be observed radiographically.

Table 28-8. Landmark definitions (After Daskalogiannakis[57] and Rakosi[58]).

Anterior Nasal Spine (ANS): The tip of the bony anterior nasal spine at the inferior margin of the piriform aperture.

Basion (Ba): The most anterior-inferior point on the margin of the foramen magnum.

Condylion (Co): The most posterior-superior point on the head of the mandibular condyle.

Gnathion (Gn): The most anterior-inferior point of the chin. Constructed gnathion is formed at the intersection of the mandibular plane (Go-Me) and the facial plane (Na-Pog). Anatomical gnathion lies on the contour of the chin at the point of intersection of the facial axis (PTM-Constructed Gn).

Gonion (Go): The most posterior-inferior point on the outline of the mandible. Constructed gonion lies at the intersection of lines tangent to the posterior margin of the ascending ramus and to the lower border of the mandible.

Menton (Me): The most inferior point of the mandibular symphysis. It is formed at the line of intersection of the mandibular plane.

Nasion (Na): The intersection of the internasal and frontonasal sutures.

Orbitale (Or): Lowermost point on the inferior orbital margin.

Pogonion (Pog): Most anterior point of the bony chin. Formed at the point of contact of the facial plane with the chin contour.

Point A: The deepest point in the curved bony outline from the base to the alveolar process of the maxilla. Usually found adjacent to the maxillary incisor root apex.

Porion (Por): The most superior point on the outline of the external auditory meatus.

Pterygomaxillary Fissure (Ptm): A bilateral inverted teardrop-shaped radiolucency, whose anterior border represents the posterior surfaces of the tuberosities of the maxilla. The landmark is taken on the posterior-superior point on the contour of the pterygomaxillary fissure.

Analysis of Serial Films

As mentioned earlier, the four-point superimposition of Ricketts[27,28] is used in the analysis of longitudinal records. The sequence of superimposition is important, as each superimposition acts as a check to make sure that the tracings are completed correctly. It also is important that the two films are traced at the same time, so that tracing standardizations can be imposed.

The first superimposition is based on the internal structures of the maxilla (Fig. 28-44). This superimposition determines the amount of tooth movement relative to the skeletal part of the maxilla, and it ensures that the maxillary teeth have been traced similarly in the two films. For example, intrusion of the maxillary molars would not be observed in the second film unless therapy undertaken involves intrusion; however, improper tracing of the position of the molars in either film may not be evident unless this type of superimposition is carried out first.

The amount of maxillary displacement is determined next by superimposing along the basion-nasion line at nasion (Fig 28-45). In this type of superimposition, both the anteroposterior and the vertical displacement of the maxilla become evident.

The next step in the analysis is to superimpose the tracings on the internal structures of the mandible (Fig. 28-43). Usually, the inferior alveolar canal or the lingual border of the symphysis (or, in young patients, the third molar crypt) can be identified.

Only after the first three regional superimpositions have been completed is the overall cranial base superimposition attempted (Fig. 28-42). This composite tracing is carried out by superimposing along the basion-nasion line at PTM point, located arbitrarily at the posterosuperior aspect of the pterygomaxillary fissure. In addition, it is extremely important that the operator concurrently examine the superimposition of the anterior and posteroinferior outlines of the skull from one tracing to another to make sure that the identification of basion and nasion is correct. The cranial base superimposition allows for an overall visualization of the skeletal and dental changes that occur between the two films. Knowledge of normative growth increments allows for precise measurement of the treatment effects that have occurred in the given patient.

CONCLUDING REMARKS

This chapter has attempted to provide the rationale for the cephalometric analysis used routinely in diagnosis and treatment planning. Although the text and figures in the chapter are extensive, the actual analysis, once understood, can be performed relatively quickly, in perhaps 3–5 minutes. The information derived from this analysis appears to provide a reasonable baseline to which other measures can be added, depending on the need of the particular patient.

One point must be stressed here again. This analysis has been presented verbally and published for more than 20 years, and it has been incorporated into most comercially available cephalometric software programs. Yet, many practitioners still do not understand the correct use of the composite norms (Table 28-5). *These norms are not age or gender specific.* Rather, the length and sagittal position of the midface determines a range of mandibular lengths and lower anterior facial heights. The composite norms, however, originally were *derived* in part from values that are age and gender related, as is seen in several of the tables within the chapter.

There is a wide range of facial sizes and shapes that are only generally related to age and gender (*e.g.*, adult males with small facial dimensions, adult females with large facial dimensions). The composite norms simply represent ratios, rather than specific values globally applicable. Thus, when performing the analysis, the position and size of the midface is determined first and adjusted, if necessary; then the other legs of what can be called the diagnostic triangle can be determined. If this analysis is applied properly, that part of the orthodontic diagnosis based on the lateral cephalometric headfilm is straightforward.

REFERENCES

1. McNamara JA, Jr. Components of Class II malocclusion in children 8–10 years of age. Angle Orthod 1981;51:177–202.
2. Ellis E, McNamara JA, Jr. Components of adult Class III malocclusion. J Oral Maxillofac Surg 1984;42:295–305.
3. Ellis E, McNamara JA, Jr. Components of adult Class III open-bite malocclusion. Am J Orthod 1984;86:277–90.
4. Ellis E, McNamara JA, Jr. Cephalometric evaluation of incisor position. Angle Orthod 1986;56:324–44.
5. Ellis E, McNamara JA, Jr. Cephalometric reference planes sella nasion vs. Frankfort horizontal. Int J Adult Orthod Oral Surg. 1988;3:81–87.
6. Ellis E, McNamara JA, Jr, Lawrence TM. Components of adult Class II open-bite malocclusion. J Oral Maxillofac Surg 1985;43:92–105.
7. Lawrence TN, Ellis E, McNamara JA, Jr. The frequency and distribution of skeletal and dental components in Class II orthognathic surgery patients. J Oral Maxillofac Surg 1985;43:24–34.
8. Guyer EC, Ellis E, McNamara JA, Jr, Behrents RG. Skeletal and dental morphological variability in juveniles and adolescents with Class III malocclusions. Angle Orthod. 1986;56:7–30.
9. McNamara JA, Jr, Ellis E. Cephalometric analysis of untreated adults with ideal facial and occlusal relationships. Int J Adult Orthod Orthognath Surg 1988;3:221–31.
10. McNamara JA, Jr, Brust EW, Riolo ML. Soft tissue evaluation of individuals with an ideal occlusion and a well-balanced face. In: McNamara JA, Jr, ed. Esthetics and the treatment of facial form. Ann Arbor: Monograph 28, Craniofacial Growth Series, Center for Human Growth and Development, University of Michigan, 1993.
11. McNamara JA, Jr, Bookstein FL, Shaughnessy TG. Skeletal and dental changes following functional regulator therapy on Class II patients. Am J Orthod 1985;88:91–110.
12. McNamara JA, Jr, Howe RP, Dischinger TG. A comparison of the Herbst and Fränkel appliances in the treatment of Class II malocclusion. Am J Orthod Dentofac Orthop 1990;98:134–44.
13. Chang JY, McNamara JA, Jr, Herberger TA. A longitudinal study of skeletal side-effects induced by rapid maxillary expansion. Am J Orthod Dentofac Orthop 1997;112:330–337.
14. McGill JS, McNamara JA, Jr. Treatment and post-treatment effects of rapid maxillary expansion and facial mask therapy. In: McNamara JA, Jr, ed. Growth modification: what works, what doesn't and why. Ann Arbor: Monograph 36, Craniofacial Growth Series, Center for Human Growth and Development, University of Michigan, 1999.
15. Bussick TJ, McNamara JA, Jr. Dentoalveolar and skeletal changes associated with the pendulum appliance. Am J Orthod Dentofac Orthop 2000;117:333–343.
16. Toth LR, McNamara JA, Jr. Treatment effects produced by the twin block appliance and the FR-2 appliance of Frankel compared to an untreated Class II sample. Am J Orthod Dentofac Orthop 1999;116:597–609.
17. McNamara JA, Jr. Influence of respiratory pattern on craniofacial growth. Angle Orthod 1981;51:269–300.
18. Long RE, Jr., McNamara JA, Jr. Facial growth following pharyngeal flap surgery: skeletal assessment on serial lateral cephalometric radiographs. Am J Orthod 1985;87:187–96.
19. Downs WB. Variation in facial relationships: Their significance in treatment and prognosis. Am J Orthod 1948;34:812–840.
20. Downs WB. The role of cephalometrics in orthodontics case analysis and diagnosis. Am J Orthod 1952;38:162–182.
21. Downs WB. Analysis of the dento-facial profile. Angle Orthod 1956;26:191–212.
22. Steiner CC. Cephalometrics for you and me. Am J Orthod 1953;39:729–755.
23. Steiner CC. Cephalometrics in clinical practice. Angle Orthod 1959;29:8–29.
24. Steiner CC. The use of cephalometrics as an aid to planning and assessing orthodontic treatment. Am J Orthod 1960;46:721–735.
25. Tweed CH. Evolutionary trends in orthodontics: Past, present, and future. Am J Orthod 1953;39:81.
26. Tweed CH. The Frankfort-mandibular incisor angle (FMIA) in orthodontic diagnosis, treatment, planning, and prognosis. Angle Orthod 1954;24:121–169.

27. Ricketts RM. The influence of orthodontic treatment on facial growth and development. Angle Orthod 1960;30: 103–133.
28. Ricketts RM. Perspectives in the clinical application of cephalometrics. The first fifty years. Angle Orthod 1981; 51:115–50.
29. Ricketts RM, Bench RW, Hilgers JJ, Schulhof R. An overview of computerized cephalometrics. Am J Orthod 1972;61:1–28.
30. Jenkins DH. Analysis of orthodontic deformity employing lateral cephalostatic radiography. Am J Orthod 1955; 41:442–452.
31. Johnston LE, Jr. A statistical evaluation of cephalometric prediction. Angle Orthod 1968;38:284–304.
32. Jacobson A. The "Wits" appraisal of jaw disharmony. Am J Orthod 1975;67:125–38.
33. Jacobson A. Application of the "Wits" appraisal. Am J Orthod 1976;70:179–89.
34. Wylie WL, Johnson EL. Rapid evaluation of facial dysplasia in hte vertical plane. Angle Orthod 1952;22:165–181.
35. Coben SE. The integration of facial skeletal variants. Am J Orthod 1955;41:407–434.
36. Sassouni V. A classification of skeletal facial types. Am J Orthod 1969;55:109–23.
37. Sassouni V. The Class II syndrome: differential diagnosis and treatment. Angle Orthod 1970;40:334–41.
38. Jarabak JR, Fizzel JA. Technique and treatment with lightwire edgewise appliance. St Louis: CV Mosby, 1972.
39. Bimler HP. The Bimler cephalometric analysis. Wiesbaden: 1973.
40. Enlow DH, Moyers RE, Hunter WS, McNamara JA, Jr. A procedure for the analysis of intrinsic facial form and growth. An equivalent-balance concept. Am J Orthod 1969;56:6–23.
41. McNamara JA, Jr. A method of cephalometric evaluation. Am J Orthod 1984;86:449–69.
42. Baumrind S, Frantz RC. The reliability of head film measurements. 1. Landmark identification. Am J Orthod 1971; 60:111–27.
43. Harvold EP. The activator in interceptive orthodontics. St. Louis: CV Mosby, 1974.
44. Woodside DG. Cephalometric roentgenography. In: Clark J, ed. Clinical Dentistry. Philadelphia: WB Saunders, 1975.
45. Broadbent BH, Sr, Broadbent BH, Jr, Golden WH. Bolton standards of dentofacial developmental growth. St. Louis: CV Mosby, 1975.
46. Scheideman GB, Bell WH, Legan HL, Finn RA, Reisch JS. Cephalometric analysis of dentofacial normals. Am J Orthod 1980;78:404–20.
47. Miyajima K, McNamara JA, Jr, Kimura T, Murata S, Iizuka T. Craniofacial structure of Japanese and European-American adults with normal occlusions and well-balanced faces. Am J Orthod Dentofac Orthop 1996; 110: 431–8.
48. Behrents RG, McNamara JA, Jr. Cephalometric values derived from the Bolton Standards. Unpublished data, 1978.
49. Linder-Aronson S, Woodside DG, Daigle DJ. A longitudinal study of the growth in length of the maxilla in boys between ages 6–20 years. Trans Eur Orthod Soc 1975;51: 169–179.
50. Linder-Aronson S. Respiratory function in relation to facial morphology and the dentition. Br J Orthod 1979;6:59–71.
51. Vig PS, Spalding PM, Lints RR. Sensitivity and specificity of diagnostic tests for impaired nasal respiration. Am J Orthod Dentofac Orthop 1991;99:354–60.
52. Trotman CA, McNamara JA, JR, Dibbets JMH, Van der Wheele LT. Association of lip posture and the dimensions of the tonsils and sagittal airway with facial morphology. Angle Orthod 1997;67:425–432.
53. Warren D. Personal communication, 1987.
54. Warren D. In: McNamara JA, Jr, ed. The enigma of the vertical dimension. Monograph 37, Craniofacial Growth Monograph Series, Center for Human Growth and Development, The University of Michigan, Ann Arbor, 2000.
55. McNamara JA, Jr. Dentofacial adaptations in adult patients following functional regulator therapy. Am J Orthod 1984;85:57–71.
56. McNamara JA, Jr. An orthopedic approach to the treatment of Class III malocclusion in young patients. J Clin Orthod 1987;21:598–608.
57. Daskalogiannakis J. Glossary of orthodontic terms. Chicago: Quintessence, 2000.
58. Rakosi T. An atlas and manual of cephalometric radiography. London: Wolfe Medical Atlases, 1982.

Chapter 29

ORTHODONTICS, OCCLUSION, AND TEMPOROMANDIBULAR DISORDERS

With Donald A. Seligman and Jeffrey P. Okeson

In 1987, the orthodontic community was shocked and dismayed at the outcome of a malpractice trial in Michigan in which the jury held that the treatment of a 16-year-old female by an orthodontist* led to temporomandibular (TM) dysfunction in the patient, resulting in a million dollar judgment against the clinician.[1] This event, together with the outcomes of several other jury trials throughout the United States in the late 1980s dealing with the same issue, raised the awareness of the dental profession in general and the specialty of orthodontics in particular to the rela-tionship of orthodontic treatment and occlusal factors to temporomandibular disorders (TMD).

Although temporomandibular joint disorders had long been recognized by orthodontists as clinical problems, relatively little emphasis had been placed on this subject by the practicing orthodontist until the occurrence of this series of events. This litigious climate stimulated the *American Association of Orthodontists* not only to sponsor a series of risk management teleconferences and newsletters, but also to underwrite research concerning the relationship of orthodontic treatment and related occlusal factors to TMD. The last decade has seen rapid increase in both the number and quality of clinical studies dealing with the relationship between orthodontics, occlusion, and TMD.

This chapter represents an evolution of a solicited manuscript first presented at the *International Workshop on the TMDs and Related Pain Conditions*, which was sponsored by the National Institutes of Health in 1994. The original version of this review[2] considered the broad topic of the relationship of occlusal factors and orthodontic treatment to temporomandibular disorders. A second iteration of this effort,[3] which focused only on the orthodontic/TMD interface, was presented at the *1996 NIH Technology Assessment Conference on the Management of Temporomandibular Disorders*. This work has been expanded further and, by request, has been published in other areas of dentistry as well.[2,4] This review has been updated further as the basis of this chapter.

The purpose of this chapter, therefore, is to explore the topic of TMD as it relates to orthodontic treatment and the occlusion. An attempt also is made to correct some occlusal misconceptions about TMD and orthodontics/orthognathic treatment. These misconceptions have been maintained by popular beliefs that are not sustained in current literature. Thus, it is the intent of this chapter to put the subject of occlusion into its proper perspective relative to current knowledge about role of occlusal factors in TMD.

ORTHODONTIC TREATMENT AND TMD

During the last half century, a number of prominent orthodontic clinicians and researchers have had a keen interest in the diagnosis and treatment of temporomandibular disorders, primarily as specific clinical entities, rather than simply as an aspect of routine orthodontic

---

*It should be remembered that the original complaint also included an oral and maxillofacial surgeon who had extracted the patient's four third molars and who settled out of court before the trial.

treatment. Thompson[5-7] was one of the earliest pioneer orthodontists in TMD recognition and therapy. He noted that patients with disturbances in the vertical dimension appeared to be more prone to temporomandibular joint problems. Thompson stressed the establishment of normal vertical dimensions, especially in deep bite patients, and advocated the elimination of all interferences in the "freeway space" envelope of mandibular movement.

Graber[8,9] was one of the first to call attention to the multifactorial nature of TMD, with occlusion being only one factor. Graber cited stress and uncontrolled nocturnal parafunction as contributing factors. He cautioned against treatments using strict gnathological concepts, stating that the articulator cannot properly emulate TMJ function and condylar position. His treatment recommendations extended beyond the narrow confines of the dentition, with stress control and psychological counseling being components of the therapy.

Ricketts,[10-13] who developed a cephalometric laminographic technique to evaluate the temporomandibular articulation, conducted one of the largest early patient studies. He evaluated the temporomandibular joint regions of over 400 individuals and used the range of variation found in 50 patients with "satisfactory occlusions" as a basis for comparison of individual pathologic conditions. Ricketts also stressed the role of the musculature in the determination of condylar position relative to the glenoid fossa.[13]

In spite of the interest in TMD among a few prominent orthodontic clinicians, prior to the late 1980s orthodontists typically did not focus on TMD problems in their patients, except in instances of severe clinical problems. Traditionally, scant mention was made of TMD treatment in the curricula of graduate programs in orthodontics, and only cursory examinations of the temporomandibular joint region were conducted in routine orthodontic clinical examinations. In addition, before the mid-1980s only a limited number of methodologically sound clinical studies regarding the relationship between orthodontic treatment and the TMDs had been published, at least as judged by current standards of clinical research. The last decade of the twentieth century, however, saw an explosion of new information regarding orthodontics and TMD.

Early Clinical Studies

In a comprehensive review of the literature on this subject published between 1966 and 1988, Reynders[14] divided 91 publications into three categories: viewpoint articles, case reports, and sample studies. The most numerous were *viewpoint articles* (N=55), publications that usually were anecdotal in nature, stating the opinion of the author regarding the orthodontic-TMD relationship. Little or no data were presented to support the author's opinion. Further, Reynders[14] notes that 23 of the 55 viewpoint articles were published in *The Functional Orthodontist*, with articles advancing the concept that orthodontic treatment can either cause or cure TMD.

The second most frequent type of article (N=30) was the *case report*, a category of publication that described the influence of certain orthodontic treatment modalities used in one or more patients on the signs and symptoms of TM dysfunction. The least numerous (N=6) were in the third category of *sample studies*, investigations that reported data from large sample groups. These studies were of variable quality, often having the same methodological problems and limitations as discussed previously for studies of occlusal factors. Since 1988, however, a substantial number of clinical investigations have considered the association of orthodontics and temporomandibular disorders.

Recent Clinical Studies

Viewpoint articles, of course, are not suitable for critical evaluation of associations between two entities such as orthodontic treatment and TMD; they are, however, useful in identifying questions that may be worthy of scientific investigation. Although the literature is not as extensive on the relationship of orthodontics to TMD as it is to the occlusal factors/TMD relationship, the questions discussed below have been addressed in a substantial number of recent studies. These reports are discussed in detail below, with many of the investigations considering more than one question.

1. What is the prevalence of signs and symptoms of TMD in orthodontically treated populations?

Numerous epidemiological studies have examined the prevalence of signs and symptoms associated with TMD in a wide variety of subject populations. In general, the prevalence has been shown to be of significance, with an average of 32% reporting at least one symptom of TMD, and an average of 55% demonstrating at least one clinical sign (Table 29-1).

Cross-sectional epidemiological studies of specific adult non-patient populations indicate that at any given time, between 40% and 75% have at least one sign, and about one third report at least one symptom of TMD.[15-20] According to Montegi and co-workers,[21] the point prevalence of symptoms in children and teenagers is lower, about 12–20%.

Table 29-1 Epidemiologic studies of the signs and symptoms of TMD in untreated populations. (Adapted and expanded from Okeson[136])

Author	No. of individuals	No. of women/men	Age (yr)	Population	Prevalence (%) At least one symptom	At least one clinical sign
Nilner and Lassing, 1981[199]	440	218/222	7–14	Swedish children	33	72
Egermark-Eriksson et al., 1981[85]	136	74/62	7	Swedish children	39	33
	131	61/70	11	Swedish children	67	46
	135	59/76	15	Swedish children	74	61
Gazit J et al., 1984[200]	369	181/188	10–18	Israeli children	56	44
Nilner, 1981[201]	309	162/147	15–18	Swedish children	41	77
Swanljung and Rantanen 1979[202]	583	341/256	18–64	Finnish workers	58	86
Solberg et al., 1979[203]	739	370/369	19–25	American University Students	26	76
Pullinger et al., 1988[164]	222	102/120	9–40	Dental hygiene, dental students	39	48
Rieder et al., 1983[204]	1040	653/387	13–86	American private practice	33	50
Ingervall et al., 1980[205]	389	0/389	21–54	Swedish reservists	15	60
Osterberg and Carlsson 1979[206]	384	198/186	70	Retired Swedish	59	37

Because of the longitudinal nature of orthodontic treatment (*e.g.*, 2–3 years for adolescents; 5–7 years for patients starting a two-phase treatment protocol in the early mixed dentition), an understanding of the changes in the signs and symptoms of TMD in a healthy population is essential. Several investigators have reported that signs and symptoms of TMD generally increase in frequency and severity, beginning in the second decade of life.[22–24] Wänman and Agerberg[25] have noted that the incidence of joint sounds (*e.g.*, clicking, popping, crepitus) in young adults in their late teens can be as high as 17.5% over a two-year period. Thus, the occurrence of joint sounds during orthodontic treatment must be considered within the context of longitudinal changes in a comparable untreated population studied during the same time interval.

2. Does orthodontic treatment lead to a greater incidence of TMD?

Two of the first investigations sponsored by the *National Institutes of Health* to consider the relationship between orthodontics and TMD were initiated about 15 years ago (Table 29-2). These research efforts considered the prevalence of TMD and the status of the "functional occlusion" (to be discussed later) in large groups of subjects who had undergone orthodontic treatment at least ten years previously.

Sadowsky and Begole[26] reported on the findings from a University of Illinois study of 75 adult subjects who at least ten years previously had been treated as adolescents with full orthodontic appliances. The treated group was compared to a group of 75 adults with untreated malocclusions. In a subsequent article by Sadowsky and Polson,[27] the sample from the Illinois study (increased to 96 treated and 103 controls) was compared to a treatment group of 111 subjects who had been treated at least 10 years previously at the Eastman Dental Center and a control group of 111 individuals with untreated malocclusions. In the two studies, 15–21% of the subjects presented with one or more sign of TMD and 29–42% had at least one or more symptom of TMD, usually joint sounds. There were no statistically significant differences between the treated and untreated groups.[28] The results of these two studies provide evidence in support of the concept that orthodontic treatment performed during adolescence generally does not increase or decrease the risk of developing TMD later in life.

Another study of the long-term effects of orthodontic treatment was conducted by Larsson and Rönnerman.[29] They evaluated 23 adolescent patients who had been treated orthodontically at least ten years earlier. Eighteen of the patients were treated with fixed appliances, while five patients received activator treatment. Using an index* developed by Helkimo[30] as an evalua-

*Intended as a measure of severity, the Helkimo Dysfunction Index[30] originally was designed to quantify mandibular dysfunction based on subjective and objective measures, lumping all forms of TMD under the umbrella term "TMJ muscle pain dysfunction." Its construct, however, has never been validated. Specifically, the impact of normative data on the dysfunction spectrum captured by the index was not appreciated fully by the field at the time when the index was constructed. Given the heterogeneity of TMD conditions, including the fact that the validity of many of its index items and their measurement reliability are in question, the index no longer receives the attention it once did previously.

Table 29-2 Major studies of the relationship between orthodontic treatment and signs and symptoms of TMD.

Authors	Sample	Appliance	Ext. vs Non-ext.	Relationship
Sadowsky and BeGole, 1980[26]	75 treated 75 untreated	Fixed	No	No
Larsson and Rönnerman, 1981[29]	23 treated	Fixed	No	Improvement
Janson and Hasund, 1981[45]	60 treated 30 untreated	Fixed and Functional	Yes	Improvement
Sadowsky and Polson, 1984[27]	207 treated 214 untreated	Fixed	No	No
Pancherz, 1985[46]	22 treated	Functional	No	No
Dibbets and Van der Weele, 1987[57]	135 treated	72 Fixed 63 Functional	Yes	No
Dahl et al., 1988[31]	51 treated 47 untreated	Fixed Functional	No	No
Smith and Freer, 1989[35]	87 treated 28 untreated	Fixed	No	No
Sadowsky et al., 1991[53]	160 treated	Fixed	Yes	No
Dibbets and Van der Weele, 1991[43]	109 treated	Fixed Functional	Yes	No
Kundlinger et al., 1991[59]	29 treated	Fixed	Yes	No
Luecke and Johnston, 1992[67]	42 treated	Fixed	Yes	No
Årtun et al., 1992[69]	63 treated	Fixed	Yes	No
Kremenak et al., 1992[36]	65 treated	Fixed	Yes	No
Kremenak et al. 1992[37]	109 treated	Fixed	No	No
Egermark and Thilander 1992[84]	402 mixed	Fixed Functional	No	Improvement
Rendell et al., 1992[32]	462 treated	Fixed	No	No
Hirata et al., 1992[39]	102 treated 41 untreated	Fixed	No	No
Wadhwa et al., 1993[33]	31 treated 71 untreated	Fixed	No	No
O'Reilly et al., 1993[207]	60 treated 60 untreated	Fixed	Yes	No
Olsson and Lindqvist, 1995[87]	210 treated	Fixed?	No	Improvement

tive tool, mild dysfunction was recorded in eight patients, whereas one patient had severe dysfunction. Comparing their results to published epidemiological studies, Larsson and Rönnerman[29] stated that comprehensive orthodontic treatment could be undertaken without fear of creating TMD problems.

Dahl and co-workers[31] examined 51 subjects five years after the completion of orthodontic treatment. Signs and symptoms of TMD were noted and compared to the findings from a similar group of 47 untreated individuals. According to the authors, "nobody really had craniomandibular disorders" in either group. Severe symptoms (e.g., difficulties in wide opening, locking, pain on mandibular movement) typically were not observed; however, mild symptoms (e.g., joint sounds, muscle fatigue, stiffness of the lower jaw) were noted more frequently in the untreated group than in the treated group, a difference that was statistically significant. Dahl and co-workers[31] reported that the number of subjects in both groups who had at least one mild symptom was relatively high (70% in the treated group, 90% in the untreated group), especially in comparison to the previously mentioned investigation of Larsson and Rönnerman,[29] who reported a 27% occurrence of mild dysfunction in their treated patients. They stated that differences between samples might be due as much to measuring differences (e.g., lack of factor definition, differences in the interpretation of the criteria of the Helkimo Index) as to a true reflection of differences between groups.

Rendell and colleagues[32] examined 462 patients receiving treatment in an orthodontic graduate clinic (90% adolescents, 10% adults), using a modification of the Helkimo Index. Eleven of the patients presented with TMD signs/symptoms before treatment. During the 18-month study period, none of the patients who had been sign-/symptom-free at the beginning of treatment developed signs or symptoms of TMD. No clear or consistent changes in the levels of pain and dysfunction occurred during the treatment period in those patients with preexisting signs or symptoms. Rendell and co-workers[32] concluded that a relationship could not be established in their patient population between orthodontic treatment and either the onset or the change in severity of TMD signs and symptoms.

Wadhwa and co-workers,[33] also using the Helkimo Index,[30] compared the status of signs and symptoms of TM disorders in three groups of adolescents and young North Indian adults. The groups consisted of 30 persons with normal occlusions, 41 with untreated malocclusions, and 31 with treated malocclusions. The results showed that the normal occlusion group had the maximum number of persons free from any dysfunction, but the differences between the groups in the distribution of persons according to the anamnestic (*i.e.,* health history) and clinical dysfunction indices were not significant. The only statistically significant finding was the difference in the clinical dysfunction index scores of the persons with normal occlusions and untreated malocclusions. According to the anamnestic portion of their study, the most frequently reported symptoms were related to periods of stress. Among the clinical signs and symptoms, the most commonly occurring were crepitations on palpation and sounds on stethescopic auscultation of the joints in all three groups.

Seligman and Pullinger[34] examined two female populations in a multifactorial discriminant analysis that included orthodontic treatment history along with 16 other occlusal, trauma, and demographic variables. Orthodontic treatment history was not a significant contributor to defining the five differentiated patient groups compared to asymptomatic controls.

One of the few clinical studies to report positive findings is the investigation of Smith and Freer[35] who examined 87 patients treated with full orthodontic appliances during adolescence. About two-thirds of the sample had permanent teeth removed as part of the treatment protocol. The treated group was compared to an untreated control group of 28 individuals. Four years following the end of retention, symptoms were found in 21% of the treated group and 14% of the controls, a difference that was not significant statistically. The investigators, however, did note that a single sign was statistically significant, the exception being the association between what they termed "soft clicks" and previous treatment. Soft clicks were found in 64% of the treatment group and 36% of the untreated group. They did not find any difference in joint sounds (*i.e.,* crepitus as determined by stethoscopic examination) between the two groups. In apparent contrast to their findings, the authors concluded the article by stating: "The null hypothesis that there is a significant association between orthodontic treatment and occlusal or joint dysfunction has been rejected by nearly all previously reported studies and continues to be rejected by the present study."

Relatively few prospective studies have examined the relationship of orthodontics to TMD. The two major investigations have been conducted at the University of Groningen in the Netherlands (to be discussed later) and at the University of Iowa.[36-38] In the latter ongoing study, 30 new orthodontic patients have been enrolled annually since 1983. The method of Helkimo[30] was used to collect TMD data prior to orthodontic treatment and at yearly intervals following the completion of treatment. Patients were treated using comprehensive edgewise appliances with and without extractions. No longitudinal data on a comparable untreated population were obtained.

Kremenak and co-workers[37] have reported data from pre-treatment and post-treatment examinations from 109 patients. Data on follow-up examinations from one to six years post-treatment were available on declining sample sizes of 92, 56, 33, 19, 11, and 7 individuals. No significant differences were noted between mean pre-treatment and post-treatment Helkimo Index scores for any of the various groupings. Ninety percent of the patients had Helkimo scores that remained the same or improved, and 10% had scores that worsened (an increase of 2–5 Helkimo points.[30]). Kremenak and colleagues[36-38] concluded that the orthodontic treatment experienced by their sample was not an important etiologic factor for TMD.

Hirata and co-workers[39] examined 102 patients before and after orthodontic treatment for signs of TMD. Findings from this group were compared to findings from 41 untreated subjects matched for age. The incidence of TMD signs for the treatment and control groups was not significantly different.

Pocock and colleagues,[40] using an anamnestic questionnaire, similarly found no differences between an orthodontically treated population when compared with various normative populations. Further, they noted no significant differences between scale scores of various combinations of malocclusions or treatment subgroups of the treated patients.

3. Does the type of appliance (e.g., fixed vs. functional; orthodontic vs. orthopedic) make a difference?

In the other major longitudinal study of this subject, Dibbets and colleagues[41-44] followed 171 patients, 75 of whom were treated using the Begg technique (most patients had extractions as part of their treatment protocol). Sixty-six patients were treated using activator therapy, and 30 patients were treated with chin cups. The *pretreatment* records revealed a strong dependence of the prevalence of signs and symptoms on age: from 10% at age 10 years, signs increased to 30%, while symptoms increased to over 40% at age 15 years. They also noted that at the end of treatment, the fixed appliance group had a higher percentage of objective symptoms than did the functional group, but no differences existed at the twenty-year follow-up.[44]

Janson and Hasund[45] conducted a similar study of adolescent patients with Class II, division 1 malocclusion who were examined five years out of retention. Thirty patients underwent a two-phase treatment regimen (headgear/activator therapy followed by fixed appliances) without the removal of teeth, whereas thirty patients were treated with fixed appliances following the removal of four premolars. An additional thirty untreated subjects were used as controls. One or more symptoms were reported in about 42% of the subjects overall (treated and untreated), with similar findings for the clinical dysfunction index.

One prospective study examined the effect of functional mandibular advancement in patients with Class II, division 1 malocclusions. Pancherz[46] used the banded Herbst appliance alone in 22 adolescent patients with Class II, division 1 malocclusions during a treatment period of six months. Following an initial incisal edge-to-edge bite registration, Pancherz reported that a number of patients complained of muscle tenderness during the first three months of treatment. At 12 months following treatment, however, the number of subjects with symptoms was the same as before treatment.

4. Does the removal of teeth as part of an orthodontic protocol lead to a greater incidence of TMD?

Viewpoint articles and texts, publications that are long on opinion and short on data, have strongly associated the extraction of premolars with the occurrence of TMD in orthodontic treatment.[47-52] In contrast, the clinical studies that have dealt with this issue have not shown a relationship between premolar extraction and TMD. For example, Sadowsky and co-workers[53] reported findings on 160 patients, 54% of whom were treated using extraction treatment strategies. Joint sounds were monitored before and after treatment in 87 extraction patients and 68 non-extraction orthodontic patients. Before treatment, 25 percent of patients had joint sounds whereas 17 percent had sounds after treatment. Similarly, 14 percent of patients had reciprocal clicking; only eight percent had clicking after treatment. The investigators concluded that their findings did not indicate a progression of signs and symptoms to more serious problems during treatment. They also reported no increase in the risk of developing joint sounds regardless of whether teeth were removed or not.

The long-term effect of extraction and non-extraction edgewise treatments were compared in 63 patients from St. Louis University with Class II, division 1 malocclusions who were identified by discriminant analysis as being equally susceptible to the two treatment strategies.[54,55] In terms of a menu of 62 signs and symptoms (*e.g.*, muscle palpation, joint function) that commonly are thought to be characteristic of TMD, there were no differences between extraction and non-extraction samples. A follow-up study by Luppanapornlarp and Johnston[56] that examined an additional 62 "clear-cut" patients (those in the tails of the distribution) also noted that both extraction and non-extraction samples demonstrated similar findings.

The longitudinal studies at the University of Iowa also have addressed the extraction/non-extraction question. Kremenak and colleagues[36] followed three groups of patients: 26 patients treated non-extraction, 25 patients with four premolars extracted and 14 patients with two maxillary premolars extracted. No significant intergroup differences between mean pretreatment or post-treatment Helkimo Index[30] scores were noted. A small but statistically significant improvement in Helkimo scores was observed post-treatment in both the non-extraction group and the four premolar extraction group.

Dibbets and Van der Weele[43] followed 111 of the original 172 orthodontic patients in the University of Groningen study over a fifteen-year period. In this group, a non-extraction approach was used in 34% of the patients, four premolars were extracted in 29% and other extraction patterns were used in the remaining 37%. Functional appliances were used in 39%, fixed appliances (Begg) were used in 44%, and chin cups were used in 17% of the patients. Symptoms increased from 20% to 62%; signs of clicking and crepitus increased from 23% to 36% after four years and then stabilized. In contrast to the finding from the first ten years,[57] during which there was no difference between the three treatment groups with regard to clicking, after 15 years[43] this symptom was seen more often in the premolar extraction group. The authors noted, however, that clicking was higher in the premolar extraction group before treatment was started and concluded that the original growth pattern, rather than the extraction protocol, was the most likely factor responsible for the TMD complaints seen many years post-treatment. These investigators also noted that for a substantial number of patients, symptoms of TMD appeared and disappeared during the course of study. At the twenty-year follow-up,[44] however, the difference between groups had disappeared completely. They also noted that even though the overall incidence of symptoms increased with time, many previously symptomatic children were found to have become asymptomatic at the time of subsequent evaluations.

O'Reilly and co-workers[58] examined 60 treated patients and 60 untreated subjects who were the siblings nearest in age to the orthodontic patients. The patients underwent fixed orthodontic treatment that included extraction and the wearing of Class II intermaxillary elastics. No differences were seen between the treated and untreated groups. Kundlinger and colleagues[59] compared 29 extraction-orthodontically treated and 29 untreated subjects with regard to condylar position, using tomograms and electromyography of some of the muscles of mastication. No differences were observed between groups.

Another specific concern expressed in viewpoint articles is that orthodontic treatment involving the extraction of first premolars causes a decrease in the vertical dimension of occlusion. Staggers[60] examined the records of 45 Class I non-extraction patients and 38 Class I first premolar extraction patients. The pre-treatment and post-treatment cephalograms were analyzed to evaluate the vertical changes occurring as a result of orthodontic treatment. Statistical analysis of the data revealed no significant differences between the vertical changes occurring in the extraction and non-extraction groups. On average, the vertical dimension increased in both extraction and non-extraction treatment groups.

Although not a study that specifically concerned orthodontic patients, the previously cited investigation of Pullinger and colleagues[61] also considered the association of missing teeth to signs and symptoms of TMD. The interaction of eleven occlusal factors, including missing teeth, was evaluated in five randomly collected but strictly defined diagnostic groups compared to asymptomatic normals. A multiple logistic regression model was used for simultaneous assessment of the relative odds of each potential occlusal factor, with the outcome always the disease classification compared to the asymptomatic controls. Based on this analysis, Pullinger and co-workers[62] reported that the contribution of the extraction of two to four teeth *per se*, for example as part of an orthodontic treatment protocol, was negligible in most patients when other variables were controlled.

5. Can orthodontic treatment lead to a posterior displacement of the mandibular condyle?

A number of viewpoint articles have asserted that a wide variety of traditional orthodontic procedures (*e.g.*, premolar extraction, extraoral traction, retraction of maxillary anterior teeth) cause TMD signs and symptoms by producing a distal displacement of the condyle.[47,63–65] This allegation is contradicted by the gnathologist's view of condylar position, a topic that will be considered in the next section.

Gianelly and co-workers[66] used corrected tomograms to evaluate condylar position prior to beginning orthodontic treatment in 37 consecutive patients ages 10 to 18 years and compared them with tomograms from 30 consecutively treated patients treated with fixed appliances (edgewise or Begg) and the removal of four premolars. No differences in condylar position were noted between groups. The position of the condyle tended to be centered within the glenoid fossa, but wide variation in condylar position was noted in both groups.

Luecke and Johnston[67] evaluated the pre-treatment and post-treatment cephalograms of 42 patients treated with fixed appliances in conjunction with the removal of two maxillary premolars. The results of this study indicated that the majority of patients (about 70%) undergo a forward mandibular displacement and a slight opening rotation of the mandible. The remainder of the sample had distal movement of the condyle. Incisor changes were essentially unrelated to condylar displacement during treatment. Luecke and Johnston[67] stated that a change in the spatial position of the mandible is a function of changes in the anteroposterior position of the occluding buccal segments, rather than the relatively non-occluding incisors. These observations also are supported by the findings of Tallents and co-worker.[68]

The recall studies of Beattie and co-workers[55] and Luppanapornlarp and Johnston[56] reported no differences between groups with regard to TMD signs and symptoms. They also noted that both extraction and non-extraction treatments produced a mean anterior displacement of the mandible.

Årtun and colleagues[69] also investigated the relationship of orthodontic treatment to posterior condylar displacement. Sixty-three female patients were evaluated after comprehensive fixed appliance treatment (29 with extraction, 34 without extraction). Condylar position was measured in percent anterior and posterior displacement from absolute concentricity, based on sagittally corrected tomograms. The investigators noted a mean difference in condylar position between the two treatment groups, but the difference was due mainly to the occurrence of *presumed* anteriorly displaced condyles in the non-extraction group (data on the pre-treatment position of the condyles were not obtained). They also noticed that the condyles in patients with clicking were in a more posterior position, although there was a wide variation of condylar position in all samples. This variation also extended to different tomographic sections within the same condyle. These researchers concluded that posterior condyle position was not a result of orthodontic treatment.

6. Should the occlusions of orthodontic patients be treated to specific gnathologic standards?

Several viewpoint articles, including those by Roth,[70-73] and Williamson[74] have maintained that temporomandibular disorders may result from a failure to treat orthodontic patients to gnathologic standards that include the establishment of a "mutually protected occlusion" and proper seating of the mandibular condyle within the glenoid fossa (in contrast to the more anterior position of the condyle advocated by the so-called "functional orthodontists"). The gnathologists claim that non-functional occlusal contacts, when introduced through orthodontic treatment, can lead to signs and symptoms of TMD.

The discussion of the relationship of occlusion and malocclusion to TMD presented earlier in this paper illustrates the lack of association between most occlusal factors and TMD. Pullinger and co-workers[61] reported that small occlusal slides, mostly less than one millimeter, are common in asymptomatic subjects as well as TMD patients. Only when a slide between retruded contact position (RCP) and intercuspal position (ICP) becomes extreme (5 mm or greater) does the odds ratio (*i.e.*, chance) for TMD become elevated. Thus, a modest slide following orthodontic treatment typically is within the adaptive capabilities of most patients.

Sadowsky and Begole[26] and Sadowsky and Polson[27] evaluated the prevalence of non-functional occlusal contacts in patients at least ten years after orthodontic treatment. They noted a high incidence of such occlusal contacts in both orthodontic and control groups. Similar findings have been reported by Cohen[75] and Rinchuse and Sassouni,[76] among others.

Hwang and Behrents[77] investigated the effects of orthodontic treatment on centric discrepancy between ICP and RCP. Thirty-six individuals who had received orthodontic treatment were compared to 30 subjects who had received no treatment. After using a leaf gauge to record centric position, centric slide and centric prematurity were recorded using an articulator and a mandibular position indicator. No differences were noted in the amount or direction of centric slide between the orthodontic and control groups. The authors concluded that orthodontic treatment generally does not result in an increase in centric discrepancy.

It probably is prudent to establish morphological treatment goals that mimic what is observed in untreated occlusions that have been judged normal or ideal, such as the "six keys of ideal occlusion" advocated by Andrews,[78,79] and to treat a patient so that there is a minimal (<2 mm) slide between RCP and ICP. The establishment of an occlusion that meets gnathologic ideals, however, probably is unnecessary, particularly in adolescent patients. Sometimes the attainment of a gnathologic ideal may be impossible in certain adult patients.

7. Does orthodontic treatment prevent TMD?

This last topic is the most difficult to investigate, given the prevalence of signs and symptoms of TMD in healthy individuals and the many types of orthodontic treatment philosophies, goals, and techniques in existence today. The question of whether orthodontic treatment can prevent TMD is complicated further by many of the unsubstantiated viewpoint articles that claim preventive capabilities of non-extraction treatment, functional appliances, and some of the more non-traditional orthodontic treatment protocols (*e.g.*, second-molar extraction and third-molar "replacement") that have been advocated vigorously.[49,51,63,80-82]

As discussed above, most studies that have compared treated and untreated populations have found no differences between groups in the occurrence of TMD signs and symptoms. One of the few investigations that found improved TMD health in a treated group was the sample studied by Magnusson and co-workers[83] and Egermark and Thilander.[84] These investigators re-evaluated at five and ten years, respectively, a group of 402 children and adolescents who originally had been evaluated cross-sectionally by Egermark-Eriksson.[85,86] The sample originally was divided into three groups according to age (7, 11, and 15 years). About one-third of the sample had received orthodontic treatment at the end of the final examination period. Bruxism awareness and subjective symptoms of TMD increased in all age groups, with symptoms slightly more pronounced in untreated individuals. The investigators also noted that clicking recorded at the first examination sometimes disappeared at subsequent examinations and that clicking sometimes appeared at subsequent intervals, regardless of whether or not the subject underwent orthodontic treatment. As in many previous studies, the Helkimo Index[30] was used to measure clinical signs of TMD. The clinical dysfunction index outcome was lower in those undergoing orthodontic treatment than those who had not.

Olsson and Lindqvist[87] conducted a longitudinal study on 245 consecutive prospective patients before and after orthodontic treatment. Of the 245 referred patients, eight declined treatment and 27 moved before the treatment was completed, leaving a sample of 210 patients. Symptoms of temporomandibular disorders were found in 17% of the patients before treatment and in 7% after treatment. The number of subjects without signs or symptoms of TMD increased from 27% before treatment to 46% afterward. According to the scores from the Helkimo Index, 32% of the patients had a moderate and 14% a severe mandibular dysfunction before the start of orthodontic treatment. After treatment, the corresponding figures were 14% and 6%, respectively. The authors concluded that "orthodontic treatment can to some extent prevent further development of and cure temporomandibular disorders."

As mentioned above, a trend toward decreased prevalence of TMD signs and symptoms in treated patients also was noted by Sadowsky and Polson[27] and Dahl and co-workers.[31] The signs and symptoms of TMD in the previously treated orthodontic patients very seldom were so severe that it could be said that these patients suffered from TMD (even if they had signs and symptoms).

Only a very few reports of positive associations between TMD and Class II malocclusions have appeared in the literature.[87-89] A much larger body of research has not identified an association between Angle classification and TMD.[33,90-98] Pullinger and co-workers reported a risk for disc displacement only when the mandibular first molar is at least 9 mm retrusive relative to the maxillary first molar.[61]

Finally, one clinical condition that may be worthy of further investigation is unilateral posterior crossbite in growing children. The relationship of unilateral posterior crossbite to TMD has been studied from several perspectives. Pullinger and co-workers[61] examined five strictly defined patient groups in comparison to asymptomatic controls (the so-called "gold standard"). For a clinically perceptible influence to be significant, Pullinger and co-workers stated that an occlusal feature would need at least to double the risk (*i.e.*, chance) of disease (at least a 2:1 mean odds ratio). Five occlusal conditions reached this threshold, including unilateral posterior crossbite. This occlusal feature, occurring in about 10% of the adult population, posed a greater risk for TMJ derangement. Nearly one-fourth of the non-reducing disc displacement patients included this feature, and the chance that an individual with this type of crossbite also would have TMJ disc displacement *with* reduction was over 3:1. Similar odds ratios were seen for the disc displacement group *without* reduction and in the osteoarthrosis with disc-displacement history patients. The association, however, vanished in two later populations of only female patients,[92] suggesting that the associations may represent another confounding variable.

Nevertheless, Pullinger and co-workers[99] note that the persistence of an elevated risk for disease association into adulthood indicates that the adaptive response in a small percentage of subjects may be less than optimal. This observation leads to the suggestion that functional adaptation to a unilateral posterior crossbite in childhood may occur at the expense of the articular disc through the development of internal derangement, eventually progressing to arthrosis in a small number of patients. These investigators believe that a case can be made for the treatment of children with unilateral crossbites to reduce the adaptive demands on the masticatory system. Conversely, the orthodontic correction of unilateral crossbite in adults to prevent TMJ derangement development probably is not warranted, because skeletal adaptation already has occurred.

Thilander[100,101] has recommended the treatment of posterior crossbite at a young age in order to prevent not only asymmetrical facial growth, but also to prevent unilateral posterior condylar displacement. Based on the results of electromyographic studies of patients with unilateral crossbite that demonstrated muscular hyperactivity on the crossbite side,[102,103] Thilander hypothesized that this condition may influence craniofacial and temporomandibular joint growth unfavorably, the latter region readily affected by changes in the functional environment at a young age. Thilander and colleagues,[104] on the basis of a longitudinal study of early interceptive treatment in children with unilateral crossbite, recommend selective equilibration of the deflecting supracontacts in the deciduous dentition or aggressive expansion treatment in patients with more severe maxillary transverse discrepancies. Although there appears to be some rationale for early correction of unilateral posterior crossbites in growing children, no prospective clinical trial of this type of treatment efficacy has been conducted to date.

OCCLUSAL FACTORS AND TMD

The diagnosis and treatment of temporomandibular disorders (TMD) has been a focus of many in dentistry for much of this century, due in part to the presumed association of TMD to occlusion of the teeth. The assumed strong association between TMD and occlusion has been a major reason that the diagnosis and treatment of these disorders have remained within the purview of dentistry. Numerous etiologic and therapeutic theories are based either partly or completely on this presumed connection and have justified many of the most common treatment approaches.[105] These include occlusal appliance therapy, occlusal adjustment, restorative procedures and combined orthodontic/orthognathic surgical treatment. On the other hand, many types of dental interventions, including routine orthodontic treatment, have been alleged to be causes of TMD.[106]

This emphasis on occlusion is carried over to the most recent Medicare guidelines, which list "malocclusion" as one of the covered temporomandibular joint (TMJ) diagnoses,[107] implying that the occurrence of occlusal variation is itself a disease. Despite much recent debate that suggests a more limited role for occlusal factors in temporomandibular joint pain and dysfunction, the question remains open for many in the field.[3]

There is general agreement among TMD experts that occlusion only has a relatively small role in the etiologically diverse and multifactorial origins of TMD.[107,108] Nevertheless, the influence of occlusion continues to be greatly overrated by practicing dentists and specialists outside the TMD expert circle.[109] This considerable discrepancy between the opinions of practicing dentists and TMD experts on the role of occlusion in the pathophysiology of TMD impacts greatly on the contemporary quality of diagnosis and treatment for these chronic conditions.

Historical Perspective

One of the first practitioners to call attention to the possible relationship of occlusion to temporomandibular joint problems was Costen,[110] an otolaryngologist who noted that many of his patients who had pain in the temporomandibular joint region seemed to benefit from therapeutic alteration of their occlusion, particularly in the vertical dimension. This apparently logical association of mandibular dysfunction to occlusion stimulated some interest within the dental community in the diagnosis and treatment of temporomandibular joint-related problems. Even though most of Costen's original concepts have been discredited, his suggestion of using bite-opening appliances became the treatment protocol of choice for many clinicians.[111,112] During the next decade, however, others began to question the effectiveness of bite-raising appliances,[113–115] and alternative treatments were sought.

In the 1950s and 1960s, there was an increased interest in the treatment of TMD through permanent adjustments of the occlusion.[116–119] At this time, emphasis shifted to masticatory pain disorders, with the etiology of these disorders often related to occlusal "disharmony."[9,120–122]

The diversity and multifactorial nature of the TMDs began to be recognized in the 1960s and 1970s, with the role of stress and other psychological states being acknowledged as contributing factors.[123–126] Later, the role of intracapsular problems, specifically disc interference disorders, was described and clarified,[127–129] as improved diagnostic methodologies (*e.g.*, CT scans, magnetic resonance imaging) became available.

It was only in the 1980s that the breadth of the multifactorial nature of the TMDs was appreciated. Attempts were made to bring together basic scientists and clinicians in interdisciplinary symposia.[130–132] The *American Academy of Orofacial Pain* published and subsequently revised a so-called "white paper" entitled *Craniomandibular* (later *Temporomandibular*) *Disorders: Guidelines for Classification, Assessment, and Management*.[106,133,134] Gradually categories of TMD were defined, and masticatory muscle pain, internal (disk) derangement, and degenerative joint disorders became recognized as distinct and sometimes coexisting conditions.

Thus, the emphasis on occlusal therapies (*e.g.*, occlusal appliances, occlusal adjustment) as singular treatments for TMD gradually has given way to the recognition that temporomandibular disorders are a cluster of related conditions of the temporomandibular joint and the masticatory musculature that have many overlapping symptoms and signs. TMD may be classified further as one of a musculoskeletal disorder subgroup of orofacial pain disorders.[135–137] Orofacial pain patients may suffer from a variety of conditions, including systemic-related problems as well as articular, neuromuscular, neurologic, neurovascular, and behavioral disorders.[106]

Past Clinical Studies

Numerous clinical studies have investigated the relationship of occlusal factors and the signs and symptoms associated with the TMDs in relatively large patient and non-patient (*i.e.*, control) populations (Table 29-3). Some studies reported statistically significant associations, whereas others did not, and few common trends were apparent. For example, Nilner[138] examined 749 juveniles and adolescents and reported that TMD signs and symptoms were associated with centric slides and balancing-side contacts. Egermark-Eriksson and colleagues,[139] after examining a random sample of 402 children, reported that occlusal supracontacts as well as many characteristics of unusual occlusion (*i.e.*, anterior crossbite, anterior open bite, Class II malocclusion, Class III malocclusion) were associated with signs and symptoms of TMD. Similarly, Brandt[140] in a study of 1,342 children noted a positive correlation of overbite, overjet, and anterior open bite with TMD.

In contrast, other investigators have found no such

Table 29-3. Previous studies of the relationship between occlusal factors and TMD. (Adapted and expanded from Okeson[136])

Author	No. of individuals	No. of women/men	Age (yr)	Population	Relationship between occlusion and TMD	Type of occlusal condition related
Williamson and Simmons, 1979[208]	53	27/26	9–30	Orthodontic patients	No	None
DeBoever and Adriaens, 1983[141]	135	102/33	12–68	TMJ pain/dysfunction patients	No	None
Egermark-Eriksson et al., 1983[139]	402	194/208	7–15	Random sample of children	Yes	Occlusal interferences, anterior open bites, anterior crossbite, Class II & Class III
Gazit et al., 1984[200]	369	181/188	10–18	Israeli school children	Yes	Class II, III, crossbite, open-bite, crowding
Brandt, 1985[140]	1342	669/673	6–17	Canadian school children	Yes	Overbite, overjet, open-bite
Nesbitt et al., 1985[209]	81	43/38	22–43	Growth study patients	Yes	Class II, open bite, deep bite
Thilander, 1985[101]	661	272/389	20–54	Random sample in Sweden	Yes	Class III, crossbite
Budtz-Jorgenson et al., 1985[178]	146	81/65	>60	Elderly	Yes	Lost teeth
Bernal and Tsamtsouris, 1986[210]	149	70/79	3–5	American pre-school children	Yes	Anterior cross-bite
Nilner, 1986[102]	749	380/369	7–18	Swedish children adolescents	Yes	Centric slides, non-working contacts
Stringert and Worms, 1986[211]	62	57/5	16–55	Subjects with structural and functional changes of TMJ vs. control	No	None
Riolo et al., 1987[212]	1342	668/667	6–17	Random sample of children	Yes	Class II
Kampe et al., 1987[151]	29		16–18	Adolescents	Yes	Unilateral RCP
Kampe and Hannerz, 1987[93]	225			Adolescents	Yes	Occlusal interferences
Gunn et al., 1988[142]	151	84/67	6–18	Migrant children	No	None
Dworkin et al., 1990[143]	592	419/173	18–75	HMO members	No	None
Pullinger, Seligman and Solberg, 1988[164]	222	102/120	19–41	Dental and dental hygiene students	Yes	Class II div. 2, lack of RCP-ICP slide, asymmetrical slide
Seligman and Pullinger, 1989[191]	418	255/159	18–72	Patients and non patient controls	Yes	Class II div 1, asymmetrical slide, RCP-ICP slides >1 mm, Anterior open bite
Linde and Isacsson, 1990[213]	158	127/137	15–76	Patients with disc displacement and myofascial pain	Yes	Asymmetric RCP-ICP slide, unilateral RCP
Kampe et al., 1991[179]	189		18–20	Young adults	No	None
Steele et al., 1991[96]	72	51/21	7–69	Migraine headache patients	No	None
Takenoshita et al., 1991[214]	79	42/37	15–65	TMD patients	No	None
Pullinger and Seligman, 1991[160]	319	216/103	18–72	Patients and asymptomatic controls	Yes	Increased overjet and anterior open-bite with osteoarthrosis
Wänman and Agerberg, 1991[25]	264	Not given	19	Swedish young adults	Yes	Reduced number of occlusal contact in ICP, long slide length

Table 29-3. (Continued)

Author	No. of individuals	No. of women/ men	Age (yr)	Population	Relationship between occlusion and TMD	Type of occlusal condition related
Cacchiotti et al., 1991[215]	81	46/35	19–40	Patients and non-patient controls	No	None
Egermark and Thilander, 1992[84]	402	194/208	7–15	Swedish students	Yes	RCP-ICP slide length, unilateral RCP, occlusal interferences
Glaros et al., 1992[149]	81		12–36	matched non-TMD patients	No	None
Huggare and Raustia, 1992[150]	32	28/4	14–44	TMD patients and controls	No	None
Kirveskari et al., 1992[187]	237	115/122	5, 10	Finnish children	Yes	Occlusal interferences
Könönen, 1992[95]	104	0/104	18–70	Finnish men with Reiter's Disease and matched controls	Yes	Loss of teeth
Könönen et al., 1992[183]	244	117/127	21–80	Matched groups of rheumatoid arthritis, psoriatic arthritis, ankylosing spondylitis patients and controls	Yes	Longer RCP-ICP slide length, mediotrusive interferences, lost teeth, asymmetric slide
List and Helkimo, 1992[216]	74	58/22	19–71	Myofascial pain patients	No	None
Shian and Chang, 1992[188]	2033	872/1161	17–32	Taiwanese university students	Yes	Balancing interferences, group function, presence of restorations
Al Hadi, 1993[97]	600	189/311		Dental students	Yes	Group function, occlusal interferences, overjet>6 mm
Pullinger and Seligman, 1993[99]	418	287/131	18–72	Patients and asymptomatic controls	No	None (attrition)
Pullinger et al., 1993[61]	560	403/157	12–80	TMD patients differentiated into five disease groups and asymptomatic controls	Yes	Unilateral lingual crossbite, >4 missing posterior teeth, RCP-ICP slide>4 mm, first molars retrusive >8 mm, anterior open bite, overjet >5 mm
Scholte et al., 1993[168]	193	152/41	mean: 33	random TMD patients	Yes	lost molar support
Tanne et al., 1993[154]	305	186/119		Orthodontic patients	Yes	Anterior open bite, crossbite, deep overbite
Wadhwa et al., 1993[33]	102	69/33	13–25	Teenagers and young adults	No	None (Angle Classification)
Keeling et al., 1994[91]	3428	1789/1639	6–12	Florida grade schoolers	No	None
Magnusson et al., 1994[186]	12	78/46	25	Former Swedish students	Yes	Attrition, balancing contacts
Tsolka et al., 1994[152]	61	61/0	20–40	Female TMD patients and matched controls	Yes	Overjet
Vanderas, 1994[153]	386		6–12	Caucasian children	No	None
Bibb et al., 1995[171]	429	249/180	>65	Random elderly	No	None (posterior tooth support)

Table 29-3. (Continued)

Author	No. of individuals	No. of women/men	Age (yr)	Population	Relationship between occlusion and TMD	Type of occlusal condition related
Castro, 1995[148]	63	34/29		TMD patients	Yes	Balancing side interferences
Hochman et al., 1995[184]	96		20–31	Israeli young adults	No	None
Lebbezzo-Scholte et al., 1995[174]	522	423/99	Mean: 34	TMD patients	Yes	Balancing side interferences
Olsson and Lindqvist, 1995[87]				Orthodontic patients	Yes	Angle Class II, div 1, deep bite, anterior open bite
Mauro et al., 1995[98]	125		Mean: 36	TMD patients	No	None
Tsolka et al., 1995[88]	2	80/12	Age matched	TMD patients and controls	Yes	Angle Class II, div 1
Westling, 1995[181]	193	96/97	17	Swedes	Yes	RCP-ICP slides >1 mm
Raustia et al., 1995[217]	49	34/15	Mean: 24	TMD patients and non-patient controls	Yes	Overbite, Asymmetric RCP/ICP slides, midline discrepancy
Seligman and Pullinger, 1996[92]	567	567/0	17–78	Two sets of female TMD patients and asymptomatic controls	Yes	Anterior open bite, unreplaced missing posterior teeth, RCP-ICP slide length, large overjet, laterotrusive attrition
Conti et al., 1996[185]	310	52/48	Mean: 20	High school and university students	No	None
Ciancaglini et al., 1999[175]	483	300/183	Mean: 45	Epidemiological non-patient survey	No	None (posterior support)
Seligman and Pullinger, 2000[145]	171	171/0	Mean: 35	Female patients with intracapsular TMD and asymptomatic controls	Yes	Anterior open bite, crossbite, anterior attrition, RCP/ICP slide length, overjet

associations (Table 29-3), including DeBoever and Adriaens[141] in 135 TMD patients, Gunn and coworkers[142] in 151 migrant children and Dworkin and colleagues[143] in 592 health maintenance organization participants.

Problems with Previous Study Design

The above-mentioned studies exemplify the lack of universal agreement as to the relationship of occlusal factors to the TMDs. These differences in findings can be explained in part, however, by problems in study design. According to Seligman,[144] some of the problems are as follows:

1. *Symptoms are not disease states.* The most common type of study used in TMD research is an investigation of *symptoms*. This approach is problematic because isolated symptoms are not the same as disease. Any actual association of a symptom to a specific disease state may be obscured when only isolated symptoms are monitored. For example, the report of joint clicking would not differentiate disc displacement due to osteoarthrosis from simple soft tissue internal derangement. Similarly, latent muscle tenderness to palpation may reflect problems within a specific muscle group or may be an indication of global chronic fibromyalgia. If the differences among symptoms are subtle, overlapping symptoms can mask distinguishing morphological differences by including too many different pathological processes in the analysis.

2. *Lack of differential diagnosis.* Most investigations have grouped subjects into a single disease *category*

without differentially diagnosing each *patient*. Thus, often it is unclear as to which disease process is being studied. Further, many patient studies are purely descriptive and do not compare patient populations with equivalent populations of healthy individuals.

3. *Unrepresentative samples.* In some studies, the sample population does not represent the target population, particularly with regard to age and gender. For example, it is inappropriate to extrapolate to adults with osteoarthritis or fibromyalgia findings from children who rarely appear as patients with these conditions. The sample should match the target population as much as possible, especially with regard to age and gender.

4. *Lack of factor definition.* The factors being studied must be defined in operational terms, with specific criteria established for each variable. For instance, when multiple occlusal factors are grouped together into an overall variable termed "malocclusion," it is difficult to determine exactly which factors are being investigated. For example, it is risky to assume that factor such as posterior crossbite in one patient has the same impact on the analysis as does a deep overbite in another patient. And if the efficacy of poorly defined occlusal treatments is examined (*e.g.,* occlusal equilibration) and the treatment is focused on the correction of a wide range of occlusal conditions rather than on the elimination of a single condition (*e.g.,* slides between centric occlusion and centric relation), it is impossible to identify which occlusal treatment is responsible for any therapeutic effect.

5. *Inappropriate groupings of data.* Every attempt should be made to consider continuous variables over the entire range of their occurrence. Otherwise, there may be an artificial or arbitrary skewing of the results. Further, the transformation of real data to unvalidated severity scales should be avoided. If a transformation is to be performed, the individual measures in the severity scale must be shown to be roughly equivalent. For example, the number of muscles tender to palpation can be quantified. For this information to be useful, it must be shown that that a certain number of tender muscles is of greater concern than another number, and that there is no threshold of a minimum number of muscles before an effect is noted.

If two or more unrelated symptoms are included in a severity scale (*e.g.,* clicking, crepitus, muscle tenderness), the investigator must prove that the weighted input ascribed to each variable is valid. In addition, if one sign or symptom is emphasized in a given scoring system (*e.g.,* muscle tenderness over clicking), this preference for one type of factor also must be shown to be valid.

6. *Multifactorial analysis not used.* Perhaps the greatest deficiency of past research has been the failure to consider in the methodology the well regarded biophysical tenets of multifactorial influence, multiple factor interactions, and multiple pathways to disease.[109,145] Combinations of factors must be studied together (*i.e.,* multifactorial analysis) rather than separately. Isolated pair-wise or sensitivity-specificity analyses attribute either major responsibility or no significant role to the occlusal factors that they examine. It is obvious that individual occlusal factors do not act in isolation from one another, and without multiple factor analysis, no estimate can be made of the relative impact of each factor in characterizing the condition. This failure has resulted in overly simplistic occlusal models that only explain a small proportion of the disease development or the treatment efficacy.

Conclusions. These observations of Seligman[144] illustrate the necessity of examining previous studies not necessarily on the basis of the conclusions stated by the authors, but rather by the groups studied, the criteria used, and the methods of analysis employed.

Critical Reviews of the Literature

Two of the most comprehensive reviews that have considered the relationship of occlusion to the TMDs have been published by Seligman and Pullinger, one considering *morphological* occlusal relationships[90] and the second *functional* occlusal relationships.[146] These reviews were compiled in an attempt to determine consensus on the roles of various occlusal factors on the pathophysiology of temporomandibular disorders. These investigators considered only original research articles and emphasized those that used appropriate methodology, in particular research that evaluated diagnostic groups or disease states rather than symptoms. The reader is referred to these articles for an in-depth literature review on each subject.

Univariate Analyses of Occlusal Factors: Morphological Occlusal Relationships.

Seligman and Pullinger[90] considered five identifiable factors related to the static occlusion.

1. *Overbite/openbite.* The vertical overlap of the teeth should be considered as a continuous variable. Deep overbite is common in non-patient populations[147] and thus cannot be used to define a patient population. Studies that do not consider overbite as a continuous variable report mixed results, with nearly all reporting no[89,91,92,148–153] or very selective[87,154,155] associations.

There is consensus that minimal overbite in adults is associated with osteoarthrosis.[148] A reduced overbite may be a result of osseous changes in the joint, rather than *vice versa*.

Skeletal anterior openbite is of particular significance. This condition is characterized as a negative vertical overlap of the anterior teeth that often is combined with occlusal contacts only in the molar region. Skeletal openbite is not common in asymptomatic subjects[147,148] and usually is associated with disease states demonstrating intracapsular changes (*e.g.*, osteoarthrosis[92,148,156]). Larheim and co-workers[157] among others have noted that these occlusal changes may be a result, rather than the cause, of these osseous changes. Skeletal anterior open bite in adults should be distinguished from anterior open bite in children that may arise from different causes (*e.g.*, thumb sucking, abnormal tongue posture).

2. *Overjet*. The common dimension of horizontal overlap of the teeth does not seem to be associated with TMJ symptoms or disease.[88,90,93,150,152,158,159] Seligman and Pullinger[90,92,160] note one exception, namely the higher prevalence of large overjet in patients with osteoarthropathies of the temporomandibular joint. Pullinger and Seligman[92,160] found that although larger overjets were associated with osteoarthrosis patients having a prior history of disc derangement, no such association was evident in derangement patients without osteoarthrosis. Despite the association with osteoarthrosis, large overjet is common in non-patient populations as well, and thus this measure lacks specificity in defining patient groups.

3. *Crossbite*. Most previous univariate studies of crossbite have considered younger patient populations.[89,93,103,153,154,161,162] Although asymmetrical muscle activity has been reported in children with unilateral posterior crossbite,[163,164] there is little evidence in pairwise analysis that this type of morphologic relationship leads to TMJ symptomatology.[62,93,153,165] Most patient studies report no greater prevalence of crossbite in patients as compared to non-patients.[89,92,94,152,166,167] Seligman and Pullinger[90] note that crossbites persisting in adults typically are skeletal in origin and do not appear to provoke TMD symptoms or disease. Thus, the correction of crossbite in adults to prevent potential TMD problems does not appear to be warranted.

4. *Posterior occlusal support*. Loss of posterior tooth support has been associated with osteoarthrosis,[92,94,167,168] or inflammatory TMJ arthritis,[95] but this association becomes questionable when the evaluation is controlled for age effects.[169–171] Associations to other patient populations are denied in recent patient studies.[92,168,172–175]

Two of the few researchers to consider the longitudinal relationship of the loss of posterior teeth to the health of the masticatory system have been Käyser[176] and Witter.[177] They have shown that the adaptive capacity of the masticatory system is great, and that most people with loss of molar support have acceptable masticatory function and no increased TMD signs and symptoms. Thus, no conclusions can be drawn regarding the benefits of prosthetically replacing missing posterior teeth as a preventive measure for TMD.

5. *Asymmetrical contact in retruded contact position*. If imbalances of tooth contacts exist in retruded contact position (RCP)/centric relation, they may be most obvious in younger patient populations,[139] and as with a loss of posterior dental support, may be associated with age. Few associations of this occlusal factor and TMD have been reported in older populations.[84,90,93,94,96,153,159,174,178–182] Prophylactic adjustment of the natural occlusion is not indicated on the basis of published studies, but the establishment of bilateral contact in RCP may be a prudent restorative goal.

Functional Occlusal Relationships

Seligman and Pullinger[146] reviewed published research concerning the relationship of the functional movements of the mandible to the TMDs.

1. *Balancing and working occlusal contacts*. Most controlled surveys have failed to demonstrate any association between occlusal supracontacts and TMD signs or symptoms in symptomatic non-patients or in populations of TMD patients,[84,95,96,146,151,152,159,168,174,179,182–185] although a few recent reports of associations to symptoms[97,148,151,186–188] and specific types of arthritis[95,174] have appeared. The consensus of the literature is that an association to disease is absent. Occlusal supracontacts are so common and variable[189] that they lack the sensitivity and specificity for defining a present or potential TMD population. Further, a precise and reproducible method for determining the presence of occlusal supracontacts does not exist.

2. *Slides between centric occlusion and centric relation*. The majority of past univariate research found little association between the length of the slide between RCP/centric relation and ICP/centric occlusion and signs or symptoms of disorders in asymptomatic individuals[92,96,98,152,174,182,183,185] or most TMJ disease.[84,93,153,159,178,179,188] Studies of patients with radiographically-determined osteoarthrosis report longer slides in arthrosis patients than in controls,[92,183,190,191] a finding that indicates that osseous remodeling or condylar lysis can be accompanied by an increased

slide. In most of the studies, the amount of the slide is not handled as a continuous variable, thus adding bias to the interpretation of the data. By consensus, the RCP-ICP slide asymmetry, while more common in patients,[146,155] is not associated with TMJ symptoms[146,153,159,178,179,188] or disease.[92,94,190]

3. *Occlusal guidance pattern.* Whereas there is evidence that occlusal guidance patterns can alter muscle activity levels,[192,193] there is little evidence to suggest that a given guidance pattern can provoke TMD symptomatology.[146,185] Little is known concerning the influence of specific guidance patterns in differentiated patient populations.

4. *Parafunction.* Bruxism and clenching often are cited as etiologic factors in the development of TMD, but similar to occlusal interferences, these activities (especially bruxism) seem to be endemic in the general population.[194] Furthermore, comparisons of groups identified according to self-reports of parafunctional activities are suspect because of the universality of this activity and the lack of agreement about severity measures. Seligman and Pullinger[146] state that there is increasing evidence that parafunction is not associated with chronic TMD, and thus reversible rather than non-reversible treatment should be provided in attempts to prevent or minimize possible harmful effects of this activity.[195]

5. *Dental attrition.* There is no evidence from most non-patient univariate studies that dental attrition is associated with signs or symptoms of TMD[25,93,151,88] or disease.[88,92,96,146] Men show greater attrition severity than women,[196] yet they have fewer TMD symptoms. Once again, patients with osteoarthrosis have the most notable occlusal changes, often demonstrating advanced rates of attrition.[99] These changes may be secondary to the occlusal changes resulting from the arthrosis.

Table 29-4. Occlusal variables considered by Pullinger and co-workers[61]

Anterior open bite
Maxillary lingual posterior crossbite
RCP-ICP slide length
RCP-ICP slide asymmetry
Unilateral RCP contact
Overbite
Overjet
Dental midline discrepancy
Number of missing posterior teeth
First molar relationships (the greater of the mesiodistal maxillary discrepancies at the first molar location)
Right vs. left first molar position asymmetry[145]
Anterior attrition severity
Mediotrusive attrition severity
Laterotrusive attrition severity

Multiple Analysis of Occlusal Factors

The studies cited above considered the significance or non-significance of occlusal factors relative to TMD as isolated factors. Pullinger, Seligman and Gornbein[61,197] used a blinded multifactorial analysis, later confirmed in two independent experimental female populations,[92] to determine the *weighted influence* of each factor acting in combination with the other factors. The interaction of eleven occlusal factors (Table 29-4) was considered in randomly collected but strictly defined diagnostic groups (Table 29-5) compared to asymptomatic controls.

The asymptomatic controls were considered the "gold standard," in that the subjects in this group were without signs and symptoms and had no history of TMD. The samples were representative demographically, and the occlusal factors studied were collected blindly and strictly defined. A multiple logistic regression model was used for simultaneous assessment of the relative odds of each potential occlusal factor. The outcome always was a specific disease classification compared to the asymptomatic controls.

Findings in Healthy Subjects

Wide variation in occlusal features was noted in the asymptomatic control group, including overjet from −1 mm to 6 mm, overbite from −2 mm to 10 mm, midline discrepancies to 5 mm, anteroposterior molar relationships from −6 mm to 6 mm, molar asymmetries from 0 to 6 mm, and RCP-ICP slides up to 2 mm in length. In addition, a wide variety of crossbites, asymmetrical slides, retruded posterior contacts, and severe attrition facets were observed. Skeletal anterior open bite relationships were not observed. Thus, variations in occlusal morphology were found to be the norm in healthy individuals, indicating the capacity of the human masticatory system to adapt to a wide variety of morphological and functional occlusal features.

Pullinger and co-workers[61] proposed a new definition of "normal" within the context of TMD, based on those occlusal features that exist without significant elevated risk of disease. Such "normal" features include RCP-

Table 29-5. The diagnostic groups of Pullinger and co-workers[61]

1. Disc displacement with reduction (N=81)
2. Disc displacement without reduction (N=48)
3. TMJ Osteoarthrosis with disc displacement history (N=75)
4. Primary osteoarthrosis (N=85)
5. Myalgia only (N=124)
6. Asymptomatic normals (N=147)

ICP slides of two millimeters or less, deep overbite to 10 mm, and minimal overjet from 6 mm retrusive to 1 mm protrusive. They also noted midline discrepancies from 0–5 mm, all Angle classifications of malocclusion, moderate to severe attrition facets in all dental locations, less than five missing posterior teeth, and mandibular first molar positions from 6 mm retrusive to 6 mm protrusive of a neutral position. Further, in asymptomatic normals, they found the presence all types of crossbite, asymmetric RCP-ICP slides and unilateral contact in RCP. These factors alone cannot define either TMD patients or asymptomatic normals, because they also are seen in both groups.

Findings in Patient Populations

No single occlusal factor was sufficient to differentiate patients from healthy subjects. There were four occlusal features, however, that occurred mainly in TMD patients and were rare in normals:

- The presence of a skeletal anterior open bite;
- RCP-ICP slides of greater than two millimeters;
- Overjets of greater than four millimeters; and
- Five or more missing and unreplaced posterior teeth.

Unfortunately, all of these signs are rare not only in healthy individuals, but in patient populations as well, indicating the limited diagnostic usefulness of these features.

Pullinger and co-workers[61,92,197] concluded that many occlusal parameters that traditionally were believed to be influential actually accounted for only a minor increase in risk in the multiple factor analysis used in their studies. They reported that although the relative chance of disease was elevated with several occlusal variables, clear definition of disease groups was evident only in selective extreme ranges and involved only a few subjects. Furthermore, the contribution of the occlusal factors diminished in the later study that included additional non-occlusal variables.[61,92] Thus, they concluded that occlusion cannot be considered the most important factor in the definition of TMD.

Pullinger and colleagues[61,92,197] noted, however, that the results of their study indicated that occlusal factors may make a limited contribution to TMD. Combinations of between two and five of the occlusal parameters, involving eight of the eleven factors, contributed to risk for disease, when other non-occlusal factors are not included. These investigators stated that more commonly used statistical methods, such as robust pair-wise testing, would have ignored some of these variables. The minor elevation in the odds ratio revealed by the multiple factor analysis indicates that specific occlusal factors are making some biological contribution and thus cannot be ignored. Pullinger and colleagues[61,92,197] stated further that a biological system must adapt to its various morphological features until stability is achieved, and some occlusal features may place greater adaptive demands on the system. While most individuals compensate without problems, adaptation in others may lead to an increased risk of dysfunction.

Occlusal Risk Factors for TMD

Some occlusal differences between diagnostic groups were reported.[164,197] For a clinically perceptible influence to be significant, Pullinger and co-workers[61] stated that an occlusal feature would need at least to double the risk of disease (at least a 2:1 mean odds ratio). Only the following occlusal conditions reached this threshold:

1. *Anterior open bite.* The highest odds ratio and strongest correlation to disease was for anterior open bite. This occlusal manifestation was seen predominantly in both the osteoarthrosis and the myofascial pain groups, an observation noted previously by Seligman and Pullinger[90] and Stegenga.[198] For anterior open bite to be shown as an etiologic factor in the development of osteoarthritis, some evidence of this occlusal factor should exist in other diagnostic groups thought to be conditions often preceding osteoarthrosis. Anterior open bite, however, was not common in disc displacement disorders, with or without reduction. Furthermore, Pullinger and co-workers[61] noted that most osteoarthrosis and myofascial pain patients did not present with anterior open bite.

2. *Overjets greater than 6–7 mm.* Overjets of greater than 4 mm were associated with the likelihood of osteoarthrosis, as were the anterior open-bite populations. There was no contribution to the TMJ derangement patients.[61,92,197] Pullinger and co-workers[61] stated that some large overjets in adults can be secondary to the condylar repositioning seen with advanced osteoarthrosis. An overjet of 6 mm or larger was needed for a subject to be assigned to one of these disease classifications with an odds ratio of at least 2:1. The occurrence of a progressively increasing overjet in adults should alert the clinician to evaluate a patient for other signs of TMD disease.

3. *RCP-ICP occlusal slides.* Small occlusal slides, mostly under one millimeter, were common in all patient groups and normals, but sagittal slides longer that 2 mm were found in the disease groups only. None of the asymptomatic subjects had occlusal slides greater than 2 mm.

Pullinger and co-workers[61,92,197] found that larger

slides occasionally were associated with degenerative changes within the temporomandibular joint. A slide of 5 mm or greater would be necessary to reach a 2:1 odds ratio threshold for notable risk, and this ratio never was observed in patients. Thus, the effective clinical contribution of this factor was determined to be minimal.

Because an occlusal slide in the range usually seen in patients has not been shown to be a significant contributor to the TMD equation, the prophylactic elimination of most slides through occlusal equilibration procedures is seldom if ever indicated. Even in the presence of symptoms that may appear to be associated with an occlusal slide, the removal of a large discrepancy between centric occlusion and centric relation may not be advisable because the slide may be a consequence of an articular disorder (e.g., primary arthrosis) rather than a result of occlusal factors.

It should be noted that the above three factors which have emerged from the multiple factor analysis have a primary association with diseases characterized by osseous and ligamentous changes within the articular compartments of the temporomandibular joints. Thus, these occlusal factors may in fact be a result, rather than a cause, of these joint changes.

4. *Unilateral maxillary lingual crossbite.* This occlusal feature, occurring in about 10% of the adult population,[147] poses a greater risk for assignment to the TMJ derangement groups. Nearly one-fourth of the non-reducing disc displacement patients exhibited this feature. The chance that an individual with this type of crossbite also would have TMJ disc displacement *with* reduction was over 9:1.[197] Similar odds ratios were seen for the disc displacement group *without* reduction (8:1).

5. *Missing posterior teeth.* In the samples studied by Pullinger and colleagues,[61] extensive posterior tooth loss was not common. Five or more posterior teeth needed to be missing before the odds ratio of assignment to disease groups assumed a minimal critical ratio of 2:1 for osteoarthrosis with disc displacement history and primary osteoarthrosis.[197] Age is associated with both osteoarthrosis[22] and tooth loss;[22] the increase in odds ratio in patients with osteoarthrosis and in patients with more than four missing teeth also may be a reflection of age.

Much of the tooth loss in the patients characterized by disc displacement with reduction, who generally were younger than patients in the osteoarthrosis groups, was due to premolar extraction as part of orthodontic treatment. Pullinger and co-workers[61] noted that the extraction of two to four teeth (e.g., as part of an orthodontic treatment protocol) was a negligible factor in most instances when other variables were controlled. As mentioned earlier, longitudinal studies of patients with multiple missing posterior teeth have shown acceptable masticatory function without increased signs and symptoms of TMD.[176,177]

6. *Anterior Attrition.* In a recent multifactorial study of occlusal plus attrition factors in females with undifferentiated intracapsular TMD,[145] Seligman and Pullinger reiterated that those with disease had longer slides, more unilateral crossbites, and greater anterior attrition. As with the earlier studies, however, the significant factors only accounted for about 30% of the differences; about 70% of the acting influences remained unidentified.

In a complimentary decision tree analysis, patients were defined in one model by either above average anterior attrition levels, or even average levels if below 37 years of age. A second decision tree model associated patients with anterior open bite, overjet greater than 5.25 mm, or RCP-ICP slide lengths greater than 1.75 mm. Although asymptomatic normals were identified accurately by the logistic regression and the classification tree models (specificity >90%), the overlap between diseased individuals and controls for the predominant ranges of the significant variables reduced the sensitivity to an unacceptable 51–63%.

Conclusions. The multifactorial analyses of Pullinger and co-workers[61,92,145,197] have shown that, except for a few defined occlusal conditions, there is a relatively low risk of occlusal factors associated with various types of TMD. In subsequent studies, Seligman[144,145,197] found additional support that the overall contribution of occlusal factors in defining TMD patients probably is from 5 to 30%, which leaves 70–95% of the TMD patient characteristics unexplained by the patient's occlusion.

None of these studies identifies a cause and effect relationship between occlusal factors and TMD. The fact that the correlation coefficients usually are in the 0.3 range, however, explains less than 10% of the variation. In a specific disease condition, the causative agent usually explains 80–90% of the variation.

CONCLUDING REMARKS

This chapter has attempted to review the current literature regarding the relationship of orthodontic treatment to temporomandibular disorders. Although the orthodontic community has had a persistent interest in the association between orthodontics and TMD, this association became a focus of conversation within the dental and legal communities in the late 1980s, resulting in a burst of research activity during the last decade.

The findings of current research on the relationship

of orthodontic treatment to the TMDs can be summarized as follows:

1. Signs and symptoms of TMD occur in healthy individuals;
2. Signs and symptoms of TMD increase with age, particularly during adolescence, until menopause. Thus, temporomandibular disorders that originate during orthodontic treatment may not be related to the treatment;
3. Orthodontic treatment performed during adolescence generally does not increase or decrease the chances of developing TMD later in life;
4. The extraction of teeth as part of an orthodontic treatment plan does not increase the risk of TMD;
5. There is no evidence of an elevated risk for TMD associated with any particular type of orthodontic mechanics;
6. Although a stable occlusion is a reasonable orthodontic treatment goal, not achieving a specific gnathologic ideal occlusion does not result in the development TMD signs and symptoms; and
7. Thus far, there is little evidence that orthodontic treatment prevents TMD, although the role of unilateral posterior crossbite correction in children may warrant further investigation.

In this chapter, we also reviewed the recent literature regarding the interaction of morphologic and functional occlusal factors with the TMDs. We have cited the articles of Seligman, Pullinger and colleagues[61,90,146] as comprehensive reviews of this literature on this subject. Of particular importance is the methodological weakness of previously published studies, particularly with regard to the sample groups studied, the criteria used for evaluation, and the method of analysis employed.

The multiple factor analyses of Pullinger and coworkers[61,145,197] revealed a relatively low association of occlusal factors in characterizing TMD. This association, however, is not zero; several occlusal features characterized the diagnostic groups, albeit at fairly low levels of correlation. They include:

1. Skeletal anterior open bite;
2. Overjets greater than 6–7 mm;
3. RCP/ICP slides greater than 4 mm;
4. Unilateral lingual crossbite;
5. Five or more missing posterior teeth; and
6. Above average anterior attrition.

The factors often are associated with TMJ arthropathies and may be the result of an osseous or ligamentous change within the temporomandibular articulation. Overall, Seligman and Pullinger[144,145,197] estimate that the total contribution of occlusal factors to the multifactorial characterization of TMD patients is no greater than about 5–30%, with other factors, both pronounced and subtle, interacting and providing at least 70–95% of the differences between patients and healthy subjects. These findings are strongly suggestive of multifactorial influences in TMD.

Thus, according to the existing literature, the relationship of the TMDs to occlusion and orthodontic treatment is minor and selective. The important question that remains is how this minor contribution can be identified within the population of TMD patients. Increased efforts should be made toward developing a more complete understanding of these occlusal factors so that reliable criteria can be developed to assist the orthodontist and other dental practitioners in deciding when dental therapy plays a role in the management of TM disorders. Reliable criteria likely would spare many TMD patients significant dental therapies and related health costs. Until such criteria are developed, the dental profession should be encouraged to manage TMD symptoms with reversible therapies, only considering permanently alterations of the occlusion in patients with unique circumstances.

REFERENCES CITED

1. Pollack B. Cases of note: Michigan jury awards $850,000 in ortho case: a tempest in a teapot. Am J Orthod Dentofac Orthop 1988;94:358–359.
2. McNamara JA, Jr, Seligman DA, Okeson JP. The relationship of orthodontic treatment and occlusal factors to the TMDs. In: Sessle B, Bryant PS, Dionne, RA, ed. Temporomandibular disorders and related pain conditions, in: Progress in pain research, Vol 4. Seattle: IASP Press, 1995: 399–428.
3. McNamara JA, Jr. Orthodontics and temporomandibular disorders. Oral Surg Oral Med Oral Path Oral Radiol Endod 1997;83:107–117.
4. McNamara JA, Jr, Seligman DA, Okeson JP. The relationship between occlusion, orthodontics and temporomandibular disorders: Facts and fallacies. In: Hardin JP, ed. Clark's clinical dentistry. Philadelphia: JB Lippencott, 1998.
5. Thompson JR. The rest position of the mandible and its significance to dental science. J Am Dent Assoc 1946;33: 151–180.
6. Thompson JR. Function—the neglected phase of orthodontics. Angle Orthod 1956;26:129–143.
7. Thompson JR. Abnormal function of the stomatognathic system and its orthodontic implications. Am J Orthod 1962;48:758–765.

8. Graber TM. Craniofacial anomalies in cleft lip and palate deformities. Surg Gynec Obstet 1949;88:359–369.
9. Graber TM. Temporomandibular disorders: Concordance and conflict. In: Carlson DS, ed. Craniofacial growth theory and orthodontic treatment. Ann Arbor: Monograph 23, Craniofacial Growth Series, Center for Human Growth and Development, The University of Michigan, 1990.
10. Ricketts RM. Various conditions of the temporomandibular joint as revealed by cephalometric laminography. Angle Orthod 1952;22:98–115.
11. Ricketts RM. Laminography in the diagnosis of temporomandibular joint disorders. J Am Dent Assoc 1953;46:620–648.
12. Ricketts RM. Present status of laminography as related to dentistry. J Am Dent Assoc 1962;65:56–64.
13. Ricketts RM. Occlusion—The medium of dentistry. J Prosthet Dent 1969;21:39–60.
14. Reynders RM. Orthodontics and temporomandibular disorders: a review of the literature (1966–1988). Am J Orthod Dentofac Orthop 1990;97:463–471.
15. Rugh JD, Solberg WK. Oral health status in the United States. Temporomandibular disorders. J Dent Educ 1985;49:398–404.
16. Schiffman E, Friction JR. Epidemiology of TMJ and craniofacial pain. In: Friction JR, Hathaway KM, eds. TMJ and craniofacial pain: Diagnosis and management. St Louis: IEA Publ, 1988.
17. De Kanter RJ, Truin GJ, Burgersdijk RC, Van't Hof MA, Battistuzzi PG, Kalsbeek H. Prevalence in the Dutch adult population and a meta-analysis of signs and symptoms of temporomandibular disorder. J Dent Res 1993;72:1509–1518.
18. Greene CS. Temporomandibular disorders in the geriatric population. J Prosthet Dent 1994;72:507–509.
19. Nourallah H, Johansson A. Prevalence of signs and symptoms of temporomandibular disorders in a young male Saudi population. J Oral Rehabil 1995;22:343–347.
20. Hiltunen K, Schmidt-Kaunisaho K, Nevalainen J, Narhi T, Ainamo A. Prevalence of signs of temporomandibular disorders among elderly inhabitants of Helsinki, Finland. Acta Odontol Scand 1995;53:20–23.
21. Montegi E, Miyasaki H, Oguka I. An orthdontic study of temporomandibular joint disorders. Part I: Epidemiologic research in Japanese 6–18 year olds. Angle Orthod 1992;62:249–256.
22. Pullinger AG, Seligman DA. TMJ osteoarthrosis: a differentiation of diagnostic subgroups by symptom history and demographics. J Craniomandib Disord 1987;1:251–256.
23. Egermark-Ericksson I, Carlsson GE, Magnusson T. A long-term epidemiologic study of the relationship between occlusal factors and mandibular dysfunction in children and adolescents. J Dent Res 1987;67:67–71.
24. Salonen L, Hellden L, Carlsson GE. Prevalence of signs and symptoms of dysfunction in the masticatory system: an epidemiologic study in an adult Swedish population. J Craniomandib Disord 1990;4:241–250.
25. Wänman A, Agerberg G. Etiology of craniomandibular disorders: evaluation of some occlusal and psychosocial factors in 19-year-olds. J Craniomandib Disord 1991;5:35–44.
26. Sadowsky C, BeGole EA. Long-term status of temporomandibular joint function and functional occlusion after orthodontic treatment. Am J Orthod 1980;78:201–12.
27. Sadowsky C, Polson AM. Temporomandibular disorders and functional occlusion after orthodontic treatment: results of two long-term studies. Am J Orthod 1984;86:386–90.
28. Sadowsky C. The risk of orthodontic treatment for producing temporomandibular mandibular disorders: a literature overview. Am J Orthod Dentofac Orthop 1992;101:79–83.
29. Larsson E, Rönnerman A. Mandibular dysfunction symptoms in orthodontically treated patients ten years after the completion of treatment. Eur J Orthod 1981;3:89–94.
30. Helkimo M. Studies on function and dysfunction of the masticatory system. Kungsbacka: Elanders boktryckeri AB, 1974.
31. Dahl BL, Krogstad BO, Ogaard B, Eckersberg T. Signs and symptoms of craniomandibular disorders in two groups of 19-year-old individuals, one treated orthodontically and the other not. Acta Odont Scand 1988;46:89–93.
32. Rendell JK, Norton LA, Gay T. Orthodontic treatment and temporomandibular joint disorders. Am J Orthod Dentofac Orthop 1992;101:84–87.
33. Wadhwa L, Utreja A, Tewari A. A study of clinical signs and symptoms of temporomandibular dysfunction in subjects with normal occlusion, untreated, and treated malocclusions. Am J Orthod Dentofac Orthop 1993;103:54–61.
34. Seligman DA, Pullinger AG. TMJ derangements and osteoarthrosis subgroups differentiated according to active range of mandibular opening. J Craniomandib Disord 1988;2:35–40.
35. Smith A, Freer TJ. Post-orthodontic occlusal function. Austral Dent J 1989;34:301–309.
36. Kremenak CR, Kinser DD, Harman HA, Menard CC, Jakobsen JR. Orthodontic risk factors for temporomandibular disorders (TMD). I: Premolar extractions. Am J Orthod Dentofac Orthop 1992;101:13–20.
37. Kremenak CR, Kinser DD, Melcher TJ, Wright SD, Harrison RR, Zaija RR, Harman HA, Ordahl JN, Demro JG, Menard CC, Doleski KA, Jakobsen JR. Orthodontics as a risk factor for temporomandibular disorders (TMD). II. Am J Orthod Dentofac Orthop 1992;101:21–27.
38. Kinser DD. Orthodontic treatment, orthognathic surgery, and temporomandibular disorders. In: Trotman CA, McNamara JA, Jr, eds. Orthodontic treatment: outcome and effectiveness. Ann Arbor: Monograph 30, Craniofacial Growth Series, Center for Human Growth and Development, The University of Michigan, 1995.
39. Hirata RH, Heft MW, Hernandez B, King GJ. Longitudinal study of signs of temporomandibular disorders (TMD) in orthodontically treated and nontreated groups. Am J Orthod Dentofac Orthop 1992;101:35–40.
40. Pocock PR, Mamandras AH, Bellamy N. Evaluation of an anamnestic questionnaire as an instrument for investigating potential relationships between orthodontic therapy and temporomandibular disorders. Am J Orthod Dentofac Orthop 1992;102:239–43.
41. Dibbets JHM. Juvenile temporomandibular joint dysfunction and craniofacial growth. A statistical analysis. Leiden: Stafleu en Tholen, 1977.

42. Dibbets JHM, Van der Weele LT, Boering G. Craniofacial morphology and temporomandibular joint dysfunction in children. In: Carlson DS, McNamara JA, Jr, Ribbens KA, eds. Developmental aspects of temporomandibular joint disorders. Ann Arbor: Monograph 16, Craniofacial Growth Series, Center for Human Growth and Development, University of Michigan, 1985.
43. Dibbets JM, Van der Weele LT. Extraction, orthodontic treatment, and craniomandibular dysfunction. Am J Orthod Dentofac Orthop 1991;99:210–219.
44. Dibbets JM, Van der Weele LT. Long-term effects of orthodontic treatment, including extraction, on signs and symptoms attributed to CMD. Eur J Orthod 1992;14:16–20.
45. Janson M, Hasund A. Functional problems in orthodontic patients out of retention. Eur J Orthod 1981;3:173–179.
46. Pancherz H. The Herbst appliance—Its biologic effects and clinical use. Am J Orthod 1985;87:1–20.
47. Bowbeer GRN. Saving the face and the TMJ. Funct Orthodont 1985;2:32–44.
48. Witzig JW, Yerkes IM. Functional jaw orthopedics: Mastering more technique. In: Gelb H, ed. Clinical management of head, neck and TMJ pain. 2nd ed. Philadelphia: WB Saunders, 1985.
49. Witzig JW, Spahl TJ. Volume I: Mechanics. The clinical management of basic maxillofacial orthopedic appliances. Littleton: PSG Publishing, 1987.
50. Witzig JW, Yerkes IM. Researchers question dogma of protruded maxilla: Findings hint of improper orthodontic treatment. Dentist 1988;66:23–49.
51. Broadbent JM. Crossroads: Acceptance or rejection of functional jaw orthopedics. Am J Orthod Dentofac Orthop 1987;92:75–78.
52. Covey EJ. The effects of bicuspid extraction orthodontics on TMJ dysfunction. Funct Orthod 1990;7:1–2.
53. Sadowsky C, Theisen TA, Sakols EI. Orthodontic treatment and temporomandibular joint sounds—a longitudinal study. Am J Orthod Dentofac Orthop 1991;99:441–447.
54. Paquette DE, Beattie JR, Johnston LE, Jr. A long-term comparison of nonextraction and premolar extraction edgewise therapy in "borderline" Class II patients. Am J Orthod Dentofac Orthop 1992;102:1–14.
55. Beattie JR, Paquette DE, Johnston LE, Jr. The functional impact of extraction and nonextraction treatments: a long-term comparison in patients with "borderline," equally susceptible Class II malocclusions. Am J Orthod Dentofac Orthop 1994;105:444–449.
56. Luppanornlarp S, Johnston LE, Jr. The effects of premolar-extraction: a long-term comparison of outcomes in "clear-cut" extraction and nonextraction Class II patients. Angle Orthod 1993;63:257–272.
57. Dibbets JM, Van der Weele LT. Orthodontic treatment in relation to symptoms attributed to dysfunction of the temporomandibular joint. A 10-year report of the University of Groningen study. Am J Orthod Dentofac Orthop 1987;91:193–199.
58. O'Reilly M, Rinchuse DJ, Close J. Class II elastics and extractions and temporomandibular disorders: a longitudinal prospective study. Am J Orthod Dentofac Orthop 1993;103:459–463.
59. Kundinger KK, Austin BP, Christensen LV, Donegan SJ, Ferguson DJ. An evaluation of temporomandibular joints and jaw muscles after orthodontic treatment involving premolar extractions. Am J Orthod Dentofac Orthop 1991;100:110–115.
60. Staggers JA. Vertical change following first premolar extractions. Am J Orthod Dentofac Orthop 1994;105:19–24.
61. Pullinger AG, Seligman DA, Gornbein JA. A multiple regression analysis of the risk and relative odds of temporomandibular disorders as a function of common occlusal features. J Dent Res 1993;72:968–979.
62. Runge ME, Sadowsky C, Sakols EI, BeGole EA. The relationship between temporomandibular joint sounds and malocclusion. Am J Orthod Dentofac Orthop 1989;96:36–42.
63. Spahl TJ. Problems faced by fixed and functional schools of thought in pursuit of orthodontic excellence. Funct Orthod 1988;5:28–34.
64. Bowbeer GRN. The seventh key to facial beauty and TMJ health—Part 2: Proper condylar position. Funct Orthod 1990;7:4–32.
65. Wyatt WE. Preventing adverse effects on the temporomandibular joint through orthodontic treatment. Am J Orthod Dentofac Orthop 1987;91:493–499.
66. Gianelly AA, Hughes HM, Wohlgemuth P, Gildea G. Condylar position and extraction treatment. Am J Orthod Dentofac Orthop 1988;93:201–205.
67. Luecke PE, Johnston LE, Jr. The effect of maxillary first premolar extraction and incisor retraction on mandibular position: testing the central dogma of "functional orthodontics." Am J Orthod Dentofac Orthop 1992;101:4–12.
68. Tallents RH, Catania J, Sommers E. Temporomandibular joint findings in pediatric populations and young adults: a critical review. Angle Orthod 1991;61:7–16.
69. Årtun J, Hollender LG, Truelove EL. Relationship between orthodontic treatment, condylar position, and internal derangement in the temporomandibular joint. Am J Orthod Dentofac Orthop 1992;101:48–53.
70. Roth RH. Functional occlusion for the orthodontist. J Clin Orthod 1981;15:32–40, 44–51.
71. Roth RH, Rolfs DA. Functional occlusion for the orthodontist. Part II. J Clin Orthod 1981;15:100–123.
72. Roth RH. Functional occlusion for the Orthodontist. Part III. J Clin Orthod 1981;15:174–9, 182–198.
73. Roth RH, Gordon WW. Functional occlusion for the orthodontist. Part IV. J Clin Orthod 1981;15:246–254, 259–265.
74. Williamson EH. Occlusion: Understanding or misunderstanding. Angle Orthod 1976;46:86–93.
75. Cohen WE. A study of occlusal interferences in orthodontically treated occlusions and untreated normal occlusions. Am J Orthod 1965;51:647–689.
76. Rinchuse DJ, Sassouni V. An evaluation of functional occlusal interferences in orthodontically treated and untreated subjects. Angle Orthod 1983;53:122–130.
77. Hwang HS, Behrents RG. The effect of orthodontic treatment on centric discrepancy. J Craniomandib Pract 1996;14:133–138.
78. Andrews LF. The six keys to normal occlusion. Am J Orthod 1972;62:296–309.
79. Andrews LW. Straightwire: The concept and appliance. San Diego: LA Wells, 1989.

80. Wilson HE. Extraction of second molars in orthodontics. Orthodontist 1971;3:18–24.
81. Mehta J. Incorporating functional appliances in a traditional fixed appliance practice. Funct Orthod 1984;1:30–32.
82. Stack B. Orthopedic/orthodontic case finishing techniques on TMJ patients. Funct Orthod 1985;2:28–44.
83. Magnusson T. Five-year longitudinal study of signs and symptoms of mandibular dysfunction in adolescents. Cranio 1986;4:338–344.
84. Egermark I, Thilander B. Craniomandibular disorders with special reference to orthodontic treatment: an evaluation from childhood to adulthood. Am J Orthod Dentofac Orthop 1992;101:28–34.
85. Egermark-Eriksson I, Carlsson GE, Ingervall B. Prevalence of mandibular dysfunction and orofacial parafunction in 7-, 11- and 15-year-old Swedish children. Eur J Orthod 1981;3:163–172.
86. Egermark-Eriksson I. Mandibular dysfunction in children and in individuals with dual bite. Swed Dent J, Suppl 10 1982;6:1–45.
87. Olsson M, Lindqvist B. Mandibular function before and after orthodontic treatment. Eur J Orthod 1995;17:205–214.
88. Tsolka P, Walter JD, Wilson RF, Preiskel HW. Occlusal variables, bruxism and temporomandibular disorders: a clinical and kinesiographic assessment. J Oral Rehabil 1995;12:849–856.
89. Peltola J. Radiographic structural findings in the mandibular condyles of orthodontically treated children and young adults. Dissertation. Helsinki Finland: University of Helsinki, 1995.
90. Seligman DA, Pullinger AG. The role of intercuspal occlusal relationships in temporomandibular disorders: a review. J Craniomandib Disord 1991;5:96–106.
91. Keeling SD, McGorray S, Wheeler TT, King GJ. Risk factors associated with temporomandibular joint sounds in children 6 to 12 years of age. Am J Orthod Dentofac Orthop 1994;105:279–287.
92. Seligman DA, Pullinger AG. A multiple stepwise logistic regression analysis of trauma history and 16 other history and dental co-factors in women with temporomandibular disorders. J Orofacial Pain 1996;10:351–361.
93. Kampe T, Hannerz H. Differences in occlusion and some functional variable in adolescents with intact and restored dentitions. Acta Odontol Scand 1987;45:31–39.
94. Whittaker DK, Davies G, Brown M. Tooth loss, attrition, and temporomandibular joint changes in a Romano-British population. J Oral Rehabil 1985;12:407–419.
95. Könönen M. Signs and symptoms of craniomandibular disorders in men with Reiter's disease. J Craniomandib Disord 1992;6:247–253.
96. Steele JG, Lamey PJ, Sharkey SW, Smith G. Occlusal abnormalities, pericranial muscles and joint tenderness, and tooth wear in a group of migraine patients. J Oral Rehabil 1991;18:453–458.
97. Al Hadi LA. Prevalence of temporomandibular disorders in relation to some occlusal parameters. J Prosth Dent 1993;70:345–350.
98. Mauro G, Tagliaferro G, Bogini A, Fraccari F. A controlled clinical assessment and characterization of a group of patients with temporomandibular disorders. J Orofac Pain 1995;9:101.
99. Pullinger AG, Seligman DA. The degree to which attrition characterizes differentiated patient groups of temporomandibular disorders. J Orofacial Pain 1993;7:196–208.
100. Thilander B. Treatment in the mixed dentition with special regard to the indications for orthodontic treatment. Trans Eur Orthod Soc 1975:141–154.
101. Thilander B. Temporomandibular joint problems in children. In: Carlson DS, McNamara JA, Jr, Ribbens KA, eds. Developmental aspects of temporomandibular joint disorders. Ann Arbor: Monograph 16, Craniofacial Growth Series, Center for Human Growth and Development, University of Michigan, 1985.
102. Nilner M. Functional disturbances and diseases of the stomatognathic system. A cross-sectional study. J Pedodont 1986;10:211–238.
103. Troelstrup B, Moller E. Electromyography of the temporalis and masseter muscle in children with unilateral crossbite. Scand J Dent Res 1970;78:425–430.
104. Thilander B, Wahlund S, Lennartsson B. The effect of early interceptive treatment in children with posterior cross-bite. Eur J Orthod 1984;6:25–34.
105. Kirveskari P. The role of occlusal adjustment in the management of temporomandibular disorders. J Orofacial Pain 1997;83:87–90.
106. Okeson JP, ed. Orofacial pain: Guidelines for assessment, diagnosis and management. Chicago: Quintessence 1996.
107. Social Security Administration. Revised Medicare guidelines. Washington, DC: US Government Printing Office, 1991.
108. Clark GT, Tsukiyama Y, Baba K, Simmons M. The validity and utility of disease detection methods and occlusal therapy for temporomandibular disorders. J Orofacial Pain 1997; 83:101–106.
109. Just J, Ayer W, Greene C. Treating TM disorders. A survey on diagnosis, etiology, and management. J Am Dent Assoc 1991;122:56–60.
110. Costen JB. Syndrome of ear and sinus symptoms dependent on disturbed function of the temporomandibular joint. Ann Otol Rhinol Laryngol 1934;43:1–15.
111. Bleiker RF. Ear disturbances of temporomandibular origin. J Am Dent Assoc & Dent Cosmos 1938;25:1390–1399.
112. Pippin BN. A method of repositioning the mandible in the treatment of lesions of the temporomandibular joint. Washington Univ Dent J 1940;6:107–120.
113. Harvey W. Investigation and survey of malocclusion and ear symptoms, with particular reference to ototic barotrauma (pains in ears due to change in altitude). Brit Dent J 1940;85:219–225.
114. Harvey W. Investigation and survey of malocclusion and ear symptoms with particular reference to ototic barotrauma. Br Dent J 1948;85:249–255.
115. Brussels IJ. Temporomandibular joint disease: Differential diagnosis and treatment. J Am Dent Assoc 1949;39:532–554.
116. Gerry RG. The clinical problems of the temporomandibular articulation. J Am Dent Assoc 1947;34:261–269.
117. Ramfjord SP. Dysfunctional temporomandibular joint and muscle pain. J Prosthet Dent 1961;11:353–374.
118. Krogh-Poulsen WG, Olsson A. Occlusal disharmonies

118. and dysfunction of the stomatognathic system. Dent Clin North Am 1966:627–635.
119. Ramfjord SP, Ash MM. Occlusion. Philadelphia: WB Saunders, 1971.
120. Perry HT, Harris SC. The role of the neuromuscular system in functional activity of the mandible. J Am Dent Assoc 1954;48:665–673.
121. Jarabak JR. An electromyographic analysis of muscular and temporomandibular joint disturbances due to imbalance in occlusion. Angle Orthod 1956;26:170–190.
122. Shore NA. Occlusal equilibration and temporomandibular joint dysfunction. Philadelphia: JB Lippincott, 1959.
123. Moulton RE. Psychiatric considerations in maxillofacial pain. J Am Dent Assoc 1955;51:408–414.
124. Laskin DM. Etiology of the pain-dysfunction syndrome. J Am Dent Assoc 1969;79:147–153.
125. Solberg WK, Flint RT, Brantner JP. Temporomandibular joint pain and dysfunction: a clinical study of emotional and occlusal components. J Prosthet Dent 1972;28:412–427.
126. Rugh JD, Solberg WK. Psychological implictions in temporomandibular pain and dysfunction. In: Zarb GA, Carlsson GE, eds. Temporomandibular joint function and dysfunction. St Louis: CV Mosby, 1979.
127. Farrar WB. Diagnosis and treatment of anterior dislocation of the articular disc. New York J Dent 1971;41:348–351.
128. Farrar WB, McCarty WL. A clinical outline of temporomandibular joint diagnosis and treatment. Montgomery: Walder Printing Co, 1983.
129. McCarty WL. Diagnosis and treatment of internal derangements of the articular disc and mandibular condyle. In: Solberg WK, Clark GT, eds. Temporomandibular joint problems: Biologic diagnosis and treatment. Chicago: Quintessence, 1980.
130. Laskin D, Greenfield W, Gale E, Rugh J, Neff P, Alling C, Ayer WA. The President's conference on the examination, diagnosis and management of temporomandibular disorders. Chicago: Am Dent Assoc, 1983.
131. Carlson DS, McNamara JA, Jr, Ribbens KA. Developmental aspects of temporomandibular joint dysfunction. Ann Arbor: Monograph 16, Craniofacial Growth Series, Center for Human Growth and Development, University of Michigan, 1985.
132. Stohler CS, Carlson DS. Biological and psychological aspects of orofacial pain. Ann Arbor: Monograph 29, Craniofacial Growth Series, Center for Human Growth and Development, The University of Michigan, 1994.
133. McNeill C. Craniomandibular disorders: Guidelines for classification, assessment, and management. American Academy of Craniomandibular Disorders. Chicago: Quintessence, 1990.
134. McNeill C. Temporomandibular disorders: Guidelines for classification, assessment, and management. American Academy of Orofacial Pain. Chicago: Quintessence, 1993.
135. Bell WE. Clinical management of temporomandibular disorders. Chicago: Year Book Medical Publishers, 1982.
136. Okeson JP. Management of temporomandibular disorders. St Louis: Mosby Year Book, 1993.
137. Okeson JP. Bell's orofacial pains. Chicago: Quintessence, 1995.
138. Nilner M. Functional disturbances and diseases in the stomatognathic system among 7- to 18-year-olds. Cranio 1985;3:358–367.
139. Egermark-Eriksson I, Ingervall B, Carlsson GE. The dependence of mandibular dysfunction in children on functional and morphologic malocclusion. Am J Orthod 1983;83:187–194.
140. Brandt D. Temporomandibular disorders and their association with morphologic malocclusion in children. In: Carlson DS, McNamara JA, Jr, Ribens KA, eds. Developmental aspects of temporomandibular joint disorders. Ann Arbor: Monograph 16, Craniofacial Growth Series, Center for Human Growth and Development, University of Michigan, 1985.
141. DeBoever JA, Adriaens PA. Occlusal relationship in patients with pain-dysfunction symptoms in the temporomandibular joint. J Oral Rehabil 1983;10:1–7.
142. Gunn SM, Woolfolk MW, Faja BW. Malocclusion and TMJ symptoms in migrant children. J Craniomandib Disord 1988;2:196–200.
143. Dworkin SF, Huggins KH, LeResche L, Von Korff M, Howard J, Truelove E, Sommers E.. Epidemiology of signs and symptoms in temporomandibular disorders: Clinical signs in cases and controls. J Am Dent Assoc 1990;120:273–281.
144. Seligman DA. Occlusal risk factors in craniomandibular disorders: Recommendations for diagnostic examination and treatment. Hamburg: Europ Acad Craniomand Disorders, 1994.
145. Seligman DA, Pullinger AG. An analysis of occlusal variables, dental attrition, and age for distinguishing healthy controls from female patients with intracapsular TMD. J Prosth Dent, in press.
146. Seligman DA, Pullinger AG. The role of functional occlusal relationships in temporomandibular disorders: a review. J Craniomandib Disord 1991;5:265–279.
147. Brunelle JA, Bhat M, Lipton JA. Prevalence and distribution of selected occlusal characteristics in the US population. J Dent Res 1996;75:706–713.
148. Castro L. Importance of the occlusal status in the research diagnostic criteria of craniomandibular disorders. J Orofac Pain 1995;9:98.
149. Glaros AG, Brockman DL, Ackerman RJ. Impact of overbite on indicators of temporomandibular joint dysfunction. Cranio 1992;10:277–281.
150. Huggare JA, Raustia AM. Head posture and cervicovertebral and craniofacial morphology in patients with craniomandibular dysfunction. Cranio 1992;10:173–177.
151. Kampe T, Carlsson GE, Hannerz H, Haraldson T. Three-year longitudinal study of mandibular dysfunction in young adults with intact and restored dentitions. Acta Odontol Scand 1987;45:25–30.
152. Tsolka P, Fenlon MR, McCullock AJ, Preiskel HW. A controlled clinical, electromyographic, and kinesiographic assessment of craniomandibular disorders in women. J Orofac Pain 1994;8:80–89.
153. Vanderas AP. Relationship between craniomandibular dysfunction and malocclusion in white children with and without unpleasant life events. J Oral Rehabil 1994;21:177–183.
154. Tanne K, Tanaka E, Sakuda M. Association between malocclusion and temporomandibular disorders in orthodontic patients before treatment. J Orofacial Pain 1993;7:156–162.

155. Raustia AM, Pirttiniemi PM, Pyhtinen J. Correlation of occlusal factors and condylar position asymmetry with signs and symptoms of temporomandibular disorders. Cranio 1995;13:152–156.
156. Piper MA, Omlie MR. Facial skeleton remodeling due to temporomandibular degeneration: An imaging study of 100 patients. J Craniomand Pract 1992;10:248–259.
157. Larnheim TA, Storhaug K, Tveito L. Temporomandibular joint involvement and dental occlusion in a group of adults with rheumatoid arthritis. Acta Odontal Scand 1983;41:301–309.
158. Keeling SD, Gibbs C, Hall MB, Lupkiewicz S. Internal derangement of the TMJ: changes associated with mandibular repositioning and orthodontic therapy. Am J Orthod Dentofac Orthop 1989;96:363–374.
159. Wanman A, Agerberg G. Etiology of craniomandibular disorders: Evaluation of some occlusal and psychological factors in 19-year-olds. J Oral Rehabil 1991;5:35–44.
160. Pullinger AG, Seligman DA. Overbite and overjet characteristics of refined diagnostic groups of temporomandibular disorder patients. Am J Orthod Dentofac Orthop 1991;100:401–415.
161. Lieberman MA, Gazit E, Fuchs C, Lilos P. Mandibular dysfunction in 10–18 year old schoolchildren as related to morphological malocclusion. J Oral Rehabil 1985;12:209–214.
162. DeBoever JA, van den Berghe L. Longitudinal study of functional conditions in the masticatory system in Flemish children. Comm Dent Oral Epidemiol 1989;15:100–103.
163. Ingervall B, Thilander B. Activity of temporal and masseter muscles in children with a lateral forced bite. Angle Orthod 1975;45:249–258.
164. Pullinger AG, Seligman DA, Solberg WK. Temporomandibular disorders Part II: Occlusal factors associated with temporomandibular joint tenderness and dysfunction. J Prosthet Dent 1988;59:363–367.
165. Helöe B, Helöe LA. Characteristics of a group of patients with temporomandibular joint disorders. Comm Dent Oral Epidemiol 1975;3:72–79.
166. Mohlin B, Kopp S. A clinical study on the relationship between malocclusion, occlusal interferences and mandibular pain and dysfunction. Swed Dent J 1978;2:105-112.
167. Granados J. The influence of the loss of teeth and attrition on the articular eminence. J Prosthet Dent 1979;42:78–85.
168. Scholte AM, Steenks M, Bosman F. Characteristics and treatment outcome of diagnostic subgroups of CMD patients. A retrospective study. Comm Dent Oral Epidemiol 1993;21:215–220.
169. Whittaker DK, Jones JW, Edwards PW, Molleson T. Studies on the temporomandibular joints of an 18th century London population (Spitalfields). J Oral Rehabil 1990;17:89–97.
170. Leake JL, Hawkins R, Locker D. Social and functional impact of reduced posterior dental units in older adults. J Oral Rehabil 1994;21:1–10.
171. Bibb CA, Atchison KA, Pullinger AG, Bittar GT. Jaw function status in an elderly community sample. Comm Dent Oral Epidemiol 1995;23:303–308.
172. Takenoshita Y. Development with age of the human mandibular condyle: histological study. Cranio 1987;5:317–23.
173. Sato H, Osterberg T, Ahlqwist M, Carlsson GE, Grondahl H-G, Rubenstein B. Temporomandibular disorders and radiographic findings of the mandibular condyle in an elderly population. J Orofacial Pain 1996;10:180.
174. Lebbezoo-Scholte AM, DeLeeuw JRJ, Steenks MH, Bosman F, Buchner R, Olthoff LW. Diagnostic subgroups of camiomandibular disorders. Part 1: Self-report data and clinical findings. J Orofac Pain 1995;9:24–36.
175. Cianciaglini R, Gherlone EF, Radaelli G. Association between loss of occlusal support and symptoms of functional disturbances of the masticatory system. J Oral Rehabil 1999;26:248–253.
176. Käyser AF. Shortened dental arches and oral function. J Oral Rehabil 1981;8:457–462.
177. Witter DJ. A 6 year follow-up study of the oral function in shortened dental arches. Nijmegen: Thesis, University of Nijmegen, 1993.
178. Budtz-Jorgensen E, Luan W-M, Holm-Pedersen P, Fejerskov O. Mandibular dysfunction related to dental, occlusal and prosthetic conditions in a selected elderly population. Gerodontics 1985;1:28–33.
179. Kampe T, Hannerz H, Strom P. Five-year longitudinal recordings of functional variables of the masticatory system in adolescents with intact and restored dentitions: A comparative anamnestic and clinical study. Acta Odontol Scand 1991;49:239–246.
180. Magnusson T. Signs and symptoms of mandibular dysfunction in complete denture wearers five years after receiving new dentures. Cranio 1985;3:267–72.
181. Westling L. Occlusal interferences in retruded contact position and temporomandibular joint sounds. J Oral Rehabil 1995;8:601–606.
182. Könönen M, Murtomaa H, Ylipaavalniemi P. Craniomandibular disorders and general health in psoriatics. J Craniomandib Disord 1987;1:179–184.
183. Könönen M, Wenneberg B, Kallenberg A. Craniomandibular disorders in rheumatoid arthritis, psoriatic arthritis, and ankylosing spondylitis: A clinical study. Acta Odontol Scand 1992;50:281–287.
184. Hochman N, Ehrlich J, Yaffe E. Tooth contact during dynamic lateral excursion in young adults. J Oral Rehabil 1995;22:221–224.
185. Conti PCR, Ferreira PM, Pegoraro LF, Conti JV, Salvatore MCG. A cross-sectional study of prevalence and etiology of signs and symptoms of temporomandibular disorders in high school and university students. J Orofacial Pain 1996;10:254–262.
186. Magnusson T, Carlsson GE, Egermark I. Changes in clinical signs of craniomandibular disorders from the age of 15 to 25 years. J Orofac Pain 1994;8:207–215.
187. Kirveskari P, Alanen P, Jamsa T. Association between craniomandibular disorders and occlusal interferences in children. J Prosthet Dent 1992;67:692–696.
188. Shian W, Chang C. An epidemiological study of temporomandibular disorders in university students of Taiwan. Comm Dent Oral Epidemiol 1992;20:43–47.
189. Agerberg G, Sandstrom R. Frequency of occlusal interferences: A clinical study in teenagers and young adults. J Prosthet Dent 1988;59:212–217.

190. Akerman S, Kopp S, Nilner M, Petersson A, Rohlin M. Relationship between clinical and radiologic findings of the temporomandibular joint in rheumatoid arthritis. Oral Surg Oral Med Oral Pathol 1988;66:639–643.
191. Seligman DA, Pullinger AG. Association of occlusal variables among refined TM patient diagnostic groups. J Craniomandib Disord 1989;3:227–236.
192. Shupe RJ, Mohamed SE, Christensen LV, Finger IM, Weinberg R. Effects of occlusal guidance on jaw muscle activity. J Prosthet Dent 1984;51:811–818.
193. Belser UC, Hannam AG. The influence of altered working side occlusal guidance on masticatory muscle and related jaw movement. J Prosthet Dent 1985;53:406–413.
194. Seligman DA, Pullinger AG, Solberg WK. The prevalence of dental attrition and its association with factors of age, gender, occlusion and TMJ symptomatology. J Dent Res 1988;67:1323–1333.
195. Okeson JP, Kemper JT, Moody PM. A study of the use of occlusion splints in the treatment of acute and chronic patients with craniomandibular disorders. J Prosthet Dent 1982;48:708–712.
196. Steigman S, Barad A, Michaeli Y. The effect of load duration on long-term recovery of the eruptive function in the rat incisor. Am J Orthod Dentofac Orthop 1988;93:310–314.
197. Pullinger AG, Seligman DA. Quantification and validation of predictive values of occlusal variables in TMD using multifactorial analysis. J Prosth Dent, in press.
198. Stegenga B. Temporomandibular joint osteoarthrosis and internal derangement: Diagnostic and therapeutic outcome assessment. Groningen, The Netherlands: Drukkerij Van Denderen BV, 1991.
199. Nilner M, Lassing MA. Prevalence of functional disturbances and diseases of the stomatognathic system in 7–14 year olds. Swed Dent J 1981;5:173–187.
200. Gazit E, Lieberman M, Eini R, Hirsch N, Serfaty V, Fuchs C, Lilos P. Prevalence of functional disturbances in 10–18 year old Israeli school children. J Oral Rehab 1984;11:307–317.
201. Nilner M. Prevalence of functional disturbances and diseases of the stomatognathic system in 15–18 year olds. Swed Dent J 1981;5:189–197.
202. Swanljung O, Rantanen T. Functional disorders of the masticatory system in Southwest Finland. Comm Dent Oral Epidemiol 1979;7:177–182.
203. Solberg WK, Woo MA, Houston J. Prevalence of mandibular dysfunction in young adults. J Am Dent Assoc 1979;98:25–34.
204. Rieder CE, Martinoff JT, Wilcox SA. The prevalence of mandibular dysfunction. Part I: Sex and age distribution of related signs and symptoms. J Prosthet Dent 1983;50:81–88.
205. Ingervall B, Mohlin B, Thilander B. Prevalence of symptoms of functional disturbances of the masticatory system in Swedish men. J Oral Rehabil 1980;7:185–197.
206. Osterberg T, Carlsson GE. Symptoms and signs of mandibular dysfunction in 70-year-old men and women in Gothenburg, Sweden. Comm Dent Oral Edpdemiol 1979;7:315–321.
207. O'Reilly MT, Rinchuse DJ, Close J. Class II elastics and extractions and temporomandibular disorders: A longitudinal prospective study. Am J Orthod Dentofac Orthop 1993;103:459–463.
208. Williamson EH, Simmons MD. Mandibular asymmetry and its relation to pain dysfunction. Am J Orthod 1979;76:612–617.
209. Nesbitt BA, Moyers RE, TenHave TR. Adult temporomandibular joint disorder symptomatology and its association with childhood occlusal relations: A preliminary report. In: Carlson DS, McNamara JA, Jr, Ribbens KA, eds. Developmental aspects of temporomandibular joint disorders. Ann Arbor: Monograph 16, Craniofacial Growth Series, Center for Human Growth and Development, The University of Michigan, 1985.
210. Bernal M, Tsamtsouris A. Signs and symptoms of temporomandibular joint dysfunction in 3- to 5 year old children. J Pedodont 1986;10:127–140.
211. Stringert HG, Worms FW. Variations in skeletal and dental patterns in patients with structural and functional alterations of the temporomandibular joint: A preliminary report. Am J Orthod 1986;89:285–297.
212. Riolo ML, Brandt D, TenHave TR. Associations between occlusal characteristics and signs and symptoms of TMJ dysfunction in children and young adults. Am J Orthod Dentofac Orthop 1987;92:467–477.
213. Linde C, Isacsson G. Clinical signs in patients with disk displacement versus patients with myogenic craniomandibular disorders. J Craniomandib Disord 1990;4:197–204.
214. Takenoshita Y, Ikebe T, Yamamoto M, Oka M. Occlusal contact area and temporomandibular symptoms. Oral Surg Oral Med Oral Pathol 1991;72:388–394.
215. Cacchiotti DA, Plesh O, Bianchi P, McNeill C. Signs and symptoms in samples with and without temporomandibular disorders. J Craniomandib Disord 1991;5:167–172.
216. List T, Helkimo M. Acupuncture and occlusal splint therapy in the treatment of craniomandibular disorders: II. A 1-year follow-up study. Acta Odontol Scand 1992;50:275–285.
217. Raustia AM, Pyhtinen J. Direct sagittal computed tomography as a diagnostic aid in the treatment of an anteriorly displaced temporomandibular joint disk by splint therapy. Cranio 1987;5:240–245.

Chapter 30
STUDY MODELS

One aspect of orthodontic diagnosis that is part of the common knowledge of the profession and yet has not been described often in the literature is the fabrication of study models (Fig. 30-1). This final chapter will describe a technique for study model fabrication that can be used on a routine basis.

One of the sources of information regarding the proper trimming of study models is the document issued by the *American Board of Orthodontics*[1] (ABO) that suggests standards for study model fabrication. The style of trimming described in this chapter is based on ABO recommendations.

IMPRESSIONS

Well-fitting standard aluminum trays or disposable plastic trays can used to obtain accurate impressions of the dentition and associated soft and hard tissue structures. The edges of the trays can be lined with a border of wax that prevents the edge from impinging on the soft tissue. Care should be taken to ensure that the trays are neither too wide nor too narrow, so that minimal soft tissue distortion occurs. The areas of tissue attachment, particularly in the region of the labial frenum and in areas of soft tissue attachment adjacent to the upper first premolars, should be reproduced in the impression. Obtaining a proper impression of the hard and soft tissue of the dentoalveolar region is critical for the efficient fabrication of diagnostic study models.

After the impression has been made with alginate, it should be checked thoroughly. The impression should appear smooth with no major voids, and the borders of the impression should be rolled with good extension into the vestibular areas. The impression also should extend posteriorly in the palatal area and lingually in the mandibular region. Finally, the impression should be checked for the presence of any large air bubbles, especially on the occlusal surfaces of the teeth. After obtaining the impression, it should be disinfected to prevent possible contamination of the laboratory area (to be discussed later).

WAX BITE REGISTRATION

Clinicians use a wide variety of substances to record the orientation of the upper and lower dental arches. Normally, the bite registration is taken in centric occlusion, a tooth-guided position. In instances in which there is a substantial difference between centric occlusion and centric relation, an additional bite registration should be taken in centric relation. The clinician then must decide whether the study models are to be trimmed in centric occlusion or centric relation.

Most study models are trimmed to a centric occlusion bite registration. In instances in which a centric relation registration is desired, it often is useful to mount the models on an appropriate articulator, utilizing a face-bow transfer.

For routine procedures, one or two thicknesses of yellow bite registration wax (Great Lakes Orthodontic Products, Tonawanda NY) are used. The horseshoe-shaped wafers of wax are softened first in warm water

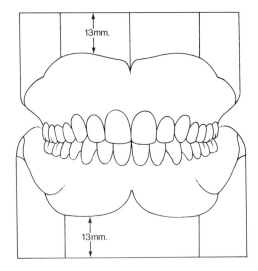

Figure 30-1. Frontal view of a well-trimmed set of study models.

and then placed on the maxillary dental arch. The patient then closes his or her mouth so that the lower teeth bite into the softened wax. The patient should be instructed to bite through the wax, to avoid producing study models that "rock" or are unstable when trimmed. Using finger pressure, the clinician then presses the wax against the facial surfaces of teeth to achieve a three-dimensional registration of the bite. Many clinicians advocate keeping the labial surfaces of the upper and lower anterior teeth free of wax when obtaining the bite registration. The incisal edges can be registered in the wax, but the midlines should be kept visible so that the transverse orientation of the wax bite (using the midlines) can be determined.

After the impression and wax bite have been taken, they are wrapped in moistened paper toweling and placed in a sealable plastic bag.

DISINFECTING THE IMPRESSION

A thorough rinsing of the impressions both before and following disinfection is necessary for adequate disinfection and to avoid possible adverse effects on the study model.[2] Rinsing before disinfection reduces the number of microorganisms on the surface of the impressions by removing plaque and secretions. Rinsing after disinfection removes residual disinfectant that may affect the surface of the poured stone adversely.

Immersion disinfection usually will not distort or otherwise harm the impression if care is taken in the selection of the appropriate disinfectant, limiting immersion time to that recommended by the product manufacturer for TB and viral disinfection and thoroughly rinsing the impression following removal from the disinfectant solution.[2] Products that are accepted by the *American Dental Association* and that require no more than 30 minutes for disinfection are preferred.

The impressions should be immersed in a commercially availalbe idsinfectant for approximately 10 minutes. A 1:10 solution of chlorine bleach and water also can be used as a disinfecting solution. The impressions then are rinsed in lukewarm water and rebagged until the time they are poured.

POURING THE IMPRESSIONS

The first step in pouring the impressions is to fill in the area occupied by the tongue in the mandibular impression. Filling the tongue region before pouring the model makes finishing the model much easier.

This modification of the lower impression can be accomplished initially by placing a thumb or piece of moistened paper towel or tissue in the tongue space. One scoop of alginate is mixed to normal consistency and placed in the area normally occupied by the tongue. As the alginate begins to harden, the laboratory technician dips his or her finger in water and uses it to smooth the alginate into the existing impression. After the initial set is completed, the impression is put aside until a final set is attained. After that time, the impression should be checked for accuracy, making sure that the alginate addition does not obstruct the anatomical structures in the lingual region of the mandibular impression.

The impressions are poured using white orthodontic stone (or plaster). The impression should have been rinsed previously, not only to eliminate the residue of the disinfectant but also to eliminate traces of saliva that otherwise might affect the integrity of the finished surface of the stone. The stone is mixed in a vacuum mixer to eliminate bubbles that otherwise would be trapped in the stone. The stone is poured in the tooth portion of the impression first, using a vibrator and a waxing instrument or spatula. Additional stone is added with the spatula to form the anatomical portion of the impression.

After the pouring of the anatomical portion of the impression is completed, the remaining stone is poured into a large base former (TP Laboratories, La Porte IN), again using the vibrator. The impression tray is turned upside down and pushed into the stone in the base former. Care should be taken to verify that the occlusal surface of the impression remains parallel to the bottom surface of the base former. In addition, the impression tray should not be pushed into the plaster in the base former. If the impression tray becomes trapped in the plaster, difficulties will be encountered

STUDY MODELS

in removing the tray, and the vertical thickness of the study model may be reduced.

The impression tray is removed from the poured stone after it is hardened. Usually, the stone goes through a period in which heat is generated during setting. Ordinarily, a wait of 30–60 minutes after the onset of the mix is adequate to make sure that the orthodontic stone is set. Care should be taken in removing the impression from the set stone so that the teeth (particularly the upper and lower incisors) are not fractured during tray removal.

TRIMMING THE STUDY MODEL

The trimming of the poured stone is an arduous task that needs to be performed slowly and carefully. It is advisable to soak the cast in water for approximately 10 minutes to facilitate the trimming of the stone. Leaving the cast in water for longer periods may result in pitting and dissolution of the stone or plaster.

As a first step in the procedure, a laboratory knife is used to remove any large or small chunks of plaster that interfere with the occlusion of the cast when the two parts of the study models are placed together initially. Such interferences include bubbles on the occlusal surfaces as well as lateral extensions in the posterior regions, particularly behind the last erupted molar.

Rough Trimming the Maxillary Model

The maxillary model is trimmed symmetrically with the top of the model parallel to the occlusal plane (Fig. 30-2). The back of the model is trimmed perpendicular to the midline of the palate, as indicated by the orientation of the midline palatal raphe (Fig. 30-3). Rough trimming of the stone bases first can be accomplished free hand, using the platform on the model trimmer as a guide.

After the model is rough trimmed, the model is placed on its posterior surface so that the top of the cast can be trimmed. The teeth rest against the attachment of the model trimmer that slides into the groove on the trimming platform.

The anatomical base of the maxillary model (Figs. 30-1 and 30-2) should be about 1.5 cm thick (the ABO recommendation is 13 mm). If the maxillary base has been poured to an inadequate thickness, or if the base has been trimmed excessively, the finished study models will look uneven. The total height of each cast should measure approximately 3.5–4.0 cm from the occlusal surface to the top of the model.

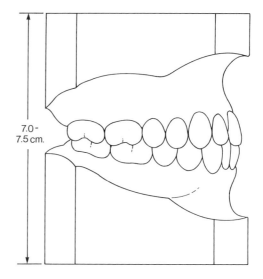

Figure 30-2. Lateral view of a well-trimmed set of study models.

Trimming the Backs of the Models

Once the top of the cast has been trimmed flat, it is placed with its top surface against the trimming platform. The cast then is oriented so that the palatal raphe is perpendicular to the wheel of the model trimmer. It is advisable to use the palatal raphe as a guide, because the dental midlines often are not coincident with the skeletal midlines.

The cast is trimmed so that there is about 5 mm of stone distal to the most posterior tooth. In instances of severe Class II malocclusion, additional space (*e.g.*, 5-10 mm) should be allotted in the posterior region until the final occlusion is determined.

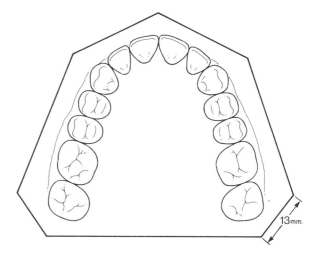

Figure 30-3. Maxillary view of well-trimmed study model. The palatal raphe is represented by the vertical line in the middle of the hard palate.

Establishing the Interarch Relationship

The upper and lower casts are placed together, and the operator checks for any interference that might prevent a proper occlusion from being established. The wax bite registration is placed on the maxillary cast, and the mandibular cast is occluded into the wax indentations.

The models then are placed on the trimming table with the casts in occlusion and the maxillary model on the bottom, with the backs of the casts facing the trimming wheel. The casts are held together firmly, and the back surfaces of the models are trimmed. At this point, only the mandibular cast touches the trimming wheel. The casts should be held gently but firmly together as the casts are pushed into the coarse grinding wheel. Trimming continues until both the upper and lower casts are touching the trimmer.

After it has been determined that the backs of the casts have been trimmed in a parallel fashion, the models are removed from the trimmer, and the backs of the casts placed on a flat surface. At this point, the models should lie flush on the surface with the wax bite in place. If this is not the situation, the models should be placed back in the trimmer with the wax bite in place and retrimmed until both surfaces are flush against the trimmer.

At this point, the wax bite is removed and the casts occluded in a hand-held fashion. Once again, the models should be checked for the appropriate bite orientation by placing the backs of the models on a flat surface. If the backs of the models are not flush, they should be retrimmed without the wax bite in place. If there is any uncertainty concerning the accuracy of the wax bite, a new bite should be obtained.

Rough Trimming the Mandibular Model

With the models in occlusion and the wax bite in place, the models are placed on the trimming table with the lower base against the trimming wheel. Using the perpendicular attachment of the trimming table against the top surface of the upper cast, the bottom of the lower cast is trimmed parallel to the top of the upper cast. The cast is trimmed so that the base of the lower model is equal in thickness to that of the upper model (Figs. 30-1 and 30-2). The total height of both casts in occlusion should be about 7–7.5 cm.

FINAL TRIMMING

Maxillary Model

The precise angulations of the study models are determined using an angulator that can be screwed into the trimming table. The angulator allows the operator to set the correct angle for each surface. By placing the back of the cast against the flat surface of this device, an angle is formed between the surface of the cast and the trimming wheel surface that allows for the correct angulation to be determined. The screw on the angulator should be tightened firmly to prevent slipping of the device that could result in trimming errors.

First, the angulator is set at 70° (Fig. 30-4). The cast is placed in the appropriate position, and the first side is trimmed until the deepest extent of the vestibule is reached. The thickness of the initial trim should be roughly the thickness of a standard wooden pencil, as measured from the alveolus facially to the trimmed sides of the model. It is best to be cautious at this point, because it is, of course, possible to retrim any surface. The opposite side also is trimmed at 70°.

The angulator then is set to 25°, and the front of the maxillary cast trimmed so that both sides meet anteriorly. The tip of the cast should approximate the midline as determined by the palatal raphe. The anterior borders of the maxillary cast are equal in length.

The last portions of the maxillary cast to be trimmed are the back edges. These edges are trimmed perpendicular to a line drawn from the intersection of the lateral and posterior borders of the cast and the intersection point of the lateral and frontal surfaces of the cast on the opposite side (Fig. 30-4). The length of the corner segments should be 13–15 mm. Care should be taken to avoid trimming this area too quickly, or excess stone may be removed.

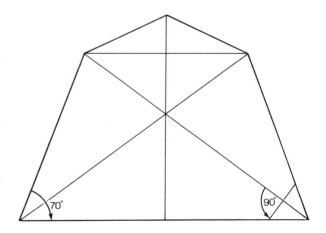

Figure 30-4. Trimming of the maxillary cast. The lateral surfaces of the maxillary cast is trimmed at a 70° angle to the posterior surface. The posterior corners of the cast are trimmed perpendicular to a line formed between the intersection point of the posterior and lateral surfaces and the intersection point of the lateral and frontal surfaces of the cast on the opposite side.

Mandibular Model

The angulator is set at 65° when initially trimming the lower model (Fig. 30-5). Each side is trimmed to the depth of the vestibule, again with the width of a standard wooden pencil as an initial guide.

The next step in trimming is to establish the posterior angles of the mandibular cast. As with the maxillary model, the posterior edges of the mandibular model are trimmed perpendicular to a line bisecting the angle formed by the lateral aspect of the cast and the posterior aspect of the cast (Fig. 30-5). The length of this posterior surface should be 13–15 mm (Fig. 30-6).

The anterior contour of the cast is not angled, but rather is rounded, according to convention. The determination of the curvature is accomplished free hand through gentle movement of the cast in a smooth arcing fashion. The anterior curvature is trimmed to the depth of the vestibule in most instances. In instances of dentoalveolar protrusion, care must be taken to avoid damaging the teeth during the trimming process.

FINISHING PROCEDURES

Filling Voids

The casts are inspected carefully and any remaining bubbles removed with a cleoid-discoid or waxing instrument. Particular attention is paid to the gingival margin as well as to other soft tissue areas. Any air holes or voids are filled with stone, and the surface is smoothed carefully, using either a finger or small brush to add plaster to the model. All voids are filled, regardless of whether they are on the anatomical or non-anatomical (artistic) portions of the model.

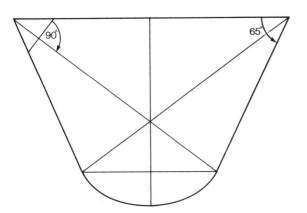

Figure 30-5. Trimming of the mandibular cast. The lateral surfaces of the cast are trimmed to a 65° angle to the posterior surface. The posterior corners are trimmed perpendicular to a line bisecting the associated angle.

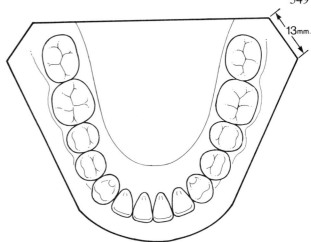

Figure 30-6. Occlusal view of the mandibular cast. The width of the posterior corners should be 13–15 mm.

Finishing

The edges of the dental cast are smoothed slightly with a laboratory knife so that they are smooth and even. If there are obvious asymmetries in the extension of the vestibule that are due to impression technique rather than anatomical variation, these areas may be modified using a plaster knife or a rotary instrument.

The fine polishing of the artistic portions of the dental cast is initiated using a piece of fine-grained sand paper. The edges of the study models are smoothed under warm water. In addition, the flat surfaces of the model are smoothed in areas of voids that previously have been filled with plaster.

The edges of the models should not be rounded. The finished models should have sharp angles but generally should be smooth in appearance. The models are set aside in an area to dry and allowed to do so for at least 24 hours.

Polishing the Study Models

The casts are placed in a soaping solution for one hour. The casts then are removed from the soap bath, rinsed under warm water, and allowed to dry for approximately 20 minutes. Using a soft rag, the bases are buffed until the casts are smooth and shiny. The casts are labeled in the appropriate manner, noting the name and age of the patient, as well as the date of the impression.

CONCLUDING REMARKS

The quality of a clinician's routine study models often is used, whether justified or not, as an indicator of the overall quality of orthodontics in a given practice. The procedure outlined in this chapter allows for a relatively consistent protocol for the routine fabrication of diagnostic casts.

In this era of increased litigation, the existence of diagnostic casts, both pre- and post-treatment, is an integral part of risk management procedures. Not only should the study models appear well finished and polished, but also the accuracy of the bite registration is of critical importance when determining the pre-treatment and post-treatment occlusion. Care should be taken to make routine study models not only artistically pleasing but also anatomically accurate so that proper diagnosis and treatment planning can be completed for the routine orthodontic patient.

REFERENCES CITED

1. American Board of Orthodontics. Specific instructions for candidates. St. Louis, 1990.
2. Molinari JA, Merchant VA, Gleason MJ. Update on disinfection of impressions and prostheses. Monitor 1991;8:1–4.

INDEX

ACCO appliance, 70–71
Activator, 3
Acid etch, 171–172
Acrylic splint expanders, 215–229
    Appliance removal, 227–229
    Clinical management, 218–229
    Home care instructions, 225–226
    Maintenance plate, 229
Active vertical corrector, 133–134
Adhesion booster, 173
Adult dentition, 34
Adult treatment, 5
Airway obstruction, 122–128
    Clinical studies, 125–128
    Experimental studies, 123–125
    Naso-respiratory physiology, 122–123
Aligners, 479–486
American Board of Orthodontics criteria, 454–455
Anterior bite plate, 137
Anterior bracket placement, 51–52
Apically positioned flap, 395
Arch dimension, 35
Archwires, 158–164
    Chrome cobalt archwires, 160
    Gold-nickel archwires, 159
    Stainless steel archwires, 159–160
    Titanium alloy archwires, 160–164
Asymmetrical facebow, 364–365
Axial inclination of teeth, 104–106

Band cementation, 178–180
Bionator, 77–78, 319–331
    Bite registration, 322–324
    Clinical management, 329–330
    Construction, 324–329
    Impression technique, 322
    Preparation of work models, 322
    Types of bionators, 320–322
Bonded lingual retainers, 459–461
Bonding, 169–186
    Acid etch, 171–172
    Adhesion booster, 173
    Acrylic jacket, 181–182
    Bonding adhesives, 174–178
    Composite restoration, 181–182
    Dual-cure systems, 178
    Isolation, 170–171
    Light-cure adhesives, 176–178
    Lingual retainer, 183–185
    Metal, 182
    Mixed adhesives, 174–176
    No-mix adhesives, 176
    Plastic bracket, 183
    Porcelain crown, 181–182
    Prophylaxis, 169–170
    Rebonding bracket, 182–183
    Rinsing and drying, 172–173
    Wet field, 180
Bonding adhesives, 174–178
Bonding to surfaces, 180–185
Broadening the smile, 107–108
Buffalo elastics, 455–456

Care call, 28
Cephalometric evaluation, 487–517
    Airway analysis, 508–510
    Analysis of single film, 488–510
    Analysis of serial films, 510–512
    Basis of analysis, 488
    Composite norms, 492, 497
    Development of analysis, 487–488
    Hard tissue analysis, 490–510
    Maxilla to cranial base, 488–495
    Maxillary incisor to maxilla, 503–505
    Mandible to midface, 495–503
    Mandibular incisor to mandible, 505–508
    Soft tissue evaluation, 489–491
Cervical-pull facebow, 68, 361–365
Cervical vertebral maturation, 78–80
Chin cup, 91–93, 134–136
Chrome cobalt archwires, 160
Circumferential retainer, 457–458
Class II malocclusion, 9, 63–84
    Components, 63–66
    Sagittal components, 63–65
    Spontaneous correction, 55–56
    Transverse components, 67
    Vertical components, 65–66
Class III malocclusion, 4, 85–95
    Components, 85–87
    Growth, 87
    Spontaneous correction, 56–57
    Treatment strategies, 87–92
Clinical examination, 13–30
    Care call, 28
    Dental and TMJ history, 22

Digital imaging, 20
Examination by orthodontist, 26
Examination by treatment coordinator, 22
Explanation by treatment coordinator, 28
Family history, 21
Initial contact with office, 14
Initial examination protocols, 16
Health history, 16
New patient letter, 15
Oral measurements, 25
Oral questions, 22
Panoramic radiograph, 27
Personal history, 21
Practice demographics, 13
Radiographic examination, 19
Respiratory history, 22
Risk management, 29
Telephone interaction, 15
TMJ examination, 22–25
Treatment coordinator, 13–30
Clinical examination form, 23
Cool tool, 166
Combi facebow, 364
Comprehensive orthodontic therapy, 130–131, 137–138, 149
   Archwire selection, 158–164
   Appliance selection, 149
   Bans selection, 156–158
   Bracket placement, 152–156
   Sequence of treatment, 150–152
Compressed springs, 356
Congenitally missing mandibular second premolars, 427–434
Congenitally missing maxillary lateral incisors, 434–444

Damon bracket, 165–167
Deciduous dentition, 7
Deep bite, 115–116, 137–141
Deflection of straight wires, 356–357
Dental cast analysis, 102–104
Dentitional development, 31–39
Distal Jet appliance, 350–353
Digital habits, 129–130
Dual-cure systems, 178

Early mixed dentition, 8
Electromyographic studies, 243–247
Enamoplasty, 463
Eruption facets, 327
Expansion, 40
   Orthodontic expansion, 40
   Passive expansion, 40
   Orthopedic expansion, 41
Experimental studies, 243–247
Extraction, 39
Extraoral traction, 68–69, 131, 138, 361–373
   Facebows, 361–365
   Historical perspective, 361
   J-hook headgears, 365–368
   Kloehn facebow, 361–363
   Treatment effects, 368–371

Facebows, 68–69
Facial mask, 88–90, 375–385
   Components, 377–380
   Clinical management, 380–383
   Treatment effects, 375–376
   Treatment timing, 376377
Flap/closed eruption technique, 395–396
Function regulator (FR-2) of Fränkel, 74–75, 265–284
   Advancement, 282–283
   Appliance delivery, 277
   Clinical management, 273–283
   Bite registration, 274–276
   Fabrication, 277
   Home care instructions, 280–281
   Impression technique, 273–274
   Intraoral evaluation, 278–281
   Laboratory instructions, 277
   Lip seal exercises, 281
   Notching of the teeth, 277–278
   Parts of appliance, 267
   Preparation of work models, 275–276
   Pterygoid response, 281
   Treatment effects, 267–273
   Types of appliances, 267
Function regulator (FR-3) of Fränkel, 90–91, 387–394
   Activation, 393
   As a retainer, 393–394
   Bite registration, 390–391
   Clinical management, 390–394
   Impression technique, 390
   Parts of the appliance, 387–390
   Preparation of work models, 391
   Treatment effects, 390
Functional jaw orthopedics, 3, 73–78, 131–132, 138–139
Functional protrusion experimental studies, 243–247

Gingivectomy, 395, 462
Gold-nickel archwires, 159

Hawley retainer, 456–457
Health history, 17–18
Herbst appliance, 76–77
   Advancement, 300, 308
   Acrylic splint type, 76–77, 303–308
   Banded type, 289–291
   Historical perspective, 285–286
   Role of expansion, 288–289
   Stainless steel crown type, 76–77, 291–303
   Treatment effects, 286–288, 308–315
High-pull facebow, 364
Histological studies, 243–247

Inactive retention status form, 471
Impacted teeth, 395–422
   Mandibular canine, 411–413
   Mandibular first molar, 414–418
   Mandibular second molar, 418
   Mandibular second premolar, 413–414
   Maxillary canines, 397–411
   Maxillary central incisors, 396–397
   Potential problems, 418–421
   Surgical techniques, 395–396
Initial contact with office, 14
Interdental spacing, 31–34

INDEX

Interdisciplinary treatment, 4
Interocclusal acrylic, 328
Interproximal reduction, 39, 45, 463–465
Invisible retainers, 470, 475–479
Invisalign system, 4, 479–486
Interlandi headgear, 70

J-hook headgear, 69
Jasper Jumper, 333–342
    Additional applications, 340–341
    Clinical management, 337–340
    Method of attachment, 334–335
    Parts of appliance, 333–334
    Treatment effects, 335–337

Keys to optimal occlusion, 453–454
Kloehn headgear, 361–363

Late mixed dentition, 8
Light-cure adhesives, 176–178
Lingual arch, 53–54
Lingual retainer, 183–185
Lip bumper, 51
Lip seal exercises, 128–129

Maintenance plates, 52–53, 229
Magnetic appliances, 357–358
Malformed maxillary incisors, 423–426
Mandibular dental decompensation, 48
Maxillary skeletal protrusion, 68
Maxillary skeletal retrusion, 68–69
Microetcher, 178–180
Mini-distalization appliance, 349–350
Mixed adhesives, 174–176
Mixed dentition treatment, 5
Molar distalization appliances, 343–359
Multiple malformed incisors, 426

Nasal resistance, 107
Naso-respiratory function, 122–128
    Clinical studies, 125–128
    Experimental studies, 123–125
    Naso-respiratory physiology, 122–123
New patient letter, 15
No-mix adhesives, 176
NiTi coils, 72–73, 356
Non-occlusion, 112

Occlusal factors and TMD, 527–537
Occlusal keys, 453–454
Occlusal table, 327–328
Open bite, 112
    Anterior open bite, 113
    Overview, 112
    Posterior open bite, 114
    Treatment, 128–137
Open gingival embrasures, 448–452
Oral measurements, 25
Orthodontic expansion, 40
Orthodontics and TMD, 519–527
Orthopedic expansion, 41, 45–48
Orthopedic facial mask, 88–90

One-phase treatment, 5
Orthognathic surgery, 136–137, 139

Passive expansion, 40
Pendex appliance, 3, 71–72, 343–349
    Clinical management, 344–348
    Treatment effects, 348–349
Pendulum appliance, 3, 71, 343–349
    Clinical management, 344–348
    Treatment effects, 348–349
Permanent dentition, 9
Phases of treatment, 5
Positioner, 465–468
Posterior bite blocks, 132–133
Practice demographics, 13
Pterygoid response, 281–282

Quadhelix appliance, 54

Rapid maxillary expansion, 2, 99–108, 211–231
    Acrylic expanders, 215–229
    Banded expanders, 212–215
    Bonded expanders, 215–229
    Clinical management, 214–215
    Clinical studies, 99–104
    Haas-type, 212–213
    Hyrax-type, 213–214
    Mechanism of action, 211–212
Rebonding bracket, 182–183
Repelling magnets, 357–358
Restorative treatment, 423–452
    Congenitally missing mandibular second premolars, 427–434
    Congenitally missing maxillary lateral incisors, 434–444
    Malformed maxillary incisors, 423–426
    Multiple malformed incisors, 426
    Open gingival embrasures, 448–452
    Traumatic fracture of teeth, 445–447
    Uneven gingival margins, 447–448
Retention, 453–474
    Bonded lingual retainers, 459–461
    Circumferential retainer, 457–458
    Enamoplasty, 463
    Gingivectomy, 462
    Hawley retainer, 456–457
    Inactive retention status form, 471
    Interproximal reduction, 463–465
    Invisible retainers, 470
    Positioner, 465–468
    Protocols, 4, 455–472
    Ricketts retainer, 458
    Serpentine wires, 466–467
    Spring retainer, 470, 472
    Supracrestal fiberotomy, 461
    Transpalatal ("Buffalo") elastics, 465–466
    Van der Linden retainer, 458–459
    Vertical ("spaghetti") elastics, 467–468
Ricketts retainer, 458
Risk management, 29

Schwarz appliance, 49–51, 233–241
    Uses, 234

Schwarz appliance (*continued*)
  Clinical management, 237–239
  Clinical studies, 235–237
Self-ligating brackets, 164–167
Serial extraction, 42–45
Serpentine wires, 466–467
Soft tissue, 120–122, 489–491
Spaghetti elastics, 467–468
Spontaneous correction of sagittal malocclusion, 54–57
  Class II malocclusion, 55–56, 106
  Class III malocclusion, 56–57
Spring retainer, 470, 472
Stainless steel archwires, 159–160
Straight-pull facebow, 70
Stress-strain curves, 160–162
Study models, 545–551
Superelasticity, 163

Telephone interaction, 15
Temperature sensitivity, 163–164
Temporomandibular disorders, 4, 519–543
  Orthodontics and TMD, 519–527
  Occlusal factors and TMD, 527–537
Thumb contract, 129–130
Thumb sucking, 114
Titanium alloy archwires, 160–164
Tooth-size relationships, 31, 34
Transitional appliances, 53
Transitional dentition, 36
Transpalatal arch, 53, 199–209
  Activation, 205–208
  Clinical problems, 208
  Contraindications, 203–204
  Fabrication, 204–205
  Fixed type, 205–208
  Indications, 203–204
  Removable, type, 204
  Uses, 199–203
Transpalatal ("Buffalo") elastics, 465–466
Transpalatal width, 25, 35–37
Transverse dimension, 97–110
Traumatic fracture of teeth, 445–447
Treatment coordinator, 13–30
Treatment options, 1, 27
Treatment possibilities, 4

Treatment strategies, 39, 67–78, 87–92
  Mixed dentition, 42
  Permanent dentition, 39
Treatment timing, 7, 78–80
  Deciduous dentition, 7
  Early mixed dentition, 8
  Late mixed dentition, 8–9
  Permanent dentition, 9–10
TMJ examination, 22–25
Twin block appliance, 75–76, 243–263
  Appliance delivery, 255–256
  Biological basis, 243–247
  Bite registration, 252–254
  Clinical management, 251–259
  Contouring the acrylic, 256–257
  Historical perspective, 243
  Impression technique, 252
  Laboratory prescription, 254
  Parts of appliance, 247–251
  Reactivation, 257
  Support phase, 258–259
  Treatment effects, 259–261
Two-phase treatment, 6

Uneven gingival margins, 447–448
Utility arches, 187–197
  Basic components, 187
  Clinical problems, 196
  Instruments, 188
  Intrusion, 69, 190–193
  Passive, 188–190
  Protraction, 69, 195–196
  Retraction, 69, 193–195
  Wire selection, 188

Van der Linden retainer, 458–459
Vertebral maturation, 78–80
Vertical dimension, 111–148
  Types of vertical malocclusions, 111
Vertical dysplasia, 116–119
Vertical ("spaghetti") elastics, 467–468

Wet field bonding, 180
Wilson distalizing appliance, 353–356
Wire stiffness, 160

ABOUT THE AUTHOR

James A. McNamara, Jr., a graduate of the University of California Berkeley with a degree in Speech, received his dental and orthodontic education at the University of California, San Francisco, and a Doctorate in Anatomy from the University of Michigan. He serves as the Thomas M. and Doris Graber Endowed Professor of Dentistry in the Department of Orthodontics and Pediatric Dentistry, School of Dentistry, the University of Michigan. He also is Professor of Cell and Developmental Biology in the University of Michigan Medical School and Research Scientist at the Center for Human Growth and Development, an interdisciplinary research unit located on the Ann Arbor campus. Dr. McNamara is the curator of the *University of Michigan Elementary and Secondary School Growth Study*.

The author was the recipient of the Milo Hellman Research Award given by the American Association of Orthodontists in 1973 and was the E. Sheldon Friel Memorial Lecturer of the European Orthodontic Society in 1979. He also was given the Research Recognition Award of the American Association of Oral and Maxillofacial Surgeons in 1983. He received the Jacob A. Salzmann Award at the 1994 meeting of the American Association of Orthodontists. He also is the 1997 recipient of the BF Dewel Biomedical Research Award of the American Association of Orthodontists Foundation. He is the 2001 recipient of the James E. Brophy Distinguished Service Award, the highest award given by the American Association of Orthodontists.

Dr. McNamara has maintained a practice limited to orthodontics in Ann Arbor since 1971. He is a Diplomate of the American Board of Orthodontics and a Fellow of the American College of Dentists. He also served as a member of the Oral Biology and Medicine Study Section of the National Institutes of Health from 1978–1981 (chairman, 1978–1980). He is President-elect of the Midwestern Component of the Edward H. Angle Society of Orthodontists. In addition, Dr. McNamara served as the Chairman of the Council on Scientific Affairs of the American Association of Orthodontists from 1993–1996 and is Editor-in-Chief of the 38 volume *Craniofacial Growth Monograph Series* published through the University of Michigan. Dr. McNamara has published over 160 scientific articles in refereed journals, has written, edited or contributed to 48 books, and has presented courses and lectures in 27 countries.

ABOUT THE ARTIST

William L. Brudon is an Associate Professor Emeritus in the School of Art and an Associate Professor Emeritus of Medical and Biological Illustration in the Department of Anatomy and Cell Biology in the School of Medicine at The University of Michigan.

A self-trained artist, Mr. Brudon came to the University of Michigan in 1948, after having served in World War II, and became staff artist for the Museum of Zoology, a position he held until 1960. He then became senior medical illustrator and staff artist in the Department of Anatomy within the School of Medicine, a position that he held until his retirement in 1985.

Mr. Brudon has been a principal illustrator for a number of well-known texts in the medical and dental fields including *The Human Face* by Donald Enlow, *Essentials of Human Anatomy* by Russell Woodburne, *Occlusion* by Sigurd Ramfjord and Major Ash and *Wheeler's Atlas of Tooth Form*, edited by Major Ash.

Mr. Brudon received the Fine Arts Award from the American Association of Medical Illustrators in 1971 and 1981. He served as President of the Association of Medical Illustrators from 1981 to 1982.